Trauma Nursing Core Course (TNCC)

Provider Manual

Sixth Edition

Emergency Nurses Association
Des Plaines, IL

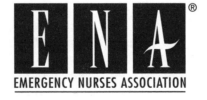

EMERGENCY NURSES ASSOCIATION

Printed in the United States of America
ISBN 0-935890-98-X
ISBN 978-0-935890-98-3

The official Trauma Nursing Core Course of the Emergency Nurses Association (ENA) (United States)

The official Trauma Nursing Core Course of Stichting Ziekenverpleging Aruba operator of Dr. Horacio E. Oduber Hospital.

The official Trauma Nursing Core Course of the Australian College of Emergency Nursing (Australia)

The official Trauma Nursing Core Course of the National Emergency Nurses' Affiliation, Inc. (NENA) (Canada)

The official Trauma Nursing Core Course of the Trauma Nursing Committee of Greece.

The official Trauma Nursing Core Course of the Hong Kong Emergency Nurses Association

The official Trauma Nursing Core Course of the Sistema de Urgencias del Estado de Guanajuato (SUEG) (Mexico)

The official Trauma Nursing Core Course of the Foundation of Trauma Nursing Netherlands (STNN)

The official Trauma Nursing Core Course of the College of Emergency Nursing New Zealand (CENNZ)

The official Trauma Nursing Core Course of the Anestesisykepleiernes Lansgruppe av Norsk Sykepleierforbund (ALNSF) (Norway)

The official Trauma Nursing Core Course of the Associacao Portuguesa de Enfermeiros de Urgencia (Portugal)

The official Trauma Nursing Core Course of the Trauma Committee of South Africa

The official Trauma Nursing Core Course of the Swedish Association of Trauma Nurses (RST)

The official Trauma Nursing Core Course of the Tadreeb National Training-Trauma Council

The official Trauma Nursing Core Course of the Trauma Nursing Limited (United Kingdom)

The official Trauma Nursing Core Course of the Western Australia Trauma Education Committee of the Department of Health, Western Australia

ENA accepts no responsibility for course instruction by the course director or any course instructors. Because implementation of this course of instruction involves the exercise of professional judgment, ENA shall not be liable for the acts or omissions of course participants in the application of this course of instruction.

The authors, editors, and publisher have checked with reliable resources in regards to providing information that is complete and accurate. Due to continual evolution of knowledge, treatment modalities, and drug therapies, ENA cannot warranty that the information, in every aspect, is current. ENA is not responsible for any errors, omissions, or for the results obtained from use of such information. Please check with your health care institution regarding applicable policies.

Medication dosages are subject to change and modification. Please check with your local authority or institutional policy for the most current information.

Table of Contents

The Emergency Nurses Association (ENA) would like to extend its appreciation to the TNCC Sixth Edition Revision Workgroup for the development and implementation of the Trauma Nursing Core Course (TNCC).

TNCC Revision Workgroup Chairperson

Beth Broering, RN, MSN, CEN, CCRN
Trauma Coordinator
Vanderbilt University Medical Center
Nashville, TN

TNCC Sixth Edition Revision Workgroup Members

Melody Campbell, RN, MSN, CEN, CCRN, CCNS
Trauma Program Manager/CNS
Good Samaritan Hospital
Dayton, OH

Laura Favand, RN, MS, CEN
Commander
67th Forward Surgical Team
Miesau, Germany

Andrew Galvin, APRN, BC, CEN
Emergency Nurse Practitioner
and Clinical Nurse Specialist
Emergency Physicians Medical Group, PC
Montgomery Regional Hospital
Blacksburg, VA

Reneé Holleran, RN, PhD, CEN, CCRN, CFRN, CTRN, FAEN
Nurse Manager, Adult Transport Services
Intermountain Life Flight
Salt Lake City, UT

TNCC Sixth Edition Revision Curriculum Consultant

Vicki Patrick, MS, APRN, BC, ACNP, CEN, FAEN
Instructor, Acute Care and Emergency Nurse
Practitioner Program
University of Texas at Arlington
School of Nursing
Arlington, TX

TNCC Revision Workgroup ENA Board Liaisons

Chris Gisness, RN, MSN, CEN, BC, FNP
Nurse Practitioner
Department of Emergency Medicine
Emory University
Atlanta, GA

Michael Moon, RN, CNS-CC, MSN, CEN
Instructor
School of Nursing and Health Professions
University of the Incarnate Word
San Antonio, TX

Staff Support

Education Officer: **Donna Massey, RN, MSN**

Nursing Education Editor:
Sharon Graunke, RN, APN, MS, CEN

Editorial Project Coordinator: **Jennifer Lucas**

Developmental Editor: **Linda Conheady**

Marketing Officer: **Stuart Meyer**

Cover Designer & Senior Graphic Designer:
Leslie Arendt

Indexer: Composition by **Kevin Campbell**

Contributing Authors

Cynthia Blank-Reid, RN, MSN, CEN
Clinical Nurse Specialist
Division of Trauma
Temple University Hospital and Temple University
Children's Medical Center
Philadelphia, PA

John Fazio, RN, MS, FAEN
Emergency Clinical Nurse Specialist
San Francisco General Hospital
San Francisco, CA

Teresa D. Fulwood, RN, CCRN, CFRN, NREMT
Flight Nurse
Vanderbilt University Medical Center
Nashville, TN

Barbara Bennett Jacobs, RN, MPH, PhD
West Hartford, CT

Patricia Manion, RN, MS, CCRN, CEN
Trauma Program Director
Genesys Regional Medical Center
Grand Blanc, MI

Paul C. Reid, Sr. RN, MSN, CEN
Clinical Nurse Level III,
Department of Emergency Medicine
Hospital of the University of Pennsylvania
Philadelphia, PA

Kimberly K. Smith, RN, MS, CCRN
Critical Care Clinical Nurse Specialist
Brooke Army Medical Center
Fort Sam Houston, TX

Louis R. Stout, LTC, RN, MS, CEN
Chief, Professional Programs
Defense Medical Readiness Training Institute
Fort Sam Houston, TX

Jeffery Strickler, RN, MA, CFRN, EMT-P
Director Emergency Services
University of North Carolina Hospitals
Chapel Hill, NC

Jennifer Ezell Wilbeck, MSN, APRN, CEN
Assistant Professor, Acute Care Nurse
Practitioner Program
Coordinator, FNP/ACNP-ED Program
Vanderbilt University School of Nursing
Nashville, TN

Content Reviewers

Linda S. Arapian, RN, MSN, RN,C, CEN
Emergency Department Education Coordinator
Children's National Medical Center
Washington, DC

Andreas Åström, RN, CRNA
Karolinska University Hospital, Huddinge
Stockholm, Sweden

Ray Bennett, RN, BSN, CEN, NREMT-P
SCTU/EMS Education Coordinator
Robert Wood Johnson University Hospital
New Brunswick, NJ

Agneta Brandt, RN, CRNA, MSN
Danderyd University Hospital
Stockholm, Sweden

Eric Christensen, RN, BSN, CEN, CLNC
Emergency Department Clinical Nurse Educator
Denver Health Medical Center
Denver, CO

Liz Cloughessy, AM, RN, MHM
Executive Director
Australian College of Emergency Nursing
Toongabbie, New South Wales, Australia

Nancy J. Denke, RN, MSN, FNP-C, CCRN
Trauma Nurse Practitioner
Scottsdale Healthcare – Osborn
Scottsdale, AZ

Kathleen L. Emde, RN, MN, CEN, FAEN
Director of Emergency Services
Auburn Regional Medical Center
Auburn, WA

John Fazio, RN, MS, FAEN
Emergency Clinical Nurse Specialist
San Francisco General Hospital
San Francisco, CA

James Gillam, RN, CEN
Staff Nurse, Emergency Trauma Center
Saint John's Medical Center
Springfield, MO

Grethe Kjeilen, CRNA
Nurse Anaesthetist/Development Nurse
Section for Anaesthetics
Vestfold Central Hospital
Tønsberg, Norway

Karen Latoszek, RN, ENCc
Senior Manager
University of Alberta/Stollery Children's Hospital
Emergency Department
Edmonton, Alberta, Canada

Dawn McKeown, RN, CEN
Staff Nurse and Emergency Department Educator
LSU Health Sciences Center – Shreveport
Shreveport, LA

Leanne Norrena, RN, BScN
Emergency AACN Sessional Instructor
Emergency Staff Nurse
Calgary Health Region
Calgary, Alberta, Canada

Vicki Patrick, MS, APRN, BC, ACNP, CEN, FAEN
Instructor, Acute Care and Emergency Nurse
Practitioner Program
University of Texas at Arlington
School of Nursing
Arlington, TX

Carole Rush, RN, M.Ed., CEN
Injury Prevention Specialist
Emergency Staff Nurse
Calgary Health Region
Calgary, Alberta, Canada

Jeffrey A. Solheim, RN, CEN
Consultant
Solheim Enterprises
Keizer, OR

Louis R. Stout, LTC, RN, MS, CEN
Chief, Professional Programs
Defense Medical Readiness Training Institute
Fort Sam Houston, TX

Robert Timmings, RN, BHScN, MEmergN, PhD(c)
Nurse Educator
Cunningham Center, Southern Area Workforce Unit
Toowoomba, Queensland
Lecturer – Clinical Skills
School of Medicine
University of Queensland, Australia

Mary Ellen Wilson, RN, MS, FNP, CEN, FAEN
Health Services Manager
Avery Dennison
Strongsville, OH

Jill Windle, RN, BA
Lecturer Practitioner in Emergency Nursing
Hope Hospital
Salford, Manchester, United Kingdom

A special thanks to the following who worked on the previous editions of TNCC.

TNCC Fifth Edition

Liz Cloughessy, AM, RN, MHM

Mary E. Fecht Gramley, RN, PhD, CEN

K. Sue Hoyt, RN, MN, CEN

Barbara Bennett Jacobs, RN, MPH, MS

Louise LeBlanc, RN, BSCN, ENC(c)

Ginger Morse, RN, MN, CEN, CCRN, CS, PhDc

Vicki Patrick, RN, MS, CS, ACNP, CEN

Jill Windle, RN, BA

TNCC Fourth Edition

Barbara Bennett Jacobs, RN, MPH, MS

Pam Baker, RN, BSN, CEN, CCRN

Peggy Hollingsworth-Fridlund, RN, BSN

Ginger Morse, RN, MN, CEN, CCRN

Vicki Patrick, RN, MS, CEN

Mark Parshall, RN, MSN, CS, CEN

Jean Proehl, RN, MN, CEN, CCRN

TNCC Third Edition

LTC Ruth Rea, RN, PhD, CEN

Karen Kernan Bryant, RN, MSN, CEN

Sharon Gavin Fought, RN, PhD

Jane Goldsworth, RN, BSN, CEN

Mary Martha Hall, RN, MSN,CEN

K. Sue Hoyt, RN, MN, CEN

Barbara Bennett Jacobs, RN, MPH

Linda Larson, RN, MS, ENP, CEN

Marguerite Littleton, RN, DNSc

Lynne Nemeth, RN, MS, CEN

Cecelia Irene Paige, RN, MSN, CEN

Vicki Patrick, RN, MS, CEN

Jacqueline Rhoads, RN, PhD, CEN, CCRN

Judy Selfridge, RN, MSN, CEN

Jill Schoerger Walsh, RN, MS

TNCC First and Second Editions

Ruth Rea, RN, MS, CEN

Sharon Gavin Fought, RN, PhD

Mary Martha Hall, RN, MSN, CEN

Linda Larson, RN, MS, ENP, CEN

Marguerite Littleton, RN, DNSc

Lynne Nemeth, RN, MS, CEN

Cecelia Irene Paige, RN, MSN, CEN

Judy Selfridge, RN, MSN, CEN

In the United States, trauma remains the leading cause of death and disability in persons younger than 45 years of age and is the fifth leading cause of death for all ages. Traumatic injury places a considerable burden on individuals, health care institutions, and society. Approximately one third of all ED visits and more than 8% of all hospitalizations are due to injuries. Additionally, traumatic injuries often have long-term consequences. It is estimated that 5.3 million people in the United States have long-term disabilities from traumatic brain injury and 200,000 from spinal cord injury. It is essential that the emergency care of the trauma patient is organized and collaborative to ensure the best possible outcomes.

Since 1986, the Emergency Nurses Association's *Trauma Nursing Core Course* (TNCC) has served as the standard of nursing practice for providing trauma care to patients who have sustained injuries. This sixth edition of TNCC represents ENA's continued commitment to providing an educational program for nurses that teaches a standardized approach to the initial assessment and management of the injured patient and fosters collaboration and communication among all members of the heath care team. TNCC provides a common framework of communication and collaboration that can ultimately save lives and improve outcomes. The TNCC course has been taught to thousands of nurses in the United States and around the world.

This new edition has been updated by members of the TNCC Revision Workgroup and trauma nursing experts both in the United States and internationally. Although there are some significant changes in the structure of the TNCC course, the basic tenets of providing safe, high-quality trauma nursing care have not changed since the publication of the fifth edition in 2000. More sophisticated technology continues to be developed, and more evidence-based guidelines are being used to direct both diagnostic and therapeutic decision making during the initial resuscitation and throughout the trauma care continuum.

Many of the changes in the sixth edition were suggested by TNCC instructors and course participants. Several of these changes include a new chapter (Chapter 14) on disaster management and triage priorities with multiple casualty scenarios for group discussion and a new chapter (Chapter 4) on airway and ventilation with Airway Skill Station scenarios that reflect the didactic content. Information on trauma and pregnancy, pediatric trauma, and trauma in older adults, presented in three separate chapters in the fifth edition, has been combined into a single chapter (Chapter 13) on special populations. A new chapter on ocular, maxillofacial, and neck trauma (Chapter 7) likewise incorporates existing sections of three chapters from the fifth edition. In Chapter 2, Epidemiology, Biomechanics, and Mechanisms of Injury, the epidemiology information on countries other than the United States has been expanded and appears in an appendix to the chapter. Material on soft tissue trauma has been moved from the musculoskeletal trauma chapter (Chapter 11) to Chapter 12, Surface and Burn Trauma. Finally, all chapters have been updated to reflect the latest research in assessment and management.

For the Skill Stations, new Trauma Nursing Process scenarios for both teaching and evaluation and a new Spinal Immobilization station have been added. Also, components of the Selected Interventions station have been incorporated into other stations. Specifically, chest trauma and chest drainage system management and problem solving are now part of the Airway and Ventilation Skill Station. One of the biggest changes to the course, however, is the elimination of the Airway and Ventilatory Management and Spinal Immobilization as evaluation stations. These two stations will be taught during the teaching day of the course with emphasis on a "hands-on approach," and each participant will actively engage in the scenarios. The Physical Assessment station has minor changes and remains an optional station for courses held both in the United States and internationally.

TNCC continues to provide core-level knowledge, in terms of both cognitive and psychomotor skills, based on the nursing process as the standard of care. Although TNCC provides the scientific or empirical knowledge as the foundation of our practice, each of us contributes unique qualities to the relationship between the nurse and the patient/family. Our past experiences, the moral and ethical framework on which we base our practice, and influences from other disciplines complement the scientific foundation. It is through our commitment to trauma nursing, communication, and collaboration that patients and their families will benefit.

Beth Broering, RN, MSN, CEN, CCRN
TNCC Revision Workgroup Chairperson

Sample Questions

1. The correct sequence for the primary assessment of the trauma patient is:

   a. airway, breathing, circulation, cervical spine protection, neurological, remove clothes.

   b. circulation, airway, breathing, cervical spine protection, neurological, remove clothes.

   c. airway, cervical spine protection, breathing, circulation, neurological, remove clothes.

   d. remove clothes, neurological, airway, cervical spine protection, breathing, circulation.

Reference: Chapter 3, Initial Assessment

2. The proper sequence of interventions for a patient whose only injury is a deformed, swollen, and painful thigh is:

   a. administration of high-flow oxygen via nonrebreather mask, initiation of two large-caliber IVs, and application of a traction splint.

   b. application of a backboard, initiation of two large-caliber IVs, and application of a posterior long leg splint.

   c. application of a traction splint, administration of high-flow oxygen via a nonrebreather mask, and initiation of two large-caliber IVs.

   d. administration of high-flow oxygen via nonrebreather mask, initiation of two large-caliber IVs, and application of a backboard.

Reference: Chapter 11, Musculoskeletal Trauma

3. The position that best optimizes the microcirculation to an extremity with a suspected compartment syndrome is:

   a. elevation of the extremity above the level of the head.

   b. turning the patient to the unaffected side.

   c. elevation of the extremity to the level of the heart.

   d. placing the patient in Trendelenburg position.

Reference: Chapter 11, Musculoskeletal Trauma

4. Your emergency department is receiving 44 casualties following a tornado strike. A patient with no pulse or respirations should be triaged to which area?

   a. Emergency department for life-saving measures

   b. Holding area/hospital morgue for non-salvageable injuries.

   c. Minor care area for minimal patient care

   d. Off-site clinic for walking wounded

Reference: Chapter 14, Disaster Management

5. A gastric tube is inserted in a trauma patient to:

   a. administer drugs until peripheral access is established.

   b. decompress the stomach to prevent vomiting and aspiration.

   c. test the gag reflex.

   d. lavage suspected toxic substances.

Reference: Chapter 3, Initial Assessment

Questions 6 and 7 refer to the information below.

An unrestrained passenger involved in a front-end collision arrives in a private vehicle. The patient has pale, cold, moist skin and is very restless. Blood pressure is 90/70 mm Hg, pulse 120 beats/minute, and respirations are 24 breaths/minute. Breath sounds are equal bilaterally, abdomen is rigid, and bowel sounds are absent.

6. Based on the assessment findings, the emergency nurse should suspect a:

   a. ruptured spleen.

   b. contused kidney.

   c. pericardial tamponade.

   d. tension pneumothorax.

Reference: Chapter 9, Abdominal Trauma

7. The patient suddenly becomes more restless and complains of increased difficulty breathing. Current vital signs are blood pressure of 90/76 mm Hg, pulse of 140 beats/minute, and respirations of 32 breaths/minute. The priority nursing intervention is:

   a. obtaining baseline laboratories/radiographs.

   b. initiation of high-flow oxygen via nonrebreather mask.

   c. preparation of the patient for peritoneal lavage.

   d. insertion of a gastric tube.

Reference: Chapter 3, Initial Assessment

8. The basis for the physiologic responses of the body to shock is:

   a. ventilation/perfusion abnormalities.

   b. pump or left ventricular failure.

   c. anaerobic cellular metabolism due to inadequate tissue perfusion.

   d. vasodilation and clotting abnormalities.

Reference: Chapter 5, Shock

9. An unconscious trauma patient is unable to maintain his airway. Endotracheal intubation was unsuccessful. The priority intervention for this patient is:

   a. blind nasotracheal intubation.

   b. insertion of a dual-lumen, dual-cuff airway.

   c. surgical cricothyrotomy.

   d. ventilation with a bag-mask device.

Reference: Chapter 4, Airway and Ventilation

10. A trauma patient becomes restless and agitated with circumoral cyanosis. Further assessment reveals diminished breath sounds bilaterally and no jugular venous distension. The priority intervention for this patient is:

    a. obtain a chest radiograph.

    b. apply high-flow oxygen using a non-rebreather mask.

    c. insert 2 large-caliber IVs and infuse fluid at a rapid rate.

    d. administer pain medication.

Reference: Chapter 4, Airway and Ventilation.

11. The physiologic responses producing clinical findings specific to tension pneumothorax are:

    a. decreasing intrathoracic pressure and increased cardiac output.

    b. rising intrathoracic pressure and increased cardiac output.

    c. decreasing intrathoracic pressure and decreased cardiac output.

    d. rising intrathoracic pressure and decreased cardiac output.

Reference: Chapter 8, Thoracic Trauma

12. A 22-year-old female was found unconscious with a penetrating stab wound to the left chest at the level of the 5th rib from an ice pick. The emergency nurse should suspect which of the following injuries?

    a. Pericardial tamponade

    b. Laceration of the peroneal artery

    c. Liver laceration

    d. Diaphragmatic hernia

Reference: Chapter 8, Thoracic Trauma

13. The two components of cerebral perfusion pressure (CPP) are:

    a. mean arterial pressure (MAP) and intracranial pressure (ICP).

    b. systolic blood pressure and cardiac output.

    c. stroke volume and peripheral vascular resistance.

    d. PaO_2 and $PaCO_2$.

Reference: Chapter 6, Brain and Cranial Trauma

14. Which of the following interventions is the initial priority for a patient with a suspected cervical spine injury?

    a. Initiation of intravenous fluids for volume replacement

    b. Administration of supplemental oxygen

    c. Protection and/or immobilization of the cervical spine

    d. Insertion of a gastric tube

Reference: Chapter 10, Spinal Cord and Vertebral Column Trauma

15. The priority nursing intervention for a patient with facial trauma is:

    a. application of a dressing to uncontrolled facial bleeding.

    b. stabilization of the cervical spine.

    c. clearing the airway of debris.

    d. administration of intravenous fluids.

Reference: Chapter 7, Ocular, Maxillofacial, and Neck Trauma

16. A 50 kg patient sustained deep partial thickness burns covering 40% of the body surface area at 10:00 p.m. By 6:00 a.m. the patient should receive how many ml of fluid? (Use 4 ml/kg/% burn as a basis to calculate fluid administration).

    a. 4000 ml

    b. 2000 ml

    c. 8000 ml

    d. 500 ml

Reference: Chapter 12, Surface and Burn Trauma

17. If peripheral venous access cannot be readily established in a pediatric trauma patient in shock, the nurse should:

    a. continue peripheral venous access attempts.

    b. initiate intraosseous access.

    c. assist with central line placement.

    d. stop all attempts and call the intravenous team.

Reference: Chapter 13, Special Populations: Pregnant, Pediatric, and Older Adult Trauma

18. The primary epidemiologic cause of injury to the elderly patient is:

    a. poisoning.

    b. motor vehicle crashes.

    c. suicide.

    d. falls.

Reference: Chapter 13, Special Populations: Pregnant, Pediatric, and Older Adult Trauma

19. For an individual experiencing grief precipitated by the death of a family member, the nurse should support the process by:

    a. using words like "expired" or "left us" when referring to the incident.

    b. never using silence after notification of death.

    c. reinforcing reality and showing acceptance of the body, even if severely injured.

    d. using statements such as "It was really for the best."

Reference: Chapter 15, Psychosocial Aspects of Trauma Care

20. Prior to interfacility transfer, nursing interventions should include:

    a. administering prescribed analgesic and antianxiety medications.

    b. covering large burn areas with cool saline dressings.

    c. advising the family to closely follow the ambulance to the receiving hospital.

    d. irrigating thermal burn areas with antibiotic solution.

Reference: Chapter 16, Transition of Care for the Trauma Patient

TNCC Sample Questions Answer Key

1. C
2. A
3. C
4. B
5. B
6. A
7. B
8. C
9. D
10. B
11. D
12. A
13. A
14. C
15. C
16. A
17. B
18. D
19. C
20. A

TNCC Overall Course Objectives

On completion of this chapter/lecture, the learner should be able to:

- Identify the common mechanisms of injury associated with trauma.

- Describe the pathophysiologic changes as a basis for signs and symptoms.

- Describe the nursing assessment of patients with trauma.

- Describe the appropriate interventions for patients with trauma.

- Describe mechanisms for evaluating the effectiveness of nursing interventions for patients with trauma.

TNCC Psychomotor Skill Station Objectives

On completion of this course, the learner should be able to:

- Demonstrate a standardized, systematic, and organized approach to assessment, planning, intervention, and evaluation.

- Perform primary and secondary assessments.

- State patient problem based on assessment data.

- Identify an appropriate plan of care.

- Identify priorities for nursing interventions based on assessment data.

- Describe appropriate interventions for a plan of care.

- Identify patients' potential responses to nursing interventions.

Chapter 1

The Trauma Nursing Core Course and Trauma Nursing

Objectives

On completion of this chapter/lecture, the learner should be able to:

1. Define trauma nursing.

2. Discuss the team approach to trauma nursing.

3. Describe the purpose of the Trauma Nursing Core Course.

4. Identify four roles associated with trauma nursing.

Preface

It is strongly suggested that the learner read the following chapter before attending the Trauma Nursing Core Course (TNCC). This chapter will be referred to during the introduction and before the other lectures. Knowledge of the nursing process serves as the foundation for understanding the format of the TNCC and the nursing approach used to address the care of trauma patients.

Introduction

Trauma is a major threat to the immediate and often long-term health of individuals. In the United States, despite efforts at public awareness and injury prevention, trauma remains the <u>first</u> leading cause of death for persons younger than age 44. Nurses, working in a variety of settings, play an integral role in the assessment and management of patients with traumatic injuries. The *Trauma Nursing Core Course,* developed by the Emergency Nurses Association, serves as the basis for a standardized approach to initial trauma care. This chapter describes trauma nursing philosophy, the roles and responsibilities of a trauma nurse, as well as the background and organization of the TNCC and manual.

The discipline of trauma nursing encompasses the different roles nurses have throughout the continuum of care: from the initial encounter with the trauma patient through the resuscitative, acute, intermediate, and postacute phases. Knowledge is the core of any discipline. Nursing uses knowledge from science, technology, and nonscientific disciplines as well as intuition and past nursing experience. Nursing makes use of knowledge while maintaining respect and balance for the uniqueness of the individual and the responses of that individual to the traumatic event.

Ethics, or moral knowledge, helps the trauma nurse distinguish right from wrong. Esthetic knowledge gives meaning as trauma nurses engage in situations, intuitively process, and ultimately envision solutions and responses to a trauma patient's experience.[1,2]

Personal knowledge is the knowledge of self and others that is accumulated over time and enhances trauma nurses' ability to use their personal selves therapeutically. The four patterns of knowing with corresponding questions they may answer are:[1,3]

- Empirics—What is the scientific basis for my action?
- Ethics—Is there an ethical principle to guide my action?
- Esthetics—Do my actions create artistry?
- Personal Knowing—Do I know what I do; do I do what I know?

The 2003 American Nurses Association *Nursing's Social Policy Statement* avoids a single definition of nursing. It does suggest that the following four features be identified in any definition of nursing:[4]

- Recognition of all responses a person may have to illness (injury) experiences
- Integration of both subjective and objective data
- Use of empirical or scientific knowledge to diagnose and intervene
- Use of a caring relationship to promote health and healing

Belief Statements

After analyzing the impact of traumatic injury nationally and internationally and the potential for positive contributions by professional nurses in the care of the trauma patient, the Emergency Nurses Association formulated the following belief statements:

1. The optimal care of the trauma patient is best accomplished within a framework in which all members of the trauma team use a systematic, standardized approach to the care of the injured patient.

2. Emergency nurses are essential members of the trauma team. Morbidity and mortality of trauma patients can be significantly reduced by educating nurses to competently provide care to trauma patients.

3. The Emergency Nurses Association and its constituents have the responsibility to facilitate trauma-related continuing education opportunities for nurses who provide care to trauma patients.

4. The Emergency Nurses Association supports injury prevention and control that is collaborative, identifies specific problems within specific populations, utilizes databases, and addresses the three approaches to prevention (engineering/technology, enforcement/legislation, and education/behavioral).

Trauma Nursing Roles and Responsibilities

The scope of trauma nursing encompasses nursing assessment, interventions, and evaluation of patients in a variety of settings including the prehospital environment, community hospitals, and designated trauma centers. Regardless of the setting, trauma nursing is collaborative and involves different roles and responsibilities. The roles and responsibilities the trauma nurse assumes include the following:

1. **Designs, manages, and coordinates care.**

   In some settings, the nurse is the first health professional to interact with the trauma patient and may be solely responsible for completing the initial patient assessment and developing a plan of care. In other settings, the nurse functions as a member of a trauma team that may include emergency physicians, general surgeons, or both; residents; and ancillary care providers, each with institutional-specific responsibilities during trauma resuscitations.

   The trauma nurse is responsible for the clinical leadership and direction of nursing activities for the trauma patient. The trauma nurse is also responsible for communicating with health care team members outside the emergency setting (e.g., the intensive care unit, operating room, general acute care units) and medical and nursing staff at other facilities where a patient may be transferred. The trauma nurse is often the team coordinator responsible for organizing, through effective communication skills, the care of the trauma patient.[5]

2. **Engages in and promotes a nurse–patient relationship to provide care.**

A nurse-patient relationship not only results in direct patient care but also promotes patient advocacy and patient education. Trauma nurses may be responsible for communicating the overall plan of care, providing psychosocial support, and educating the patient and family. The nurse-patient relationship suggests that the "professional power" the relationship generates for the nurse is actually being given by the patient in exchange for knowledgeable and safe care. With a holistic view, the trauma nurse engages in relationships with individual patients, families, and often communities.

3. **Documents the care of the trauma patient.**

Documentation of care provided and patient response during the acute resuscitation or emergency department (ED) phase is an essential part of the communication necessary to ensure a seamless transition of the patient from the ED to the inpatient unit or to another facility. Timely, accurate, and appropriate documentation is important throughout the entire trauma care continuum because patients frequently return to the emergency care setting after diagnostic procedures or later for follow-up care. The nurse's documentation of care provides a significant source of information for databases (such as trauma registries) as well as for evaluation of the extent, appropriateness, quality, and timeliness of care. Analysis of the trauma team's performance serves as an important resource for identifying educational needs of the staff, practice changes, research topics, and injury prevention opportunities.

4. **Evaluates research and incorporates appropriate findings into practice.**

As with all areas of nursing, trauma nursing should be evidence-based. Trauma nurses should be involved in ensuring that diagnostic and therapeutic interventions are based on the latest research recommendations. In some settings, nurses may have the opportunity to participate in trauma care research. Roles of the trauma nurse may include helping to obtain informed consent from a patient or family member, participating in the administration of specific research protocol interventions, assisting with the collection and analysis of data for a protocol, or presenting or publishing research.

Trauma Nursing Core Course

In response to the belief statements listed in the Trauma Nursing Philosophy section of this chapter, the Emergency Nurses Association developed the Trauma Nursing Core Course (TNCC) for national and international dissemination as a means for identifying standards of nursing care based on current knowledge related to trauma. The first TNCC was presented in 1986. Currently, the TNCC is offered in the United States and more than eleven other countries.

Purpose

The purpose of the TNCC is to present core-level knowledge and psychomotor skills for the initial assessment and management of patients with traumatic injury. Emphasis is placed on the standardized and systematic process for initial assessment. Psychomotor skill stations facilitate integration of cognitive knowledge and psychomotor abilities in a setting that simulates trauma patient situations. The Trauma Nursing Process Skill Station was developed to reinforce the systematic assessment of a trauma patient.

It is the intent of the TNCC to enhance the nurse's ability to rapidly and accurately assess the patient's responses to the trauma event and to work within the context of a trauma team. It is anticipated that the knowledge and skills learned in the TNCC will ultimately contribute to a decrease in the morbidity and mortality associated with trauma.

Course Description

The *Trauma Nursing Core Course* (TNCC) is designed to provide the learner with cognitive knowledge and psychomotor skills. The trauma nursing process is reflected throughout the chapters and in the psychomotor skill stations. Participants receive continuing education credit hours (CECHs) for attending the course.

Lectures and psychomotor skill stations are presented by verified TNCC instructors and TNCC instructor candidates. The lecture content is organized to provide the learner with substantive knowledge for use in the psychomotor skill stations. Participation in all psychomotor skill stations is required for successful completion of the course. The skill stations presented are

- Trauma nursing process
- Airway and ventilation
- Spinal protection, helmet removal, and splinting

Evaluation of learners includes a written multiple-choice examination and the Trauma Nursing Process Psychomotor Evaluation Station. These evaluations are designed to assess acquisition of cognitive knowledge, important skills, and critical thinking.

To successfully complete the TNCC, the learner must achieve a minimum 80% on the written examination, actively participate in all skill stations, and demonstrate all critical criteria and at least 70% of all steps in the Trauma Nursing Process Psychomotor Evaluation Station.

Course Participants

Nurses interested in the initial care of the trauma patient will benefit from participating in the TNCC. It is recommended that a nurse have at least 6 months of clinical nursing experience in an emergency care setting before taking the course. It is assumed that the course participant has an understanding of initial trauma care terminology and is familiar with standard emergency trauma equipment. If the participant is a novice in trauma nursing, the course content and psychomotor skill stations will provide valuable information and practice within a supportive learning environment.

The TNCC may be officially attended only by registered nurses (RNs). Emergency medical technician-paramedics, physician assistants, or licensed practical nurses may desire, and are encouraged, to attend the TNCC; however, they are not eligible for evaluation or verification.

Organization of the TNCC Manual

The TNCC manual is designed to reinforce and supplement lectures and psychomotor skill content. To enhance learning, chapters (where relevant) are presented in a consistent format throughout the manual, as follows:

- **Objectives**—To emphasize the most important concepts, several objectives that learners should be able to attain at the completion of each chapter/lecture are listed.

- **Introduction**—The introduction covers information regarding epidemiology, mechanisms of injury, and biomechanics as well as an overview of the usual and concomitant injuries.

- **Anatomy and Physiology Review**—In most chapters, a brief review of relevant anatomy and physiologic concepts is presented to enhance the understanding of the injury process for specific injuries described. This material will not be discussed during lectures or evaluated in the multiple-choice examination.

- **Pathophysiology as a Basis for Signs and Symptoms**—Pathophysiologic concepts are presented to explain the body's physiologic responses to injury and associated signs and symptoms.

- **Selected Injuries**—The most frequently occurring or life-threatening injuries associated with a particular body system are described, along with their signs and symptoms.

- **Nursing Care**—The basic sequence of the nursing process is used to organize the nursing care principles to include assessment, analysis, planning, implementation, and evaluation and ongoing assessment.

- **Summary and References**—Each chapter closes with a brief statement of chapter highlights and a section of updated references, including Web sites.

- **Analysis, Nursing Diagnoses, Interventions, and Expected Outcomes**—Each chapter has a detailed appendix specific to the injury or topic covered.

The TNCC manual also includes the following resources:

- **Skill Stations**—Templates for the psychomotor skill stations of airway and ventilation; spinal protection, helmet removal, and splinting; and the trauma nursing process are presented. Each station presents core objectives for use in the care of the trauma patient and the steps in skill performance.

- **Index**—The index helps learners find topics quickly.

Summary

Trauma is a major threat to the health and socioeconomic well-being of individuals, communities, and countries around the world. A coordinated, collaborative, and systematic approach to the initial assessment and management of trauma is essential to ensure optimal outcomes and minimize morbidity and mortality. The Emergency Nurses Association believes that the knowledge and skills presented in the *Trauma Nursing Core Course* will assist professional nurses to systematically assess the trauma patient, to intervene or assist with interventions, and to function within the context of a trauma team.

Despite significant progress in injury control and prevention, trauma remains a leading cause of disability. Ongoing commitment and efforts to improve injury surveillance, research, trauma system development, and governmental support for trauma care and injury prevention remain a top priority.

References

1. Chin, P. L., & Kramer, M. K. (1999). *Theory and nursing: Integrated knowledge development* (5th ed.). St. Louis, MO: Mosby.

2. Schwirian, P. M. (1998). *Professionalization of nursing: Current issues and trends* (3rd ed.) Philadelphia: Lippincott.

3. Brencick, J. M., & Webster, G. A. (2000). *Philosophy of nursing: A new vision for health care*. Albany, NY: State University of New York Press.

4. American Nurses Association. (2003). *Nursing's social policy statement*. Silver Spring, MD: Author.

5. American Association of Colleges of Nursing. (1998). *The essentials of baccalaureate education for professional nursing practice* (pp. 4–6). Washington, DC: Author.

Chapter 2

Epidemiology, Biomechanics, and Mechanisms of Injury

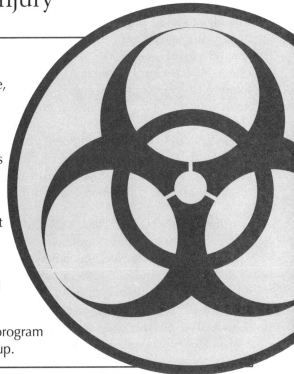

Objectives

On completion of this chapter/lecture, the learner should be able to:

1. Define the term "trauma."

2. Identify epidemiologic characteristics associated with trauma.

3. Describe the body's response to energy transfer from the environment and the effects on human tissues.

4. Identify potential injuries that may occur from specific mechanisms and patterns of injury.

5. Describe how an injury prevention program can decrease injuries in a select group.

Introduction

Trauma is defined as injury to human tissues and organs resulting from the transfer of energy from the environment. Injuries are caused by some form of energy that is beyond the body's resilience to tolerate.[1,2] Trauma epidemiology is the study of the distribution of trauma in populations, the determinants of injury, and the associated causes and risk factors.[1]

Traumatic events are rarely "accidental," and as such the term "accident" is no longer being used in the trauma literature. Most traumatic deaths and injuries do not happen by chance and are preventable. As a result of this shift in thinking, the phrase "motor vehicle crash" (MVC) has replaced the phrase "motor vehicle accident" (MVA), and injuries are now classified as intentional (suicide or homicide) or unintentional (MVC or falls).

Epidemiology of Trauma

The following section of this chapter, Epidemiology of Trauma (which deals only with the United States) will not be covered during the lecture. However, it is strongly suggested that the learner read this section (or the relevant section in Appendix 2-A) before the TNCC to gain knowledge about the epidemiologic issues associated with the incidence of trauma. Please see Appendix 2-A, Epidemiology of Trauma in Selected Countries, at the end of this chapter, for information submitted from countries other than the United States.

Incidence in the United States

Unintentional injury is the fifth leading cause of death for all ages combined in the United States and the leading cause of death for those aged 1 to 44 years.[1,2] Annually, approximately 164,112 deaths result from trauma.

Many injuries do not result in death, but nonetheless place a considerable burden on individuals, the health care system, and society. Approximately one third of all ED visits and 8% of all hospital stays are due to injuries.[3] There were an estimated 40.2 million injury-related ED visits during 2003. In addition, many injuries have consequences well beyond the discharge from the hospital. It is estimated that 5.3 million people in the United States have long-term disabilities from traumatic brain injury. Approximately 2.6 million persons are hospitalized each year as a result of injuries, poisonings, or both.[3]

Human Characteristics

The Subcommittee on Epidemiology of the American Trauma Society has guidelines that are used to monitor the epidemiology of trauma. The guidelines suggest that demographic data elements such as age, gender, and ethnicity be collected to link particular populations with specific mechanisms of injury. These data can be used for planning injury prevention programs.

Age

Injuries result in the death of more persons between the ages of 35 and 44 than in any other age group. Although the actual number of individuals who die of injuries is highest in the age group from 15 to 64 years, those older than age 85 have a greater likelihood of dying.[2] Age-related risk factors that make older adults more prone to injury include decreases in vision, hearing, and cognitive function as well as physical impairments. In addition, the comorbid conditions that many older adult patients have increase the likelihood of them having significant mortality and morbidity. The leading cause of death for every age group from 5 to 24 years is MVC.[2,5]

Gender

There are differences between male and female death rates from injury, depending on the cause of the injury. The overall death rate from injuries is 2.3 times greater for males than females.[4] Exposure to injury-producing events, the amount of risk involved, occupation, and cultural norms have been considered reasons for the gender difference in these rates.

The mechanisms of injury also vary significantly between genders. Men are more likely to be a fatality in an MVC, but women sustain 80% of all hip frac-tures.[5] Men are also more likely than women to sustain a penetrating injury and die of it. However, when data from intimate partner violence (IPV) are examined, 20% of nonfatal violence is against women and 3% against men.[6] However, 76% of all IPV homicides were female and 24% were male.[7]

Race

The causes of death from injury and subsequent death rates vary by race:

- Caucasians

  Motor vehicle crashes remain a leading cause of death for Caucasian males. When one compares the fatality rates of Caucasian females from MVCs against those of Caucasian males, the death rate for women is lower (9.8% versus 22.2%).[2,8]

- African Americans

  Intentional trauma is the leading cause of death for those aged 10 to 24 years. African-American women are considered to be in the higher-risk category for IPV.[9,10]

- Hispanics

  Intentional trauma is the second leading cause of death for those aged 10 to 24 years. Hispanic women are considered to be in the higher-risk category for IPV.[9,10] Hispanics have the highest fatality rate of fatal work injuries.[11,12] This rate has been attributed to the large number of low-paying agricultural and industrial positions worked because of illegal immigration.

- Asians

  Asians have the lowest rate of firearm injury and death among all races.[5,11,12] They also have the lowest fatality rate of all races in MVCs.[5]

- Native Americans

  Injuries are the leading cause of death for Native Americans aged 1 to 44 years and the third leading cause of death overall. Injuries and violence account for 75% of all deaths among Native Americans aged 1 to 19 years. Native Americans have the highest injury-related fatality rate for MVCs, pedestrian events, and suicide when compared to similar age groups of African Americans and Caucasians (frequently 2 to 3 times greater). Women of this minority are considered to be in the higher-risk category for IPV.[6,10,13-15]

Alcohol

Alcohol plays a role in almost all types of traumatic injury. Alcohol influences cognitive functions as well as balance, coordination, and judgment. The effects of alcohol are heightened by sun exposure, heat, and dehydration. The National Highway Traffic Safety

Administration (NHTSA) has reported that fatalities in alcohol-related crashes have been trending downward for a few years.[16] Although fatalities have declined by 1.8% in crashes where the highest blood alcohol concentration was 0.08 grams per deciliter (g/dl) or higher, the use of alcohol remains a problem for young drivers.

With any level of blood alcohol concentration, the risk of involvement in an MVC is greater for teens than for older drivers.[17] Studies have shown that 25% of drivers aged 15 to 20 years who died in MVCs had a blood alcohol concentration of 0.08 g/dl or higher.[17] Among teenaged drivers who were killed in MVCs after drinking and driving, 74% were unrestrained. More than 50% of teenage deaths tended to occur on Friday, Saturday, and Sunday between 9:00 p.m. and 6:00 a.m.[17]

Alcohol is involved in 25 to 50% of adolescent and adult fatalities associated with water recreation.[18] Alcohol use also contributes to an estimated 40% of residential fire deaths.[19,20]

Tobacco

Tobacco plays a role in trauma in several ways. Smoking causes significant health issues, which greatly increases the morbidity and mortality associated with trauma. In addition, smoking is the leading cause of fire-related deaths.[19,20]

Drugs

It is difficult to accurately report the link between drug use (illicit, over-the-counter, and prescription) and trauma. Substance abuse reaches across all socioeconomic and educational boundaries. Some of the more common substances include marijuana, cocaine, amphetamines, painkillers, and diet pills. All medications need to be factored in when contemplating the contributing causes to a trauma, whether the trauma is an MVC, fall, drowning, suicide, or occupational or intentional injury.

Violence

Violence, a public health problem with multiple aspects, includes but is not limited to assault; homicide; IPV; and physical, sexual, and psychological abuse. Homicide is the leading cause of death among young people aged 10 to 24 years.[21] It is estimated that assaultive violence leads to the deaths of 19,000 to 23,000 persons a year in the United States. Firearm injury in the United States has averaged 32,608 deaths annually from 1970 to 2001.[12] It is the second leading cause of death from injury after MVCs and is the leading cause in several states.[12] Firearms are involved in approximately 70% of homicides, 60% of suicides, 40% of robberies, and 20% of aggravated assaults.[12,13]

The correlation between firearm availability and rates of homicide is consistent across high-income industrialized nations: Where there are firearms, there are higher rates of homicide overall.[22] The United States has the highest rates of both firearm homicide and private firearm ownership. The death rate for American children younger than 16 years was nearly 12 times higher than for children in 25 other industrialized countries combined.[21,22]

Among all industrialized countries, more men than women are killed by firearms. However, women in the United States die of firearm injuries in a higher proportion than in most other high-income countries.[21] Each year, 5.3 million incidents of IPV occur among American women aged 18 and older, and 3.2 million occur among men. Most assaults are relatively minor and consist of pushing, grabbing, shoving, slapping, and hitting.[9,10]

Data on the confirmed number of U.S. child maltreatment cases are available from child protective services agencies but are generally considered underestimates. It is estimated that between 1 and 3 million children per year are victims of intentional trauma, and this results in the deaths of at least three children per day.[23] There has been an escalation of abuse against older adults; estimates range from 700,000 to 1.1 million older adults abused annually.[24]

Injury Prevention/Control

Injury prevention focuses on reducing the incidence of injury events. Injury control is a broader concept that not only includes reducing the incidence but also reducing the severity of injuries.[1] Today's health care professionals no longer treat just the injury—they are part of a concerted effort to understand the precipitating factors that contribute to the occurrence of trauma and are taking steps toward the prevention of injury through anticipatory guidance. Because so many traumatic injuries are preventable, one of the most important aspects of trauma nursing is prevention. It is essential that we all learn various safety skills to prevent trauma in our own lives, in those we care about, and in society as a whole. This effort requires a significant commitment to education and behavior modification. Ultimately, nurses can make valuable contributions to a safer environment and a healthier population.

The Committee on Injury Prevention and Control convened by the Institute of Medicine of the National Academy of Sciences has made the following recommendations for promoting injury prevention. This approach is being done through injury prevention research and health care science research.[25]

- Enhance injury surveillance systems, including the development of a national intentional injury surveillance system.

- Enhance the research of biomechanics for high-risk populations.

- Continue to use animals and cadavers for model testing.

- Enhance research related to pathophysiology and reparative processes.

- Develop a national policy addressing the prevention of firearm injuries.

- Authorize the Health Resources and Services Administration to fund trauma care systems' planning, development, and outcomes research.[5]

The annual estimate of "costs" for both fatal and nonfatal injuries is difficult to assess. Such costs include those associated with medical care (including acute and long-term care), indirect morbidity (costs reflective of lost productivity), and indirect mortality (costs reflective of lost productivity because of life years lost).[26,27]

Injury prevention is a systematic approach with the primary purpose of finding solutions that will eliminate or decrease the factors that cause injuries. If injuries occur despite this approach, there will be a high-quality system for prehospital and hospital care to decrease the human effects of trauma.[26]

Injury prevention programs should be based on data that specifically indicate what behavior or situation requires a change. Programs should be determined, designed, and evaluated based on the following steps:[26]

1. Collect data on trauma-related injuries.

2. Analyze the data.

3. Identify specific concerns.

4. Target the population at risk.

5. Identify the population characteristics.

6. Develop prevention strategies (e.g., cost-effectiveness).

7. Implement a prevention plan.

8. Evaluate behavioral changes in the target population.

Injury prevention efforts are primary, secondary, or tertiary. Each phase has its own goal that will ultimately have an impact on reducing or eliminating the injury:

1. Primary: The elimination of trauma-related injuries.

2. Secondary: The reduction of the severity of injury during the incident.

3. Tertiary: All efforts after trauma to improve the outcome.

For an injury prevention program to succeed, educational, legislative, and technologic strategies need to be used. The Centers for Disease Control and Prevention (CDCP) has officially designated the National Center for Injury Prevention and Control a "center" within the CDCP. The agency has devised a strategy whereby most injury control interventions can be classified as one of the following, sometimes referred to as the three "Es." [27,28]

- Engineering and technologic interventions

  These include animal barriers along highways, separation barriers along highways (can be cement, grass, or guardrails), high-mounted rear brake lights, driver vision enhancements, and automated collision notification.

- Enforcement and legislative interventions

  These include seat belt laws, helmet laws, laws against drunk driving, laws forbidding drivers to use handheld cell phones when driving, gun control laws, and the use of cameras at busy intersections to capture photographs of license plate numbers and drivers who run through red lights.

- Education and behavioral interventions

  These include school-based injury prevention programs, driving education programs for new drivers as well as older adults, EN CARE (an injury and violence prevention program of the Emergency Nurses Association), Advanced Trauma Life Support® courses, the Trauma Nursing Core Course from the Emergency Nurses Association, and Prehospital Trauma Life Support courses.

Biomechanics and Mechanisms of Injury

The terms "biomechanics," "kinematics," and "mechanism of injury" are often used interchangeably, although they really have different meanings. The broadest term, biomechanics, refers to the "study of the principles of the action of forces and their effects."[26,27]

Kinematics is a branch of mechanics (energy transfer) that refers to motion and does not consider the concepts of force and mass of the object or body.[29] It is the process of determining which injuries may conceivably have resulted from the forces and motion involved. This concept is based on fundamental principles of physics.

- Newton's First Law: A body at rest will remain at rest. A body in motion will remain in motion until acted on by an outside force.

- Law of Conservation of Energy: Energy can neither be created nor destroyed. It is only changed from one form to another.
- Newton's Second Law: Force equals mass multiplied by acceleration or deceleration.
- Kinetic Energy (KE): KE equals ½ the mass (M) multiplied by the velocity squared (V^2).

Mechanism of injury refers to the transfer of energy from an external force to the human body. The extent of injury is determined by the type of energy applied (blunt, penetrating, thermal, etc.), how quickly it is applied, and to what part of the body it is applied. Energy is the agent that causes physical injury. Energy sources are mechanical/kinetic, thermal, chemical, electrical, and radiant. Drowning is a special circumstance whereby the agent or cause of the injury or death or both is lack of oxygenation (**Table 2-1** and **Figure 2-1**). Mechanical energy is the most common agent of injury in MVCs, motorcycle crashes, falls, and penetrating trauma.

The medical care of a trauma patient can be divided into three phases (precrash, crash, and postcrash). This model is also called a trimodal distribution of how an injury occurs.[26] The term "crash" does not refer to an MVC but rather the moment that energy is transmitted to the patient and an injury occurs.

- Precrash

  All the events that lead up to the incident. This can involve substance abuse, preexisting medical conditions, weather conditions, use of poor judgment, etc.

- Crash

  The transfer of energy. It begins with the first impact and continues until all the impacts are done and the full amount of energy has been dissipated.

- Postcrash

  This begins as soon as the energy has been absorbed and the patient has been injured. It also involves the prehospital provider who renders care to the injured patient.

Mechanical Energy

Injuries sustained from MVCs, falls, gunshots, or any other moving source result from the mechanical energy that is loaded onto the victim and the body's response to that energy. Energy that is beyond the body's resistance to tolerate may cause injury to one of the four types of body tissues: epithelial, connective, muscle, and nerve tissue (**Table 2-2**).[30] The type of tissue injured is important because each type of tissue and structure has a different response and tolerance to the energy load.

Table 2-1: Energy Sources and Mechanisms of Injury

Energy Agent	Mechanism of Injury
Mechanical or kinetic energy	• Motor vehicle crashes • Motorcycle crashes • Firearms, falls, assaults
Thermal energy	• Heat, steam, fire
Chemical energy	• Plant and animal toxins • Chemical substances
Electrical energy	• Lightning • Exposure to wires, sockets, plugs
Radiant energy	• Rays of light (sun rays) • Sound waves (explosions) • Electromagnetic waves (x-ray exposure) • Radioactive emissions (nuclear leak)
Oxygen deprivation (cause, not agent)	• Drowning • Asphyxiation from inhalation of toxic substances (e.g., carbon monoxide, heat, soot)

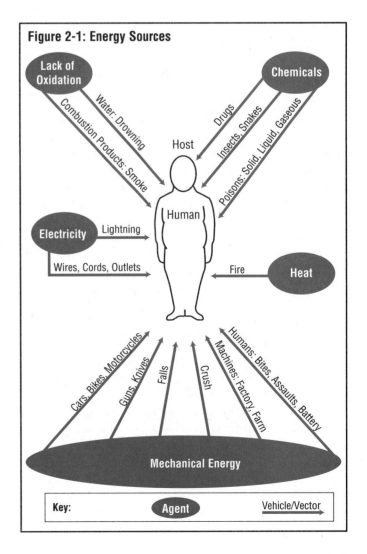

Figure 2-1: Energy Sources

Table 2-2: Types and Examples of Body Tissues

Type	Example
Epithelial tissue	Skin, trachea, mucous membranes, linings of blood vessels and body cavities
Connective tissue	Cartilage, bone, and joint structures
Muscle tissue	Cardiac, skeletal, and smooth (blood vessels, viscera)
Nerve tissue	Neurons and supporting (glial) cells

External Forces Associated with Mechanical Energy and Moving Objects

Mechanical energy from an MVC or fall affects the body through deceleration forces, acceleration forces, or a combination of both. The amount of force an object or body produces depends on the mass of the object or body and the velocity at which it is moving. Both animate objects, such as occupants of a moving motor vehicle, and inanimate objects, such as a motor vehicle or motorcycle traveling at any speed, have energy. Although both mass and velocity contribute to the amount of energy a moving object has, velocity has the greater influence. If the mass of an object is doubled, the energy is doubled. However, if the velocity is doubled, the energy is quadrupled; therefore, the faster the victim or object is moving (velocity), the greater the energy on impact.

Deceleration Forces

Deceleration, or drag, is the force that stops or decreases the velocity of a moving person or object.[26] When a moving object decelerates or decreases its velocity to zero, the energy on impact is dissipated and absorbed around the site of impact. When a person falls from a height and strikes the ground, body tissues partially absorb the sudden change in velocity (deceleration) on impact.

When a body in motion comes to a stop, such as during a fall or MVC, the energy load on human tissue can cause injuries mainly because of deceleration forces. The motor vehicle decelerates and comes to a complete stop as a result of the vehicle's impact. The victim will also come to a stop, dissipating additional energy, once he or she comes in contact with an immovable surface such as the steering column or windshield. During a crash or fall, the body decelerates, yet not all anatomic structures decelerate at the same time. The relative fixation of certain anatomic structures predisposes them to deceleration-type injuries. Two anatomic locations susceptible to deceleration injury are the descending thoracic aorta and the duodenum.

The descending thoracic aorta is partially fixed to the left pulmonary artery by the ligamentum arterio-

sum (a remnant of fetal circulation) and is therefore more likely to be partially or completely transected because of deceleration forces.

Similar forces may cause injury to the retroperitoneal duodenum (portion of the second section, third and fourth sections), or the jejunum near the ligament of Treitz (a fibrous band at the duodenojejunal flexure). If the ligament of Treitz is stressed at the same time the pylorus of the stomach closes, the C-loop of the duodenum (the area where the duodenum leaves the stomach) may sustain an increase in its intraluminal pressure, resulting in perforation of the small bowel.[27]

Acceleration Forces

Acceleration is an increase in speed. A stationary or slow-moving pedestrian who is struck by a car, or an occupant of a slow-moving car who is struck from the rear by another faster-moving car, may sustain injuries from the acceleration of his or her body. Some injury events, like certain MVCs, may lead to injuries that result from a combination of acceleration and deceleration forces.

Other Forces

Bullets, fists, and stabbing instruments are all examples of objects in motion with varying amounts of energy. The amount of energy is dependent on the velocity at which the object strikes the victim and the object's mass. Blasts and explosions are other forces that cause human tissue damage. The injuries are a result of contact with light, heat, or pressure (or all three). Blast forces may lead to blunt, penetrating, and burn injuries.

Internal Forces Associated with Mechanical Energy and Moving Objects

As energy is loaded onto the body, the internal forces of stress and strain are exerted within the body as the body tissues change their dimensions.[27] Stresses are defined as "the forces applied to deform the body or the equal and opposite forces with which the body resists."[29] The degree to which specific tissues are injured is dependent on the resistance of the tissues to energy loads. Stress can be

- Tensile stress, whereby the tissue cells are separated (e.g., stretch on the splenic capsule)
- Compressive stress, whereby they are pressed together (e.g., comminuted bone fracture)
- Shearing stress, whereby the stress results from a tangential force (e.g., tearing of the aorta)[1]

Strain is the tissue damage or deformation that results from the stress.[28] Strain, among other things, is dependent on the properties of the particular tissue involved. For example, because of their elastic fibers, muscles may be stretched and deformed as a result of energy loads. Certain organs, such as the spleen and liver, have minimal elastic ability and are much more susceptible to rupture.[30]

Certain bones can resist energy loads and forces better than others. The femur, sternum, scapula, and the first and second ribs fall into this category. The contents of the cranium are somewhat protected by the meninges and the bony skull. However, the rigidity and internal bony protuberances of the skull may injure the cortex or surface of the brain. This is especially true during injury events that cause the brain to rebound in the cranial vault in a contrecoup fashion.[31] A blow to the back of the head may cause frontal contusions as the brain strikes the internal portion of the anterior skull.

Types of Injuries

One method to categorize injuries resulting from the transfer of mechanical energy is determining whether the energy causes disruption of the skin. Penetrating or open injuries disrupt the skin, whereas in blunt or closed injuries, the skin surface remains intact. The energy associated with blunt trauma is more widespread around the impact point, but it can be absorbed by the underlying structures.

A second method to categorize injuries is determining whether the insult to the body tissues was primary or secondary. Primary injury is a direct result of the impact of energy (thermal, electrical, mechanical, etc.) on the tissue or organ. Secondary injury results from ischemia, swelling, or bleeding that develops as a result of the primary injury.

Blunt Trauma

Blunt injuries tend to be associated with MVCs, motorcycle crashes, assaults, and falls. Because of the vastness of these mechanisms, many variables can contribute to increasing or decreasing the severity of the injury. For example, injuries sustained from an MVC will vary depending on an individual's location in the vehicle, the speed at impact, the stopping distance, the type of vehicle, the point of impact, road or highway barriers, and the use of restraint systems.

Penetrating Trauma

A penetrating injury occurs when there is only an entrance wound. A perforating injury occurs when the object passes completely through the body, resulting in both an entrance and an exit wound. Seventy-eight percent of all penetrating trauma mortality in the United States occurs in urban communities.[32] Most penetrating trauma in urban settings is the result of firearms or sharp objects that either cut or have a

point. In rural settings, the vehicles of energy transfer include animals, machinery, motorized vehicles, missiles launched by machinery, high-pressure equipment, firearms, and sharp objects or materials.[33] The Regional Rural Injury Study found that lacerations were the most common injury, followed by punctures, amputations, and lacerations and punctures combined.[34]

Drowning and Water-Related Injuries

Drowning is the third leading cause of unintentional death in the United States. Males account for 78% of all drowning incidents. Although drowning rates have slowly declined, drowning remains the second leading cause of injury-related death for children aged 1 to 14 years.[5] Most children younger than 1 year drown in bathtubs, buckets, or toilets.[5] Children aged 1 to 4 years who drowned in residential swimming pools had been out of sight less than 5 minutes and were in the care of one or both parents at the time.[5]

Drowning is defined as death by suffocation after submersion. Near drowning has been defined as happening to those who survive, at least temporarily, after submersion. Secondary drowning refers to the deterioration of a seemingly well patient after submersion. Drowning can be classified by the type of water (fresh versus salt) or the amount of water in the lungs (wet versus dry). Whenever a near-drowning patient presents to the emergency department, the possibility of a traumatic injury needs to be ruled out. The most common injuries associated with drownings are spinal cord and head injuries from diving into shallow areas.

Most boating fatalities (70%) are caused by drowning and the remainder by trauma, hypothermia, carbon monoxide poisoning, or other causes. Open motor boats were involved in 41% of all reported incidents, and personal watercraft (i.e., jet skis, windsurfing) were involved in another 28%.[18]

Burns

Tissue injury in burns is related to the coagulation of cellular protein as a result of heat produced by thermal, chemical, electrical, or radiant energy. For a more comprehensive description of burns, please see Chapter 12, Surface and Burn Trauma.

Blast Injuries

Although blast injuries are often associated with the military and terrorism, they are found in a wide variety of settings. They can occur in industrial settings (mining, grain storage, etc.) as well as under circumstances involving explosives (e.g., fireworks, military situations, terrorism). Explosives can be defined as materials that are rapidly converted into gases when detonated. Blast and blast injury describe the gaseous decomposition and the damage occurring to an organism that is subjected to the pressure field produced by an explosion. Blasts are characterized by the release of large quantities of energy in the form of pressure and heat. The blast wave is the result of the expanding gases that displace air, causing it to move away at a very high velocity.

The most common cause of blast injury seen in the United States occurs from fireworks. Although fireworks injuries tend not to be fatal, it is estimated that approximately 9,300 injuries occur each year, and 45% of those injured are children aged 14 years and younger. Children between the ages of 5 and 9 years have the highest injury rate for fireworks-related injuries.[35] Most of these injuries occur at home and usually involve burns to the hands, fingers, eyes, and face. Sparklers are associated with most injuries for children younger than 5 years, and those older than 5 years were injured by fireworks, rockets, and other devices.

When larger explosive situations from bombs and industrial situations occur, the amount of energy released can be tremendous. The four mechanisms that affect individuals who are involved in a blast situation are described in **Table 2-3**, along with the causes and primary organs affected.[26,27]

Motor Vehicle-Related

The pattern of injury for each trauma patient is different. The pattern of injury is a combination of the patient's age, mechanism of injury, anatomic structures involved, and preexisting factors (e.g., alcohol ingestion and restraint systems). Knowing the pattern of injury can guide the trauma nurse to predict and be prepared for the manifestations of certain injuries. The history of the injury event may reveal information leading to early identification and treatment of injuries.

Factors contributing to the pattern of injury sustained by persons involved include the use or nonuse of restraint systems, the position of the victim in the vehicle, and the type of collision or impact. The five types of collisions are frontal, or head-on; rear impact; lateral, or side impact; angular; and rollover.[26,27] **Table 2-4** describes patterns of injury in unrestrained occupants of MVCs.[26,36]

Table 2-5 describes injuries that may occur when pedestrians or motorcyclists are struck by motor vehicles.[26] When a pedestrian or motorcyclist is struck, different injuries may be sustained during impact or when the victim is thrown on top of the vehicle, sliding from the vehicle to the ground, or dragged under the vehicle.

Table 2-6 reflects percentages of injuries sustained by unrestrained occupants and drivers involved in nonfatal MVCs.[31]

Vehicular Occupant Protection

Familiarity with vehicular occupant protection technology will assist in the trauma nurse's understanding of patterns of injury. Vehicle crash-worthiness, "friendly" interiors, and restraint systems are the three main occupant protection concepts.[37] An example of increased crash-worthiness is improved construction

Table 2-3: Mechanisms of Blast Injuries

Mechanism	Causation	Primary Organs Affected
Primary	Initial blast or air wave. It is important to try to determine what type of blast occurred (steam, chemical, gas, electrical, etc.) so that prehospital providers can be safe and secondary complications can be avoided with the patients.	Affects primarily air-filled organs: • Tympanic membranes—Rupture and permanent deafness can occur • Lungs—Pneumothorax, alveolar rupture, air embolus • GI—Intestinal and stomach contusions and rupture • CNS—Concussion syndrome, various types of focal and diffuse cerebral hemorrhage, cerebral air embolism
Secondary	Flying debris, which act as projectiles	Injuries will vary depending on the size of the projectiles and what and where they hit
Tertiary	The distance an individual's body travels from the blast and where it has an impact	Injuries are similar to those in an individual who has been ejected from a motor vehicle crash or fallen from a great height
Miscellaneous	Inhalation of dust or toxic gases, thermal burns, radiation, etc.	Lungs, skin, eyes

Reprinted with permission from P.C. Reid

of the vehicle's front end so that during an impact, intrusion into the occupant's compartment is minimized. Examples of friendly interiors are cars equipped with energy-absorbing steering systems or high-penetration-resistant windshields.

Restraint systems used in modern cars include safety belts, inflatable restraints (i.e., air bags), and car seats for infants and children. Safety belts include shoulder and lap belts. Improper placement of safety belts or not wearing them can result in higher morbidities and mortalities for the occupants. Adults older than 55 years wear safety belts more often than any other age group except infants and preschool children.[38]

Dual air bags became a federal standard requirement in 1997 in all passenger cars sold in the United States.[39] The air bag is a passive restraint system, meaning the occupant does not have to engage the system for it to be effective.

The rapid inflation of the air bag (which uses a pyrotechnic mechanism to fill the bag with nitrogen) and occasional debris from the air bag pose some risk to the occupant.

Air bags do not replace safety belts. Because the air bag immediately deflates, safety belt restraints should be worn to protect the occupant from vehicular ejection. Proper positioning of an occupant in a vehicle equipped with front air bags is important. There should be at least 10 inches between the occupant and the location of the air bag. The force of a deployed air bag can injure or kill a young child, even in a slow-speed crash. Children aged 12 years and younger, including infants, should never be placed in a seat in front of an air bag.[40]

Table 2-4: Patterns of Injury in Unrestrained Occupants of Motor Vehicles

Type of Impact	Predicted Injuries
Frontal impact (down-and-under trajectory)	• Chest (ribs, heart, and aorta most vulnerable) • Abdomen (liver and spleen most vulnerable) • Posterior dislocation of hip • Point of impact (e.g., knee, femur, ankle)
Frontal impact (up-and-over trajectory)	• Head and neck • Chest and upper abdomen
Lateral impact (T-bone impact)	• Head and face if thrust forward • Cervical spine • Same side shoulder, clavicle • Lateral abdomen (liver of right-side occupant, spleen of left-side occupant)
Rear impact	• Head and neck

The National Highway Traffic Safety Administration (NHTSA) has concluded that air bags:

- Reduce fatality risk for drivers by 31% in "purely frontal crashes."
- Reduce fatality risk for unbelted drivers by 13% in all crashes.

Table 2-5: Patterns of Injury Related to Pedestrians and Motorcyclists Struck by Motor Vehicles

Mechanism of Injury	Possible Injuries
Adult pedestrian struck by motor vehicle	
When struck	• Knees • Tibia, fibula, femur • Pelvis
When thrown on top of a vehicle (hood or windshield)	• Depends on victim's position when struck • If struck from the front, truncal injury (e.g., ribs, spleen) • If struck from the back, vertebral column injury
When sliding from vehicle to ground	• Cranial and spinal injuries
When dragged under the vehicle	• Pelvis
Motorcyclist	
Head-on collision	• Ejected over the motorcycle • May strike face and chest on handlebars
Angular collision	• Lower legs may become trapped
Ejection	• Cranial injuries and cervical injuries
Lay bike down on side	• Inside leg fractures and soft-tissue injuries

Table 2-6: Injuries (Percent) of Occupants and Drivers Injured in Nonfatal Motor Vehicle Crashes

Position in Vehicle	Injuries
Unrestrained front-seat passenger (right side of car)	• Pelvic fractures (46%) • Femur fractures (41%) • Cranial injuries (24%) • Abdominal injuries (13%)
Unrestrained driver (left side of car)	• Femur fracture (65%) • Pelvic fracture (46%) • Chest injury (46%) • Ankle fractures (39%) • Facial bone fractures (37%) • Cranial injuries (16%)

- Reduce overall injury risk by 60% with use of air bags and lap-shoulder belts.[41]

In January 1998, NHTSA allowed "repair shops and dealers to install on–off switches that allow air bags in passenger cars and light trucks to be turned on and off in appropriate circumstances." The installation of these switches requires written authorization from NHTSA.[41] Actual air bag deactivation (if the car manufacturer has no available on–off switch) may be authorized by NHTSA if:

- "A rear-facing infant restraint must be placed in the front seat of a vehicle because there is no back seat or the back seat is too small for the child-restraint (passenger air bag only);
- A child age 12 or younger must ride in the front seat because the child has a condition that requires frequent medical monitoring in the front seat (passenger air bag only);
- An individual who drives (or rides in the front seat of) the vehicle has a medical condition that makes it safer to have the air bag(s) turned off (driver and/or passenger air bag, as appropriate); each request based on a medical condition must be accompanied by a written statement from a physician unless the request is based on a medical condition for which the National Conference on Medical Indications for Air Bag Deactivation recommends deactivation;
- Drivers who must sit with their breast bone less than 10 inches from the air bag. These are usually individuals who cannot adjust their position to greater than 10 inches from the steering wheel."[41]

The deployment mechanism may differ, and the "switch-off" may not be available in all countries.

All 50 states and the District of Columbia have some form of child-restraint law.[41] Many varieties of car seats for infants and children are available. The use of different styles of infant and child car seats is based on the weight and age of the occupant. All children should be placed in an age- and weight-appropriate restraint system.[38] Rear-facing child car seats should not be used in front passenger seats equipped with air bags. Studies have shown that the most common misuse of child-restraint systems involved

- Loose vehicle safety belt attachment to the child-restraint system
- Loose harness securing

School bus-related fatalities have, over the past few years, influenced several political, civic, and professional groups to advocate the installation of safety belts in school buses. Considerable information related to seat belt installation is available from NHTSA.

The following is current statistical information about school bus-related fatalities:[42]

- "An average of 30 children die in school-bus related traffic crashes each year—Nine school bus occupants and 21 pedestrians."
- Fifty percent of all pedestrians fatally injured in school bus-related crashes were between 5 and 7 years old.

These statistics show that school bus safety is a multifaceted issue. Some experts suggest that more impact may be achieved by focusing injury prevention strategies on pedestrians around school buses than on their occupants. An entire school bus safety program for children is available free from NHTSA.

Falls and Jumps

Falling or jumping from a height that results in the person landing on his or her feet or head is termed "axial loading" because the energy on impact is applied to the axial skeleton. Fractures of the lower extremities and vertebral column are associated with individuals who land on their feet. Head and cervical spine injuries can result from axial loading onto the head (e.g., diving into a pool).

The pattern of injury related to falls or jumps from heights is a consequence of the following:

- Age of the person
- Distance from which the person fell or jumped
- Energy absorbency of the surface on which the person fell
- Preexisting conditions of the person
- Preexisting conditions of the environment
- Anatomic point of impact
- Energy (deceleration) loaded onto the person at the time of impact

More than one third of adults aged 65 years and older fall each year.[43] Falls are the leading cause of traumatic death and the most common cause of non-fatal injuries and hospital admissions for older adults. Among individuals aged 75 years and older, those who fall are four to five times more likely than other patients to be admitted to a long-term care facility after discharge. The most common bone fractures in falls are the vertebrae, hip, forearm, leg, ankle, pelvis, upper arm, and hand.[43]

Young children are also prone to falls, especially on the playground. About 45% of playground-related injuries involve fractures, internal injuries, concussions, dislocations, and amputations. About 75% of nonfatal injuries related to playground equipment occurred on public playgrounds and were on equipment that involved climbing. Most fatal injuries occurred on home playgrounds and involved swings.[44,45]

Stab Wounds

Stab wounds result from pointed or sharp objects (or both) being forced inward by a thrust, movement, or fall. Damage to underlying tissues occurs as structures in the path of the wounding instrument are punctured. Injury depends on the anatomic area involved. Wounds are commonly caused by knives, but other types of objects may also cause stab-type injuries (e.g., scissors, knitting needles, and nail guns). Tissue injury is related to the length of the instrument, the velocity at which the force was applied, and the angle of entry. Although the puncture site may follow a straight path, this is not always true. Tissues may be disrupted and pushed aside by the penetrating instrument, thus causing damage to adjacent structures. It is important to try to determine the blade length, whether the blade was smooth or serrated, and the angle of penetration.[46]

A narrow, pointed instrument (e.g., an ice pick) would cause microscopic tissue damage, and the damage would be confined to the path of the instrument's point. If the instrument were tapered and flat (as in a dagger), there would be fraying and crushing of the tissues as they stretched to accommodate the wide edge of the blade close to the shaft. If a blunter instrument (such as an ax) is used, there will be greater crushed tissue, and the force applied to achieve the same degree of penetration will introduce a component of "blunt" injury.[46]

Firearm Injuries

Firearms include handguns, rifles, and shotguns. Handguns are classified as revolvers or autoloading pistols and are mostly low- to medium-velocity weapons. Rifles are high-velocity weapons that can release a single shot, be semiautomatic, or be fully automatic (i.e., holding down the trigger releases more than one bullet). Shotguns are classified by the gauge (diameter of the barrel) and may be loaded with either pellets or powder shells. The tissue damage inflicted by bullets is related to their velocity, shape, construction, and mass. Tissue properties (e.g., elasticity) that contribute to cavitation and the amount of the kinetic energy on impact also are related to the degree and type of tissue damage.[27,46]

The range, or the distance, between the weapon's barrel and the victim, affects the velocity at which the bullet strikes the body tissues. The impact velocity at which the bullet strikes the victim more closely approximates the actual bullet velocity the closer the range is. A projectile missile, and its fragments in the case of a bullet, can cause direct injury to any type of tissue in its path. The indirect consequences of the penetration that contribute to the type of wound are because of shock waves that lead to compression from longitudinal displacement and shear waves that lead to cavitation from transverse displacement.[27,46]

Factors that contribute to damage are

- Missile size

  Larger bullets have greater resistance and leave a larger permanent track in the body. Caliber is the internal diameter of the gun barrel, which corresponds to the type of ammunition used.

- Missile deformity

  Hollow-point and soft-nose bullets flatten on impact, creating larger surface areas that are damaged.

- Semijacket

  The jacket expands and adds to the surface area damaged.

- Tumbling

  Tumbling causes a wider path.

- Yaw

  Yaw is the degree of rotation in the missile's flight pattern (either vertically or horizontally about its axis). This creates a larger surface area presenting to the tissue.

Bullets can be classified in various ways; the most common ways are by their composition (**Table 2-7**) and shape (**Table 2-8**).[46]

Summary

Epidemiology defines the scope of injuries in terms of their incidence and identifies associated factors and determinants of specific types of injury.[47]

Statistics and quantitative data are only a portion of the epidemiologic view of the injury problem. The epidemiologic foundation can, however, help direct program planners to form injury prevention and control programs.

Energy is the agent of injury. The type and severity of injuries that result from the transfer of energy from the environment to the human host depend on the types of external forces applied, internal forces, characteristics of the anatomic structures affected, and the pattern of injury. Even though a certain pattern of injury may be predictable for specific incidents, every trauma victim must be assessed according to the principles outlined in the primary and secondary assessment to be sure that all injuries are identified.

Table 2-7: Classification of Bullets by Their Composition

Composition of Bullets	Characteristics
Homogeneous	Made of a single substance, such as lead.
Coated	Usually have a lead core but are coated with a thin layer of another metal, usually steel.
Jacketed	Have a heavy metal core of lead or steel. Steel is used when a high muzzle velocity is anticipated, because lead has a tendency to melt while the bullet is still in the barrel due to the heat produced by high velocities. The core then has a thick covering of "gliding metal," which is usually copper, copper alloy, or steel.
Semijacketed	Same as a jacketed bullet but instead of a "full metal jacket," a portion of the bullet's core is exposed (usually the nose). This design allows the jacket to strip off, fragment within the target, and cause more serious damage. Used primarily for sport game hunting. Outlawed for use by the military (Hague Convention of 1899, Geneva Convention of 1949, and the International Committee of the Red Cross in 1974).
Rubber	There are several different kinds. Original British rubber bullets were made of rubber and designed to be fired at the ground so that they would bounce up and hit the legs of demonstrators. They were intended to inflict superficial painful injuries. Now rubber bullets are metal bullets coated in rubber or rubber plugs, plastic bullets called baton rounds, and beanbag rounds (fabric bean bags about the size of a tea bag filled with lead pellets). Each type has a different effect on the human body under different circumstances. All the bullets are designed to break apart after they are fired and inflict injury to several people with one bullet.
Exploding bullets	The nose is filled with explosive substances such as black powder (Pyrolex) or a synthetic powder, lead azide (Devastator). These bullets increase destruction by causing a secondary explosion within the tissue. These bullets can also be dangerous to health care workers, who might be injured attempting to remove them.

Reprinted with permission from P.C. Reid

Table 2-8: Classification of Bullets by Shape

Shape	Composition
Pointed nose	
Round nose	Certain kinds are called "soft points" and on impact will flatten and "mushroom" back on themselves, increasing the amount of damage.
Hollow-pointed nose	Made with a depression at the tip of their noses and deform on impact. It is thought that by becoming deformed, these bullets will increase the amount of damage.
Flat nose	One type is "Dum-Dum" bullets, which were developed by the British in 1897 at their garrison in Dum Dum, India. The Hague Convention outlawed them for military use.

Reprinted with permission from P.C. Reid

References

1. National Center for Health Statistics (NCHS). (2005). *Health, United States, 2005 with chartbook on trends in the health of Americans.* Hyattsville, MD: Author.

2. Anderson, R. N., & Smith, B. L. (2005). Deaths: Leading causes for 2002. *National Vital Statistics Reports, 53*(17), 1–10.

3. McCaig, L. F., & Burt, C. W. (2005, May 26). *National Hospital Ambulatory Medical Care Survey: 2003 Emergency department summary.* Retrieved December 20, 2006, from http://www.cdc.gov/nchs/data/ad/ad358.pdf

4. Kochanek, K. D., Murphy, S. L., Anderson, R. N., & Scott, C. (2004). Deaths: Final data for 2002. *National Vital Statistics Reports, 53*(5), 1–13.

5. Centers for Disease Control and Prevention (CDC). (2003). *Web-based injury statistics query and reporting system (WISQARS).* Retrieved December 20, 2006, from http://www.cdc.gov/ncipc/wisqars

6. Rennison, C. (2003). *Intimate partner violence, 1993–2001.* Retrieved December 20, 2006, from http://www.ojp.usdoj.gov/bjs/abstract/ipv01.htm

7. Fox, J. A., & Zawitz, M. W. (2004). *Homicide trends in the United States.* Retrieved December 20, 2006, from http://www.ojp.usdoj.gov/bjs/homicide/homtrnd.htm

8. Insurance Institute for Highway Safety (IIHS). (2003). *Fatality facts: Older people.* Arlington, VA: Author.

9. Tjaden, P., & Thoennes, N. (2000). *Extent, nature and consequences of intimate partner violence: Findings from the national violence against women survey.* Retrieved December 20, 2006, from http://www.ojp.usdoj.gov/nij/pubs-sum/181867.htm

10. Tjaden, P., & Thoennes, N. (2000). *Full report on the prevalence, incidence and consequences of violence against women: Findings from the national violence against women survey.* Retrieved December 20, 2006, from www.ncjrs.org/txtfiles1/nij/183781.txt

11. U.S. Department of Labor. (2004). *Census of fatal occupational injuries (revised data).* Retrieved December 20, 2006, from http://www.bls.gov/iif/oshcfoi1.htm

12. Federal Bureau of Investigation (FBI). (2004). *Crime in the United States, 2003: Uniform crime reports.* Washington, DC: U.S. Government Printing Office.

13. Centers for Disease Control and Prevention (CDC). (1997). *Fatal firearm injuries in the United States, 1962–1994.* Retrieved December 20, 2006, from http://www.cdc.gov/ncipc/pub-res/firarmsu.htm

14. Centers for Disease Control and Prevention (CDC). (2003). Injury mortality among American Indian and Alaska Native children and youth—United States, 1989–1998. *Morbidity and Mortality Weekly Report, 52*(30), 697–701.

15. Centers for Disease Control and Prevention (CDC). (2002). Traumatic brain injury among American Indians/Alaska Natives, 1992–1996. *Morbidity and Mortality Weekly Report, 51*(14), 301–305.

16. National Highway Traffic Safety Administration (NHTSA). (2005). *2004 traffic safety annual assessment—Early results* (DOT HS 809 897). Retrieved December 20, 2006, from http://www-nrd.nhtsa.dot.gov/pdf/nrd-30/NCSA/RNotes/2005/809897.pdf

17. Insurance Institute for Highway Safety (IIHS). (2005). *Fatality facts: Teenagers 2005.* Retrieved December 20. 2006, from http://www.iihs.org/research/fatality_facts/teenagers.html#sec1

18. U.S. Coast Guard. (2002). *Boating statistics—2002.* Retrieved December 20, 2006, from http://www.uscgboating.org/statistics/Boating_Statistics_2002.pdf

19. Ahrens, M. (2005). *The U.S. fire problem overview report: Leading causes and other patterns and trends.* Quincy, MA: National Fire Protection Association.

20. Centers for Disease Control and Prevention (CDC). (1998). Deaths resulting from residential fires and the prevalence of smoke alarms—United States 1991–1995. *Morbidity and Mortality Weekly Report, 47*(38), 803–806.

21. Anderson, R. N., & Smith, B. L. (2003). Deaths: Leading causes for 2001. *National Vital Statistics Report, 52*(9), 1–86.

22. Krug, E. G., Powell, K. E., & Dahlberg, L. L. (2000). Firearm availability and homicide rates across 26 high-income countries. *Journal of Trauma, 49*(6), 985–988.

23. McCurdy, M., & Daro, P. (1994). *Current trends in child abuse reporting and fatalities: The results of the 1993 annual fifty-state survey.* Chicago: National Committee to Prevent Child Abuse.

24. American Nurses Association. (1998). *Culturally competent assessment for family violence.* Washington, DC: Author.

25. Bonnie, R. J., Fulco, C. E., Liverman, C. T. (Eds.), & Committee on Injury Prevention and Control, Institute of Medicine. (1999). *Reducing the burden of injury: Advancing prevention and treatment.* Washington, DC: The National Academies Press.

26. McSwain, N. E., Frame, S., & Salomone, J. P. (Eds.). (2003). *PHTLS: Basic and advanced pre-hospital trauma life support* (pp. 10–61). St. Louis, MO: Mosby.

27. McSwain, N. E. (2000). Kinematics of trauma. In D. V. Feliciano, E. E. Moore, & K. L. Mattox (Eds.), *Trauma* (4th ed., pp. 127–152). Philadelphia: McGraw-Hill.

28. The National Committee for Injury Prevention and Control. (1989). Injury prevention: Meeting the challenge. *American Journal of Preventive Medicine, 5*(3), 1–303.

29. Illingworth, V. (Ed). (1991). *The penguin dictionary of physics* (2nd ed.). London: Penguin Books.

30. Porth, C. M. (1998). Cell and tissue characteristics. In C. M. Porth (Ed.), *Pathophysiology concepts of altered health states* (5th ed., pp. 3–32). Philadelphia: Lippincott.

31. Ommaya, A. K. (1985). Biomechanics of head injury: Experimental aspects. In A. M. Nahum & J. Melvin (Eds.), *The biomechanics of trauma* (pp. 245–270). Norwalk, CT: Appleton-Century-Crofts.

32. Fingerhut, L. A. (1996). Epidemiology: Urban mortality. In R. R. Ivatury & C. G. Cayten (Eds.), *The textbook of penetrating trauma* (pp. 17–31). Baltimore: Williams & Wilkins.

33. Gerberich, S. G., Gibson, R. W., & Olson, D. K. (1996). Epidemiology: Rural trauma. In R. R. Ivatury & C. G. Cayten (Eds.), *The textbook of penetrating trauma* (pp. 32–47). Baltimore: Williams & Wilkins.

34. Gerberich, S. G., Gibson, R. W., French, C. R., Carr, P., Renier, C. M., Gunderson, P. D., et al. (1993). *Regional rural injury study-I (RRIS-I): A population-based effort, a report to the Centers for Disease Control.* Minneapolis, MN: University of Minnesota Regional Injury Prevention Research Center. (NTIS No. PB 94-134848).

35. Greene, M. A., & Joholske, J. (2003, June). *2003 fireworks annual report: Fireworks-related deaths, emergency department treated injuries, and enforcement activities during 2003.* Retrieved December 20, 2006, from http://www.cpsc.gov/library/2003fwreport.pdf

36. American College of Surgeons Committee on Trauma. (2001). Appendix 2: Biomechanics of injury. In *Advanced trauma life support for doctors: Instructor course manual* (7th ed., pp. 417–438). Chicago: Author.

37. Viano, D. C. (1988). Cause and control of automotive trauma. *Bulletin of the New York Academy of Medicine, 64*(5), 376–421.

38. National Highway Traffic Safety Administration (NHTSA). (1999). *Fourth report to Congress: Effectiveness of occupant protection systems and their use* (DOT HS 808 919). Retrieved December 20, 2006, from http://www-nrd.nhtsa.dot.gov/Pubs/808-919.PDF

39. Daffner, R. H., & Lupetin, A. R. (1988). Patterns of high-speed impact injuries in motor vehicle occupants. *Journal of Trauma, 28*(4), 498–501.

40. National Highway Traffic Safety Administration (NHTSA). (2004). *Child passenger safety 2004* (DOH HS 809 231). Retrieved December 20, 2006, from http://www.nhtsa.dot.gov/people/injury/childps/safetycheck/OccProtetcFor_Children1.pdf

41. National Highway Traffic Safety Administration (NHTSA). (2002). *Occupant protection for children safety information* (DOT HS 809 575). Retrieved December 20, 2006, from http://www.nhtsa.dot.gov/people/injury/airbags/airbags03/images/Air%20Bags0307.pdf

42. National Highway Traffic Safety Administration (NHTSA). (1999). *Traffic safety facts 1998: School buses* (DOT HS 808 959). Retrieved December 20, 2006, from http://www-nrd.nhtsa.dot.gov/pdf/nrd-30/NCSA/TSF98/Schbus98.pdf

43. Centers for Disease Control and Prevention (CDC). (2001). *Web-based injury statistics query and reporting system (WISQARS).* Retrieved December 20, 2006, from Retrieved December 20, 2006, from http://www.cdc.gov/ncipc/wisqars

44. Tinsworth, D. K., & McDonald, J. E. (2001). *Special study: Injuries and deaths associated with children's playground equipment.* Retrieved December 20, 2006, from http://www.cpsc.gov/library/playgrnd.pdf

45. Phelan, K. J., Khoury, J., Kalkwarf, H. J., & Lanphear, B. P. (2001). Trends and patterns of playground injuries in United States children and adolescents. *Ambulatory Pediatrics, 1*(4), 227–233.

46. McSwain, N. E. (1996). Ballistics. In R. R. Ivatury & C. G. Cayten (Eds.), *The textbook of penetrating trauma* (pp. 105–119). Baltimore: Williams & Wilkins.

47. National Highway Traffic Safety Administration (NHTSA). (2005). *Safety rulemaking and supporting research priorities, 2005–2009.* Retrieved December 20, 2006, from http://www.nhtsa.dot.gov/nhtsa/announce/NHTSAReports/ PriorityPlan-2005.html

Web sites

- American Trauma Society—www.americantraumasociety.org
- Centers for Disease Control and Prevention—www.cdc.gov
- Department of Transportation—www.dot.gov
- Federal Bureau of Investigation—www.fbi.gov
- Mothers Against Drunk Driving (MADD)—www.madd.org
- National Center for Injury Prevention and Control—www.cdc.gov/ncipc
- National Highway Transportation Safety Administration—www.nhtsa.dot.gov
- National Institutes of Health—www.nih.gov
- United States Department of Labor—www.bls.gov
- University of Pennsylvania Firearms Injury Center—www.universityofpennsylvania/hospital/surgery/traumacenter/research

Australia (for presentation in Australia)

Introduction

Data collected on injury and traumatic death in Australia is sporadic and not well compiled to produce nationally reflective statistics. However, the Australian Bureau of Statistics publishes the most recent epidemiologic information on the health status of the Australian population. In 2001, a National Health Survey involving close cooperation with major agencies in the health field, particularly the Institute of Health and Welfare, the Department of Health and Ageing, and the State and Territory Government Health Authority, allowed the development of a snapshot of trauma statistics in Australia. Some of the following information is derived from that survey.

Incidence

The 2003 National Health Survey indicated that 2.3 million Australians had sustained an injury in the 4 weeks leading up to the survey. Extrapolated from these data is the notion that approximately 12% of the population may sustain an injury in any given month. That amounts to more than 75,000 injuries daily, or about 52 Australians injured every minute.[1]

Trauma is the fourth leading cause of death after neoplasm, ischemic heart disease, and respiratory disease. Trauma as a cause of death relates to accidents, poisonings, and violence and has consistently been between 5 and 6% over the past 5 years.

Of all traumatic deaths, suicide remains the leading cause, accounting for 3 of 10 (30%) trauma-related deaths. Transport-related mortality causes a quarter (24.9%) of trauma deaths, followed by poisoning (10%), falls (7%), assaults (4%), and drowning (2.8%).[2]

Transport accident statistics, from 26.7 per 100,000 population in 1993 to 24.1 per 100,000 in 2003, indicated a fall in the standardized death rate from vehicle trauma.

The Australian road traffic deaths rate of 8.9 road deaths per 100,000 persons in 2001 compares favorably with the rates of France (13.8), the Republic of South Korea (17.2), and the United States of America (14.8), but is higher than the rate for Sweden (6.2) and the United Kingdom (6.1).[3]

The standardized death rate in 2003 from intentional self-harm (suicide) was 17.7 per 100,000 males and 4.7 per 100,000 females, which were both decreases from the respective rates recorded in 2002 (18.8 per 100,000 males and 5.0 per 100,000 females).

In 2003, 2,213 deaths attributed to suicide were registered, 4.6% less than in 2002 and 13% lower than the 1997 record.[2]

Human Characteristics

Age

Injury remains the primary cause of death among young people. Older Australians are injured at a lower rate than other age groups but are more likely to die as a result of their injuries. Data suggest that the age group most likely to sustain an injury within any given time period is the 5- to 14-year-old age group, making this group a target area for injury prevention campaigns.

1 to 14 Years

The most common causes of unintentional death in children are motor vehicle crashes, drowning, and inhalation of foreign bodies.

Trauma accounts for 40% of all deaths in young children, with more than half of the deaths being attributed to transport injuries. Drowning is still responsible for 1 death in every 100,000 children, which is equivalent to 16% of all traumatic child deaths.[2]

15 to 24 Years

Thirty-seven (37.1) of every 100,000 young adults die as a result of trauma. This constitutes more than 69.5% of all trauma-related deaths. Transport injuries are responsible for 45% of those (16.7 per 100,000), and self-harm and substance abuse for almost 30% (11.5 per 100,000).[2]

25 to 34 Years

This age group has the highest number of traumatic deaths, with 42.6 per 100,000. Forty percent of these are the result of suicide, and more than one quarter are from transport injuries.[2]

35 to 44 Years

In this age group, suicide was the leading cause of traumatic death, with 16.2 deaths per 100,000 (40.3%). Transport injury was identified as a marginally lower cause of traumatic death, with 9.2 deaths per 100,000 population.[2]

45 to 64 Years

Similar trauma rates are reported for the fifth and sixth decades of life (32 per 100,000 and 30.2 per 100,000, respectively), with suicide only getting a mention in the statistics (14.7 per 100,000) in the 45- to 54-year-old age bracket.[2]

65 to 84 Years

The next two age groups show a steady increase in traumatic death, but not one that is disproportionate from other mortality figures. In the 75- to 84-year-old age group, falls became a highlighted issue. Although trauma was the cause of death in less than 2.2% of this older adult group, falls contributed to more than 20% of traumatic deaths.[2]

> 85 Years

In this age group, 2 to 3% of individuals (mean, 2.54%) die of trauma, with falls making up more than 27% of that trauma.[2]

Race

External causes (trauma) were a major contributor to death among indigenous Australians and ranged from approximately 12% in New South Wales to 20% in South Australia. The death rate of Aboriginal people from road crashes is 35 per 100,000 of the Aboriginal population, compared with only 14 per 100,000 population for non-Aboriginal people.[4]

Aboriginal people also have higher rates of hospitalization from road crashes across all age groups compared with non-Aboriginal people. For those aged 45 to 64 years, the rate is more than 4 times that for non-Aboriginal people, and for those aged up to 14 years, the rate is nearly 3 times as high. For those aged 65 years and older, the rate is double, although the numbers involved are small.[4]

Road crashes involving Aboriginal people have the following characteristics:

- Many are single-vehicle crashes, most of which happen in country areas.
- Many do not involve a collision (e.g., rollovers).
- High numbers of pedestrians are struck and killed or injured, with most crashes occurring in country areas.
- Many of those killed or hospitalized are passengers.
- Alcohol is a significant factor, particularly in single-vehicle crashes and crashes involving pedestrians.
- Vehicles are often overloaded.
- Seat belts are often not worn.[4]

Alcohol

Drunk driving has been one of the largest single contributors to road trauma. Twenty-five years ago, 44% of drivers and motorcycle riders killed in transport accidents had more than the legal concentration of alcohol recorded in their blood. In 1995, that proportion was 30%. The most recent national figure, for 1997, is 28%.[5]

Improvements have probably come about through a combination of reducing the permissible blood alcohol limit to 0.05 g/100 ml of blood (0.05%), introducing and maintaining a high level of random breath testing, and giving heavy penalties reinforced with publicity and information measures (e.g., the distribution of millions of "standard drink" cards, media advertising) aimed at making drunk driving socially unacceptable.

Violence

Approximately three quarters of all alcohol-related violence is committed by young persons aged 14 to 24 years, and about half of the violence committed by this age group is committed by just 6% of young persons. This violence can take many forms, from property damage to verbal abuse, from physical assault to homicide.[6]

Violence is more likely to occur in the presence of alcohol consumption. We know that levels of alcohol consumption are higher among younger people than older people, and particularly among young males. It is no surprise, then, that alcohol-related violence is concentrated among young people and particularly among young males.[6]

Suicide

In 2001, suicide became the leading cause of death from injury in Australia, accounting for 31% of all injury-related deaths.[7]

From 1993 to 2003, the male age-standardized suicide death rate was approximately four times higher than the corresponding female rate. Of all suicide mechanisms, 46% are attributed to suffocation or hangings, making this mechanism of injury the most common successful method.[2]

Age standardization allows comparison of rates between populations with different age structures. The age-standardized suicide rate for persons in 2003 was 6% lower than the corresponding rate for the previous year and 24% lower than the peak for the period 1993 to 2003, which occurred in 1997.[2]

For males in many age groups, there was a decline in age-specific suicide rates after peaks in the years 1997 and 1998. The age-standardized suicide rate for males (17.7 per 100,000) in 2003 was lower than in any year in the previous decade (1993 to 2002).[2]

Similarly, for females there were declines in rates for some age groups over this period, and the age-standardized suicide rate for females (4.7 per 100,000) in 2003 was the lowest since 1994.

The highest age-specific suicide death rate for both males and females in 2003 was observed in the 30- to 34-year-old age group (30.1 per 100,000 for males and 9.1 per 100,000 for females).

The lowest age-specific suicide death rate for males in 2003 was observed in the 15- to 19-year-old age group (12.7 per 100,000). For females, low rates occurred in the 75 years-and-older age group and in the 15- to 24-year-old age group.

Prevention

Road Safety Changes and Initiatives

Despite an increase in the number of motor vehicles, the introduction of road safety initiatives and increased public awareness have contributed to a reduction in road fatalities since the 1970s.[8]

These initiatives include the following:

- Improvements to roads, such as separated dual-lane highways, major road bypassing of towns and suburbs, use of audible edge lining, and removal of roadside hazards
- Changes to vehicles in line with the Australian Design Rules standards, including child-restraint anchorages and seats, head restraints, air bags, and increased impact resistance
- Legislation requiring the compulsory restraint of children in cars
- Legislation requiring the fitting and wearing of seat belts and motorcycle and bicycle helmets
- Initiatives against drunk driving, such as random breath testing and public education campaigns
- Enhanced police enforcement aided by technology such as red light and speed cameras

Falls

Most jurisdictions in Australia have fall prevention strategies in place in health care facilities. Community support organizations are committed to raising awareness and providing assistance to modify public areas to reduce the risk of falls. Local council playgrounds use safer play equipment, place soft-fall technology under play gym equipment, and govern public facilities with respect to workplace health and safety (falls-risk management). Examples of workplace health and safety initiatives include handrails and nonslip flooring.

Drowning

Teaching children how to swim has been heavily promoted by celebrities in the media for the past half decade. Swimming lessons have also been modified to include not only swimming technique but also contingency training, such as being able to locate a pool edge and learning how to climb out of a pool.

Instances of childhood drowning decreased in the 1990s after legislation to make swimming pool fencing compulsory was passed. When one state relaxed its policy on swimming pool fencing in the late 1990s, there were resultant increases in childhood drowning in that state.[9]

Schools continue to increase awareness of water safety. Community organizations such as the Royal Surf Life Savers launch school and media campaigns to increase water safety issues. These are seasonal initiatives to help reduce immersion injuries.

Poisoning

The media has assisted with the increase of community awareness of the dangers of both intentional and unintentional poisoning. First-aid courses now focus on prevention of poisoning (and other injuries) as a major component of the curriculum. Legislation has been introduced to require manufacturers of poisonous substances to have specific labeling requirements, with first-aid management and National Poisons Information Centre (PIC) phone numbers printed on every container. Childproof packaging for poisonous substances (including medications) and childproof locking devices for cabinets are now less expensive and more accessible.

References

1. Australian Bureau of Statistics. (2005). *Causes of death, Australia, 2003*. Retrieved October 17, 2005, from http://www.abs.gov.au/AUSSTATS/abs@.nsf/ProductsbyReleaseDate/DF33BD7579B1CB35CA25713000705177?OpenDocument

2. Australian Bureau of Statistics. (2003). *2003 Year book Australia 2003—Health, injuries and deaths due to external causes*. Retrieved October 17, 2005, from http://www.abs.gov.au/Ausstats/abs@.nsf/Previousproducts/15085C8D57AA7610CA256CAE000FC5B6?opendocument

3. Australian Bureau of Statistics. (2003). *Year book Australia 2003—Accidents involving fatalities*. Retrieved October 17, 2005, from http://www.abs.gov.au/Ausstats/abs@.nsf/Previousproducts/3875170E8478D171CA256CAE0016268F?opendocument

4. Western Australian Government. (2000). *The way ahead—Road trauma and Aboriginal people*. Retrieved October 17, 2005, from http://www.police.wa.gov.au/Services/pdf/Discussion_Paper.pdf

5. Australasian College of Road Safety. (2004). *Alcohol—ACRS policy statement*. Retrieved October 17, 2005, from http://www.acrs.org.au/collegepolicies/people/alcohol.html

6. Australian Institute of Criminology. (2001). *Alcohol and violence—The missing link.* Retrieved October 17, 2005, from http://www.aic.gov.au/media/2001/20010227.html

7. Australian Bureau of Statistics. (2003). *Australian social trends, 2003—Mortality and morbidity: Injuries.* Retrieved October 17, 2005, from http://www.abs.gov.au/AUSSTATS/abs@.nsf/2f762f95845417aeca25706c00834efa/1a0ecc988f5f1d50ca2570eb008398cd!OpenDocument

8. Australian Bureau of Statistics. (2005). *Year book Australia, 2005—Road fatalities and fatality rates 1925–2003.* Retrieved October 17, 2005, from http://www.abs.gov.au/Ausstats/abs@.nsf/Previousproducts/1301.0Feature%20Article302005?opendocument&tabname=Summary&prodno=1301.0&issue=2005&num=&view=

9. Australian Bureau of Statistics. (2001). *Year book Australia 2001—Child health since federation.* Retrieved October 17, 2005, from http://www.abs.gov.au/ausstats/abs@.nsf/0/3CE0381F7CBAB608CA2569DE0024ED6D?Open

Canada (for presentation in Canada)

Introduction

Injuries, both unintentional and intentional, are a significant public health problem in Canada.[1] During 2003–2004, 9,892 major injury (Injury Severity Scale > 12) cases were reported.[1] These injuries accounted for 162,082 hospital days; 1,369 (14%) of those injured died either in the emergency department or after admission.[1]

There are a number of sources for injury data in Canada. These include:[2]

- The Canadian Institute for Health Information (CIHI), created in 1994, is a national agency responsible for coordinating the development and maintenance of a comprehensive and integrated health information system. CIHI receives information related to 78% of all acute care discharges. The database utilizes "E codes" from the International Classification of Diseases (ICD) that relate to the external cause of injury (e.g., motor vehicle crashes, poisonings, and homicides). Information from the database can be used to quantify both the financial and human costs of injuries. CIHI coordinates Canada's National Trauma Registry (http://secure.cihi.ca/cihiweb/splash.html).

- The Canadian Hospitals Injury Reporting and Prevention Program (CHIRPP) is a major program of the Injury Section of the Health Surveillance and Epidemiology Division of Health Canada. CHIRPP is an injury surveillance system based on data gathered from 15 hospital emergency departments. The primary purpose of this data source is injury surveillance. Other purposes include research and reporting (Web site: http://www.phac-aspc.gc.ca/injury-bles/).

- First Nations and Inuit Health Information System (FNIHIS) is part of the First Nations and Inuit Health Branch's (FNIHB) Community Health Program Directorate, which is responsible for the delivery of health programs and services. Their mandate is to work with FNIHB Regions and First Nations and Inuit organizations to assist their people to maintain and improve their health (Web Site: http://www.hc-sc.gc.ca/fnih-spni/index_e.html).

- The Statistics Canada Vital Statistics—Death Database is primarily used for population estimates. In 1921, a central repository of all vital statistical data was established in collaboration with provincial/territorial vital statistic registries. Data are used to generate tables and reports to support surveys and program work, and to link with other internal databases for specific studies (Web site: http://www.statcan.ca/cgi-bin/imdb/p2SV.pl?Function=getSurvey&SDDS=3233&lang=en&db=IMDB&dbg=f&adm=8&dis=2).

- The Transport Canada, Traffic Accident Information Database is used to support the regulatory activity of the Motor Vehicle Safety Act and to provide national figures, both to Canada and the international community, of all reported traffic collisions in the country. These data are primarily used to identify issues/characteristics related to traffic crashes, develop countermeasures, analyze trends, and generate reports.

- The Canadian Agricultural Injury Surveillance Program (CAISP) became a national collaborative program in 1995 with funding from Agriculture and Agri-Food Canada, 10 provincial organizations, and the Ontario Farm Safety Association. The main purpose of the data source is for research. It supports injury surveillance with the collection, integration, interpretation, and dissemination of injury data to public health professionals and safety promotion organizations (Web site: http://meds.queensu.ca/~emresrch/caisp/welcome-english.html).

- The Canadian Surveillance System for Water-Related Fatalities tracks drownings and other water-related deaths, and disseminates the information through public education. The database is jointly owned, managed, and maintained by the Canadian Red Cross. The primary purpose of this data source is to support prevention training programs, public education campaigns, and drowning research projects (Web site http://www.redcross.ca/article.asp?id=000881&tid=024).

Incidence

In 2003 to 2004, the main categorical breakdowns of injuries were blunt trauma (94%), penetrating trauma (4%), and burns (2%). Head injuries stand out as being the most commonly reported (65%) medical diagnosis.[1]

The most prevalent mechanisms of injury in 2003 to 2004 were:[1]

- Motor vehicle crashes (MVCs)—47%

- Unintentional falls—29%

- Homicide and injury purposefully inflicted—8%

- Other incidents (includes being unintentionally struck by object or person, being unintentionally struck by falling object, and incidents caused by machinery)—6%

Because MVCs caused the most injuries, it is not surprising that they accounted for almost half (42%) of all injury-related deaths.[1] The most frequently injured person in an MVC was the driver (54%), including those on motorcycles, followed by their passengers (28%).[1] Pedestrians accounted for 16% of those injured, but 28% of those killed. Cyclists made up 4% of injury-related deaths, while another 4% had major injuries.[1]

Causes of unintentional falls correlated to age and illustrate important focus areas for injury prevention. Falls from one level to another (including playground equipment) accounted for 24% of those injured through this mechanism in the under 20-year-old age group. Significant in the 20- to 34-year-old age group were falls from buildings/structures (27%). Falls on or from stairs were the most common mechanism for those aged 35 to 64 years (20%) and older than 65 years (24%).[1]

Human Characteristics

Age

MVCs are the leading cause of injury for all age groups except seniors, where unintentional falls are more numerous. During 2003 to 2004, the mean age for sustaining a major injury (ISS > 12) was 43 years, and the leading mechanisms were

- Under 20 years: MVCs 53% (excluding cyclists for this age group only), Unintentional falls 16%, Other 8%, Cyclist 7%

- 20 to 34 years: MVC 58%, Homicides 15%, Unintentional falls 12%, Other 10%

- 35 to 64 years: MVC 47%, Unintentional falls 28%, Other 12%, Homicide 8%

- 65 years and older: Unintentional falls 62%, MVCs 30%, Other 4%, Fire and flames 1%[1]

Gender

Males accounted for 72% of those sustaining major injuries. This is consistent for most injury causes, except for homicide and intentional injuries where males accounted for 90% of those injured.[1] Males (68%) were also more likely than their female counterparts to die as a result of an MVC.

Race and Geographical Considerations: Aboriginal Peoples

Similar to the nonnative population in Canada, injury is the leading cause of death for Aboriginal people, but the injury rate is significantly increased in this group:[3]

- The injury death rate among Aboriginal teens is almost four times that of Canadians overall.

- Aboriginal disability rates are reported at 31%, double the national rate, with a large proportion attributed to injuries.

- First Nations and Inuit suicide rates are almost three times higher than those of Canadians overall.

Substance Abuse

Alcohol plays a significant role in trauma. From 2003 to 2004, 13% of those injured had blood alcohol levels above the Canadian legal limit (0.08 mg/dl).[1] Almost half (43%) of people who consumed more than eight alcoholic drinks per week admitted to driving after consuming more than two consecutive drinks.[1] Men were three times more likely to report such drinking and driving activities.[1] Alcohol is not the only substance that can lead to injury. Many illicit, as well as prescription, drugs can also alter decision-making skills and lead to both intentional and unintentional injury. Evidence is clear that a moderate or higher dose of cannabis will impair driver performance.[4] After alcohol, cannabis is the most widely used psychoactive drug in Canada. A recent study of Ontario students found that during the previous year, 19.3% of drivers in high school reported driving within an hour of using cannabis.[4] Two recent studies detected cannabinoids in 13.9% and 19.5% of samples of seriously injured and fatally injured drivers, respectively.[4]

Violence and Self Inflicted Injury

In 2003 to 2004, homicides and intentional injuries accounted for 8% of all major injury cases.[1] They were primarily male (90%), and the mean age of those involved was 31 years.[1] Blunt trauma injuries (66%) were predominately featured, followed by penetrating trauma at 34%.[1] Where reported, mechanisms of intentional injuries included fights (28%), stabbings (25%), and gunshot wounds (13%).[1] Twenty percent were due to other causes or the cause was not reported.[1] Suicide continued to be a problem and primarily affected younger adults (mean age, 38 years), accounting for 3% of the total injuries reported, not including data related to poisonings.[1]

Injury Prevention

Injury prevention is the practice of assessing and managing risk, with the goal of instituting injury-preventing behaviors or, simply, living in healthy ways that minimize the risk of injury.[5] At all levels, the social, economic, political, cultural, educational, and environmental conditions that support injury-preventing behaviors must be in place for prevention to become a reality. Injury prevention means making positive choices about minimizing risk at all levels of society while maintaining healthy, active, and safe communities and lifestyles. These choices are strongly influenced by the environments where one lives, works, learns, and plays. Injury-prevention programs cost money, and the outcomes are not quickly measured. For example, it may take 10 years for a bicycle helmet program to significantly show the trend of reduction in head injuries. Funding for acute trauma care versus injury prevention is not equitable. Injury prevention practitioners use financial data to demonstrate the stark contrast between the cost of preventing injuries and the cost of treating injuries; prevention always costs less. A study by the Centers for Disease Control and Prevention (CDC)[6] is used in both Canada and the United States to illustrate these facts:

- $1 spent on smoke alarms saves $69
- $1 spent on bicycle helmets saves $29
- $1 spent on child safety seats saves $32
- $1 spent on road safety improvements saves $3
- $1 spent on prevention counseling by pediatricians saves $10
- $1 spent on poison control services saves $7

Canada has governmental and nongovernmental groups working toward the prevention of injuries. **Table 2-9** provides a list of some of the key agencies involved with injury prevention and control. In the provinces, several injury prevention and control centers have been established. The purpose of these centers is to develop regional programming and research infrastructure. The centers work with government departments, local organizations, and injury coalitions to establish educational programs, environmental modifications, and legislative and policy changes designed to prevent injuries. **Table 2-10** provides contact information for these provincial organizations.

There is a movement to create and implement a National Strategy for Injury Prevention. The SMARTRISK

Foundation serves as the coordinating agency for these efforts. The initial workbook document, *Developing an Integrated Canadian Injury Prevention Strategy,* and updates on the progress of this strategy can be obtained through the Web site (http://www.injury preventionstrategy.ca/downloads/IP_Strat_bckgrnd.pdf).

Costs

Injury costs Canadians about $12.7 billion each year.[7] A document released in November 1998, *The Economic Burden of Unintentional Injury in Canada,*[8] is filled with compelling statistics and highlights the economic impact to Canadians. Similar studies have since been completed in various Canadian provinces. All documents can be downloaded from the SMARTRISK Web site (http://www.smartrisk.ca/).

References

1. Canadian Institute for Health Information. (2006). *National trauma registry report: Major injury in Canada.* Toronto, ON: Author.

2. Health Surveillance Working Group, Injury Surveillance Sub-Group. (2002). *Inventory of Injury Data Sources and Surveillance Activities.* Ottawa: Health Canada.

3. SmartRisk. (2005). *Ending Canada's invisible epidemic: A strategy for injury prevention.* Toronto: Author. Retrieved September 26, 2006, from http://www.injurypreventionstrategy.ca

4. Mann, R. E., Brands, B., Macdonald, S., & Stoduto, G. (2003, May). *Impacts of cannabis on driving: An analysis of current evidence with an emphasis on Canadian data.* Ottawa: Transport Canada. (TP14179E).

5. SmartRisk. (2005) *What is injury prevention?* Retrieved September 28, 2005, from http://www.injurypreventionstrategy.ca/whatis.html

6. Centers for Disease Control and Prevention. (2000). *Working to prevent and control injury in the United States—Fact book for the year 2000.* Atlanta, GA: National Center for Injury Prevention and Control.

7. SmartRisk (2005). *Why is injury a problem?* Retrieved September 28, 2005, from http://www.injurypreventionstrategy.ca

8. SmartRisk. (1998). *The economic burden of unintentional injury in Canada.* Retrieved September 28, 2005, from http://www.smartrisk.ca

Table 2-9: Key Canadian Agencies for Injury Prevention and Control

Agency Name	WEB SITE for Data, Resources, Handouts
Agriculture Canada (Farm Safety Surveillance System and Injury Prevention)	http://www.agr.gc.ca
Block Parents of Canada	http://www.blockparent.ca/english/main.html
Canada Safety Council	http://www.safety-council.org
Canadian Association for Suicide Prevention	http://www.thesupportnetwork.com/CASP/main/html
Canadian Association of Poison Control Centers	http://www.napra.org/practice/Toolkits/Toolkit6/poison_control.html
Canadian Centre of Occupational Health and Safety	http://www.canoshweb.org
Canadian Centre on Substance Abuse	http://www.ccsa.ca
Canadian Firearms Center	http://www.cfc.gc.ca
Canadian Institute of Child Health	http://www.cich.ca
Canadian Institute of Health Information (CIHI)—National Trauma Registry	http://secure.cihi.ca/cihiweb/dispPage.jsp?cw_page=home_e
Canadian Parks and Recreation Association (Playground Safety)	http://www.cpra.ca
Canadian Pediatric Society	http://www.cps.ca
Canadian Public Health Association	http://www.cpha.ca
Canadian Red Cross Society	http://www.redcross.ca
Centre for Suicide Prevention	http://www.suicideinfo.ca
Fire Prevention Canada	http://www.fiprecan.ca
Health Canada—Seniors Injury Prevention (Aging and Seniors Section)	http://www.phac-aspc.gc.ca/seniors-aines/pubs/injury_prevention
Health Canada (Many divisions and departments with Injury Prevention Information)	http://www.hc-sc.gc.ca
Lifesaving Society of Canada	http://www.lifesaving.ca
MADD Canada	http://www.madd.ca
Public Health Agency of Canada	http://www.phac-aspc.gc.ca/new_e.html Includes Emergency Preparedness, Child, Adult, and Seniors Injury Prevention
Rick Hansen Man in Motion Foundation (Spinal Cord Injury Prevention)	http://www.rickhansen.com
SAFEKIDS Canada (Unintentional injury prevention for children Birth–14 yrs.)	http://www.sickkids.ca/safekidscanada
Safe Communities Foundation	http://www.safecommunities.ca
Statistics Canada (Injury hospitalization & mortality data)	http://www.statcan.ca/
St. John Ambulance (First Aid training and prevention of injuries)	http://www.sja.ca
ThinkFirst Foundation (Head and spinal injury prevention)	http://www.thinkfirst.ca
Transport Canada (Road, rail, air, marine)	http://www.tc.gc.ca/en/menu.htm
War Amps of Canada	http://www.waramps.ca

Table 2-10: Provincial Injury Prevention and Control Centers

Regional Center	Web Site
British Columbia Injury Prevention & Research Unit	http://www.injuryresearch.bc.ca
Alberta Center for Injury Control and Research, Edmonton, AB	http://www.med.ualberta.ca/acicr
KIDSAFE Connection, Stollery Children's Health Centre, Capital Health, Edmonton, AB Calgary Health Region	http://www.capitalhealth.ca/YourHealth/Campaigns/KidSAFE http://www.calgaryhealthregion.ca/hecomm/IPC/ipc
Saskatchewan Prevention Institute, Saskatoon, SK	http://www.preventioninstitute.sk.ca
IMPACT, the Injury Prevention Centre of Children's Hospital Winnipeg, MB	http://www.hsc.mb.ca/impact
SMARTRISK Foundation, Toronto, ON	http://www.smartrisk.ca
Plan-it Safe, Children's Hospital of Eastern Ontario, Ottawa, ON	http://www.plan-itsafe.com
Quebec WHO Collaborating Center for Safety Promotion and Injury Prevention	http://www.inspq.qc.ca/
Child Safety Link, IWK Children's Health Centre, Halifax, NS	http://www.childsafetylink.ca
Nova Scotia Health Promotion	http://www.gov.ns.ca/ohp/injuryPrevention/ns_strategyl
Atlantic Network for Injury Prevention	http://www.anip.ca

Norway (for presentation in Norway)

Incidence

Trauma is the third leading cause of death in Norway after cardiovascular disease and cancer. Since 1985, Norway has had an injury registry in several trauma centers, which collected data from other hospitals' databanks on diagnosis, treatment, "E codes," etc. In 2006, Norway implemented a new national system of accidents and injury registration in which all Norwegian hospitals caring for trauma patients will participate. This system will enable the country to carry out a continuous surveillance of information related to trauma and trauma care. One of the main reasons for compiling these data was to intensify preventive work throughout Norway.

Characteristics

Age

In Norway, the most common places where injuries occur for pediatrics were classified as (1) home, (2) traffic, (3) sports, (4) other leisure activities, and (5) school. The mechanisms were identified as a fall on the same level, high falls, being hit by sharp or blunt objects, and collisions. The most common places where injuries occur for older adults are (1) home, (2) streets (not traffic), (3) leisure, (4) work-hobby, and (5) traffic. Injuries are most likely caused by falls on the same level, falls down, hit by blunt or sharp objects, and high-energy collisions.

Sweden (for presentation in Sweden)

Incidence

Trauma is a serious threat to the well-being of the inhabitants of Sweden. It is the fourth leading cause of death, behind heart and vascular disease, respiratory organ disease, and cancer. Young healthy persons often are involved in trauma, which causes a loss of their productive years. Suicide remains a significant problem in Sweden. Since the 1970s, the incidence of suicide has continued to increase. Suicide fatality rates are higher in men, but women are more likely to attempt it. Sweden has become more proactive in injury prevention over the past few years. In January 2005, Sweden enacted a law that made it mandatory for all children younger than 15 years to wear a helmet when on a bicycle.

Human Characteristics

Age

Most injuries leading to death caused by trauma occur between the ages of 15 and 44 years. Most of the deaths between 16 and 64 years of age are associated with suicide and traffic accidents, whereas falls are more common in older adults.

Gender

For men up to the age of 45 years, trauma is the most common cause of death. In women up to the age of 45 years, it is the second most common cause of death. Men tend to be involved more with motor vehicle crashes and suicide, whereas women sustain falls and hip fractures. There are significant gender differences between people injured in the large cities and people injured in sparsely populated areas. For those aged 20 to 44 years, the frequency of injuries for men is 80% higher in sparsely populated areas than in large cities. For women, the difference is lower, at 60%. In the 45- to 64-year-old age group, there is the greatest difference. More than 60% more injuries occur in sparsely populated areas among men and 30% more among women than in large cities.

Violence

Violence is not very common in Sweden. It was estimated that in Sweden in 1996, assaults resulted in the deaths of 150 persons and the hospitalization of 2,278 persons. In data released in 2002, the number of homicides was roughly the same.

References

1. National Board of Health and Welfare/ Epidemiologic Center. (2002). *Causes of death 1999.* Andersson.

2. Ponzer, S. (1996). *Psychological factors in trauma patients. Studies on trauma recurrence and trauma recovery.* Doctoral dissertation, Karolinska Institute. Stockholm, Sweden: Author.

3. The Centre for Epidemiology at the National Board of Health and Welfare. (1996). *The Swedish hospital discharge register.* Stockholm, Sweden: Author.

4. WHO Collaboration Centre on the Community Safety Promotion, Karolinska Institute, Stockholm, Sweden.

United Kingdom (for presentation in the UK)

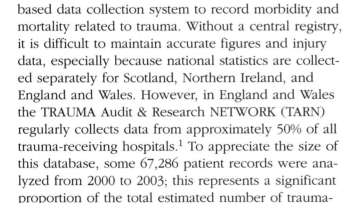

Introduction

In the United Kingdom (UK), there is no centrally based data collection system to record morbidity and mortality related to trauma. Without a central registry, it is difficult to maintain accurate figures and injury data, especially because national statistics are collected separately for Scotland, Northern Ireland, and England and Wales. However, in England and Wales the TRAUMA Audit & Research NETWORK (TARN) regularly collects data from approximately 50% of all trauma-receiving hospitals.[1] To appreciate the size of this database, some 67,286 patient records were analyzed from 2000 to 2003; this represents a significant proportion of the total estimated number of trauma-related deaths annually across the UK. The Scottish Trauma Audit Group (STAG) collates similar information from all major trauma units in Scotland.

The trauma audit networks aim to improve the management of the seriously injured trauma patient through data analysis of patient demography, the nature and severity of injury, and the clinical management of the patient. Through audit and research of trauma patients and their outcomes, data can be used to inform and improve trauma care across the UK.

Incidence

Trauma is the fourth leading cause of death for all ages combined in the UK, but it is the most common cause of death for those younger than 40 years.[1,2] Taking a global view of "life years lost" through premature death and disability, injury will be in second place by 2020.[1]

The annual UK figures for trauma-related deaths are estimated to be between 14,500 and 18,000 people. The cost to the British taxpayer is around £2.22 billion per annum, which represents about 1% of the gross national product.[3]

The latest review from the Office for National Statistics on causes of mortality in England and Wales (2004) states the following common causes of traumatic death:[4]

- Motor vehicle crashes (36%)
- Falls (16%)
- Intentional self-harm/suicide (20%)
- Exposure to smoke, fire, and flames (2%)
- Assault (2%)
- Drowning and submersion (1%)
- All other trauma events and their adverse effects (33%)

The Office of National Statistics classifies deaths attributed to all other trauma causes to include environmental and industrial accidents and overdoses.[4]

The incidence of life-threatening injuries in different body systems is

- Head—30 to 70%
- Chest—20 to 35%
- Abdomen—10 to 35%
- Spine—5%

More than 40% of trauma victims have a concurrent orthopaedic injury, which is usually not life threatening.[3] Ninety percent of trauma deaths in children occur in the context of head injury. Sixty-four percent of all deaths on the TARN database occur in head-injured patients, even though it is known that only 13% of this group have a significant (CT positive) head injury.[5]

Human Characteristics

Age

National statistics reveal that although the incidence of trauma deaths is greatest from 15 to 54 years (**Table 2-11**), the death rate, per head of population, is greatest for those older than 85 years. The leading cause of death for ages 15 to 44 years remains motor vehicle crashes.[4]

According to TARN data (**Table 2-12**), 11% of injuries occur in the 0- to 15-year-old age group, 65% in the working adult (16- to 64-year-old) age group, and 24% in those older than 65 years.

Mortality rates climb from about 3% in children to 11% in older adults, even though the injury severity score (ISS) is 9, which is equivalent to a moderate brain injury OR (not *and*) a displaced limb fracture in each age group. This seems to reflect our increasing vulnerability to injury with age (**Table 2-13**).[1]

Gender

There are differences in male to female injury death rates, depending on the cause of the injury. The overall death rate from injury is twice as high for males as females. Exposure to the injury-producing event, the amount of risk involved, the occupation, and cultural norms are possible reasons for the gender differences.

Alcohol

The number of alcohol-related deaths in England and Wales, which rose throughout the 1980s and 1990s, has continued to rise in more recent years. It increased from 5,970 in 2001 to 6,580 in 2003. Alcohol-related deaths are much more common for males than females. In 2003, males accounted for almost two thirds of the total number of alcohol-related deaths.[4]

There is a growing recognition that the use of illegal substances, either in conjunction with alcohol ingestion or not, is a factor related to trauma deaths. The true picture of deaths as a result of substance abuse is difficult to capture and calculate at this time because random drug testing is not a routine feature of traffic policing, and blood alcohol testing is illegal. Having blood alcohol levels or a blood alcohol concentration of 80 mg/100 ml or higher is illegal.

Suicide

In 2003 there were 5,755 recorded adult suicides (18.1 deaths per 100,000 population) in the UK, the lowest figure since 1973. Suicide is much more common in men than in women, with three quarters of the 2003 deaths being male. Despite the figures, the suicide rates for both sexes have decreased steadily since 1998.[4]

Violence

In British society, the presence of violence is becoming increasingly more common. Violent incidents can be classified as assaults (with or without weapons), rape, and sexual assault. Violent assault "includes both nonfatal and fatal interpersonal violence where physical force or other means is used by one person with the intent of causing harm, injury, or death to another."[6] However, according to TARN data, only 2% of trauma deaths are attributed to penetrating trauma in great contrast to the United States. In the United States, the use of firearms is related to both violence and suicide. The firearm death rate for United States teenagers (ages 15 to 19) rose at the alarming rate of 77% from 1985 to 1990.[7]

The increasing incidence of violence as a public health problem in the UK is raising the awareness of the general public and government. The risks and predetermining factors that need to be investigated include gang culture, lack of nonviolent male role models, drug culture, and unemployment.

References

1. TRAUMA Audit & Research NETWORK. (2005). Retrieved from www.tarn.ac.uk

2. The Scottish Trauma Audit Group (STAG). (2005). Retrieved from www.1shtm.ac.uk

3. Gwinnutt, C., & Driscoll, P. (Eds.). (2003). *Trauma resuscitation: The team approach* (2nd ed.) Oxford, England: BIOS Scientific Publishers Ltd.

4. Office for National Statistics. (2004). *Mortality statistics: Cause 2003*. Series DH2 no.30. HMSO. London: Author. Retrieved from www.statistics.gov.uk

5. Patel, H.C., Bouamra, O., Woodford, M.W., King, A.T., Yates, D.W., & Lecky, F.E. (2005). Trends in head injury outcome from 1989 to 2003 and the effect of neurosurgical care: An observational study. *Lancet, 366,* 1538-44.

6. Rosenberg, M. L., & Fenley, M. A. (1991). *Violence in America: A public health Approach.* New York: Oxford University Press.

7. Fingerhut, L. A. (1993). Firearm mortality among children, youth, and young adults 1 to 34 years of age, trends and current status: United States 1985–90. *Advance Data from Vital and Health Statistics, 231,* 1–20.

Table 2-11: External Causes of Morbidity and Mortality—Accidents in the United Kingdom (Death rates per million population)

Age (years)	< 1	1–4	5–14	15–24	25–34	35–44	45–54	55–64	65–74	75–84	> 85
Male	60	40	25	229	208	193	183	182	258	782	2,946
Female	46	26	15	53	45	48	74	85	155	692	3,118

Reprinted with permission from the Office for National Statistics (2004). *Mortality statistics: Cause 2003*. Available at www.statistics.gov.uk

Table 2-12: Mortality by Year and Age in the United Kingdom (excluding transfers out)

Year of admission	Number	Median	25th Percentile	75th Percentile
Age Group 0 – 15				
2000	2,034	9	9	13
2001	1,937	9	9	11
2002	1,896	9	9	11
2003	1,704	9	9	11
Total	**7,571**	**9**	**9**	**12**
Age Group 16 – 64				
2000	11,028	9	9	10
2001	11,085	9	9	10
2002	10,799	9	9	11
2003	11,292	9	9	13
Total	**44,204**	**9**	**9**	**10**
Age Group 65+				
2000	4,152	9	9	9
2001	3,787	9	9	9
2002	3,810	9	9	9
2003	3,762	9	9	9
Total	**15,511**	**9**	**9**	**9**

The TRAUMA Audit & Research NETWORK Prepared September 2005

Table 2-13: Injury Severity Score by Year and Age in the United Kingdom

Year of admission	Number	Median	25th percentile	75th percentile
2000	17,214	9	9	10
2001	16,809	9	9	10
2002	16,505	9	9	10
2003	16,758	9	9	10
Total	**67,286**	**9**	**9**	**10**

The TRAUMA Audit & Research NETWORK Prepared September 2005

Chapter 3

Initial Assessment

Introduction

A systematic process for initial assessment of the trauma patient is essential for recognizing life-threatening conditions, identifying injuries, and determining priorities of care based on assessment findings.[1,2,3] The initial assessment is divided into two phases, primary and secondary assessments. Both phases can be completed within several minutes unless resuscitative measures are required. Within an organized team approach to trauma care, this first step of the nursing process (assessment) is often simultaneously conducted with the identification of nursing diagnoses that require immediate intervention. Utilizing an organized, systematic approach when one assesses each trauma patient helps to ensure that injuries will not be missed and that priorities can be set for each intervention based on the life-threatening potential of each injury.

Standard Precautions

Nurses involved in trauma resuscitation must follow Occupational Safety and Health Administration (OSHA), Centers for Disease Control and Prevention (CDC), and institutional guidelines to protect themselves and the patient from any unnecessary risk of exposure to infectious diseases. Adherence to "Standard Precautions" (precautions for care of all patients in hospitals) and "Transmission-based Precautions" (precautions for care of patients who are known or suspected of being infected or colonized by certain pathogens transmitted by air or contact with skin or droplet) are indicated for use by the trauma team. All trauma team members should be provided with personal protective equipment (PPE). This equipment should include gloves, gowns/aprons, masks and respirators (if indicated), and goggles and face shields.[4] Factors that influence the type of PPE to be used during trauma resuscitation include the type of exposure anticipated, the durability and appropriateness for the task, and the fit of the equipment. Trauma team members should be taught how to use PPE appropriately. Personal protective equipment should be put on before contact with the patient, used carefully so that contamination is not spread, and then removed and carefully discarded. After removal of PPE, hand hygiene should be immediately performed.

A Guide to Initial Assessment

Initial assessment provides the nurse with subjective and objective data that are analyzed, interpreted, and documented. The following mnemonic may assist nurses during the initial assessment of a trauma patient:

- Primary Assessment

  A—Airway with simultaneous cervical spine protection

  B—Breathing

  C—Circulation

  D—Disability (neurologic status)

  E—Expose/environmental controls (remove clothing and keep the patient warm)

- Secondary Assessment

  F—Full set of vital signs/focused adjuncts (includes cardiac monitor, urinary catheter, and gastric tube)/family presence

  G—Give comfort measures (verbal reassurance, touch, and pharmacologic and nonpharmacologic management of pain)

  H—History and Head-to-toe assessment

  I— Inspect posterior surfaces

Primary Assessment and Resuscitation

The primary assessment begins immediately on the patient's arrival at the hospital, with collection of primarily objective information. The extent and timing of obtaining information related to both the injury event and the patient's past medical history depend on the severity of the patient's condition. Subjective information from prehospital personnel, family, or the patient at this point of the assessment process is limited to a brief statement composed of the patient's major injuries or chief complaints and the mechanism of

injury. A more detailed history is obtained during the secondary assessment.

Airway with simultaneous cervical spine protection,[5] breathing, circulation, disability (neurologic status), and expose/environmental control are the A-B-C-D-E of the primary assessment. Remove only those clothes necessary to expose the patient to conduct the primary assessment. If any life-threatening injuries or circumstances are determined, implement interventions to correct them immediately. Additional assessment steps are not taken until the primary assessment is completed.

Airway with Cervical Spine Protection

Assessment

Open and inspect the patient's airway while initiating or maintaining cervical spine protection. Because partial or total airway obstruction may threaten the patency of the upper airway, observe for the following:

- Vocalization

  Is the patient able to talk? Is the patient crying or moaning?

- Tongue obstructing the airway
- Loose teeth or foreign objects
- Blood, vomitus, or other secretions
- Edema

If the patient has been intubated or an alternative airway has been inserted before arrival at the hospital, confirm that the airway device is in the correct place by

- Observing for equal rise and fall of the chest with ventilation.
- Listening over the epigastrium (nothing should be heard) and then over the lung fields (breath sounds should be heard equally bilaterally).
- Using a specific device to confirm tube placement:
  - Exhaled CO_2 detector
  - Esophageal detection device (EDD)
- Obtaining a chest radiograph.

Interventions

Airway Patent

- Maintain cervical spine protection for any patient whose mechanism of injury, symptoms, or physical findings suggest a spinal injury.
- If the patient is awake and breathing, he or she may have assumed a position that maximizes the ability to breathe. Before proceeding with cervical spine protection, ensure that interventions do not compromise the patient's breathing status.

Airway Totally Obstructed or Partially Obstructed

- Place the patient in a supine position.

  If the patient is not already supine, logroll the patient onto his or her back while maintaining cervical spine protection. Remove any headgear such as a football helmet, if necessary, to allow access to the airway and cervical spine. Removal of such gear should be done carefully and gently to prevent any manipulation of the spine. Penetrating wounds may cause disruption of the integrity of the airway, and blunt trauma may lead to injury of the larynx or other upper structures, causing partial or complete obstruction.

- Protect the cervical spine.

  - If the patient is already in a rigid cervical collar and strapped to a backboard, do not remove any devices until directed by an appropriate care provider. Check that the devices are placed appropriately.

  - If the patient has not been immobilized, perform in-line manual stabilization of the patient's head. Complete spinal immobilization includes application of a rigid cervical collar, placing the patient on a backboard, and having the patient appropriately strapped to the backboard. Complete spinal immobilization should be done at the completion of the secondary assessment, depending on the degree of resuscitation required and the availability of team members.

  - Cervical spine protection is a concept that includes in-line manual stabilization and complete spinal immobilization. During the primary and secondary assessments, the patient may only have in-line manual stabilization as a means to protect the cervical spine until the resuscitation and assessment are completed.

- Open and clear the airway.

(Read Chapter 4, Airway and Ventilation, for an expanded discussion on airway management.)

  - Techniques to open or clear an obstructed airway during the primary assessment include

    - Jaw thrust
    - Chin lift
    - Removal of loose teeth or foreign objects
    - Suctioning

  - Maintain the cervical spine in a neutral position. Do not hyperextend, flex, or rotate the neck during these maneuvers.

  - Suctioning and other manipulation of the oropharynx must be done gently to prevent stimulation of the gag reflex and subsequent vomiting, aspiration, or both.

- Insert an oropharyngeal or nasopharyngeal airway.

- Prepare for endotracheal intubation.

  - Ventilate the patient with a bag-mask device before endotracheal intubation.

  - Administer medications to facilitate endotracheal intubation.

  - Use an alternative airway if the patient's airway cannot be managed with endotracheal intubation.

    Some injuries or problems with patient anatomy may restrict passage of an endotracheal tube. Continue to ventilate the patient with a bag-mask device with supplemental oxygen until an alternative airway can be established. Numerous alternative airway devices are available, including the esophageal-tracheal Combitube®, laryngeal mask airway, and surgical airways.

If there are any life-threatening compromises in airway status, stop and intervene to correct the problem before proceeding to breathing assessment. Examples of life-threatening airway conditions are partial or complete obstruction of the airway by the tongue; loose teeth or foreign objects; blood, vomitus, or other secretions; edema; or all of these.

Breathing

Assessment

Life-threatening compromises in breathing may occur with a history of any of the following:

- Blunt or penetrating injuries of the thorax
- Acceleration, deceleration, or a combination of both types of forces (e.g., motor vehicle crashes, falls, crush injuries)

Once the patency of the airway is ensured, assess for the following:

- Spontaneous breathing
- Rise and fall of the chest
- Rate and pattern of breathing
- Use of accessory muscles, diaphragmatic breathing, or both
- Skin color
- Integrity of the soft tissues and bony structures of the chest wall
- Bilateral breath sounds

  - Auscultate the lungs bilaterally at the second intercostal space midclavicular line and at the fifth intercostal space at the anterior axillary line.

- Tracheal deviation and jugular venous distention (JVD) are considered late signs of breathing compromise. Identification of airway issues should be made based on the assessment parameters just listed.

Interventions

(Read Chapter 4, Airway and Ventilation, for an expanded discussion on interventions that improve breathing effectiveness.)

Breathing Present: Effective

All trauma patients should receive oxygen, regardless of their preexisting history. Although various oxygen delivery methods are available, it is best to use a tight-fitting nonrebreather mask for alert patients. Supplemental oxygen should be administered at a flow rate sufficient to keep the reservoir bag inflated during inspiration. Proper administration via a nonrebreather mask usually requires a flow rate of at least 12 liters/minute and may require 15 liters/minute or more.[5]

Breathing Present: Ineffective

When spontaneous breathing is present but ineffective, the following signs may indicate a life-threatening condition:

- Altered mental status (e.g., restless, agitated)
- Cyanosis, especially around the mouth
- Asymmetric expansion of the chest wall
  - Paradoxical movement of the chest wall during inspiration and expiration
- Use of accessory or abdominal muscles or both or diaphragmatic breathing
- Sucking chest wounds
- Absent or diminished breath sounds
  - Administer oxygen via a nonrebreather mask or assist ventilations with a bag-mask device, as indicated.
  - Anticipate definitive airway management to support ventilation.

Breathing Absent

- Ventilate the patient via a bag-mask device with an attached oxygen reservoir system.
- Assist with definitive airway management to support ventilation.

If there are any life-threatening injuries that compromise breathing, stop and intervene before proceeding to circulation assessment. Examples of life-threatening injuries that may compromise breathing are tension pneumothorax, open pneumothorax, flail chest with pulmonary contusion, and hemothorax. These conditions may require simultaneous assessment and immediate intervention (e.g., needle thoracentesis or covering an open chest wound).

Circulation

Assessment

- Palpate a central pulse (carotid, femoral, or brachial in infants under one year of age) for strength (normal, weak, or strong) and rate (normal, slow, or fast).
- Inspect and palpate the skin for color, temperature, and moisture.
- Capillary refill is used to assess perfusion in the pediatric patient. Blanch the nail bed for a few seconds and then release the pressure. The time it takes for the nail to return to its original color is the capillary refill time. Normal capillary refill takes two seconds or less in a warm ambient environment. Factors that may affect capillary refill, not related to an alteration in general tissue perfusion, include a cool ambient temperature and injury with vascular compromise.[6]
- Inspect for any obvious signs of uncontrolled external bleeding.
- Auscultate blood pressure.

  If other members of the trauma team are available, auscultate the blood pressure. If not, proceed with the primary assessment and auscultate the blood pressure at the beginning of the secondary assessment.

Interventions

Circulation: Effective

If the circulation is effective, proceed with assessment. Obtain vascular access with a large-caliber intravenous catheter and administer warmed isotonic crystalloid solution at a rate appropriate for the patient's condition.

Circulation Present: Ineffective

Although the pulse is present, other signs may indicate inadequacy of circulation, such as

- Tachycardia
- Altered level of consciousness or mental status (e.g., agitated, confused, decreased arousability)
- Uncontrolled external bleeding
  - Pale, cool, moist skin
- Distended or abnormally flattened external jugular veins
- Distant heart sounds

Circulation: Effective or Ineffective

- Control any uncontrolled external bleeding by
  - Applying direct pressure over the bleeding site
  - Elevating the bleeding extremity
  - Applying pressure over arterial pressure points
  - Using a tourniquet

    The use of a tourniquet is rarely indicated; however, if the preceding interventions do not control the bleeding and operative bleeding control is not readily available, a tourniquet may be the last resort.
- Cannulate two veins with large-caliber intravenous catheters, and initiate infusions of an isotonic crystalloid solution.
  - Use warmed solutions.
  - Use pressure bags to increase the speed of the infusion of the fluids.
  - Use blood administration tubing for possible administration of blood.
  - Use a rapid infusion device based on institutional protocols.
  - Use normal saline (0.9%) in the same intravenous tubing through which blood is administered.
  - Venous cannulation may require a surgical cutdown, an insertion of a central line, or both.
  - When starting intravenous lines, obtain a blood sample to determine ABO and Rh group and to facilitate any additional laboratory studies.
- Intraosseous needles may be used for access in the sternum, legs, arms, or pelvis if the patient's injuries would not interfere with the procedure.
- Administer blood or blood products, as prescribed.
  - Consider the use of a pneumatic antishock garment (PASG) for intra-abdominal or pelvic bleeding with hypotension. Despite the controversies that surround the use of PASG, the American College of Surgeons recommends their use to control bleeding from pelvic and lower extremity fractures; however, their use should not interfere with fluid resuscitation.[7]

Circulation: Absent

If a patient does not have a pulse, life-support measures should be initiated.

- In a traumatic arrest, recognition and correction of the underlying causes, such as a tension pneumothorax or exsanguination, should be addressed.
- Administer intravenous fluids and blood or blood products, as prescribed.

- Prepare for and assist with an emergency thoracotomy, as indicated, in the emergency department or resuscitation area. Open thoracotomy should be performed only in facilities with the resources to manage postthoracotomy patients. **Table 3-1** summarizes the indications for a resuscitative thoracotomy based on recommendations of the American Heart Association.
- Prepare the patient for definitive operative care after thoracotomy, if indicated.

If any life-threatening conditions compromise circulation, stop and intervene before proceeding to the neurologic assessment. Examples of life-threatening conditions that may compromise circulation are uncontrolled external bleeding, shock because of hemorrhage or massive burns, pericardial tamponade, or direct cardiac injury.

Disability—Brief Neurologic Assessment

Assessment

After the primary assessment of airway, breathing, and circulation, conduct a brief neurologic assessment to determine the degree of disability (D) as measured by the patient's level of consciousness.

- Determine the patient's level of consciousness by assessing the patient's response to verbal or painful stimuli using the AVPU mnemonic, as follows:

  A—Speak to the patient. The patient who is alert and responsive is considered **A** for **Alert.**

  V—The patient who responds to verbal stimuli is considered **V** for **Verbal.**

  P—Apply a painful stimulus. The patient who does not respond to verbal stimuli but does respond to a painful stimulus is considered **P** for **Pain.**

  U—The patient who does not respond to a painful stimulus is considered **U** for **Unresponsive.**
- The Glasgow Coma Scale (GCS) score is a quick way to measure the patient's level of consciousness. Although it is not a measure of total neurologic function, initial and serial scores provide the trauma team with a good indication as to patient outcomes. Scores range from 3 to 15. Because assessment of brain injury hinges on the GCS score, it is essential that the GCS be performed during the initial assessment. (See Chapter 6, Brain and Cranial Trauma, for an in-depth discussion of the GCS, and **Table 13-3** for a Pediatric GCS). The Revised Trauma Score (RTS) is an assessment tool that incorporates the GCS with physiologic parameters and can be associated with

patient survival (see Appendix 3-A). The recommendation of the American College of Surgeons Committee on Trauma is that patients with a GCS score of less than 14, a systolic blood pressure less than 90 mm Hg, a respiratory rate greater than 29 or less than 10, or a total Revised Trauma Score of 11 or less should be triaged to a trauma center.[5]

- Assess pupils for size, shape, equality, and reactivity to light.
- Determine the presence of lateralizing signs (neurologic assessment findings on one side of the body). These include unilateral deterioration in motor movements or unequal pupils, symptoms that help to locate the area of injury in the brain.

Interventions

- If the disability assessment indicates a decreased level of consciousness, conduct further investigation during the secondary focused assessments.
- If the patient is not alert or verbal, continue to monitor for any compromise to airway, breathing, or circulation.
- If the patient demonstrates signs of herniation or neurologic deterioration (e.g., unilateral or bilateral pupillary dilation, asymmetric pupillary reactivity, or motor posturing), consider hyperventilation.[8] The Brain Trauma Foundation guidelines recommend the use of hyperventilation **only** if the patient is exhibiting signs of herniation or neurologic deterioration that are nonresponsive to other

resuscitative measures and mannitol.[9] For further discussion on hyperventilation, refer to Chapter 6, Brain and Cranial Trauma.

Expose/Environmental Controls

Assessment

The patient's clothing should be carefully removed so that all injuries can be quickly identified. Injuries such as gunshot wounds, abdominal and pelvic trauma that can cause severe shock from blood loss, and open fractures can be missed without adequate exposure.

Interventions

- Remove the patient's clothing carefully because weapons, needles, or objects such as glass from the incident may injure trauma team members.
  - Ensure appropriate decontamination procedures if the patient has been exposed to a hazardous substance.
- Keep the patient warm by using warm blankets or heating lamps or turning up the room heat to prevent hypothermia. Hypothermia in trauma patients has been associated with increased mortality rates as a result of dysrhythmias, coma, coagulopathy, and decreased cardiac output.[5]
- Consider whether the clothing may be evidence and preserve it according to policy (see Initial Assessment and Management of the Victim of Violence, discussed later in this chapter).

Table 3-1: Suggested Indications for Resuscitative Thoracotomy in Patients with Traumatic Cardiac Arrest

Type of Injury	Assessment
Blunt trauma	Patient arrives at emergency department or trauma center with blood pressure and spontaneous respirations and then experiences cardiac arrest
Penetrating cardiac trauma	Patient experiences a witnessed cardiac arrest in the emergency department or trauma center after < 5 minutes of out-of-hospital cardiopulmonary resuscitation with positive secondary signs of life (e.g., pupillary reflexes, organized electrocardiogram activity)
Penetrating thoracic (noncardiac) trauma	Patient experiences a witnessed cardiac arrest in the emergency department or trauma center OR Patient arrives in the emergency department or trauma center after < 15 minutes of out-of-hospital cardiopulmonary resuscitation and with positive secondary signs of life (e.g., pupillary reflexes, organized electrocardiogram activity)
Exsanguinating abdominal vascular trauma	Patient experiences a witnessed cardiac arrest in the emergency department or trauma center OR Patient arrives in the emergency department or trauma center with positive secondary signs of life (e.g., pupillary reflexes, organized electrocardiogram activity) OR Resources available for definitive repair of abdominal-vascular injuries

Reprinted with permission from American Heart Association. (2005). Cardiac arrest associated with trauma. *Circulation*, 112, IV, 146–149.

Consider the Need for Transfer

Not all hospitals are able to provide the emergent care that an injured patient requires. During the primary assessment, enough information may be collected that would indicate the patient has been severely injured and requires transfer to another facility. The earlier the patient transfer is initiated, the quicker the patient can be transported to a center that can provide the most appropriate care. Indications for transfer recommended by the American College of Surgeons Committee on Trauma are summarized in **Table 3-2**. Arrangements for transfer and transport should follow Emergency Medical Treatment and Active Labor Act (EMTALA) guidelines, as discussed in Chapter 16, Transition of Care for the Trauma Patient. To safely and legally transfer a patient, there should be, at a minimum:

- An accepting physician
- An available bed **AND** resources to care for the patient
- An appropriate mode of transport used to transfer the patient based on the patient's injury and needs

Secondary Assessment

After each component of the primary assessment has been addressed and lifesaving interventions have been initiated, begin the secondary assessment. This assessment is a brief, systematic process to identify all injuries as well as collect any additional information about the patient and become aware of any comorbid factors that can affect the patient's care and resuscitation.

Full Set of Vital Signs, Focused Adjuncts, and Family Presence

The F of the assessment mnemonic stands for a full set of vital signs, focused adjuncts, and family presence.

Before initiating the head-to-toe assessment to identify other injuries, obtain a full set of vital signs, including blood pressure, pulse rate, respiratory rate, oxygen saturation, and temperature.

After the nurse completes the A-B-C-D-E of the assessment, intervenes for life-threatening conditions, and obtains a complete set of vital signs, critical decision making will determine whether to continue with the secondary assessment or perform additional interventions. The availability of other trauma team members to perform these focused interventions will influence the decision. If the patient sustained significant trauma and required lifesaving interventions during the primary assessment, assign another trauma

Table 3-2: Interhospital Transfer Criteria When the Patient's Needs Exceed Available Resources

Clinical Considerations
Central Nervous System
• Head injury
▪ Penetrating injury or depressed skull fracture
▪ Open injury with or without a cerebrospinal fluid leak
▪ GCS score < 15 or neurologically abnormal
▪ Lateralizing signs
• Spinal cord injury or major vertebral injury
Chest
• Widened mediastinum or signs suggesting great vessel injury
• Major chest wall injury or pulmonary contusion
• Cardiac injury
• Patient who may require prolonged ventilation
Pelvis/Abdomen
• Unstable pelvic-ring disruption
• Pelvic-ring disruption with shock and evidence of continuing hemorrhage
• Open pelvic injury
• Solid organ injury
Extremity
• Severe open fractures
• Traumatic amputation with potential for replantation
• Complex articular fractures
• Major crush injury
• Ischemia
Multisystem Injury
• Head injury with face, chest, abdominal, or pelvic injury
• Injury to more than two body regions
• Major burns or burns with associated injuries
• Multiple, proximal long-bone fractures
Comorbid factors
• Age > 55 years
• Children ≤ 5 years of age
• Cardiac or respiratory disease
• Insulin-dependent diabetes, morbid obesity
• Pregnancy
• Immunosuppression
Secondary Deterioration (Late Sequelae)
• Mechanical ventilation required
• Sepsis
• Single or multiple organ system failure (deterioration in central nervous, cardiac, pulmonary, hepatic, renal, or coagulation systems)
• Major tissue necrosis

Adapted with permission. *American College of Surgeons Committee on Trauma: Resources for Optimal Care of the Injured Patient*, in publication.

team member to perform the following interventions before proceeding with the secondary assessment:

- Attach ECG leads and monitor the patient's cardiac rate and rhythm.
- Attach a pulse oximeter, if available, to monitor the patient's oxygen saturation of the hemoglobin (SpO_2).
- If the patient is intubated, connect the endotracheal tube to an exhaled CO_2 detection device to monitor the patient's exhaled CO_2.
- Insert an indwelling urinary catheter to monitor urinary output. A urinary catheter provides for bladder drainage, allows for frequent monitoring of urinary output, and is necessary for any patient who is being prepared for surgery. Suspected injury to the urethra is a contraindication to catheterization through the urethra. Indications of possible urethral injury are
  - Blood at the urethral meatus
  - Palpation of a displaced prostate gland during a rectal examination
  - Blood in the scrotum
  - Suspicion of an anterior pelvic fracture
- Insert a gastric tube. Gastric distention may lead to vomiting, aspiration, or both. Distention may stimulate the vagus nerve, which can lead to bradycardia. Insertion of a gastric tube provides for evacuation of stomach contents, relieves gastric distention, and prevents vagal stimulation. Contraindications to insertion of a nasogastric tube include suspicion or definitive diagnosis of midfacial fractures. If a head injury is suspected, place an orogastric tube. After insertion of the tube, test the aspirated contents for the presence of blood and for pH. The tube must be placed carefully by
  - Maintaining protection of the cervical spine
  - Minimizing stimulation of the patient's gag reflex
  - Having suction equipment available
- Facilitate radiographic and diagnostic studies that are adjuncts to the primary assessment and the initial resuscitation of the patient.
  - Chest radiographs are done to identify
    - Life-threatening injuries such as pneumothoraces or hemothoraces
    - Position of tubes and lines
    - Presence of a widened mediastinum
    - Presence of diaphragmatic injuries
  - Pelvic radiographs are done to ascertain the presence of pelvic injury.

- Cervical spine radiographs are done to ascertain the presence of fractures or misalignment of the cervical spine.
- Diagnostic peritoneal lavage is done to aid in the diagnosis of hemoperitoneum or ruptured viscus. Once a common procedure, its use has decreased with the emergence of other types of diagnostic tests such as Focused Assessment Sonography for Trauma (FAST) and computed tomography (CT) scans. However, the American College of Surgeons Committee on Trauma still recommends the use of diagnostic peritoneal lavage for the following hemodynamically unstable patients:[5]
  - Patients with changes in sensorium related to alcohol or illicit drug use
  - Patients with changes in sensation from a spinal cord injury
  - Patients with injury to adjacent structures such as the lower ribs, pelvis, and lumbar spine
  - Patients with equivocal physical examination
  - Patients who may require lengthy diagnostic testing or surgery for other injuries
  - Patients with lap-belt sign
- Focused Assessment Sonography for Trauma can be performed rapidly in the emergency department to determine the presence of free fluid in the peritoneum.
- CT scans of the
  - Head
  - Abdomen
  - Chest
- Facilitate laboratory studies.
  - Blood typing is the highest priority. Depending on the severity of the patient's condition, blood typing studies may also include screening and crossmatching.
  - Other frequently ordered studies include hematocrit (Hct), hemoglobin (Hgb), blood urea nitrogen (BUN), creatinine, blood alcohol, toxicology screen, arterial blood gases, pH, base deficit, lactate level, electrolytes, glucose, clotting profile (platelets, prothrombin time [PT], partial thromboplastin time [PTT]), and urine or serum beta human chorionic gonadotropin (HCG) for pregnancy.
- Determine the need for tetanus prophylaxis after trauma based on the condition of the wound and the patient's past vaccination history.

The F of the mnemonic also represents family presence. Facilitate the presence of the family in the treatment area and their involvement in the patient's care. It is important to consider the diversity of both the patient and his or her family. Such things as the patient's age, culture, ethnicity, gender, nationality, race, and religion may influence both their and their family's response to injury and the interventions required.[10] For example, language and cultural barriers may cause additional stress for both the patient and staff. Inability to communicate clearly may lead to missing important pieces of patient information. Box 3-1 offers an organized way to collect information about the patient and his or her family that can contribute to better care of the injured patient.

- Assess the family's desires and needs.
- Facilitate and support the family's involvement in the care.
- Assign a health care professional to provide explanations about procedures and be with the family in the emergency department.
- Utilize resources to support the family's emotional and spiritual needs, such as a social worker or chaplain.

Give Comfort Measures

The G of the mnemonic is a reminder to the trauma team to provide comfort measures, such as touching and talking to the patient, and pharmacological and nonpharmacological pain management as needed by the patient, whether conscious or unconscious.

Box 3-1: Sample Questions to Identify Religious and Cultural Beliefs

- Why do you think you have this problem? The patient or family may believe the illness is caused by karma or evil or offended spirits, or that it has demonic origins.
- Why did it start when it did?
- In your home country, who would you see about this problem, and who would treat you? The patient or family may see a healer or a family elder. What kind of treatment would be done, and who would administer the treatment?
- How long do you think this illness or problem will last?
- What treatment have you (or your healer) tried at home or in the past?
- What results do you hope you will receive from the treatments? What treatment do you think you should receive?
- Do you plan to continue to use those treatments, or are there treatments you will use along with those prescribed in the emergency department?
- Will your healer (or others involved) work with us to make you well?

Pain Management

Pain is an unpleasant sensory and emotional experience arising from actual or potential tissue damage.[11] Pain that is not managed can cause

- Increased heart rate and force of cardiac contraction
- Peripheral vasoconstriction and pallor
- Tachypnea
- Muscle tension leading to guarding or splinting as a reflex to decrease pain
- Loss of parasympathetic tone with anorexia or nausea and vomiting
- Release of adrenal gland catecholamines resulting in an increase in blood pressure, cardiac afterload, and myocardial oxygen consumption

Assessment

There are both subjective and objective signs of pain. Because the patient's pain experience is very individualized, pain can be difficult to assess.

Consider the following in assessing pain:

- Presence of a source of pain:
  - Injuries such as fractures, lacerations, or burns
  - Procedures
    - Intravenous cannulation
    - Chest tube insertion or removal
    - Intubation
    - Wound care
    - Fracture reduction
    - Laceration repair
    - Sexual assault examination
- The treatment environment
  - Light
  - Noise
    - Cardiac monitors
    - Intravenous pumps
    - Pulse oximeter
    - Talking
- Diagnostic procedures
- Physical signs of pain:
  - Tachypnea
  - Shallow respirations
  - Nausea and vomiting
  - Diaphoresis
  - Protective behaviors—guarding, splinting
  - Pinched facial expressions
  - Clenched fist or teeth
  - Crying

A variety of pain rating scales are used to assess pain; they are outlined in Table 3-3.

Interventions

Various methods may be used to manage pain. These include analgesics, cutaneous stimulation, therapeutic touch, distraction, acupuncture, humor, and provision of comfort measures such as positioning.[12-14] Desirable properties of medications that are used in the emergency management of pain include minimal side effects, easy and painless administration, amnesic effect, short-term duration of action, few contraindications, and sedative as well as analgesic effects. The most common medications used in trauma care include opioids, benzodiazepines, local anesthetics, and some selected sedation agents for procedures or ventilatory management.

When managing a patient's pain, it is important that the trauma team remain flexible in dosing and clinical decision making related to the patient's response to pain medication. A patient's response to analgesics is not based solely on the severity and etiology of the pain. Pain management decisions should be made based on an understanding of pharmacology, appropriately timed assessments, and adjustments based on the patient's response.[14]

- Remove any pain-producing objects (e.g., shattered glass).
- Determine the level of the patient's pain.
- Administer prescribed medications.
- Monitor the patient for any side effects from the medications, such as
  - Respiratory depression
  - Hypotension
  - Nausea and vomiting
  - Bradycardia
  - Hallucinations from the medications

Table 3-3: Pain Rating Scales for Children and Adults[12,13]

Rating Scale	Description
Oucher™ scale	This tool uses six pictures of a child's face representing "no hurt" to "biggest hurt ever." It also includes a vertical scale with numbers from 0 to 100 to use with older children. The child is asked to choose the face that best describes his or her pain. This scale can be used for children 3 to 13 years of age. The numeric scale can be used if the child can count to 100.
Poker chip tool	This tool uses four red poker chips placed in front of the child. The chips are placed horizontally, and the child is told that "these are pieces of hurt." Explain to the child that each chip represents a piece of hurt. Ask the child how many pieces of hurt he or she has right now. Record the number of chips the child selected. This tool can be used for children older than 3 years of age once they can count and understand numbers.
FACES pain rating scale	This tool consists of six cartoon faces ranging from a smiling face for "no pain" to a tearful face for "worst pain." Ask the patient to pick the face that best describes his or her pain. This scale can be used for children as young as 3 years of age.
Numeric scale	This scale uses a straight line with endpoints that are labeled as "no pain" and "worst pain." Divisions with corresponding numbers from 0 to 10 are marked along the line. The patient is asked to choose the number that best describes his or her pain. This scale can be used on children older than 4 years of age once they can count and understand numbers.
Visual analogue scale	This scale uses a 10-cm horizontal line with end points marked "no pain" and "worst pain." The patient is asked to place a mark on the line that best describes the amount of his or her pain. Measure the distance with a ruler from the "no pain" end and record the measurement as the pain score. This scale can be used on children older than 4½ years of age.
Word-graphic rating scale	This scale uses descriptive words for varying intensities of pain. Examples of the words along the scale include "no pain," "little pain," "medium pain," "large pain," and "worst possible pain." This patient is asked to mark along the line the words that best describe his or her pain. Measure the distance with a ruler from the "no pain" end to the mark and record the measurement as the pain score. This scale can be used for children 5 years of age and older; however, they may need explanation of the words.
Color tool[12]	This scale uses crayons or markers for the child to construct their own scale that is used with a body outline. After having a child select four crayons that represent "no pain," "a little pain," "a little more pain," and "the worst pain you could imagine," ask the child to show on a body outline "where the hurt is" using the most appropriate crayon.

- Consider using alternative methods to manage pain, such as
  - Therapeutic touch
  - Acupressure/acupuncture
  - Positioning/splinting
  - Application of heat or cold
  - Distraction
  - Relaxation exercises
  - Guided imagery
  - Humor

History

The H of the mnemonic stands for the patient's history that can be obtained from the following:

- Prehospital information

  Obtain information from prehospital personnel as indicated by the circumstances of the injury event. The mnemonic **MIVT**—which stands for **M**echanism of injury, **I**njuries sustained, **V**ital signs, and **T**reatment—can be used as a guide to obtaining prehospital information

  - Mechanism and pattern of injury

    Knowledge of the mechanism of injury and specific injury patterns (e.g., type of motor vehicle impact) will help to predict certain injuries. If prehospital personnel transported the patient, have them describe pertinent on-scene information to the trauma team. Such information includes the location of the patient on their arrival, length of time since the injury event, and extent of extrication or reasons for extended on-scene time.

  - Injuries suspected

    Ask prehospital personnel to describe the patient's general condition, level of consciousness, and apparent injuries.

  - Vital signs
  - Treatment initiated and patient responses

- Patient-generated information

  If the patient is responsive, ask questions to evaluate the patient's level of consciousness and have the patient describe discomforts or other complaints. Elicit the patient's description of pain (i.e., location, duration, intensity, and character). If domestic violence is suspected, ask appropriate questions while providing comfort and a sense of security. Talking to the patient provides reassurance and emotional support and gives the patient information regarding upcoming procedures.

- Past medical history

  Gather information from the patient or family regarding

  - Age
  - Preexisting medical conditions
  - Current medications
  - Allergies
  - Tetanus immunization history
  - Previous hospitalizations and surgeries
  - Recent use of drugs or alcohol
  - Last normal menstrual period
  - Comorbid factors

    Comorbid factors are factors that place the patient who has sustained trauma at greater risk of having complications related to the injury. These may include:

    - History of smoking
    - History of substance abuse
    - Age > 55 years
    - Age < 5 years
    - Cardiovascular disease
    - Respiratory disease
    - Diabetes
    - Hemophilia or other blood disorders
    - Morbid obesity
    - Pregnancy
    - Immunosuppression
    - Use of anticoagulants (a significant and sometimes deadly comorbid factor)

Head-to-Toe Assessment

The H also stands for head-to-toe assessment. Information from this assessment is collected primarily through inspection, auscultation, and palpation. In specific circumstances, percussion may be indicated. The patient may focus on the more obvious distracting injury and have a decreased response to other injuries. While systematically moving from the patient's head to the lower extremities and the posterior surface, complete the assessment as described on the following pages.

General Appearance

Note the patient's body position, posture, and any guarding or self-protection movements. Observe for stiffness, rigidity, or flaccidity of muscles. Characteristic positions of limbs (flexion or extension), trunk, or head may indicate specific injuries. Note and document any unusual odors such as alcohol, gasoline, chemicals, vomitus, urine, or feces. Maintain cervical spine protection during assessment.

Head and Face

- Soft tissue injuries
  - Inspect for lacerations, abrasions, contusions, avulsions, puncture wounds, impaled objects, ecchymosis, and edema.
  - Palpate for crackling associated with subcutaneous emphysema.
  - Palpate for areas of tenderness.
- Bony deformities
  - Inspect for exposed bone.
  - Inspect for loose teeth or other material in the mouth that may compromise the airway.
  - Inspect and palpate for depressions, angulation, or areas of tenderness.
  - Inspect and palpate for facial fractures resulting in loss of maxillary, mandibular, or structural integrity.
- Observe for asymmetry of facial expressions. Also inspect the area for any exposed tissue that may indicate disruption of the central nervous system (e.g., central nervous system tissue from open wounds).
- Eyes
  - Determine gross visual acuity by asking the patient to identify how many of your fingers you are holding up. Determine whether the patient may need glasses or contacts to see.
  - Inspect for periorbital ecchymosis (raccoon eyes), subconjunctival hemorrhage, or edema. Determine whether the patient is wearing contact lenses.
  - Assess pupils for size, shape, equality, and reactivity to light.
  - Assess eye muscles by asking the patient to follow your moving finger in six directions to determine extraocular eye movements.
- Ears
  - Inspect for ecchymosis behind the ear (Battle's sign), which is a late sign of head injury.
  - Inspect for skin avulsion.
  - Inspect for unusual drainage, such as blood or clear fluid from the external ear canal. Do **NOT** pack the ear to stop drainage because it may be cerebrospinal fluid.
- Nose
  - Inspect for any unusual drainage, such as blood or clear fluid. Do **NOT** pack the nose to stop clear fluid drainage because it may be cerebrospinal fluid. If cerebrospinal fluid or drainage is present, notify the physician and do not insert a gastric tube through the nose.
  - Inspect the position of the nasal septum.
- Neck
  - Inspect for signs of penetrating or surface trauma, including presence of impaled objects, ecchymosis, edema, or any open wounds.
  - Observe the position of the trachea and the appearance of external jugular veins.
  - Palpate the trachea to determine position (i.e., midline, deviated).
  - Palpate the neck area for signs of subcutaneous emphysema, areas of tenderness, or both.

Chest

- Inspection
  - Observe breathing for rate, depth, and degree of effort required, use of accessory or abdominal muscles, and any paradoxical chest wall movement.
  - Inspect the anterior and lateral chest walls, including the axillae, for lacerations, abrasions, contusions, avulsions, puncture wounds, impaled objects, ecchymosis, edema, and scars.
  - Inspect the expansion and excursion of the chest during ventilation.
  - Observe for expressions or reactions that may indicate the presence of pain with inspiration and expiration (e.g., facial grimace).
- Auscultation
  - Auscultate lungs for breath sounds and note the presence of any adventitious sounds, such as wheezes, rales, or rhonchi.
  - Auscultate heart sounds for the presence of murmurs, friction rubs, muffled sounds, or all of these.
- Palpation
  - Palpate for signs of subcutaneous emphysema.
  - Palpate the clavicles, the sternum, and the ribs for bony crepitus or deformities (e.g., step-off, areas of tenderness).

Abdomen/Flanks

- Inspection
  - Inspect for lacerations, abrasions, contusions, avulsions, puncture wounds, impaled objects, ecchymosis, edema, and scars that may indicate previous abdominal surgery.
  - Observe for evisceration, distention, and the location of any scars.
- Auscultation
  - Auscultate for the presence or absence of bowel sounds. Auscultate before palpating

because palpation may change the frequency of bowel sounds.[15]

- Palpation
  - Gently palpate all four quadrants for rigidity, guarding, masses, and areas of tenderness; begin palpating in an area where the patient has not complained of pain or where there is no obvious injury.

Pelvis/Perineum

- Inspect for lacerations, abrasions, contusions, avulsions, puncture wounds, impaled objects, ecchymosis, edema, and scars.
- Bony deformities
  - Inspect for exposed bone.
  - Palpate for instability and tenderness over the iliac crests and the symphysis pubis.
- Inspect for blood at the urethral meatus (more common in males than females because of the length of the urethra), vagina, and rectum.
- Inspect the penis for priapism (persistent abnormal erection).
  - Assess the rectum for the presence of blood.
- Ensure that an appropriate trauma team member has performed a rectal examination to determine whether there is any displacement of the prostate gland in males (this may also be done in the posterior assessment) and to determine anal sphincter tone.
- Note pain and/or the urge, but inability, to void.

Extremities

- Inspect previously applied splints and do not remove if applied appropriately and neurovascular function is intact.
- Circulation
  - Inspect color.
  - Palpate to assess the skin temperature and for moisture.
  - Palpate pulses (always compare one side with the other and note any differences in the quality of the pulses).
  - In the lower extremities, palpate the femoral, popliteal, dorsalis pedis, and posterior tibialis; in the upper extremities, palpate the brachial and radial pulses.
- Soft tissue injuries
  - Inspect for bleeding.
  - Inspect for lacerations, abrasions, contusions, avulsions, puncture wounds, impaled objects, ecchymosis, edema, angulations, deformity, and any open wounds.
- Bony injuries
  - Inspect for angulation, deformity, and open wounds with evidence of protruding bone fragments, edema, and ecchymosis.
  - Note bony crepitus.
  - Palpate for deformity and areas of tenderness.
- Motor function
  - Inspect for spontaneous movement of extremities.
  - Determine motor strength and range of motion in all four extremities; use range of motion (ROM)/muscle strength scale 0 to 5 (**Table 3-4**).
- Sensation
  - Determine the patient's ability to sense touch in all four extremities.

Inspect Posterior Surfaces

The I of the mnemonic stands for inspection of the patient's posterior surfaces.

- Maintain cervical spine protection.
- Support extremities with suspected injuries.
- Logroll the patient with the assistance of members of the trauma team. This maneuver keeps the vertebral column in alignment during the turning process. Do not logroll the patient onto his or her side with an injured extremity. Logroll away from you (if possible) to inspect the back, flanks, buttocks, and posterior thighs for lacerations, abrasions, contusions, avulsions, puncture wounds, impaled objects, ecchymosis, edema, or scars.
- Palpate the vertebral column (including the costovertebral angles) for deformity and areas of tenderness.
- Palpate all posterior surfaces for deformity and areas of tenderness.

Table 3-4: Range of Motion (ROM)/Muscle Strength Scale

Strength Rating	Description
5	Complete ROM or active movement against gravity and full resistance
4	Complete ROM or active movement against gravity and some resistance
3	Complete ROM or active movement against gravity
2	Complete ROM or active body part movement with gravity eliminated
1	Barely detectable contraction
0	No detectable contraction

- Palpate the anal sphincter for presence or absence of tone, if not already done during the assessment of the pelvis and perineum.
- Assess the rectum for the presence of blood.

Focused Assessment

After the primary and secondary assessments and any simultaneous interventions are completed, a more detailed, focused assessment will be necessary for each area or system injured. This will further direct the priorities of care.

For details on analysis, nursing diagnoses, interventions, and expected outcomes, see **Appendix 3-B**.

Focused Adjuncts to the Secondary Assessment

Once the secondary assessment has been completed, additional interventions may be required to evaluate and manage the injured patients. These may include

- Additional laboratory studies
- Additional radiographs, (e.g., for extremity injuries)
- Angiography
- Application of PASG, pelvic orthotic device, pelvic sheet wrapping, or "beanbag" wrapping for unstable pelvic fractures
- Bronchoscopy
- Esophagoscopy
- Wound care
- Tetanus prophylaxis
- Application of traction devices
- Administration of medications, including
  - Antibiotics
  - Pain medication, such as morphine or fentanyl
  - Sedation, such as etomidate, propofol, or midazolam
  - Neuromuscular blocking agents, such as vecuronium
- Preparation for the operating room
- Preparation for admission
- Preparation for transfer and transport

Evaluation and Ongoing Assessment

The evaluation of a trauma patient is that phase of the nursing process when the nurse evaluates the patient's responses to the injury event and the effect of all interventions. The achievement of the expected outcomes is evaluated, and the treatment/ intervention plan is adjusted to enhance these out-

comes. To evaluate the patient's progress, monitor the following:

- Airway patency
- Effectiveness of breathing
- Arterial pH, PaO_2, and $PaCO_2$
- Oxygen saturation (SpO_2 or SaO_2)
- Level of consciousness
- Skin temperature, color, moisture
- Pulse rate and quality
- Blood pressure
- Urinary output

Ongoing assessment of the aforementioned parameters is an essential component of the trauma nursing process. In addition, pain and the patient's response to analgesia and sedation needs to be reassessed frequently. The goal of these interventions should be to achieve the desired level of pain management with minimal side effects (e.g., respiratory depression, hypotension), because side effects may serve to diminish the patient's response to resuscitation. Written documentation of all information generated during the trauma nursing process is an essential responsibility of the trauma nurse.

Psychosocial support of the patient should be provided. When family or friends are available, they should be allowed to stay with the patient. The patient or family may have questions and needs that should be addressed as quickly as possible by the trauma team.[2]

Selected Patient Assessments

Initial Assessment and Management of the Victim of Violence

Traumatic injuries may be the result of an act of violence. Two types of victims of violence frequently seen in the emergency department are patients who have injury as the result of intimate partner violence or who have been sexually assaulted. When injury has been sustained from an act of violence, the collection of evidence is an important part of patient care. For example, a patient who may have sustained a self-inflicted gun shot wound should have paper bags placed on the hands. However, it is important to point out that evidence collection never supersedes any interventions that are needed to save the patient's life.[16]

Assessment

History

Data collection should take place in a quiet, safe, private environment if at all possible, away from family members or individuals who may have accompanied the patient. The nurse should ascertain whether or not the victim knew the assailant.

Determination of this fact will serve as a guide to the type of questions that the nurse needs to ask to gather data. The initial questions might include

- Does the patient know his/her assailant?
- Is the patient in a relationship with someone who has hurt her or him before?
- Is the patient pregnant?
- Was the patient forced to have sexual intercourse?
- Can the patient explain the injuries he or she has sustained?

Refer to **Box 3-2** for additional screening questions that the nurse may ask in situations where intimate partner violence is suspected.

Physical Assessment

Inspection and Palpation

Assess for the presence of bruises, contusions, lacerations, and burn marks. Look for:

Box 3-2: Screening Questions for Suspected Adult Victims of Intimate Partner Violence

- Is anyone in your home being hurt, hit, threatened, frightened, or neglected?
- Do you feel safe in your current relationship?
- Do you ever feel afraid at home? Are you afraid of your children?
- Sometimes patients tell me that they have been hurt by someone close to them. Could this be happening to you?
- You seem frightened of your partner. Has he/she ever hurt you?
- Have there been times during your relationship when you have had physical fights?
- Do your verbal fights ever include physical contact?
- Have you ever been hit, punched, kicked, or otherwise hurt by someone within the past year? If so, by whom?
- You mentioned that your partner uses alcohol (drugs). How does he/she act when drinking (on drugs)?
- Sometimes when others are overprotective and as jealous as you describe, they react strongly and use physical force. Is this happening in your situation?

Reprinted from *Sheehy's Manual of Emergency Care,* 6th edition, page 904, Intimate partner violence, Copyright 2005, with permission from Elsevier.

- Contusions to the head, neck, or chest
- Bruising and contusions to the face and chest
- Bruising around wrists and ankles (signs of physical restraint)
- Burn marks on the face, chest, and genitals
- Injuries that suggest a defensive posture (bruises on the back of a patient's arms, defensive wounds)
- Injuries that do not equate with reported mechanism of injury
- Substantial delay from the time of injury to seeking treatment
- Evidence of drug or alcohol use
- Bite marks

Assess the perineum and rectum for the following:

- Bleeding
- Lacerations and tears
- Fluids
- Swelling

Assess the patient's breasts for

- Lacerations
- Bruising
- Bite marks

Palpate the patient's abdomen and rectum for tenderness and swelling.

Diagnostic Procedures

Radiographic Studies

- CT scan of the head if there is evidence of head trauma
- Radiographs of any area of injury

Laboratory Studies

Laboratory studies should be obtained based on protocols used for evidence collection related to victims of violence. Laboratory studies that may be collected include

- Tests for sexually transmitted diseases, including HIV screening
- Blood, hair, and mucosal samples for DNA evidence
- Drug screening if the patient feels that he or she may have been drugged

Other Studies

Based on each department's protocols, either the emergency staff or a forensic or sexual assault nurse examiner may perform other studies.

Planning and Implementation/Interventions

- Perform primary and secondary assessments to identify and treat any life-threatening injuries.
- Assure the patient that he or she is safe.
- Keep threatening persons away from the patient.
  - Use hospital security.
  - Call local authorities.
- Notify the forensic nurse examiner or sexual assault nurse examiner, if he or she is available, to examine and collect evidence related to the assault.[17]
- If a forensic nurse examiner or sexual assault nurse examiner is not available, collect evidence per department protocol by
  - Placing evidence in separate paper bags
  - Sealing the bag with a label that contains
    - Patient name
    - Date
    - Time
    - Location of where evidence was collected
    - Name and signature of the person collecting the evidence
- Maintain chain-of-custody of any evidence collected.
- Give the evidence to appropriate authorities and document this on the chart.
- Administer medications based on protocols, for example:
  - Treatment for sexually transmitted diseases
  - Postcoital contraception
- Obtain a patient advocate for the patient.
- Provide the patient with information about how to remain safe.
- If the patient is to be discharged from the emergency department, ensure that the patient has appropriate discharge instructions for follow-up care.

Evaluation and Ongoing Assessment

- Maintain patient safety.
- Answer the patient's questions.

Initial Assessment and Management of the Violent Patient

Patients who act violent at the scene of the injury or who are at risk of becoming violent must be carefully assessed and effectively managed so that care can be safely provided to the patient.[18] Ruling out an organic cause of the patient's violent behavior must always be done to ensure that the patient has not sustained an injury (such as head trauma) or has an illness (such as diabetes) that is causing the violent behavior.

Signs and Symptoms (Risk Factors for Violent Behavior)

- A direct threat made to a member of the trauma team, for example:
  - "If you don't stop what you are doing, you will regret it."
  - "I will hurt your family."
  - "I will kill you."
- A patient found with weapons on their person
- Previous violent behaviors
  - Intimate partner violence
  - Incarceration for physical assault
  - Incarceration for sexual assault
- A patient who is out of control because of ingestion of a substance, such as
  - Methamphetamine
  - Cocaine
  - Alcohol
- Psychiatric disorders
  - Bipolar disease
  - Paranoia
- Report of violence at the scene of the injury
  - Attempting to escape from authorities
  - Involvement in a crime such as a fight
- A patient who is being legally detained

Assessment

History

- How was the patient injured?
- Is there any history of violent or abusive behavior?
- Does the patient have a history of substance abuse?
- How was the patient transported to the emergency department?
- Did the patient require either physical or chemical restraints to be transported?
- Is the patient being legally detained?

Physical Assessment

Inspection

- Assess the patient's level of consciousness.
- Look for any evidence of substance abuse such as needle tracks or skin popping.
- Note the presence of physical restraints.

- Note violent behaviors.
  - Kicking
  - Screaming
  - Spitting
  - Biting
  - Verbal and threatening abuse
- Note evidence of self-injury.
  - Wrist lacerations
  - Scarring from previous injuries
  - Burns

Diagnostic Procedures

Radiographic Studies

- A CT scan of the head should be performed to rule out neurologic injury that may be causing the patient's violent behaviors.
- A chest radiograph should be performed to rule out a pulmonary injury that may be causing hypoxia and contributing to the patient's violent behaviors.

Laboratory Studies

- Obtain blood glucose.
- Consider obtaining arterial blood gases or a toxicology screen to ensure that the patient's behavior is not the result of an organic process.

Planning and Implementation/Interventions

- Ensure patient and staff safety by
  - Placing the patient in a safe environment
  - Applying restraints according to hospital policy
  - Administering medications
    - Neuromuscular blocking agents
    - Sedative agents
    - Antipsychotic agents
- Talk calmly to the patient.
- Allow the family to stay with the patient if they calm the patient.
- Notify the appropriate authorities if indicated.

Evaluation and Ongoing Assessment

- Continue to assess the following:
  - Changes in level of consciousness
  - Changes in circulation and sensory response to areas of the body restrained
  - Response to medications administered to manage violent behaviors
  - Changes in behavior that indicate the need for continued use of restraints

Summary

The initial assessment of the trauma patient, the first step of the trauma nursing process, includes primary and secondary assessments. If life-threatening conditions are present, the nurse must stop the assessment and intervene to correct these problems before proceeding with the assessment. Care of the seriously injured trauma patient is best accomplished through a team approach. The A through I mnemonic is

  A—Airway with simultaneous cervical spine protection

  B—Breathing

  C—Circulation

  D—Disability (neurologic status)

  E—Expose/environmental controls

  F—Full set of vital signs/focused adjuncts/family presence

  G—Give comfort measures

  H—History and head-to-toe assessment

  I—Inspect posterior surfaces

Refer to this chapter for information regarding a description of

- General information related to history, which should be collected for every trauma patient
- Assessment of the patient's airway and effectiveness of breathing and circulation
- Frequently ordered radiographic and laboratory studies
- Specific nursing interventions for patients with compromises to airway, breathing, circulation, and disability
- Ongoing evaluation of the patient's airway and effectiveness of breathing and circulation

This general information will not be repeated in the following chapters, which will focus on specific areas of injury.

References

1. McSwain, E. N., Frame, S., & Salomone, J. (2003). Patient assessment and management. In National Association of Emergency Medical Technicians, *PHTLS basic and advanced prehospital trauma life support* (revised reprint, 5th ed., pp. 64–89). St. Louis, MO: Mosby.

2. Sedlak, S. K. (2003). Patient assessment. In L. Newberry (Ed.), *Sheehy's emergency nursing principles and practices* (5th ed., pp. 84–97). St. Louis, MO: Mosby.

3. Proehl, J. (2004). Primary survey. In J. Proehl (Ed.), *Emergency nursing procedures* (3rd ed., pp. 2–4). Philadelphia: W. B. Saunders.

4. Centers for Disease Control and Prevention. (2004). *Guidance for the selection and use of personal protective equipment in health care settings* [electronic slide presentation]. Retrieved August 6, 2005, from www.cdc.gov

5. American College of Surgeons Committee on Trauma. (2004). Initial assessment and management. *Advanced trauma life support® for doctors: Instructor course manual* (7th ed., pp. 11–29). Chicago: Author.

6. Hockenberry, M. J., Wilson, D., Winkelstein, M. L, & Line, N. E. (Eds.). (2003). Physical and developmental assessment of the child. *Wong's nursing care of infants and children* (7th ed., pp. 170–239). St. Louis, MO: Mosby.

7. American College of Surgeons Committee on Trauma. (2004). Shock. *Advanced trauma life support® for doctors: Instructor course manual* (7th ed., p. 76). Chicago: Author.

8. Barker, E. (2002). Intracranial pressure monitoring. *Neuroscience nursing* (2nd ed., pp. 396–397). St. Louis, MO: Mosby.

9. Bullock, M. R., Chestnut, R. M., Clifton, G. L., Ghajar, J., Marion, D. W., Narayan, R. K., et al. (2000). *Hyperventilation. In Guidelines for the management of severe traumatic brain injury* (p. 101). New York: Brain Trauma Foundation.

10. Ruiz-Contreras, A. (2005). Diversity. In L. Newberry & L. Criddle (Eds.), *Sheehy's manual of emergency care* (6th ed., pp. 14–20). St. Louis, MO: Mosby.

11. International Association for the Study of Pain. (1979). Pain terms: A list with definitions and notes on usage. *Pain, 6,* 249.

12. Johnson, A. (2005). Pain management. In L. Newberry & L. Criddle (Eds.), *Sheehy's manual of emergency care* (6th ed., pp. 228–244). St. Louis, MO: Mosby.

13. Holleran, R. S. (2002). Problem of pain in emergency care. *Nursing Clinics of North America, 37*(1), 67–78.

14. Gordon, D. B., Dahl, J., Phillips, P., Frandsen, J., Cowley, C., Foster, R. L., et al. (2004). The use of as-needed range orders in the management of acute pain: A consensus statement of the American Society of Pain Management Nursing and the American Pain Society. *Pain Management Nursing, 5*(2), 53–58.

15. Lombardo, D. (2005). Patient assessment. In L. Newberry & L. Criddle (Eds.), *Sheehy's manual of emergency care* (6th ed., pp. 82–98). St. Louis, MO: Mosby.

16. Semonin Holleran, R. (2004). Preservation of evidence. In J. Proehl (Ed.), Emergency nursing procedures (3rd ed., pp. 816–821). Philadelphia: W. B. Saunders.

17. Semonin Holleran, R., & Hutson, L. A. (2004). Sexual assault exam. In J. Proehl (Ed.), *Emergency nursing procedures* (3rd ed., pp. 820–827). Philadelphia: W. B. Saunders.

18. Carroll, V. (2006). Violence in the healthcare workplace. In V. Lynch (Ed.), *Forensic nursing* (pp. 65–69). St. Louis, MO: Mosby.

19. Champion, H. R., Sacco, W. J., Copes, W. S., Gann, D. S., Gennarelli, T. A., & Flanagan, M. E. (1989). A revision of the trauma score. *Journal of Trauma, 29*(5), 623–629.

20. Champion, H. R., Sacco, W. J., & Copes, W. S. (1996). Trauma scoring. In D. V. Feliciano, E. E. Moore, & K. L. Mattox (Eds.), *Trauma* (3rd ed., pp. 53–67). Stamford, CT: Appleton & Lange.

The Glasgow Coma Scale score and the Revised Trauma Score are two scoring systems that measure the acuity and severity of the patient's physiologic response to injury. The Revised Trauma Score may be used by prehospital personnel and emergency staff as a triage tool. Changes in both scores will reflect the patient's ongoing response to the injury event. Scores can be calculated using a preprinted source indicating the points for each area. Data from the primary and secondary assessments can be used to determine the severity of the patient's condition and provide a baseline for ongoing evaluation of the patient's responses to the injury event and treatment.

Revised Trauma Score

The Revised Trauma Score measures the patient's physiologic response to injuries.[19,20] Measurements used to calculate the score, which ranges from 0 to 12, are the Glasgow Coma Scale score, systolic blood pressure, and the patient's respiratory rate. Coded values are used to represent ranges in each of the three measured areas.

The probabilities of survival for patients with various revised trauma scores are the following:

Score	Survivors (Percent)
12	99.5%
11	96.9%
10	87.9%
9	76.6%
8	66.7%
7	63.6%
6	63.0%
5	45.5%
3 to 4	33.3%
2	28.6%
1	25.0%
0	3.7%

Revised Trauma Score Table

Area of Measurement	Coded Value
Systolic Blood Pressure (mm Hg)	
> 89	4
76–89	3
50–75	2
1–49	1
0	0
Respiratory Rate (spontaneous inspirations/minute)*	
10–29	4
> 29	3
6–9	2
1–5	1
0	0
* Patient initiated, not artificial ventilations	
Glasgow Coma Scale score	
13–15	4
9–12	3
6–8	2
4–5	1
3	0
Total Possible Points	0–12

The primary assessment will reveal information the nurse uses to analyze the patient's responses to the injury event and determine specific nursing diagnoses. Each nursing diagnosis is derived by diagnostic reasoning, which determines the priorities of intervention. Each diagnosis represents an actual or risk health problem or one that may develop as a result of a patient being vulnerable to risk factors. The problems may be corrected by the nurse or may require a collaborative intervention with other trauma team members. The identification of specific outcomes corresponds to the goals generated by the team for the patient to correct each diagnosis or health problem.

Nursing Diagnoses	Interventions	Expected Outcomes
Airway clearance, ineffective, related to: • Edema of the airway, vocal cords, epiglottis, and upper airway • Irritation of the respiratory tract • Laryngeal spasm • Altered level of consciousness • Pain • Presence of an artificial airway • Direct trauma • Tracheobronchial secretions or obstruction • Aspiration of foreign matter • Inhalation of toxic fumes or substances	• Stabilize the cervical spine • Position the patient • Open and clear the airway • Insert oro- or nasopharyngeal airway • Consider endotracheal intubation	**The patient will maintain a patent airway, as evidenced by:** • Regular rate, depth, and pattern of breathing • Bilateral chest expansion • Effective cough and gag reflex • Absence of signs and symptoms of airway obstruction: stridor, dyspnea, hoarse voice • Clear sputum of normal amount without abnormal color or odor • Absence of signs and symptoms of retained secretions: fever, tachycardia, tachypnea

Aspiration, risk, related to:
 	
• Reduced level of consciousness secondary to injury or concomitant substance abuse
• Impaired cough and gag reflex
• Trauma to head, face, and/or neck
• Secretions and debris in airway
• Increased intragastric pressure
• Impaired swallowing
	• Stabilize the cervical spine
	• Position the patient
	• Open and clear the airway
	• Insert oro- or nasopharyngeal airway
	• Consider endotracheal intubation
	• Insert a gastric tube and evacuate the stomach contents
	• Obtain blood sample for ABGs (arterial blood gases) as indicated
		The patient will not experience aspiration, as evidenced by:
		
		• A patent airway
		• Clear and equal bilateral breath sounds
		• Regular rate, depth, and pattern of breathing
		• ABG values within normal limits
		  ▪ PaO_2 80 to 100 mm Hg (10.0 to 13.3 KPa)
		  ▪ SaO_2 > 95%
		  ▪ $PaCO_2$ 35 to 45 mm Hg (4.7 to 6.0 KPa)
		  ▪ pH between 7.35 and 7.45
		• Clear chest radiograph without evidence of infiltrates
		• Ability to handle secretions independently

Nursing Diagnoses	Interventions	Expected Outcomes

Gas exchange, impaired, related to:
 	
• Ineffective breathing pattern: loss of integrity of thoracic cage and impaired chest wall movement secondary to injury, deterioration of ventilatory efforts
• Ineffective airway clearance
• Aspiration
• Altered blood flow, oxygen-carrying capacity of the blood, oxygen supply
• Aspiration of foreign matter
• Hypo- or hyperventilation
• Inhalation of toxic fumes or substances
	• Administer oxygen via a nonrebreather mask
	• Ventilate, if needed, with 100% oxygen via a bag-mask device or with a mechanical ventilator
	• Assist with endotracheal intubation and ventilate
	• Monitor oxygen saturation with continuous pulse oximetry
	• Administer blood, as indicated
		The patient will experience adequate gas exchange as evidenced by:
		
		• ABG values within normal limits
		  ▪ PaO_2 80 to 100 mm Hg (10.0 to 13.3 KPa)
		  ▪ SaO_2 > 95%
		  ▪ $PaCO_2$ 35 to 45 mm Hg (4.7 to 6.0 KPa)
		  ▪ pH between 7.35 and 7.45
		• Skin normal color, warm, and dry
		• Level of consciousness, awake and alert, age appropriate
		• Regular rate, depth, and pattern of breathing

Fluid volume deficit, related to:
 	
• Hemorrhage
• Fluid shifts
• Alteration in capillary permeability
• Alteration in vascular tone
• Myocardial compromise
	• Control any uncontrolled bleeding by:
	  ▪ Applying direct pressure over the bleeding site
	  ▪ Elevating the extremity
	  ▪ Applying pressure over arterial pressure sites
	• Cannulate two veins with large-caliber catheters and initiate infusion of isotonic crystalloid solution
	• Administer blood as indicated
		The patient will have an effective circulating volume as evidenced by:
		
		• Stable vital signs appropriate for age
		• Urine output of 1 ml/kg/hr
		• Strong, palpable peripheral pulses
		• Level of consciousness, awake and alert, age appropriate
		• Skin normal color, warm, and dry
		• Maintenance of hematocrit of 30 ml/dl or hemoglobin of 12 to 14 g/dl or greater
		• Control of external hemorrhage

Cardiac output, decreased, related to:
 	
• Decreased venous return secondary to acute blood loss or massive peripheral vasodilatation
• Compression of heart and great vessels
• Impairment of cardiac filling and ejection
	• Control any uncontrolled bleeding by:
	  ▪ Applying direct pressure over the bleeding site
	  ▪ Elevating the extremity
	  ▪ Applying pressure over arterial pressure sites
	• Cannulate two veins with large-caliber catheters and initiate infusion of isotonic crystalloid solution
	• Consider a pneumatic antishock garment
	• Initiate cardiopulmonary resuscitation and advanced life support measures, if indicated
	• Administer blood, as indicated
		The patient will maintain adequate circulatory function, as evidenced by:
		
		• Strong, palpable peripheral pulses
		• Apical pulse rate of 60 to 100 beats/minute
		• Electrocardiogram with normal sinus rhythm, absence of dysrhythmia
		• Skin normal color, warm, and dry
		• Level of consciousness, awake and alert, age appropriate
		• Urine output of 1 ml/kg/hr

Nursing Diagnoses	Interventions	Expected Outcomes
Tissue perfusion, altered renal, cardiopulmonary, cerebral, gastrointestinal, peripheral (specific type), related to: • Hypovolemia • Interruption of flow: arterial and/or venous	• Prepare for definitive care • Control any uncontrolled bleeding • Cannulate two veins with large-caliber catheters and initiate infusion of isotonic crystalloid solution	**The patient will maintain adequate tissue perfusion, as evidenced by:** • Vital signs within normal limits for age • Level of consciousness, awake and alert, age appropriate • Skin normal color, warm, and dry • Strong and equal peripheral pulses • Urine output of 1 ml/kg/hr
Hypothermia, related to: • Rapid infusion of intravenous fluids • Decreased tissue perfusion • Exposure • Consumption of alcohol	• Administer blood, as indicated • Prepare for definitive care • Administer warm intravenous solutions • Keep the patient warm with blankets or overheard warmers • Monitor body temperature	**The patient will maintain a normal core body temperature, as evidenced by:** • Core temperature measurement of 98 °F to 99.5 °F (36 °C to 37.5 °C) • Skin normal color, warm, and dry
Pain, related to: • Effects of trauma/injury agents • Stimulation of nerve fibers • Experience during invasive procedures/diagnostic tests	• Administer analgesics, as prescribed • Use touch, positioning, or relaxation techniques to give comfort • Use ice packs, as indicated	**The patient will experience relief of pain, as evidenced by:** • Diminishing or absent level of pain through patient's self-report • Absence of physiologic indicators of pain: tachypnea, pallor, diaphoretic skin, increasing blood pressure • Absence of nonverbal cues of pain: crying, grimacing, inability to assume position of comfort, and guarding • Ability to cooperate with care as appropriate
Anxiety and fear (patient and family), related to: • Unfamiliar environment • Unpredictable nature of condition • Invasive procedures • Possible disfigurement, scarring • Effects of actual or perceived loss of significant other • Threat to or change in health status, role functions, support systems, environment, self-concept, or interaction patterns • Threat of death, actual or perceived • Lack of knowledge • Loss of control • Feelings of failure • Disruptive family life • Pain • Threat to self-concept	• Communicate with the patient and family • Facilitate family presence • Orient the patient to his or her surroundings • Establish a trusting relationship	**The patient and family will experience decreasing anxiety and fear, as evidenced by:** • Orientation to surroundings • Ability to describe reasons for equipment and procedures used in treatment • Ability to verbalize concerns and ask questions of the health care team • Use of effective coping skills • Decreased fear-related behaviors: crying, agitation • Vital signs within normal limits for age

Nursing Diagnoses	Interventions	Expected Outcomes
Powerlessness (individual and family), related to: • Loss of function • Uncontrolled pain • Lack of privacy • Lack of knowledge	• Communicate with the patient and family • Facilitate family presence • Orient the patient to his or her surroundings • Establish a trusting relationship • Maintain privacy	**The patient and family will experience an increasing feeling of control over the situational crisis, as evidenced by:** • Participation in decision-making activities • Seeking information regarding treatment and course of care • Accepting appropriate referrals and resources for support • Utilizing medical/nursing/allied staff for support and assistance

Chapter 4

Airway and Ventilation

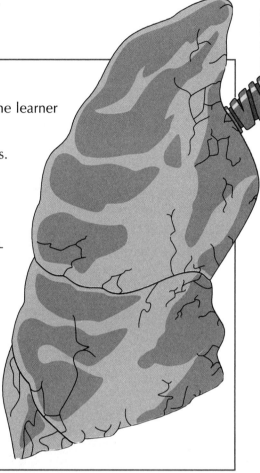

Objectives

On completion of this chapter/lecture, the learner should be able to:

1. Identify life-threatening airway problems.

2. Identify life-threatening problems with ventilation.

3. Describe the pathophysiologic changes as a basis for signs and symptoms of airway and ventilation problems.

4. Discuss the nursing assessment of patients with airway or ventilatory problems (or both).

5. Plan appropriate interventions for patients with airway or ventilatory problems (or both).

6. Evaluate the effectiveness of nursing interventions for patients with airway or ventilatory problems (or both).

Preface

Lecture begins on page 62.

Knowledge of normal physiology serves as a foundation for understanding the anatomic derangements and pathophysiologic compromises that may result from trauma. Before reading this chapter, it is strongly suggested that the learner read the following review material. Reading about the specific anatomic and physiologic concepts presented in this section will enhance the learner's ability to correlate such concepts with specific injuries. This material related to anatomy and physiology will not be covered during lectures, nor will it be evaluated by testing.

A simple and focused method of viewing the anatomy and physiology of the airway and pulmonary system is to divide it into the upper and lower airways. The upper airway is composed of the nose, the mouth, the pharynx, the larynx, and the trachea. The lower airway is composed of the bronchi and the lungs. The functional unit of the pulmonary system is the alveolus. If there is obstruction in the upper airway from such things as swelling, blood, foreign objects, or the tongue, air cannot get into the lower airway so that respiration can occur.[1-3]

Upper Airway Anatomy

Figure 4-1 shows the structures contained in the upper airway. The nose is the primary passageway for inhaled air into the lungs. It is triangular shaped and mostly composed of cartilage. The nose filters, warms, and moistens inhaled air. It also provides the sense of smell. The blood supply of the nose originates from the internal and external carotid arteries. When the nose is injured, blood can obstruct the ability to inhale adequate air.

Figure 4-2 shows the structures in the mouth, which include teeth and the tongue. The mouth is the secondary passageway for inhaled air. The tongue is one of the most common things that can obstruct the upper airway, especially in the patient who is unconscious. Broken teeth, blood, vomitus, and foreign objects can also interfere with ventilation.

The pharynx is a U-shaped fibromuscular tube that extends from the base of the skull to the lower border of the cricoid cartilage. Anteriorly, the pharynx opens into the nasal cavity, the mouth, and the lar-

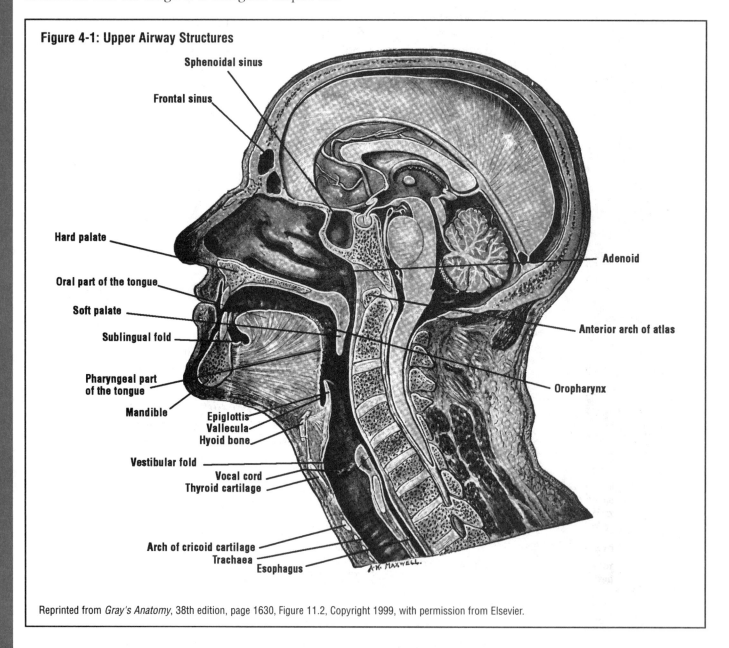

Figure 4-1: Upper Airway Structures

Sphenoidal sinus
Frontal sinus
Hard palate
Oral part of the tongue
Soft palate
Sublingual fold
Pharyngeal part of the tongue
Mandible
Epiglottis
Vallecula
Hyoid bone
Vestibular fold
Vocal cord
Thyroid cartilage
Arch of cricoid cartilage
Trachaea
Esophagus
Adenoid
Anterior arch of atlas
Oropharynx

A.K. MAXWELL.

Reprinted from *Gray's Anatomy*, 38th edition, page 1630, Figure 11.2, Copyright 1999, with permission from Elsevier.

ynx. The pharynx contains important structures that serve as a guide to locate the patient's trachea when intubation is needed to maintain a patent airway.

The larynx, which is sometimes referred to as the voice box, is a tubular structure composed of cartilage that connects the trachea to the pharynx. The epiglottis, which is a large leaflike structure, lies on top of the larynx. The primary function of the larynx is to allow air into the trachea. The larynx is the most heavily innervated sensory structure in the body. It is innervated by the vagus nerve; thus, stimulation of the larynx during intubation can cause activation of the parasympathetic nervous system increasing the patient's blood pressure and decreasing the heart rate. Below the larynx is the cricothyroid membrane **(Figure 4-3)**.

The cricothyroid membrane extends from the upper surface of the cricoid cartilage to the inferior border of the thyroid cartilage. These structures need to be quickly located when a cricothyrotomy may be required to access an emergency airway. To locate the cricothyroid membrane, find the laryngeal prominence, then note the anterior surface of the thyroid cartilage immediately caudad, usually one index finger's breadth in height. A soft indentation is caudad to the anterior surface with a very hard ridge immediately caudad to it. This is the cricothyroid membrane, and the ridge is the cricoid cartilage.[3] The cricoid cartilage is located higher in a woman's neck and is relatively smaller than a man's.

The trachea begins at the inferior border of the cricoid ring, and it is also innervated by the vagus nerve. Tracheal size is usually 9 to 15 mm in diameter and 12 to 15 cm in length.

Lower Airway Anatomy

The lower airway anatomy is composed of the thoracic cage, the bronchi, the lungs, the alveoli, and the capillaries and arterioles involved in respiration. The bronchi and the bronchioles conduct atmospheric air to the alveoli, where gas exchange takes place. The alveoli and the pulmonary capillaries are responsible for gas exchange.[4]

The thoracic cavity extends from the top of the sternum to the diaphragm **(Figure 4-4A)**. Key structures within the thoracic cavity include the lungs and the space between the lungs, termed the mediastinum **(Figure 4-4B)**.

The mediastinum is bound anteriorly by the sternum, posteriorly by the 12 thoracic vertebrae, and inferiorly by the diaphragm. The contents of the mediastinal space include the heart, thoracic aorta, esophagus, trachea, inferior and superior vena cava, vagus nerves, phrenic nerves, and other vascular structures. Correlation of anatomical structures and surface landmarks can be important in physical assessment of the chest.

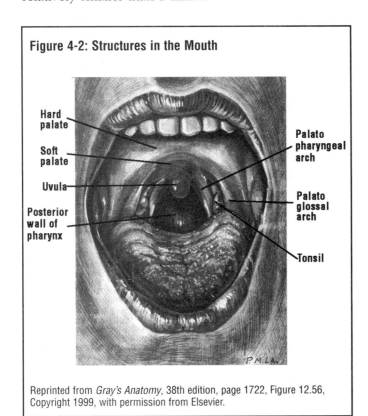

Figure 4-2: Structures in the Mouth

Hard palate

Soft palate

Uvula

Posterior wall of pharynx

Palato pharyngeal arch

Palato glossal arch

Tonsil

Reprinted from *Gray's Anatomy*, 38th edition, page 1722, Figure 12.56, Copyright 1999, with permission from Elsevier.

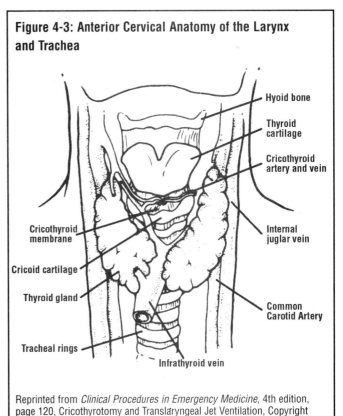

Figure 4-3: Anterior Cervical Anatomy of the Larynx and Trachea

Hyoid bone

Thyroid cartilage

Cricothyroid artery and vein

Cricothyroid membrane

Cricoid cartilage

Thyroid gland

Tracheal rings

Infrathyroid vein

Internal jugular vein

Common Carotid Artery

Reprinted from *Clinical Procedures in Emergency Medicine*, 4th edition, page 120, Cricothyrotomy and Translaryngeal Jet Ventilation, Copyright 2004, with permission from Elsevier.

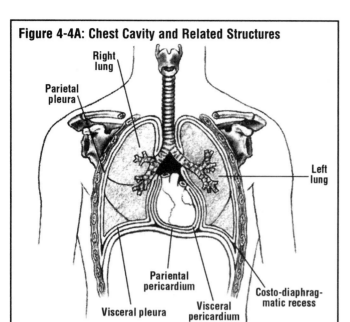

Figure 4-4A: Chest Cavity and Related Structures

Right lung

Parietal pleura

Left lung

Pariental pericardium

Costo-diaphragmatic recess

Visceral pleura

Visceral pericardium

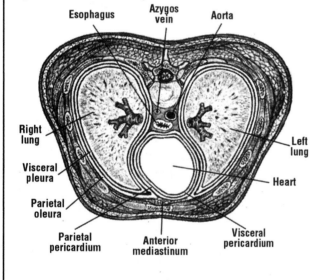

Figure 4-4B: Chest Cavity and Related Structures

Esophagus

Azygos vein

Aorta

Right lung

Left lung

Visceral pleura

Heart

Parietal oleura

Parietal pericardium

Anterior mediastinum

Visceral pericardium

Physiology

Ventilation, or breathing, begins with inhalation of air. The air is filtered, moistened, and warmed as it passes through the upper airway. If the patient is healthy and uninjured, the amount of oxygen in the air is generally adequate to ensure adequate ventilation. Ventilation is accomplished by the alternate contraction and relaxation of the diaphragm and intercostal muscles **(Figure 4-5)**. The diaphragm divides the abdominal and thoracic cavities. During inspiration, the diaphragm contracts and flattens, increasing the size of the thorax. During expiration, the diaphragm relaxes, and the lungs recoil to decrease the chest size.[4] The diaphragm rises to the 4th intercostal space during expiration and extends to the 10th or 12th intercostal space during inspiration.

The lungs are expanded and contracted by increasing and decreasing the anterior-posterior diameter of the chest cavity by elevating and lowering of the ribs.[4] The intercostal muscles contribute to increasing the anterior-to-posterior diameter of the thoracic cavity by raising the rib cage. Other muscles, such as the sternocleidomastoids and scalene, raise the sternum to the level of the first two ribs and are frequently termed accessory muscles. The muscles of expiration are the internal intercostals and the abdominal recti.

The lungs are cone shaped. The base of each lung rests against the diaphragm, and the apex of each lung extends approximately 1½ inches (4 cm) above the clavicle. The pleura are double-layered thin, transparent membranes. The outer layer, the parietal pleura, lines the thoracic cavity, and the inner layer, the visceral pleura, surrounds each lung. A potential space, the pleural space, exists between the two layers and is filled with 5 to 15 ml of lubricating fluid. The parietal and visceral pleura are in contact with each other to prevent any separation of the lungs from the chest cavity wall, yet slide smoothly over each other during breathing.

To keep the lungs fully expanded, the pressure within the pleural cavity must always remain slightly negative, –4 mm Hg, in relation to the atmospheric pressure. The lungs have an elastic tendency to recoil, whereas the thoracic cavity has an elastic tendency to expand. These opposing forces create a slight negative pressure, much like a suction cup or vacuum. This suction, or negative intrapleural pressure, keeps the two pleural membranes in contact. The negative intrapleural pressure increases during inspiration and decreases during exhalation. The intrapleural pressure may become positive during expiration.[4]

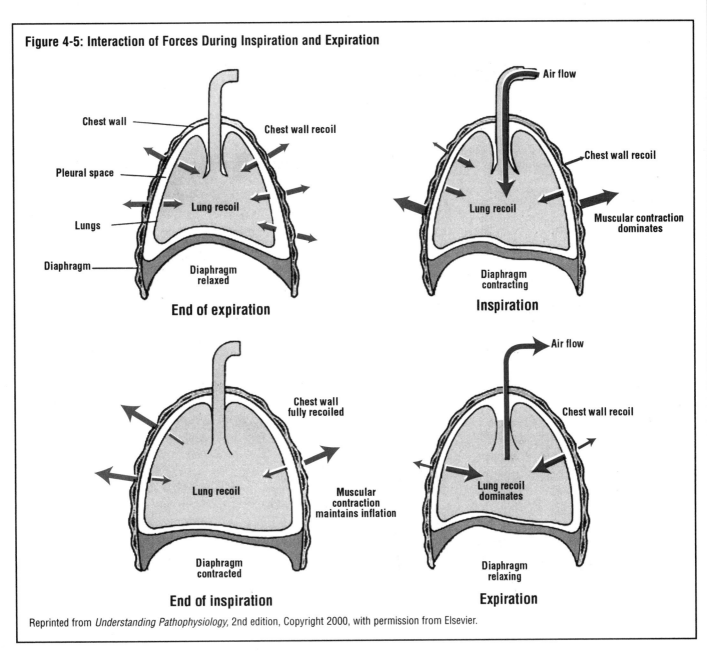

Figure 4-5: Interaction of Forces During Inspiration and Expiration

End of expiration

Inspiration

End of inspiration

Expiration

Reprinted from *Understanding Pathophysiology*, 2nd edition, Copyright 2000, with permission from Elsevier.

Introduction

The first priority in the management of an injured patient is establishing a patent airway and ensuring effective ventilation. Maintaining oxygenation and preventing hypercapnia are critical in managing the trauma patient. Hypercapnia can be very detrimental to the patient with a head injury.

Many conditions may interfere with the patient's ability to maintain a patent airway and ventilate effectively. These include an altered mental status, obstruction of the airway by the tongue or fluids, and injury to the chest.

Pathophysiology as a Basis for Signs and Symptoms

Airway Obstruction

The patient who has been injured is at great risk of airway obstruction. The patient who is unconscious, is obtunded from alcohol or drugs, or has had facial, neck, or thoracic trauma is at great risk of having an obstructed airway. One of the most common things that obstruct the airway in a trauma patient is the tongue. Blood or loose teeth from oral or facial trauma as well as an increase in secretions can contribute to the potential of not being able to keep the airway patent. It should be assumed that most trauma patients have a full stomach and will vomit. Occasionally, the patient may have actually been eating or chewing gum when the traumatic event occurred.

Loss of consciousness or an altered mental status can affect the patient's ability to keep the airway clear. Injury to the neck may cause disruption of the larynx or the trachea, initiating hemorrhage and swelling that leads to airway obstruction.

Ineffective Ventilation

The patient may have an unobstructed airway but still have problems with ventilation. Factors that may contribute to impaired ventilation include

- Altered mental status
- Loss of consciousness
- Neurologic injury
- Spinal cord injury (may result in diaphragmatic breathing and cause hypoxia)
- Intracranial injury (may cause abnormal breathing patterns and interfere with ventilation)
- Blunt trauma resulting in rib fractures and chest wall instability
- Pain caused by rib fractures (may cause shallow respirations, resulting in hypoxia)

- Penetrating trauma (may cause bleeding or a pneumothorax, which can compress the lungs and interfere with ventilation and oxygenation)
- Preexisting history of respiratory disease (e.g., chronic obstructive pulmonary disease)
- Increased age

Nursing Care of the Patient with Airway or Ventilation Problems or Both

Assessment of Airway

History

Refer to Chapter 3, Initial Assessment, for a description of general information that should be collected regarding every trauma patient. Only pertinent questions specific to patients with airway and ventilation problems are described following.

- Is there a history of facial, neck, or thoracic injury?
- Is there a history of inhalation injury that could lead to airway obstruction?
- Does the patient have a history of a loss of consciousness?
- Has the patient ingested alcohol or other drugs that could impair the ability to protect the airway?
- Is there a history of nausea or witnessed vomiting that may lead to aspiration risk?
- Does the patient have respiratory disease such as asthma or chronic obstructive pulmonary disease?
- Does the patient have a history of tobacco use? What type, how much, how long?
- What are the patient's complaints? Dyspnea, dysphagia, dysphonia?

Physical Assessment

Inspection

Inspection of the patient's airway must occur while one is maintaining cervical spine protection. Because partial or total airway obstruction may threaten the patency of the upper airway, observe for the following:

- Ability to vocalize
- Level of consciousness

  The tongue may obstruct the airway in a patient who is unresponsive or has a decreased level of consciousness. Agitation may be a sign of hypoxia, and a patient may be obtunded because of hypercapnia.
- Foreign objects, loose teeth, bleeding, or vomitus or other secretions

- Swelling or bleeding from oral or facial or neck lacerations/hematomas that may impede the airway
- Inability to open the jaw because of midface or mandibular fractures

    Facial fractures may lead to compromise of the nasopharynx or oropharynx.

- Penetrating trauma to the neck

Auscultation

Auscultate breath sounds; noisy airflow during inspiration, such as stridor or wheezing, can indicate partial or impending obstruction. Airway obstruction is more difficult to recognize in the patient who is not breathing.

Palpation

Palpate the face, neck, clavicles, and chest wall for tenderness, fractures, swelling, and subcutaneous emphysema or hematoma.

Interventions

Airway Patent

The patient is currently able to maintain his or her airway without assistance.

- Maintain cervical spine protection.
- If the patient is awake and breathing, he or she may have assumed a position that maximizes the ability to breathe. Before proceeding with cervical spine protection, be sure interventions do **not** compromise the patient's breathing status.

Airway Partially Obstructed or Totally Obstructed

The patient has shown partial or complete obstruction of the airway. This must be addressed before continuing the assessment of the patient.

- Place the patient in a supine position.
    - If the patient is not already supine, logroll the patient onto his or her back while maintaining cervical spine protection. If necessary, remove any headgear, such as a football helmet, to allow access to the airway and cervical spine; removal of such gear should be done carefully and gently to prevent any manipulation of the spine.
- Protect the cervical spine. The cervical spine must be maintained in a neutral position. Do not hyperextend, flex, or rotate the neck during any of the following procedures.
    - If the cervical spine has not been protected, manually immobilize the head.
    - If the patient is already in a rigid cervical collar and strapped to a backboard, do **NOT** remove any devices. Check that the devices are placed appropriately and are not interfering with the patient's ability to protect his or her airway.
- Open and clear the airway. Techniques to open or clear an obstructed airway during the primary assessment include the following.
    - Jaw thrust (**Figure 4-6**): The angles of the lower jaw are grasped on each side with the index fingers and thumbs on the cheekbone to move the mandible forward. This method can be used with the bag-mask device to provide a good seal for ventilation.
    - Chin lift (**Figure 4-7**): The fingers of one hand are placed under the mandible, gently lifting upward to raise the chin while the thumb pulls the lower lip to open the mouth. This maneu-

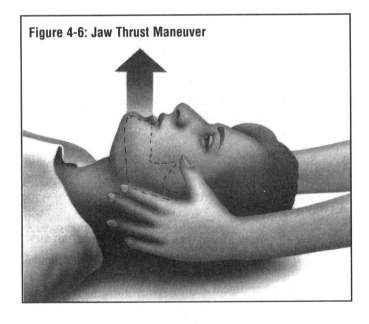

Figure 4-6: Jaw Thrust Maneuver

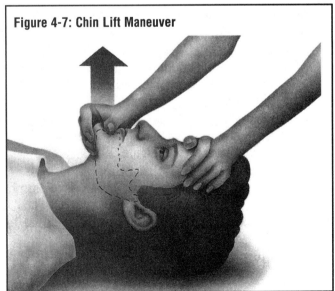

Figure 4-7: Chin Lift Maneuver

ver must be performed carefully to avoid hyperextending the neck.

- Removal of loose objects or foreign debris: Remove secretions manually or with suctioning as required.

- Suctioning and other manipulation of the oropharynx: These procedures must be done gently to prevent stimulation of the gag reflex and subsequent vomiting, aspiration, or both.

- If the patient has an altered mental status and cannot keep his or her airway open, insert an oropharyngeal or nasopharyngeal airway and begin bag-mask ventilation if the patient is not ventilating adequately.

A nasopharyngeal airway can be used in responsive or unresponsive patients, but not in patients with facial trauma or a suspected basilar skull fracture.

- Use the largest size that will fit the patient's nostril. Select the correct length of nasopharyngeal airway by holding the proximal end of the airway at the nares. The distal end should reach the tip of the earlobe.[5]

- Lubricate the airway with water-soluble lubricant before insertion.

- Insert the nasopharyngeal airway with the bevel facing the nasal septum. Direct the airway posteriorly and slightly rotate it toward the ear until the flanges rest against the nostril. Avoid inverting the airway into a nostril obstructed by septal deviation, polyps, or other similar problems. Most available nasal airways are made to insert in the right nostril.[5,6] If the left nare must be used, the airway must be turned upside down to be sure the bevel faces the septum.

- Reassess airway patency.

- An oropharyngeal airway can be used in unresponsive patients.

- Select the correct sized airway by holding the proximal end of the airway at the corner of the mouth. The distal end should reach the tip of the earlobe.

- Use a tongue depressor or a gloved finger to hold the tongue against the floor of the patient's mouth. The flange should rest against the patient's lips.

- Reassess airway patency.

- Consider the need for a definitive airway.

A definitive airway requires that a tube be placed into the trachea for the purpose of obtaining or maintaining a patent airway.[5] The decision to intubate a patient should be based on whether the patient has failed to maintain or protect the airway. Is the patient unable to adequately ventilate to remain oxygenated? What is the patient's anticipated clinical course?[7] For example, has the patient sustained a head injury that requires management of intracranial pressure, or is the patient in profound shock that requires oxygenation?

Definitive airway procedures require advanced skills, and their use should be restricted to personnel who are well trained. The emergency nurse is a member of the team that is critical to the success of these procedures. The role of the nurse is to monitor the patient throughout the procedure. In addition, the nurse should be familiar with alternative methods or resources for airway management if the operator is unable to establish a definitive airway.

- Endotracheal intubation (oral or nasal route)

- If the patient is not adequately ventilating, respirations should be supported with a bag-mask device until the airway is secured. Bag-mask ventilation is described in detail later in this chapter. Because of the risk of vomiting and aspiration with bag-mask ventilation, a tidal volume should be delivered sufficient to produce rise and fall of the chest.[6]

  - Oral endotracheal intubation is done with the patient's cervical spine in a neutral position and without any extension or flexion of the cervical spine. This requires a second person to hold the patient's head in this position.[7]

  - Blind nasotracheal intubation is **not** indicated when the patient is apneic or when there are signs of major midface fractures (e.g., maxillary fractures [LeFort II or III]). Basilar skull fractures or fractures of the frontal sinus or cribriform plate are considered relative contraindications.[7]

  - Medications—including sedatives, premedications, and neuromuscular blocking agents—may be used to facilitate intubation. The types of medications used are determined by institutional protocols and the experience level of the personnel performing the procedure. Walls[8] recommends using the **LOAD** mnemonic when describing pretreatment drugs for rapid sequence intubation: **L**idocaine; **O**pioids; **A**tropine; and **D**efasciculating agents. **Table 4-1** contains a summary of some medications that may be used to facilitate intubation.

  - If rapid-sequence intubation is to be used to facilitate intubation, it needs to be used with approved protocols in place and by skilled clinicians. Walls[8] identified seven steps that should be followed when rapid-sequence intubation is being used to manage a patient's airway. **Table 4-2** contains a summary of these steps.[8]

- Alternative airways[9,10]

When an airway cannot be obtained in the trauma patient for whatever reason, alternative airways should be available until a more definitive airway can be obtained. When an endotracheal tube cannot be passed, ventilate

Figure 4-8: Application of Bag-Mask by a Single Rescuer

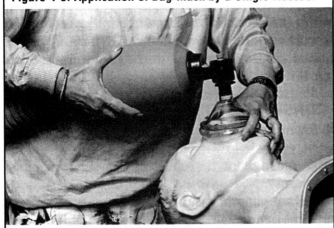

Reprinted from *Emergency Nursing Procedures,* 3rd edition, page 155, Bag-Valve Mask Ventilation, Copyright 2004, with permission from Elsevier.

Table 4-1: Medications Frequently Used to Facilitate Rapid Sequence Intubation

Premedication
- Atropine: Recommended for use in pediatric patients
- Lidocaine: Recommended for head injury patients or any patient with potentially increased intracranial pressure
- Defasciculating dose of a nondepolarizing agent

Sedation
- Benzodiazepines
  - Midazolam
  - Lorazepam
- Opioids:
  - Morphine sulfate
  - Fentanyl

Anesthesia/Induction Agent
- Etomidate
- Thiopental sodium
- Methohexital
- Propofol

Neuromuscular Blocking Agents
- Depolarizing Agent: Succinylcholine
- Nondepolarizing Agents:
  - Pancuronium
  - Vecuronium
  - Rocuronium

Table 4-2: Rapid Sequence Intubation Steps

Preparation	Gather equipment needed for the procedure. Ensure access to alternative airways, additional skilled personnel such as anesthesia staff, or an airway cart with equipment if the airway cannot be secured.
Preoxygenation	Use 100% oxygen. It is best if the patient is allowed to spontaneously breathe to prevent the risk of aspiration.
Pretreatment	This step involves the use of drugs to decrease the effects associated with intubation (Table 4-1).
Paralysis with induction	An induction agent is administered so that the patient loses consciousness. This is followed by administration of a neuromuscular blocking agent, usually succinylcholine.
Protection and positioning	Apply pressure over the cricoid cartilage (Sellick maneuver). This pressure should be continuously applied to minimize the likelihood of vomiting and aspiration.
Placement with proof	• Each attempt should not exceed 30 seconds, maximum 3 attempts. If more than one attempt is needed, ventilate patient 30 to 60 seconds between. • After intubation, inflate the cuff. • Confirm tube placement with exhaled carbon dioxide detector.
Postintubation management	• Secure endotracheal tube. • Set ventilator settings. • Obtain chest x-ray. • Continue to medicate. • Recheck vital signs and pulse oximetry.

Reprinted with permission from Walls, R. (2004). Rapid sequence intubation. In R. Walls, M. F. Murphy, R. C. Luten, & R. E. Schneider (Eds.) Manual of emergency airway management (2nd ed., pp. 22–32). Philadelphia: Lippincott Williams

the patient with a bag-mask device **(Figure 4-8)** until an alternative airway can be established. Alternative airways need to be available, and personnel should be familiar with how these devices are used in order to assist the physician or advanced practitioner.

- Combitube™

  The Combitube™ is a dual-lumen, dual-cuff airway that can be placed blindly into the esophagus to establish an airway **(Figure 4-9)**. However, if it is inadvertently inserted into the trachea, it can function on a short-term basis as an endotracheal tube. The Combitube™ comes in two sizes, one for smaller adults and one for larger adults. It allows for isolation of the airway, reduced risk of aspiration, and more reliable ventilation.[10] The Combitube™ may be used in cases where there are severe facial burns or where the patient's mouth opening is limited.

  The Combitube™ can only be used in the unconscious patient whose airway-protective reflexes are not intact. Patients with known esophageal disease, a history of caustic ingestions, and upper airway trauma caused by laryngeal injury, foreign bodies, or pathology should not have a Combitube™ placed. The Combitube™ can cause esophageal and laryngeal trauma.[10]

- Laryngeal mask airway[9]

  The laryngeal mask airway looks like an endotracheal tube but is equipped with an inflatable, elliptical, silicone rubber collar (laryngeal mask) at the distal end. The laryngeal mask airway is designed to cover the supraglottic area. It has two rubber bars that cross the tube opening at the mask to prevent herniation of the epiglottis into the tube portion of the laryngeal mask airway **(Figure 4-10)**. The intubating laryngeal mask airway (ILMA) allows the insertion of an endotracheal tube through a specially designed laryngeal mask airway.

  The laryngeal mask airway does not require laryngoscopy and visualization of the cords for insertion, which allows it to be used by nurses, respiratory therapists, and prehospital personnel with appropriate training. The laryngeal mask airway is available in sizes ranging from pediatric to adult. It can decrease the risk of regurgitation and has been shown to provide successful ventilation.[9] Some patients cannot be ventilated through the device, so another airway device should be available for them.

- Needle cricothyrotomy (percutaneous transtracheal ventilation)

  To establish an airway, a needle cricothyrotomy **(Figure 4-11)** may be performed with an over-the-needle catheter placed into the trachea through the cricothyroid membrane. This method requires a large-caliber intravenous catheter (10- to 16-gauge).

Figure 4-9: Combitube™ Airway, Distal Portion in the Esophagus

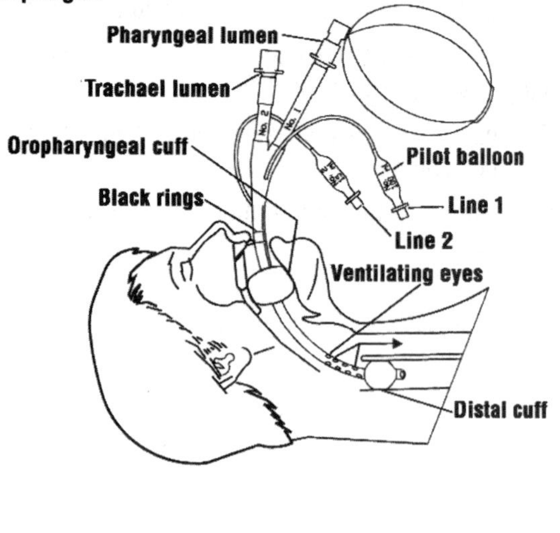

Pharyngeal lumen

Trachael lumen

Oropharyngeal cuff

Black rings

Pilot balloon

Line 1

Line 2

Ventilating eyes

Distal cuff

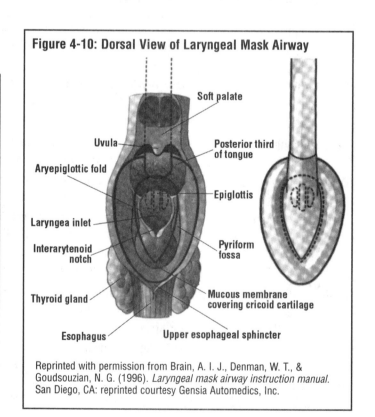

Reprinted by permission of Nellcor Puritan Bennett Incorporated, Pleasanton, California.

Figure 4-10: Dorsal View of Laryngeal Mask Airway

Soft palate

Uvula

Posterior third of tongue

Aryepiglottic fold

Epiglottis

Laryngea inlet

Interarytenoid notch

Pyriform fossa

Thyroid gland

Mucous membrane covering cricoid cartilage

Esophagus

Upper esophageal sphincter

Reprinted with permission from Brain, A. I. J., Denman, W. T., & Goudsouzian, N. G. (1996). *Laryngeal mask airway instruction manual.* San Diego, CA: reprinted courtesy Gensia Automedics, Inc.

The needle is connected to special tubing that allows oxygen (generally 50 psi) to inflate the lungs **(Figure 4-12)**. The patient then passively exhales. This is only a temporary technique; further intervention must be provided within 30 to 45 minutes. Complications related to a needle cricothyrotomy include inadequate ventilation causing hypoxia, hematoma formation, esophageal perforation, aspiration, thyroid perforation, and subcutaneous emphysema.

- Surgical cricothyrotomy[7]

A surgical cricothyrotomy is performed by making an incision in the cricothyroid membrane and placing a cuffed endotracheal or tracheostomy tube into the trachea. Percutaneous cricothyrotomy kits also are available. These kits utilize the Seldinger technique to insert an airway into the trachea through the cricothyroid membrane.

A cricothyrotomy **(Figure 4-13)** is indicated when other methods of airway management have failed and the patient cannot be adequately ventilated and oxygenated. This situation can occur as a result of edema of the glottis, fracture of the larynx, or severe oropharyngeal hemorrhage.

Only trained personnel *should* perform a surgical airway. Complications related to a surgical airway include aspiration, hemorrhage or hematoma formation or both, laceration of the trachea or esophagus, creation of a false passage, and laryngeal stenosis.

If there are any life-threatening compromises to the patient's airway, stop and intervene to correct the problem before proceeding to breathing assessment. Examples of life-threatening airway conditions are partial or complete obstruction of the airway by foreign bodies or debris (blood, mucus, and vomitus), obstruction by the tongue, or both. Penetrating wounds may cause disruption of the integrity of the airway, and blunt trauma may lead to injury of the larynx or other upper airway structures.

Confirmation of an Endotracheal Tube and Alternative Airway Placement

Whenever an endotracheal tube or alternative airway device has been placed, whether it is or is not in the trachea must be confirmed. Confirmation is accomplished by

- Visualization of the tube passing through the cords

- Using a fiberoptic bronchoscope to confirm tube placement

- Listening to breath sounds over the epigastrium and chest while ventilating the patient

---

Figure 4-11: Needle Cricothyrotomy

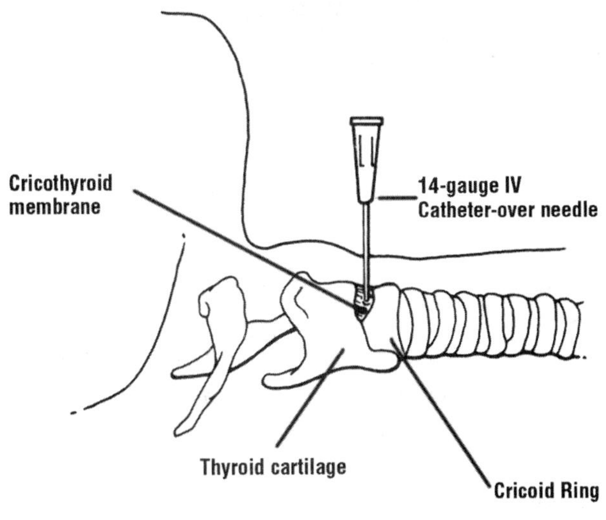

Cricothyroid membrane

14-gauge IV Catheter-over needle

Thyroid cartilage

Cricoid Ring

Reprinted from *Clinical Procedures in Emergency Medicine*, 4th edition, page 129, Cricothyrotomy and Translaryngeal Jet Ventilation, Copyright 2004, with permission from Elsevier.

Figure 4-12: One-way valve for translaryngeal ventilation during needle or surgical cricothyrotomy

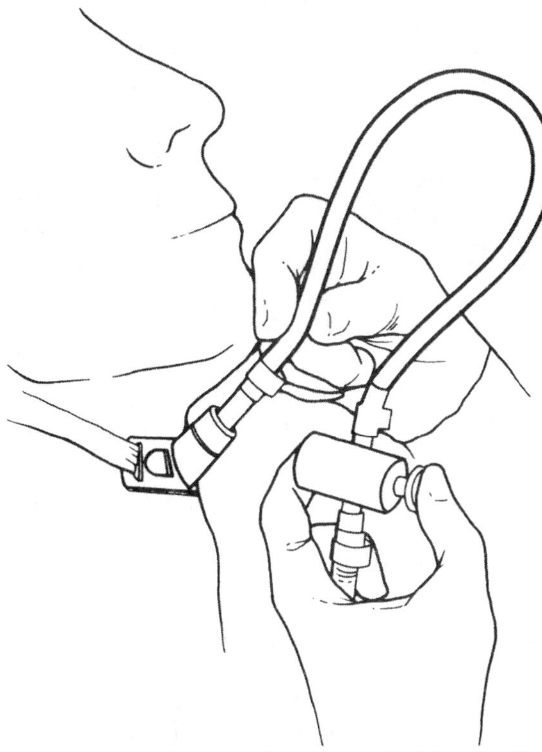

Reprinted from *Clinical Procedures in Emergency Medicine*, 4th edition, page 127, Cricothyrotomy and Translaryngeal Jet Ventilation, Copyright 2004, with permission from Elsevier.

Figure 4-13: Surgical Cricothyrotomy

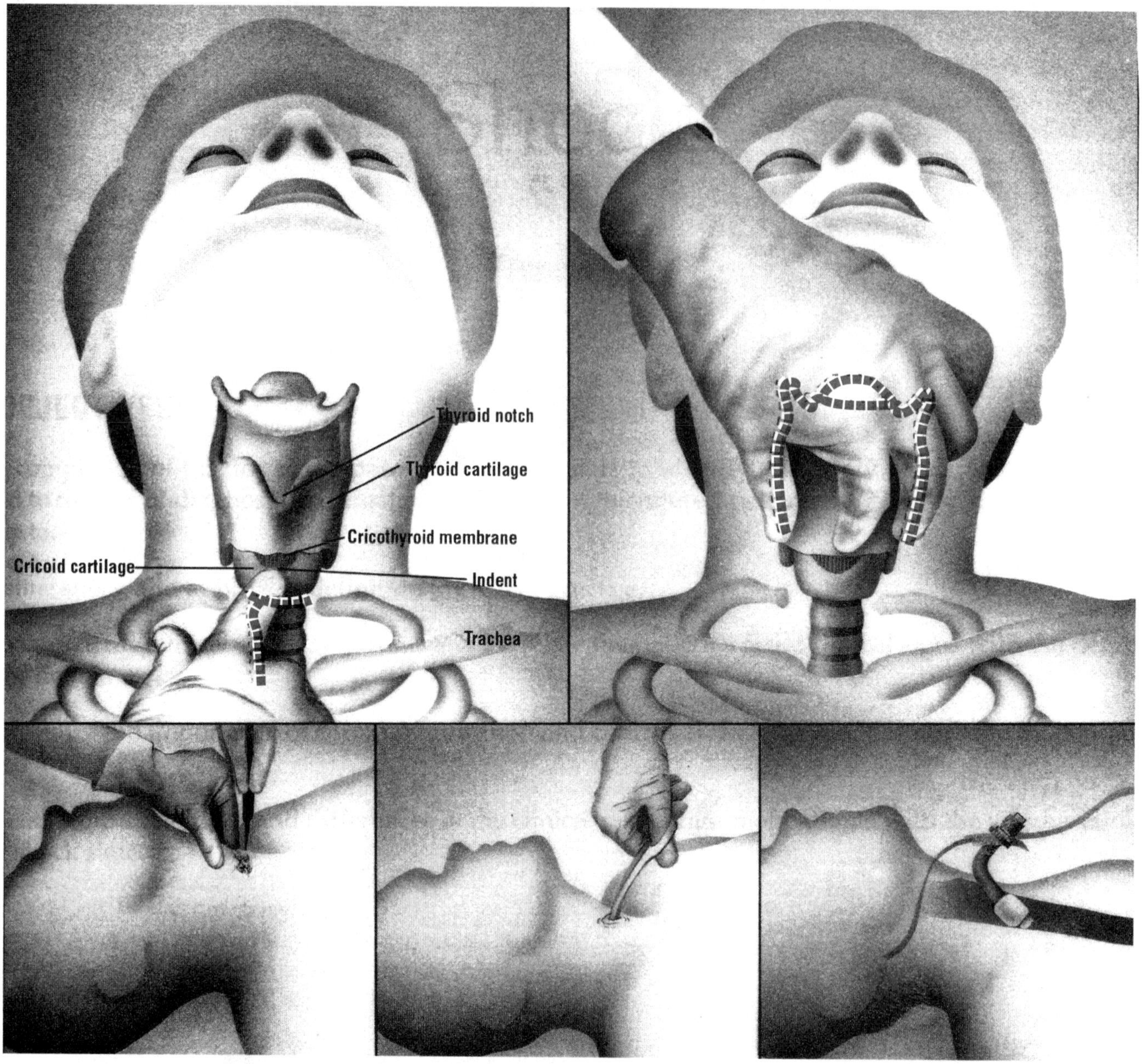

Thyroid notch
Thyroid cartilage
Cricothyroid membrane
Cricoid cartilage
Indent
Trachea

Reprinted with permission from American College of Surgeons Committee on Trauma. (2004). Airway and ventilatory management. In *Advanced trauma life support® for doctors*: Student course manual (7th ed., p. 67). Chicago: Author.

- Attaching the endotracheal tube or alternative airway device to an exhaled CO_2 detector

- Attaching an esophageal detection device (This device should be used to assess tube placement immediately after intubation. The esophageal detection device does not provide ongoing assessment of proper tube placement.)

- Obtaining a chest radiograph

Secure the endotracheal tube or alternative airway device to ensure that it does not dislodge.

Always confirm endotracheal tube or alternative airway device placement whenever there is a change in the patient's condition or the patient is moved.

Assessment of Ventilation

History

Refer to Chapter 3, Initial Assessment, for a description of general information that should be collected regarding every trauma patient. Only pertinent questions specific to patients with ventilation problems are described following.

- Are there blunt or penetrating injuries of the thorax?

- Did the patient strike an object with his or her chest?

- Did injuries result from acceleration, deceleration, or a combination of both types of forces (e.g., motor vehicle crashes, falls, and crush injuries)?
- Is the patient complaining of dyspnea?
- Have drugs or alcohol been used that may affect the level of consciousness and interfere with the patient's ventilatory efforts?
- Does the patient have any preexisting pulmonary problems?
- Has the patient been intubated before?
- Is there a history of tobacco use? What type, how much, how long?
- What is the age of the patient?

Physical Assessment

Inspection

- Observe the mental status. What is the level of consciousness, mentation? Changes in mental status can be an indication of hypoxia.
- Observe the respiratory rate and the pattern and work of breathing.
  - Is the patient spontaneously breathing?
  - Is the rate normal, slow, or fast for the age of the patient?
  - Is the pattern of breathing regular, irregular, deep, or shallow?
  - Is there use of accessory or abdominal muscles or both, or nasal flaring?
- Observe the chest wall for symmetrical movement. There will be decreased excursion on the injured side. The presence of a flail segment may produce paradoxical movement.
- Observe the chest wall for injuries that may severely impair the adequacy of breathing, such as open chest wounds. To avoid overlooking any wounds, debris or blood must first be removed from this area.
- Observe the patient's skin color. Assess for cyanosis.
- Observe for jugular vein distention (JVD) and the position of the trachea. JVD and tracheal deviation are late signs that may indicate tension pneumothorax.
- Observe for age-related changes:
  - Pediatric and geriatric patients' chests are more barrel shaped.
  - Pediatric patients utilize abdominal muscles to aid respiratory effort. Sternal or intercostal retractions in pediatric patients may be a sign of injury or respiratory distress.
  - Pediatric patients have a faster respiratory rate than adults.

Auscultation

Auscultate breath sounds bilaterally. The absence of breath sounds can indicate pneumothorax, hemothorax, or airway obstruction. Diminished sounds may occur as a result of splinting. Patients may show signs of shallow respirations as a result of pain.

Percussion

Percuss the chest. Dullness is associated with hemothorax, and hyperresonance suggests a pneumothorax.

Palpation

Palpate the chest wall, clavicles, and neck for tenderness, swelling, subcutaneous emphysema (crackling or popping sound), and step-off deformities. Subcutaneous emphysema may indicate esophageal, pleural, tracheal, or bronchial injuries.

Palpate the trachea above the suprasternal notch. Tracheal deviation may indicate a tension pneumothorax or massive hemothorax.

Interventions

Breathing Present: Effective

A patient demonstrating an effective breathing pattern will have a normal respiratory rate, depth, and oxygen saturation and will not show any respiratory problems requiring immediate intervention.

All trauma patients should receive some supplemental oxygen. Administer oxygen via a nonrebreather mask at a flow rate sufficient to keep the reservoir bag inflated; during inspiration, this usually requires a flow rate of at least 12 L/minute and may require 15 L/minute or more.

Breathing Present: Ineffective

When spontaneous breathing is present but ineffective, the following signs may indicate a potentially life-threatening condition:

- Altered mental status (e.g., restless, agitated)
- Cyanosis (especially circumoral cyanosis)
- Asymmetrical expansion of the chest wall
- Paradoxical movement of the chest wall during inspiration and expiration
- Use of accessory or abdominal muscles (or both)
- Sucking chest wounds
- Tracheal shift from the midline position

To inspect and palpate the anterior neck region (e.g., jugular veins and trachea), remove the anterior portion of the cervical collar. Another team member must hold the patient's head while the collar is being removed and replaced.

- Assess jugular veins for distention or flatness.
- Assess for absent or diminished breath sounds.

Interventions for the patient with ineffective ventilation include the following:

- Administer oxygen via a nonrebreather mask or assist ventilations with a bag-mask device, as indicated by the patient's status.
- Place the patient on a pulse oximeter.

    Pulse oximetry is a noninvasive tool that can continuously measure the oxygen saturation of arterial blood (Sp). Remember, it does not measure partial pressure of oxygen (Pa); this measurement is interpreted via arterial blood gas.

    Normal Sp is greater than 95%, meaning hemoglobin is 95% saturated with oxygen. Sp readings may not be accurate if the patient has compromised blood flow, vasoconstriction, or altered hemoglobin such as occurs with the presence of carboxyhemoglobin. Even if the patient has only a slight change in Sp readings, the change in arterial partial pressure of oxygen (Pa) is significant, especially if the Pa changes are between 100 and 60 mm Hg. The percentage of hemoglobin saturated with oxygen has a relationship to the partial pressure of oxygen, as shown by the oxygen-hemoglobin dissociation curve **(Figure 4-14)**.

    The curve plateaus when Pa levels are high, but the Sp will not significantly change at these higher ranges because essentially the hemoglobin is 100% saturated. However, at lower ranges of Pa where the curve is more sigmoidal shaped, the changes in Sp are extremely significant. For example, a 10-mm Hg drop in Pa from 90 to 80 represents only a drop in Sp from 96.5% to 94.5%. However, if the Pa drops from 50 mm Hg to 40 mm Hg, the drop in Sp is from 83.5% to 75%. The clinical significance is that patients who have pulse oximetry readings above 90% could have varying levels of Pa, and therefore, pulse oximetry alone should not be used to predict Pa levels. Oxygen saturation measurements can also be calculated from an arterial blood sample (SaO_2).[4]

- Assist with definitive airway management, as previously described.
- Perform or assist with a needle thoracentesis if the patient has signs and symptoms of a tension pneumothorax.[11]
    - Identify the insertion site. The insertion site is the second intercostal space, midclavicular line.

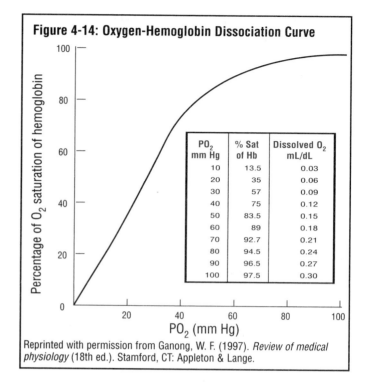

Figure 4-14: Oxygen-Hemoglobin Dissociation Curve

PO$_2$ mm Hg	% Sat of Hb	Dissolved O$_2$ mL/dL
10	13.5	0.03
20	35	0.06
30	57	0.09
40	75	0.12
50	83.5	0.15
60	89	0.18
70	92.7	0.21
80	94.5	0.24
90	96.5	0.27
100	97.5	0.30

Reprinted with permission from Ganong, W. F. (1997). *Review of medical physiology* (18th ed.). Stamford, CT: Appleton & Lange.

Insert the needle on the same side as the decreased/absent breath sounds and contralateral to the tracheal shift.

- Insert a large-caliber intravenous (10- to 14-gauge) over-the-needle catheter, 3 to 6 cm in length, over the top of the third rib into the pleural space until air escapes. Air should exit under pressure. Remove the needle and leave the catheter in place until it is replaced by a chest tube.
- If the needle is to remain in place for some time, connect the catheter to a one-way valve **(Figure 4-15)**.

- Assist with chest tube insertion.
- Monitor the chest drainage system. Types of drainage systems include the following:[12]
    - Underwater systems are those in which the water in the water seal chamber has a one-way valve that allows blood or air to escape while preventing backflow.
    - Waterless drainage systems are those in which a mechanical valve replaces water to allow drainage of blood or air (or both). The one-way valve prevents backflow.

- Assess and document fluctuation, output, color of drainage, and air leaks (FOCA).
- Monitor the patient with a thoracic injury closely when attached to a ventilator.

If there are any life-threatening injuries that could compromise breathing, stop and intervene before proceeding to assessment of circulation. Examples of

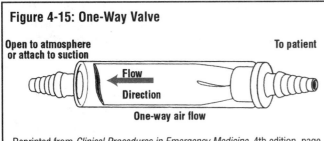

Figure 4-15: One-Way Valve

Open to atmosphere or attach to suction

To patient

Flow Direction

One-way air flow

Reprinted from *Clinical Procedures in Emergency Medicine*, 4th edition, page 201, Tube Thoracostomy, Copyright 2004, with permission from Elsevier.

life-threatening injuries that may compromise breathing are tension pneumothorax, open pneumothorax, and hemothorax. These conditions may require simultaneous assessment and immediate intervention (see Chapter 8, "Thoracic Trauma," for specific interventions). Remember that older patients may not do well even with minor chest injuries and that children may sustain significant thoracic trauma with little evidence of obvious injury.

Breathing Absent

The patient with absent ventilation requires immediate intervention and definitive management of the airway.

- Ventilate the patient via a bag-mask device with an attached oxygen reservoir system.
- Assist with endotracheal intubation; ventilate with oxygen via a bag-valve device attached to an oxygen reservoir system.
- Assess for additional life-threatening injuries that require immediate intervention.

Diagnostic Procedures

Refer to Chapter 3, Initial Assessment, for frequently ordered radiographic and laboratory studies. Additional studies for patients with airway obstruction or ineffective ventilation are listed following.

Radiographic Studies

- A chest radiograph can determine the presence of a hemothorax or pneumothorax. A chest radiograph can help to assess the position of the endotracheal tube, but it cannot exclude esophageal intubation.
- A CT scan of the chest may be ordered to discover nonobvious chest injuries.

Laboratory Studies

- Arterial blood gases are useful in evaluating the effectiveness of the patient's respiratory status.

Evaluation and Ongoing Assessment

Assessment of the patient's respiratory status should be ongoing throughout the course of care.

- Monitor respiratory rate, work of breathing, and level of consciousness frequently to identify changes in the patient's status.
- Frequently reassess breath sounds for any changes.
- Reassess interventions such as occlusive dressings and chest tube drainage to determine the amount and any change in drainage characteristics. Use the **DOPE** mnemonic to evaluate chest tube function.
- Evaluate pain status to ensure that the patient is able to take sufficiently deep breaths.
- Collaborate with other trauma team members to manage the ventilator status of the patient. Monitor patients closely on the ventilator. Utilize the mnemonic **DOPE** to troubleshoot ventilator alarms:

  D Displaced tube

  O Obstruction: Check for secretions or the patient biting the tube.

  P Pneumothorax: This condition may occur from original trauma or barotrauma from the ventilator.

  E Equipment failure: The patient may have become detached from the equipment, or there may be a kink in the tubing.

- The position of the endotracheal tube must be reassessed every time the patient is moved to ensure that adequate airway and ventilation support is provided.
- Monitor arterial blood gases.

Summary

Assessment and management of airway and ventilation for the trauma patient is an essential part of both the primary and secondary assessments of the patient. The emergency nurse must quickly recognize life-threatening airway and ventilation problems and provide appropriate interventions essential to successful resuscitation.

Early identification of all injuries requires a collaborative team approach to conduct the necessary diagnostic and therapeutic interventions. Determining the patient's need for definitive airway management and advanced ventilator support is a major consideration for members of the trauma team. The reassessment of the airway and ventilatory status of the patient is a continuous process, and the nurse must be alert to changes to ensure the optimal outcome for the patient.

References

1. Koran, Z., & Howard, P. (2003). Respiratory emergencies. In L. Newberry (Ed.), *Sheehy's emergency nursing principles and practice* (5th ed., pp. 421–449). St. Louis, MO: Mosby.

2. Olson, C. (2003). Dental, ear, nose, and throat emergencies. In L. Newberry (Ed.), *Sheehy's emergency nursing principles and practice* (5th ed., pp. 675–690). St. Louis, MO: Mosby.

3. Murphy, M. F. (2004). Applied functional anatomy of the airway. In R. Walls, M. F. Murphy, R. C. Luten, & R. E. Schneider (Eds.), *Manual of emergency airway management* (2nd ed., pp. 33–42). Philadelphia: Lippincott Williams & Wilkins.

4. Brashers, V. L. (2002). Structure and function of the pulmonary system. In K. McCance & S. Huether (Eds.), *Pathophysiology: The biologic basis for disease in adults and children* (4th ed., pp. 1082–1104). St. Louis, MO: Mosby.

5. Walls, R. (2004). The decision to intubate. In R. Walls, M. F. Murphy, R. C. Luten, & R. E. Schneider (Eds.), *Manual of emergency airway management* (2nd ed., pp. 1–7). Philadelphia: Lippincott Williams & Wilkins.

6. American Heart Association. (2005, December 13). Part 7.1: Adjuncts for airway control and ventilation. *Circulation, 112,* IV-51–IV-55.

7. American College of Surgeons Committee on Trauma. (2004). Airway and ventilatory management. *Advanced trauma life support® for doctors: Student course manual* (7th ed., pp. 41–67). Chicago: Author.

8. Walls, R. (2004). Rapid sequence intubation. In R. Walls, M. F. Murphy, R. C. Luten, & R. E. Schneider (Eds.), *Manual of emergency airway management* (2nd ed., pp. 22–32). Philadelphia: Lippincott Williams & Wilkins.

9. Murphy, M., & Schneider, R. E. (2004). Supraglottic devices. In R. Walls, M. F. Murphy, R. C. Luten, & R. E. Schneider (Eds.), *Manual of emergency airway management* (2nd ed., pp. 110–119). Philadelphia: Lippincott Williams & Wilkins.

10. York Clark, D. (2004). Combitube airway. In J. Proehl (Ed.), *Emergency nursing procedures* (3rd ed., pp. 65–68). Philadelphia: W. B. Saunders.

11. Upton, D. A. (2004). Emergency needle thoracentesis. In J. Proehl (Ed.), *Emergency nursing procedures* (3rd ed., pp. 178–181). Philadelphia: W. B. Saunders.

12. Upton, D. A., & Proehl, J. A. (2004). Management of chest-drainage systems. In J. Proehl (Ed.), *Emergency nursing procedures* (3rd ed., pp. 187–188). Philadelphia: W. B. Saunders.

The primary and secondary assessments will reveal information the nurse uses to analyze the patient's responses to the injury event and to determine specific nursing diagnoses. Each nursing diagnosis is derived by diagnostic reasoning, which determines the priorities of intervention. Each diagnosis represents an actual or risk for a health problem or one that may develop as a result of a patient being vulnerable to risk factors. The problems may be corrected by the nurse or may require a collaborative intervention with other trauma team members. The identification of specific outcomes corresponds to the goals generated by the team for the patient to correct each diagnosis or health problem.

Nursing Diagnoses	Interventions	Expected Outcomes
Airway clearance, ineffective, related to: • Edema of the airway, vocal cords, epiglottis, and upper airway • Irritation of the respiratory tract • Laryngeal spasm • Altered level of consciousness • Pain • Presence of an artificial airway • Direct trauma • Tracheobronchial secretions or obstruction • Aspiration of foreign matter • Inhalation of toxic fumes or substances	• Protect the cervical spine • Position the patient • Open and clear the airway • Insert oro- or nasopharyngeal airway • Consider endotracheal intubation	**The patient will maintain a patent airway, as evidenced by:** • Regular rate, depth, and pattern of breathing • Bilateral chest expansion • Effective cough and gag reflex • Absence of signs and symptoms of airway obstruction: stridor, dyspnea, and hoarse voice • Clear sputum of normal amount without abnormal color or odor • Absence of signs and symptoms of retained secretions: fever, tachycardia, and tachypnea

Aspiration, risk, related to:
 	
• Reduced level of consciousness secondary to injury or concomitant substance abuse
• Impaired cough and gag reflex
• Trauma to head, face, and/or neck
• Secretions and debris in airway
• Increased intragastric pressure
• Impaired swallowing
	• Protect the cervical spine
	• Position the patient
	• Open and clear the airway
	• Insert oro- or nasopharyngeal airway
	• Consider endotracheal intubation
	• Insert a gastric tube and evacuate stomach contents
	• Obtain blood sample for arterial blood gases (ABGs), as indicated
		The patient will not experience aspiration, as evidenced by:
		
		• A patent airway
		• Clear and equal bilateral breath sounds
		• Regular rate, depth, and pattern of breathing
		• ABG values within normal limits:
		  ▪ PaO_2 80 to 100 mm Hg (10.0 to 13.3 KPa)
		  ▪ SaO_2 > 95%
		  ▪ $PaCO_2$ 35 to 45 mm Hg (4.7 to 6.0 KPa)
		  ▪ pH 7.35 to 7.45
		• Clear chest radiograph without evidence of infiltrates
		• Ability to handle secretions independently

Nursing Diagnoses	Interventions	Expected Outcomes

Gas exchange, impaired, related to:
 	
• Ineffective breathing pattern: loss of integrity of thoracic cage and impaired chest wall movement secondary to injury, deterioration of ventilatory efforts
• Ineffective airway clearance
• Aspiration
• Altered blood flow, oxygen-carrying capacity of the blood, oxygen supply
• Aspiration of foreign matter
• Hypo- or hyperventilation
• Inhalation of toxic fumes or substances
	• Administer oxygen via a nonrebreather mask
	• Ventilate, if needed, with 100% oxygen via a bag-mask device or with a mechanical ventilator
	• Assist with endotracheal intubation and ventilate
	• Monitor oxygen saturation with continuous pulse oximetry
	• Administer blood, as indicated
		The patient will experience adequate gas exchange, as evidenced by:
		
		• ABG values within normal limits
		  ▪ PaO_2 80 to 100 mm Hg (10.0 to 13.3 KPa)
		  ▪ SaO_2 > 95%
		  ▪ $PaCO_2$ 35 to 45 mm Hg (4.7 to 6.0 KPa)
		  ▪ pH 7.35 to 7.45
		• Skin normal color, warm, and dry
		• Level of consciousness, awake and alert, age appropriate
		• Regular rate, depth, and pattern of breathing

Breathing pattern, ineffective, related to:
 	
• Pain
• Musculoskeletal impairment
• Unstable chest wall segment
• Lack of intact thoracic cavity wall
• Lung collapse
	• Administer oxygen via a nonrebreather mask
	• Prepare for ventilatory support with either bag-mask device or endotracheal intubation and mechanical ventilation
	• Obtain blood sample for ABGs, as indicated
	• Cover open wounds with sterile, non-porous dressing
	• If signs and symptoms of a tension pneumothorax develop:
	  ▪ After application of the dressing, remove the dressing and reevaluate the patient
	  ▪ Immediately prepare for a needle thoracentesis
		The patient will have an effective breathing pattern, as evidenced by:
		
		• Normal rate, depth, and pattern of breathing
		• Symmetrical chest wall expansion
		• Absence of stridor, dyspnea, or cyanosis
		• Clear and equal bilateral breath sounds
		• ABG values within normal limits:
		  ▪ PaO_2 80 to 100 mm Hg (10.0 to 13.3 KPa)
		  ▪ SaO_2 > 95%
		  ▪ $PaCO_2$ 35 to 45 mm Hg (4.7 to 6.0 KPa)
		  ▪ pH 7.35 to 7.45
		• Trachea midline

Chapter 5

Shock

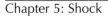

Objectives

On completion of this chapter/lecture,
the learner should be able to:

1. Define the four types of shock.

2. Describe the pathophysiologic changes as a
   basis for the signs and symptoms of shock.

3. Discuss the nursing assessment
   of the patient in shock.

4. Plan appropriate interventions
   for the patient in shock.

5. Evaluate the effectiveness of nursing
   interventions for patients in shock.

Preface

Lecture begins on page 78.

*Knowledge of normal physiology serves as a foundation
for understanding the anatomic derangements and
pathophysiologic compromises that may result from trauma. Before reading this chapter, it is strongly suggested
that the learner read the following review material.
Reading about the specific anatomic and physiologic concepts presented in this section will enhance the learner's
ability to correlate such concepts with specific injuries. This
material related to anatomy and physiology will not be covered during lectures, nor will it be evaluated by testing.*

Cell Structure and Metabolism

The body's 75 to 100 trillion cells require oxygen and nutrients to sustain function. Each cell's semi-permeable membrane takes part in complex processes that regulate both the intra- and extracellular environments. The cell's protoplasm is composed of 70 to 85% water, with the remaining 15 to 30% made up of lipids, carbohydrates (glucose), proteins, and electrolytes such as potassium, magnesium, sulfate, bicarbonate, and phosphate. The extracellular fluid contains more sodium, chloride, and bicarbonate than intracellular fluid. The cell's primary nutrients, fatty acids, oxygen, and amino acids are also in the extracellular fluid. Through active and passive transport systems, these substances can enter the cell to participate in metabolism and the production of energy.

Structurally, the cell contains lysosomes and mitochondria, which have important roles in cellular metabolism. Lysosomes contain enzymes that are responsible for ridding the cell of foreign substances such as bacteria. Mitochondria, through an oxidative process that utilizes oxygen, hydrogen ions, and stored enzymes, can extract energy from nutrients and use it to produce adenosine triphosphate (ATP). Once released from the mitochondria into the cell, ATP is the energy substance that sustains cellular metabolism.[1]

Cardiovascular System

The four-chambered heart is responsible for pumping blood into both the systemic circulation via the aorta and the pulmonary circulation via the pulmonary artery. Effective circulation depends on the following facts: (1) the flow of blood is unidirectional, (2) the output from the left and right ventricles is equal, and (3) blood flows on a pressure gradient from the arterial (high-pressure) system to the venous (low-pressure) system.[2]

The thick-walled arteries are composed of smooth muscle and an abundance of elastic fibers. The arterioles, because of their function in blood pressure control, have a predominant smooth muscle layer. The thin-walled veins are considered capacitance vessels, which are very distensible as well as collapsible. The single-cell-thick capillary is where the exchange of nutrients, gases, and byproducts of cellular metabolism occurs.

The term *microcirculation* refers to the capillaries, venules, arterioles, metarterioles (channels from arterioles to capillaries), and arteriovenous anastomoses (**Figure 5-1**). The microcirculation not only functions in the exchange of gases, nutrients, and byproducts of metabolism, but it also controls total peripheral

resistance (TPR) or systemic vascular resistance (SVR). TPR refers to the resistance in blood vessels in the entire systemic circulation. TPR is a reflection of the rate of blood flow through the vessels, which is related to the hematocrit and viscosity of the blood and the differences in pressure inside the vessels (the length, width, and radius of the vessels). The capillaries have precapillary sphincters that, under the control of the sympathetic nervous system, influence vasoconstriction and vasodilation to regulate blood flow into the capillary.[2]

In an average 70-kg person, the total blood volume is approximately 5 liters, composed of 3 liters of plasma and 2 liters of red blood cells. In addition, there are 12 liters of extracellular fluid and 23 liters of intracellular fluid for a total body fluid volume of 40 liters (**Table 5-1**).

Most systemic blood volume (64%) is in the venous capacitance system (**Table 5-2**). The arterial system functions as a pressure system to maintain blood flow to the tissues. The arterial blood pressure is a measure of cardiac output (stroke volume × heart rate) multiplied by the TPR. In the larger vessels, the radius is greater, the resistance is lower, and the flow of blood

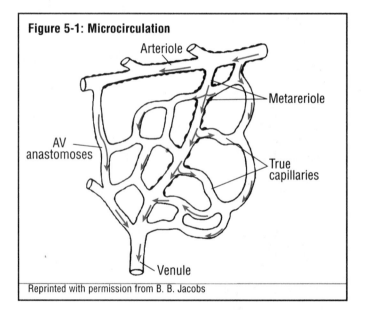

Figure 5-1: Microcirculation

Arteriole

Metarteriole

AV anastomoses

True capillaries

Venule

Reprinted with permission from B. B. Jacobs

Table 5-1: Distribution of Total Body Fluids

Fluid Compartment	Liters
Extracellular fluid (ECF)	15 L (37.5%)
Plasma	3 L
Interstitial fluid and other ECF compartments	12 L
Intracellular fluid (ICF)	25 L (62.5%)
Red blood cells	2 L
All other cells	23 L

Reprinted with permission from B. B. Jacobs

is greater than in smaller vessels. However, the actual pressure inside vessels is greatest in the larger arteries (100 mm Hg), decreases as the arterial blood flows through capillaries (35 mm Hg), and is eventually 0 mm Hg in the larger veins and the vena cavae.[2]

The systolic arterial blood pressure is more a reflection of the cardiac output (stroke volume, ejection velocity), whereas the diastolic arterial blood pressure reflects the TPR. In shock, tissue perfusion is compromised. The mean arterial pressure (MAP) will reflect the degree of tissue hypoperfusion. To calculate an estimate of the MAP, take one-third of the pulse pressure (the difference between the systolic and diastolic pressures) and add it to the diastolic pressure. **Box 5-1** provides two examples of calculating the MAP.

Nervous System Control of the Circulatory System

In general, the autonomic nervous system (ANS) is responsible for the nervous control of smooth muscle, cardiac muscle, and glands. The ANS controls the body's visceral functions. The ANS is divided into the sympathetic and parasympathetic divisions. The differences in these two subdivisions are related to the location of their nerve cell bodies, their effects on various organs, and their chemical mediators.

The sympathetic nervous system (SNS) plays an important role in shock syndromes because many of the signs that the patient demonstrates are a result of SNS stimulation. The SNS fibers originate in spinal cord segments T-1 through L-2. Because the SNS is predominantly a motor system, the sympathetic nerves travel through the anterior (motor) root of the particular spinal nerves. The postganglionic fibers eventually innervate receptor organs such as the heart, lungs, bronchi, stomach, adrenal glands, intestines, systemic blood vessels, and sweat glands. With some exceptions, the postganglionic fibers of the SNS are adrenergic, meaning that the chemical mediator they release is norepinephrine, which is a catecholamine, neurotransmitter, and powerful vasoconstrictor.[3]

Some of the effects of increased SNS stimulation are listed in **Table 5-3**. In general, when the body needs to respond to stress (e.g., shock), the SNS is stimulated.

Special pressure-sensitive receptors (baroreceptors) in the body's major arteries are innervated by ANS fibers. In the carotid sinus (wall of the internal carotid artery above the bifurcation of the common carotid artery) and in the wall of the aortic arch, there are more of these pressure-sensitive sites. When the systolic blood pressure drops below 60 mm Hg, the baroreceptors are no longer stretched, causing fewer inhibitory impulses to the vasomotor center in the brain stem. The lack of such impulses causes increased vasomotor activity, resulting in vasoconstriction and a rise in blood pressure.[4]

Table 5-2: Distribution of Blood

Location	Percentage
Systemic circulation	84%
Veins and venules	64%
Arteries and arterioles	16%
Capillaries	4%
Heart	7%
Pulmonary circulation	9%
Reprinted with permission from B. B. Jacobs	

Box 5-1: Calculation of Mean Arterial Blood Pressure (MAP)

1/3 (Systolic pressure – Diastolic pressure) + Diastolic pressure = MAP
Example 1:
120/80 mm Hg 120 mm Hg – 80 mm Hg = 40 mm Hg 1/3 of 40 mm Hg = 13 mm Hg 80 mm Hg + 13 mm Hg = 93 mm Hg
Example 2:
90/60 mm Hg 90 mm Hg – 60 mm Hg = 30 mm Hg 1/3 of 30 mm Hg = 10 mm Hg 60 mm Hg + 10 mm Hg = 70 mm Hg
Reprinted with permission from B. B. Jacobs

Table 5-3: Effects of Sympathetic Nervous System Stimulation

Organ	Effect
Heart (muscle)	Increased force of contraction (positive inotropy)
Heart (rate)	Increased heart rate (positive chronotropy)
Peripheral vessels	Vasoconstriction
Pupil	Dilation
Sweat glands (cholinergic)	Increased secretion
Adrenal glands	Increased cortical and medullary secretion
Bronchi	Dilation
Kidneys	Renin secretion increased
Liver	Glycogenolysis (breakdown of stored glycogen)
Reprinted with permission from B. B. Jacobs	

Shock is a syndrome resulting from inadequate perfusion of tissues, leading to a decrease in the supply of oxygen and nutrients required to maintain the metabolic needs of cells. When the supply of oxygen and nutrients cannot meet the demand to sustain normal cellular metabolism, the body responds initially by activating intrinsic compensatory mechanisms to improve perfusion, especially in areas of high demand such as the brain, heart, and lungs. When compensatory mechanisms fail to restore adequate perfusion, a cascade of cellular abnormalities can result in total organ dysfunction and, eventually, death.

Early recognition that the patient is in shock can assist in decreasing the mortality and morbidity associated with shock. No laboratory or radiographic test indicates a diagnosis of shock. Shock must be initially recognized by the presence of inadequate tissue perfusion, for example, cold, moist skin and an altered mental status. Once shock is recognized, the cause of shock needs to be determined so that appropriate management can be started. Hemorrhage is the most common cause of shock in the injured patient.[5]

Classification and Etiology

Numerous classification systems have been used to define shock, either by causes or by the underlying pathophysiologic effects. The following system classifies shock syndromes according to the underlying pathology[6,7] (**Table 5-4**).

Hypovolemic Shock

The most common shock syndrome to affect a trauma patient is caused by hypovolemia. Hypovolemia, a decrease in the amount of circulating blood volume, may result from a significant loss of whole blood because of hemorrhage, or it may result from the loss of the semipermeable integrity of the cellular membrane, leading to leakage of plasma and protein from the intravascular space to the interstitial space, as may occur with a burn.[6] Shock resulting from hemorrhage is classified into four groups based on the percentage of blood volume lost. The physiologic responses to the four degrees of volume loss are listed in **Table 5-5**.[5]

Cardiogenic Shock

Cardiogenic shock is a syndrome that results from ineffective perfusion caused by inadequate contractility of the cardiac muscle. Some causes of cardiogenic shock are myocardial infarction, blunt cardiac injury, mitral valve insufficiency, dysrhythmias, and cardiac failure.

Some authors use the term cardiogenic shock to refer to the shock syndrome that is actually trauma-induced cardiac insufficiency resulting from cardiac tamponade.[5] Cardiogenic shock as a result of trauma is rare. Blunt cardiac injury may lead to decreased myocardial contractility and some degree of cardiogenic shock. Assess the trauma patient for signs of a myocardial infarction, which is a more common underlying reason for cardiogenic shock. Blunt cardiac injury will be discussed in detail in Chapter 8, Thoracic Trauma.

Obstructive Shock

Obstructive shock results from an inadequate circulating blood volume because of an obstruction or compression of the great veins, aorta, pulmonary arteries, or the heart itself.[6,7] Cardiac tamponade may compress the heart during diastole to such an extent that the atria cannot adequately fill, leading to a decrease in stroke volume. A tension pneumothorax may also lead to inadequate stroke volume by displacing the inferior vena cava and

Table 5-4: Classification of Shock Etiology and Underlying Defect

Etiology	Underlying Pathology
Hypovolemic	
Hemorrhage	Whole blood loss
Burns	Plasma loss
Cardiogenic	
Myocardial infarction	Loss of cardiac contractility
Dysrhythmias	Reduced cardiac output
Blunt cardiac injury	Loss of cardiac contractility
Obstructive	
Cardiac tamponade	Compression of heart with obstruction to atrial filling
Tension pneumothorax	Mediastinal shift with obstruction to atrial filling
Tension hemothorax	Combination of preceding
Distributive	
Neurogenic shock	Loss of vasomotor tone due to decreases in sympathetic control
Anaphylactic shock	Vasodilation of vessels due to immune reaction to allergens, e.g., release of histamine
Septic shock	Mediated by systemic inflammatory response syndrome (SIRS) with hypotension and perfusion abnormalities

Reprinted with permission from B. B. Jacobs

obstructing venous return to the right atrium. An air embolus may lead to obstruction of the pulmonary artery and subsequent obstruction to right ventricular outflow during systole, with resulting obstructive shock. Signs, symptoms, and interventions for cardiac tamponade and tension pneumothorax are discussed in Chapter 8, Thoracic Trauma.

Distributive Shock

Distributive shock results from a disruption in the SNS control of the tone of blood vessels, which leads to vasodilation and maldistribution of blood volume and flow. Examples are neurogenic and septic shock. Neurogenic shock may result from injury to the spinal cord in the cervical or upper thoracic region. Autonomic sympathetic functions are lost, resulting in:

- The loss of vasomotor tone regulated by the SNS, which results in peripheral vasodilation and maldistribution of blood volume in the peripheral vessels, especially the veins, leading to hypotension.[8,9]

- The loss of cutaneous control of sweat glands, resulting in an inability to sweat, loss of thermoregulatory control, and warm and dry skin.

- Increased parasympathetic control of heart rate, resulting in bradycardia.[5,9]

Spinal shock is a phrase used to describe the areflexia and flaccidity associated with the lower motor neuron involvement in complete cord injuries; reflexes return with resolution of spinal shock.[5] Septic shock from bacteremia is another example of distributive shock. Endotoxins and other inflammatory mediators cause vasodilation, shunting of blood in the microcirculation, and other perfusion abnormalities.

Usual Concurrent Injuries

Hypovolemic shock that results from hemorrhage can occur because of a number of injuries, which are discussed in greater detail in other chapters. Injuries to the liver, spleen, major vessels in the chest, femur, multiple long bones, and the pelvis may lead to significant hypovolemia. Additionally, a combination of relatively minor injuries may also cause shock.

Pathophysiology as a Basis for Signs and Symptoms

Shock is a syndrome that involves all cells and their chemical and metabolic balance. Regardless of the underlying etiology, pathophysiologic alterations that occur during shock may be roughly divided into three stages: compensated, progressive, and irreversible.[6,8] In the compensated stage, normal physiologic compensatory mechanisms, mediated by the sympathetic nervous system, are activated to restore adequate tissue perfusion and preserve vital organ function. In nonvital tissues, cells will convert from highly efficient aerobic metabolism to anaerobic metabolism. Cellular damage occurs as lactic acid, the byproduct of anaerobic metabolism, accumulates.

In the progressive, or uncompensated, stage, compensatory mechanisms begin to fail and are unable to maintain perfusion to vital organs.[10] There is progressive tissue damage, cellular derangements, and death within all organ systems. There is further progression of lactic acidemia, activation of inflammatory processes, and deterioration of organ function.

Untreated shock can progress to irreversible stages as the body's own compensatory mechanisms fail to restore perfusion, organs become unable to maintain homeostasis, and the cellular destruction is so severe that death is inevitable.

Table 5-5: Physiologic Responses to Hemorrhage (Based on a 70-kg Male)

Class/ % Blood Loss	Pulse	Blood Pressure	Pulse Pressure (mm Hg)	Level of Consciousness	Respiratory Rate	Urinary Output
Class One (I) to 15% (up to 750 ml)	< 100	Normal	Normal or increased	Slightly anxious	14 to 20	> 30 ml/hr
Class Two (II) 15 to 30% (750 to 1,500 ml)	> 100	Normal	Decreased	Mildly anxious	20 to 30	20 to 30 ml/hr
Class Three (III) 30 to 40% (1,500 to 2,000 ml)	> 120	Decreased	Decreased	Anxious, confused	30 to 40	5 to 15 ml/hr
Class Four (IV) > 40% (> 2,000 ml)	> 140	Decreased	Decreased	Confused, lethargic	> 35	Negligible

Source: American College of Surgeons Committee on Trauma. (2004). Shock. In *Advanced trauma life support for doctors*® (Student course manual) (7th ed., p. 74). Chicago: Author.

As previously mentioned, the body responds to shock by initiating compensatory mechanisms as specific organ systems are affected. A discussion about several compensatory mechanisms and their responses follows.

Vascular Response

As blood volume decreases, the peripheral blood vessels vasoconstrict as a result of sympathetic stimulation via inhibition of the baroreceptors **(Figure 5-2)**. The arterioles constrict to increase TPR and, ultimately, blood pressure. The venous capacitance system vasoconstricts to improve venous return to the right atrium.

Chemoreceptors, located at the bifurcation of the common carotid arteries and the aortic bodies near the aorta, are sensitive to low levels of oxygen and excess levels of carbon dioxide in arterial blood. If the blood pressure is low enough, flow through the artery that supplies the chemoreceptors becomes diminished, and low oxygen and increased carbon dioxide levels stimulate these receptors. Consequently, the vasomotor center is stimulated by impulses along the same pathways as the barorecep-

tors. The result of this chemoreceptor response is vasoconstriction. Arterial blood pressure must be below 80 mm Hg to activate the chemoreceptor response that, like the baroreceptor response, is initiated within seconds of the change in blood pressure. The vascular response may be detected by a rise in the patient's diastolic blood pressure.

Cerebral Response

As shock progresses, the primary goal of the body is to maintain perfusion to the brain, heart, and lungs. Consequently, blood flow to these centers is preserved while blood flow to other organs, such as the liver, bowel, skin, and to some extent, the kidneys, may be compromised. Sympathetic stimulation (compensatory vasoconstriction) has little effect on cerebral and coronary vessels, as the brain and heart can autoregulate blood flow based on the needs of the tissues.[1] Therefore, the brain and heart are preferentially perfused during early and intermediate stages of shock. If the blood pressure drops below 50 mm Hg, cerebral ischemia occurs. The accumulation of carbon dioxide in the brain's vasomotor center will stimulate the central nervous system's ischemic response.[2] This response yields further stimulation of the SNS. Alterations in level of consciousness may indicate cerebral ischemia.

Renal Response

Renal ischemia activates the release of renin, an enzyme stored in the kidneys' juxtaglomerular cells of the arterioles. When the kidneys do not receive an adequate blood supply, renin is released into the circulation. Renin causes angiotensinogen, a normal plasma protein, to release angiotensin I. Angiotensin II is then formed from angiotensin I; the conversion to angiotensin II is enhanced by the angiotensin-converting enzyme from the lungs, where most of the conversion takes place **(Figure 5-3)**. The effects of angiotensin II are

- Vasoconstriction of arterioles and some veins
- Stimulation of the sympathetic nervous system
- Retention of water by the kidneys
- Stimulation of the release of aldosterone from the adrenal cortex (sodium retention hormone)

As powerful as the renin-angiotensin mechanism is, it does take approximately 10 to 60 minutes to fully activate.[8] Decreased urinary output may be an early sign of renal hypoperfusion, but it is also an indicator that there is systemic hypoperfusion.

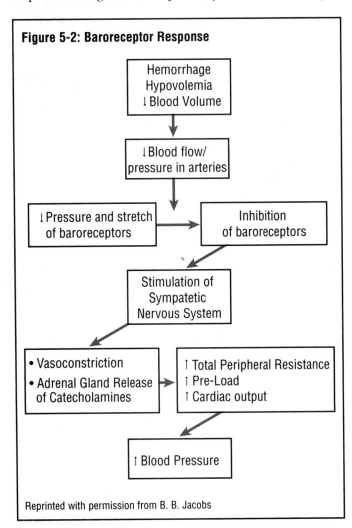

Figure 5-2: Baroreceptor Response

Hemorrhage
Hypovolemia
↓ Blood Volume

↓ Blood flow/ pressure in arteries

↓ Pressure and stretch of baroreceptors

Inhibition of baroreceptors

Stimulation of Sympatetic Nervous System

- Vasoconstriction
- Adrenal Gland Release of Catecholamines

↑ Total Peripheral Resistance
↑ Pre-Load
↑ Cardiac output

↑ Blood Pressure

Reprinted with permission from B. B. Jacobs

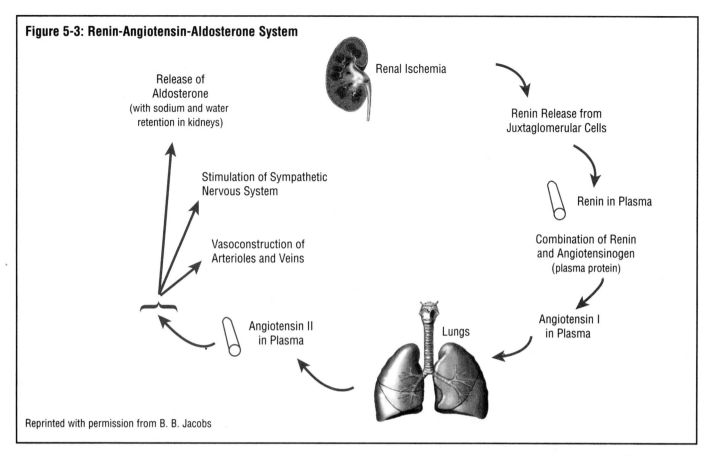

Figure 5-3: Renin-Angiotensin-Aldosterone System

Release of Aldosterone (with sodium and water retention in kidneys)

Renal Ischemia

Renin Release from Juxtaglomerular Cells

Stimulation of Sympathetic Nervous System

Renin in Plasma

Vasoconstruction of Arterioles and Veins

Combination of Renin and Angiotensinogen (plasma protein)

Angiotensin II in Plasma

Lungs

Angiotensin I in Plasma

Reprinted with permission from B. B. Jacobs

Adrenal Gland Response

When the adrenal glands are stimulated by the SNS, the release of catecholamines (epinephrine and norepinephrine) from the adrenal medulla will increase. The epinephrine stimulates receptors in the heart to increase the force of cardiac contraction (positive inotropy) and increase the heart rate (positive chronotropy) to improve cardiac output and, ultimately, improve blood pressure and tissue perfusion. Epinephrine also causes vasoconstriction. Norepinephrine promotes vasoconstriction to increase TPR and, ultimately, increase blood pressure and perfusion. The signs of shock resulting from adrenal gland release of catecholamines are tachycardia, increased anxiety, and a compensatory rise in diastolic blood pressure.

The endocrine response to shock stimulates the hypothalamus to release its corticotropin-releasing hormone that stimulates the pituitary to release adrenocorticotropin hormone (ACTH) that subsequently stimulates the adrenal gland to release cortisol. The effect of cortisol release is an elevation in blood sugar subsequent to increased insulin resistance and gluconeogenesis, the hepatic process to produce more sugar. Cortisol also causes renal retention of water and sodium, a compensatory mechanism to conserve body water.[7]

Hepatic Response

The liver can store the body's excess glucose as glycogen. As shock progresses, glycogenolysis is activated by epinephrine to break down glycogen into glucose. In a compensatory response to shock, hepatic vessels constrict to redirect blood flow to other vital areas. If, however, hepatic ischemia is too profound, the function of the liver is compromised.

Pulmonary Response

The patient in shock may have tachypnea for two reasons: (1) to maintain acid-base balance; and (2) to maintain an increased supply of oxygen. For cells to produce energy, it is essential that they have enough oxygen for oxidative processes. As the abnormal metabolic state in the shock patient persists, the resultant outcome is metabolic acidosis. Metabolic acidosis from anaerobic metabolism will be a stimulus for the lungs to increase the rate of ventilation. The increased respiratory rate is an attempt to correct the acidosis and also augments oxygen supply to maximize oxygen delivery to the alveoli.

Irreversible Shock

Untreated shock, or shock in uncompensated or irreversible stages (or both), will eventually cause compromises in most body systems. For example, prolonged hypovolemia will cause a decrease in arterial pressure because there is inadequate venous return, inadequate cardiac filling, and decreased coronary artery perfusion. Because coronary arteries are perfused during diastole, and diastolic pressure eventually falls, there will be a decrease in coronary artery perfusion with subsequent ischemia, resulting in a decrease in myocardial contractility.

The membranes of the lysosomes break down within cells and release digestive enzymes that cause intracellular damage. Other chemicals in the body, such as histamine, serotonin, and prostaglandins, are also activated. The byproducts of protein metabolism—uric acid, urea, and creatinine—are not cleared through the kidneys, but reabsorbed into the circulation. As compensatory mechanisms continue to fail, thrombi develop in the microcirculation, causing blood flow to become impeded, and most important, the tissue cells to become ischemic. The shock state becomes irreversible. Acidosis, increased capillary permeability, vasomotor failure (dilation), cardiac failure, and hepatic failure are some of the causes of a patient's demise.

Nursing Care of the Patient in Hypovolemic Shock

Assessment

A patient who arrives in the emergency department in profound shock because of trauma will require simultaneous assessment and intervention.

History

Refer to Chapter 3, Initial Assessment, for a description of general information that should be collected regarding every trauma patient. Only pertinent questions specific to patients in shock are described following.

- Does the patient have any obvious bleeding sites?
- What is the estimate of external blood loss?

Physical Assessment

Refer to Chapter 3, Initial Assessment, for a description of the assessment of the patient's airway, breathing, circulation, and disability.

Inspection

- Determine the level of consciousness.

  A patient's level of consciousness may progressively deteriorate. Restlessness, anxiety, or confusion may occur early in shock as cerebral perfusion is diminished. After 30 to 40% of the blood volume is lost, the patient may be unresponsive to verbal or painful stimuli (or both). A

loss of greater than 40% of the total blood volume generally leads to unconsciousness. The early signs of cerebral ischemia are difficult to interpret if alcohol or drug use (or both) is suspected. Consider any alteration in level of consciousness a result of cerebral ischemia until proven otherwise.

- Assess breathing effectiveness and rate of respirations.
- Identify obvious sources of uncontrolled external bleeding.
- Assess skin color and inspect for presence of moisture.

  The patient may be ashen or pale, especially around the mouth; mucous membranes may be pale. As the shock state progresses, the patient's skin will be moist to touch.

- Observe external jugular veins and peripheral veins for distention or flattening.
- Inspect the chest, abdomen, and extremities for signs of obvious bleeding, fractures, or major soft tissue injury.

Auscultation

- Obtain blood pressure.

  Because of vasoconstriction and low cardiac output, auscultated blood pressures may be difficult to obtain. A Doppler ultrasonic flow meter may assist with blood pressure measurement.

- Calculate pulse pressure.

  Trends in blood pressure are extremely important. As TPR rises in early shock, diastolic pressure rises. Early shock is characterized by a normal level or fall in systolic pressure and a rising diastolic pressure. Consequently, pulse pressure (the difference between systolic and diastolic pressures) narrows as cardiac output falls and blood vessels constrict. A narrowing pulse pressure is an ominous sign.

- Auscultate breath sounds.

  Bleeding into the thoracic cavity may lead to diminished or even absent breath sounds.

- Auscultate heart sounds.

  Heart sounds may sound distant or muffled if blood collects in the pericardial sac.

- Auscultate bowel sounds.

  The absence of bowel sounds may indicate intra-abdominal bleeding; however, even though bowel sounds are present, bleeding may still occur. Absent or hypoactive bowel sounds are common in patients in profound shock.

Percussion

- Percuss the chest and abdomen.

    Dullness of the chest or abdomen may indicate the presence of blood. Early identification of sources of internal blood loss is essential.

Palpation

- Palpate a central pulse (carotid, femoral, or brachial in infants under one year of age).

    Early in shock, tachycardia may indicate a strong positive chronotropic effect (rate) of circulating catecholamines.

    A positive inotropic effect (force of contraction) may be evidenced by a bounding central pulse.

- Palpate the peripheral pulses.

    Weak and thready pulses are caused by a decreased stroke volume as a result of hypovolemia.

- Palpate skin temperature and moisture.

Diagnostic Procedures

Refer to Chapter 3, Initial Assessment, for frequently ordered radiographic and laboratory studies. Additional studies for patients in shock are listed following.

Radiographic and Other Studies

- A chest radiograph may be done to determine the presence of a hemothorax or pneumothorax and to assess the size of the mediastinum. Widening of the mediastinum may indicate injury to the aorta or other mediastinal vessels.

- A pelvis radiograph may be done to locate fractures, which can result in significant blood loss because of disruption of pelvic veins.

- A femur radiograph may be done if fracture is suspected.

- Diagnostic peritoneal lavage (DPL), focused assessment sonography for trauma (FAST),[11] and an abdominal computed tomography (CT) scan are diagnostic studies that may be ordered if bleeding from blunt abdominal trauma is suspected.

Laboratory Studies

- Baseline levels of the patient's hemoglobin, hematocrit, serum osmolarity, electrolytes, blood urea nitrogen, creatinine, and serum lactate should be obtained.

    Serum lactate and base deficit levels are a proxy for oxygen debt in the hypoperfused shock patient. The oxygen debt (a deficit in tissue oxygenation due to poor oxygen delivery to cells and poor oxygen consumption) increases the longer the patient is hypoperfused. When serum lactate levels remain elevated, this signals that the body is attempting to produce energy through anaerobic metabolism. Mortality is increased when serum lactate levels remain high.

- Arterial pH, PaO_2, $PaCO_2$, and base deficit.

    Decreasing pH reveals a worsening of the cellular oxygen debt as metabolic acidosis develops because of anaerobic metabolism and lactic acid production. An elevated $PaCO_2$ (normal = 35 to 45 mm Hg, 4.7 to 6.0 KPa) indicates respiratory acidosis and impaired ventilation of the alveoli. A low PaO_2 (normal = 100 mm Hg, 13.3 KPa) indicates hypoxia.

    Metabolic acidosis can be measured by the base deficit. The greater the base deficit, the greater the oxygen debt. Injured patients with a severe degree of base deficit have a greater probability of decreased survival because the base deficit reflects the patient's tissue oxygen debt and poor metabolic state.[7,12]

    - Both base deficit and serum lactate are considered resuscitation end points for determining the degree of oxygen debt (lack of tissue oxygenation over resuscitation time) from shock.[7]

- Clotting studies including prothrombin time (PT) and partial thromboplastin time (PTT) may help plan for clotting factor replacement (platelets or fresh frozen plasma) and the need for ongoing monitoring of bleeding for the following:

    - Patients with head injuries

    - Patients with major bleeding

    - Patients on oral anticoagulants or oral antiplatelet agents

- Urinalysis, including specific gravity.

Planning and Implementation

Refer to Chapter 3, Initial Assessment, for a description of the specific nursing interventions for patients with compromises to airway, breathing, circulation, and disability.

- Administer oxygen via a nonrebreather mask at a flow rate sufficient to keep the reservoir bag inflated during inspiration; this usually requires a flow rate of at least 12 liters/minute and may require 15 liters/minute or more.

    Oxygen is essential for the patient in shock. Oxygen via a nonrebreather mask can deliver up to 100% O_2 with a snug fit of the mask around the nose and mouth. For the patient who requires bag-mask or bag-valve-endotracheal tube ventilation, oxygen must be delivered via a device with an appropriate oxygen reservoir.

- Control any uncontrolled external bleeding.

  Rapid control of bleeding is essential to prevent the progression of shock. Control major external bleeding by direct pressure.

- Initiate intravenous replacement of fluids and administer warmed fluids to 102.2 °F (39 °C) to prevent hypothermia.[5]

  Before the administration of blood or colloid solutions, initiate an isotonic, electrolyte-balanced, crystalloid solution via two large-caliber intravenous catheters.[5,7] The first fluid of choice is lactated Ringer's solution, which is a "near-physiologic" solution similar to the body's extracellular fluid.[12]

  Normal saline (0.9%) is considered the second fluid of choice for a hypovolemic patient.[5]

  An initial bolus of 1 to 2 liters of warmed lactated Ringer's solution may be given to adult patients as rapidly as possible.[5] The use of large-caliber, short intravenous catheters, short intravenous tubing, and a rapid infusion device will contribute to rapid infusion. It is important to observe the patient's response to the bolus by measuring blood pressure and heart rate, as well as listening to breath sounds and monitoring urinary output.

  Monitor intravenous volume replacement, especially in neurogenic shock patients. Because the patient in neurogenic shock is normovolemic, fluid overload must be avoided. The cause of hypotension may be related to hypovolemia from other injuries or neurogenic shock. Assessing the patient's pulse rate, skin temperature, and neurologic manifestations will help to differentiate between the two shock syndromes.

- Initiate blood product replacement.

  Patients who do not adequately respond to a crystalloid fluid bolus are potential candidates for blood volume replacement.

  - Type-specific and crossmatched blood.
    Type-specific and crossmatched blood is the ideal, but it may take longer to procure.

  - Type-specific blood.
    Type-specific blood is usually available within minutes from blood banks.

  - Type O-negative packed cells.
    O-negative is considered the universal donor because there are no agglutinogens (antigens) on the red blood cells of O-negative blood to possibly react with any agglutinins (antibodies) in the recipient's plasma. Rh-negative

blood has no type D antigen. O-negative blood is an option to consider.

  - O-positive packed cells.
    If O-negative packed cells are scarce, type O-positive packed cells are sometimes used for male patients because the risk of their plasma having anti-D antibodies is remote (85% of the white population and 95% of the black population is Rh positive). If O-positive packed cells are given to a premenopausal woman whose blood type is unknown, consider the need for Rh (D) immunoglobulin at a later date.

  - When large volumes of packed red cells are given, monitor for thrombocytopenia. Fresh frozen plasma, cryoprecipitate (Factor VIII), platelet administration, or all of these may be considered when coagulopathy studies are known.[5,14]

  - Administer blood through a macropore (140 to 170 microns) filtering device designed to trap any clots.[15]

  - Infuse blood through an intravenous line using normal saline.

  - Using the patient's hemoglobin level as a "transfusion trigger" is more complicated when the patient has sustained trauma requiring blood transfusions. A hemoglobin level of 8 g/dl is recommended for considering a transfusion in a patient.[14] However, if the patient has any preexisting cardiovascular or pulmonary diseases, maintaining a higher hemoglobin level is usually preferable.[14] Whether or not to give a transfusion to a trauma patient depends on physiologic measures, laboratory data, the patient's age, and preexisting comorbidities.

- Follow the facility's protocols for caring for patients who refuse allogenic blood products because of religious or other reasons.

- Consider autotransfusion for a patient with a hemothorax.

- Continue or consider application of a pneumatic antishock garment (PASG).

  - Indications for application of the PASG are controversial. Although several experts studied and commented on the use of the PASGs during the late 1980s and 1990s,[16-20] the American College of Surgeons in its Advanced Trauma Life Support® course recommends that it only be used to control bleeding in patients with pelvic or lower extremity fractures.[5] Application of the device should not delay transport time or initiation of intravenous fluid replacement.

- The pressure (tamponade) on the tissues surrounding the vessels underneath the areas of the garment causes the pressure gradient inside the vessel to decrease as well as the actual radius or size of the vessel. The PASG increases afterload (the pressure against which the heart must pump and which is predominately determined by arterial pressure), thereby improving blood flow to the brain, heart, and lungs. The controversy surrounds whether blood pressure should be "restored" before there is some control of bleeding or hemorrhage, because the increase in pressure may increase the rate of bleeding and loss of oxygen-carrying red blood cells.[17]

- Position the patient with his or her legs elevated.

  The modified Trendelenburg position may be advantageous if spinal cord or head injuries are not suspected. In this position, the patient remains supine with the legs elevated. The elevation assists venous return to the right atrium, but abdominal viscera remain in their normal position. As the patient's blood pressure is stabilized, the patient's legs may be lowered gradually while monitoring blood pressure for changes.

- Insert a gastric tube.

  Gastric distention may lead to vomiting, aspiration, or both. Distention may stimulate the vagus nerve, which may result in bradycardia. Insertion of a gastric tube provides for evacuation of stomach contents, relieves gastric distention, and prevents vagal stimulation. After the tube has been inserted, test the aspirated contents for the presence of blood.

- Insert an indwelling urinary catheter.

  A urinary catheter provides for bladder drainage, allows for frequent monitoring of urinary output, and is necessary for any shock patient who is being prepared for surgery. Suspected injury to the urethra is a contraindication to catheterization through the urethra.

- Attach monitoring leads and assess the patient's cardiac rate and rhythm.

  Electrocardiographic changes, other than sinus tachycardia, may not be apparent until very late in the course of hypovolemic shock; however, a patient with compromised coronary artery circulation may demonstrate ST changes in response to ischemia.

- Attach a pulse oximeter to assess the patient's oxygen saturation of the hemoglobin.

  Pulse oximetry readings may be inaccurate if the patient has peripheral vasoconstriction or is hypothermic.

- Peripheral vasoconstrictors are contraindicated in a hypovolemic patient, but may be considered in patients who present in neurogenic shock with no other injuries causing hypovolemia.

- Prepare the patient for surgery if bleeding (internal or external) is suspected, diagnosed, or not controlled.

Controversies in Resuscitation

- Permissive hypotension/Low-volume resuscitation

  - "Permissive hypotension" or low-volume resuscitation, a fluid resuscitation strategy for selected patients in whom bleeding has not been controlled, has been debated and studied for over a decade. The dilemma is that aggressive fluid resuscitation may be associated with hemodilution, disruption of the body's hemostatic mechanisms (clot formation) with subsequent further bleeding. However, less-than-aggressive fluid resuscitation may be associated with significant hypotension and poor tissue perfusion. Whether or not fluid resuscitation will be aggressive or not depends on a number of variables, not limited to type of trauma sustained, availability of definitive diagnosis and management of hemorrhage, time to definitive diagnosis and management, and the medical judgments and philosophy of the surgeons involved in the patient's care.[21]

- Hemoglobin-based oxygen carriers/Blood substitutes

  - Hemoglobin-based oxygen carriers (HBOCs) are being studied in clinical trials and animal models. Hemopure®, PolyHeme®, and HemoLink® are three such substances. HBOCs are solutions of a modified free-hemoglobin molecule with the ability to carry oxygen to the tissues. Some advantages of these products include longer shelf life than packed red blood cells (RBCs), the ability to store product at room temperature, absence of ABO antigens and therefore no incompatibility reactions, no disease transmission, and improved oxygen-carrying capacity to the microcirculation. Despite their potential advantages, most are still available only through research protocols.[14,22] Any experimental drug should be used with extreme caution and only in approved clinical trials.[14,22]

Evaluation and Ongoing Assessment

Refer to Chapter 3, Initial Assessment, for a description of the ongoing evaluation of the patient's airway, breathing, circulation, and disability. Additional evaluations include:

- Monitor urinary output for response to fluid resuscitation and for overall renal function. The ability of the kidneys to form urine is a reflection of the patient's overall perfusion status. An adult should produce approximately 1.0 ml/kg/hour with adequate resuscitation.

- Collaborate with other trauma team members as diagnostic studies and physical assessments help in finding the cause and source of hemorrhage.

- Monitor temperature to determine hypothermia. Hypothermia in the patient with hemorrhagic shock has serious sequelae, including:

  - Decreased tissue extraction of oxygen from hemoglobin

  - Impaired cardiac contractility and decreased cardiac output

  - Coagulopathies because of disruption of cellular enzymatic function, platelet disturbances, and increased fibrinolysis

- Coagulopathies may not develop in the first hour of resuscitation, but may develop because clotting factors are consumed, hemodilution occurs from crystalloid administration, and there is massive transfusion of blood products. Massive transfusion is described as the transfusion of large volumes (10 to 50 units) of packed red blood cells within the first 12 to 24 hours postinjury.[15] Massive crystalloid resuscitation and packed cell transfusions increase the risk for hypothermia, which is a marker for severe metabolic acidosis and a risk for progression to irreversible shock.

The combination of hypothermia, coagulopathy, and metabolic acidosis predisposes the patient to severe consequences.

Summary

Shock is a syndrome resulting from inadequate perfusion of tissues, leading to a decrease in the supply of oxygen and nutrients required to maintain the metabolic needs of the body. The four types of shock are hypovolemic, cardiogenic, obstructive, and distributive. Hypovolemic shock is the most common shock in trauma patients, caused by inadequate intravascular blood volume. The organs and certain structures of the body respond to shock in a compensatory fashion. If compensatory mechanisms fail, and treatment is not initiated, organ, tissue, and cellular ischemia ensue. Adherence to the six phases of the trauma nursing process allows for an organized approach to the assessment and management of compromises to airway, breathing, and circulation.

References

1. Carroll, E. W. (2004). Cell and tissue characteristics. In C. M. Porth (Ed.), *Pathophysiology concepts of altered states* (7th ed., pp. 69–101). Philadelphia: Lippincott Williams & Wilkins.

2. Porth, C. M. (2004). Control of cardiovascular function. In C. M. Porth (Ed.), *Pathophysiology concepts of altered states* (7th ed., pp. 449–471). Philadelphia: Lippincott Williams & Wilkins.

3. Carroll, E. W., & Curtis, R. L. (2004). Organization and control of neural function. In C. M. Porth (Ed.), *Pathophysiology concepts of altered states* (7th ed., pp. 1113–1157). Philadelphia: Lippincott Williams & Wilkins.

4. Porth, C. M. (2004). Disorders of blood pressure regulation. In C. M. Porth (Ed.), *Pathophysiology concepts of altered states* (7th ed., pp. 505–533). Philadelphia: Lippincott Williams & Wilkins.

5. American College of Surgeons Committee on Trauma. (2004). Shock. In *Advanced trauma life support® for doctors (Student course manual)* (7th ed., pp. 69–85). Chicago: Author.

6. Porth, C. M. (2004). Heart failure and circulatory shock. In C. M. Porth (Ed.), *Pathophysiology concepts of altered states* (7th ed., pp. 603–630). Philadelphia: Lippincott Williams & Wilkins.

7. Harbrecht, B. G., Alarcon, L. H., & Peitzman, A. B. (2004). Management of shock. In E. E. Moore, D. V. Feliciano, & K. L. Mattox (Eds.), *Trauma* (5th ed., pp. 201–226). New York: McGraw-Hill.

8. Guyton, A. C., & Hall, J. E. (2000). Circulatory shock and physiology of its treatment. In: A. C. Guyton & J. E. Hall (Eds.), *Textbook of medical physiology* (10th ed., pp. 253–262). Philadelphia: Elsevier.

9. Lindsey, R. W., Gugala, Z., & Pneumaticos, S. G. (2004). Injury to the vertebrae and spinal cord. In E. E. Moore, D. V. Feliciano, & K. L. Mattox (Eds.), *Trauma* (5th ed., pp. 459–492). New York: McGraw-Hill.

10. Emergency Nurses Association. (2000). *Emergency nursing core curriculum* (5th ed.). Philadelphia: W. B. Saunders.

11. Rozycki, G. S., & Dente, C. J. (2004). Surgeon-performed ultrasound in trauma and surgical critical care. In E. E. Moore, D. V. Feliciano, & K. L. Mattox (Eds.), *Trauma* (5th ed., pp. 311–328). New York: McGraw-Hill.

12. Ziglar, M. K. (2000). Application of base deficit in resuscitation of trauma patients. *International Journal of Trauma, 6*(3), 81–84.

13. Smith-Blair, N. (2003). Shock. In W. J. Phipps, J. F. Marek, F. D. Monahan, M. Neighbors, & J. K. Sands (Eds.), *Medical-surgical nursing: Health and illness perspectives* (7th ed., pp. 283–301). St. Louis, MO: Mosby.

14. Petersen, S. R., & Weinberg, J. A. (2004). Transfusion, autotransfusion, and blood substitutes. In E. E. Moore, D. V. Feliciano, & K. L. Mattox (Eds.), *Trauma* (5th ed., pp. 227–237). New York: McGraw-Hill.

15. Carrico, C. J., Mileski, W. J., & Kaplan, S. H. (2000). Transfusion, autotransfusion, and blood substitutes. In K. L. Mattox, D. V. Feliciano, & E. E. Moore (Eds.), *Trauma* (4th ed., pp. 233–244). New York: McGraw-Hill.

16. Maull, K. I. (1996). Role of military antishock trousers. In R. R. Ivatury & C. G. Cayten (Eds.), *The textbook of penetrating trauma* (pp. 170–175). Baltimore: Williams & Wilkins.

17. McSwain, N. E. (1996). Prehospital care. In D. V. Feliciano, E. E. Moore, & K. L. Mattox (Eds.), *Trauma* (3rd ed., pp. 107–121). Stamford, CT: Appleton & Lange.

18. Domier, R. M., O'Connor, R. E., Delbridge, T. R., & Hunt, R. C. (1997). National Association of EMS Physicians. Position paper: Use of the pneumatic antishock garment (PSAG). *Prehospital Emergency Care, 1*, 32–35.

19. Cayten, C. G. (1996). Commentary in Chapter 15, Role of military antishock trousers. In R. R. Ivatury & C. G. Cayten (Eds.), *The textbook of penetrating trauma* (pp. 174–175). Baltimore: Williams & Wilkins.

20. Cayten, C. G., Berendt, B. M., Byrne, D. W., Murphy, J. G., & Moy, F. H. (1993). A study of pneumatic antishock garments in severely hypotensive trauma patients. *Journal of Trauma, 34*, 728–735.

21. Revill, M., Greaves, I., & Porter, K. (2003). Endpoints of resuscitation in hemorrhagic shock. *Journal of Trauma, 54*, S53–S67.

22. Bone, H. G., & Westphal, M. (2005). The prospect of hemoglobin-based blood substitutes: Still a long stony road to go. *Critical Care Medicine, 33*, 694–695.

In addition to the nursing diagnoses outlined in Chapter 3, Initial Assessment, the following nursing diagnoses are potential problems for the patient in shock. Once a patient has been assessed, diagnoses can be defined as either actual or risk. An actual nursing diagnosis is derived from a decision based on the patient's presenting signs and symptoms. A risk nursing diagnosis is a judgment the nurse makes based on a particular patient's risk and potential for developing certain problems.

Nursing Diagnoses	Interventions	Expected Outcomes

Gas exchange, impaired, related to:
 	
• Ineffective breathing pattern: deterioration of ventilatory efforts
• Ineffective airway clearance
• Aspiration
• Altered blood flow, oxygen-carrying capacity of the blood, oxygen supply
	• Administer oxygen via a nonrebreather mask
	• Insert a gastric tube
	• Obtain blood sample for arterial blood gases (ABGs) as indicated
	• Ventilate, if needed, with 100% oxygen via a bag- mask device
	• Assist with endotracheal intubation
	• Administer blood, as indicated
	• Monitor oxygen saturation with continuous pulse oximetry
		The patient will experience adequate gas exchange, as evidenced by:
		
		• ABG values within normal limits
		  ▪ PaO_2 80 to 100 mm Hg (10.0 to 13.3 KPa)
		  ▪ SaO_2 > 95%
		  ▪ $PaCO_2$ 35 to 45 mm Hg (4.7 to 6.0 KPa)
		  ▪ pH between 7.35 and 7.45
		• Skin normal color, warm, and dry
		• Level of consciousness, awake and alert, age appropriate
		• Regular rate, depth, and pattern of breathing
		• Symmetric, bilateral breath sounds

Fluid volume deficit, related to: • Hemorrhage • Fluid shifts • Alteration in capillary permeability • Alteration in vascular tone • Myocardial compromise	• Control any uncontrolled external bleeding • Prepare for definitive care if control of internal bleeding is indicated • Cannulate two veins with large-caliber intravenous catheters and initiate infusion of an isotonic crystalloid solution • Consider autotransfusion for a patient with a hemothorax • Continue or consider application of a pneumatic antishock garment (PASG) • Position the patient with his or her legs elevated • Insert an indwelling urinary catheter • Administer blood, as indicated	The patient will have an effective circulating volume, as evidenced by: • Stable vital signs appropriate for age • Urine output of 1 ml/kg/hr • Strong, palpable peripheral pulses • Level of consciousness, awake and alert, age appropriate • Skin normal color, warm, and dry • Maintenance of hemoglobin of 8 g/dl or greater (however, this ought to be patient specific) • Control of external hemorrhage

Nursing Diagnoses	Interventions	Expected Outcomes
Cardiac output, decreased, related to: • Decreased venous return secondary to acute blood loss or massive peripheral vasodilation • Compression of heart and great vessels • Impairment of cardiac filling and ejection	• Monitor patient's cardiac rate and rhythm • Prepare for pericardiocentesis or needle thoracentesis, as indicated • Monitor hemodynamic status of patient • Control any uncontrolled external bleeding • Initiate intravenous administration of fluid and blood products • Prepare for definitive care	**The patient will maintain adequate circulatory function, as evidenced by:** • Strong, palpable peripheral pulses • Apical rate age appropriate • Normal heart sounds • Electrocardiogram with normal sinus rhythm, absence of dysrhythmias • Absence of jugular venous distention, deviated trachea • Skin normal color, warm, and dry • Level of consciousness, awake and alert, age appropriate • Urine output of 1 ml/kg/hr
Tissue perfusion, altered renal, cardiopulmonary, cerebral, gastrointestinal, peripheral (specific type), related to: • Hypovolemia • Interruption of flow: arterial and/or venous	• Control any uncontrolled bleeding • Cannulate two veins with large-caliber intravenous catheters and initiate infusion of an isotonic crystalloid solution • Administer blood, as prescribed • Prepare for definitive care	**The patient will maintain adequate tissue perfusion, as evidenced by:** • Vital signs within normal limits for age • Level of consciousness, awake and alert, age appropriate • Skin normal color, warm, and dry • Strong and equal peripheral pulses • Urine output of 1 ml/kg/hr
Hypothermia, related to: • Rapid infusion of cold intravenous fluids • Decreased tissue perfusion • Exposure • Blood loss	• Administer warmed IV fluids • Monitor body temperature • Keep the patient warm using blankets, warming lights, increased room temperature	**The patient will maintain a normal core body temperature as evidenced by:** • Core temperature measurement of 98 to 99.5 °F (36 to 37.5 °C) • Skin normal color, warm, and dry

Chapter 6

Brain and Cranial Trauma

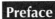

Objectives

On completion of this chapter/lecture, the learner should be able to:

1. Identify the common mechanisms of injury associated with brain and cranial injuries.

2. Describe the pathophysiologic changes as a basis for signs and symptoms.

3. Discuss the nursing assessment of patients with brain and cranial injuries.

4. Plan appropriate interventions for patients with brain and cranial injuries.

5. Evaluate the effectiveness of nursing interventions for patients with brain and cranial injuries.

Preface

Lecture begins on page 96.

Knowledge of normal anatomy serves as the foundation for understanding the anatomic derangements and pathophysiologic compromises that may result from trauma. Before reading this chapter, it is strongly suggested that the learner read the following review material. Reading about the specific anatomic and physiologic concepts presented in this section will enhance the learner's ability to correlate such concepts with specific injuries. This material related to anatomy and physiology will not be covered during lectures, nor will it be evaluated by testing.

Anatomy

Scalp

The scalp consists of five layers of tissue. They may be remembered using the mnemonic **SCALP: S**kin, **C**onnective tissue, **A**poneurotic galea, **L**oose areolar tissue, and **P**ericranium.[1] These layers provide a protective covering and may absorb some of the energy transferred during an injury event. The scalp is also highly vascular and, if lacerated or incised, may bleed profusely.

Skull

The skull, formed by the cranial bones (frontal, ethmoid, sphenoid, occipital, parietal, and temporal) and the facial bones, provides protection to the contents of the cranial vault (**Figure 6-1**). The bones of the adult skull are relatively thick (up to 6 mm), with the exception of the temporal bone. Fracture of the skull requires significant energy forces and often results in direct injury to the underlying brain parenchyma. Fractures may also lacerate underlying vascular structures, resulting in the formation of hematomas. The bones of the base of the skull form three depressions, termed fossae. They are named the anterior, middle, and posterior fossae and are often used as landmarks to identify or describe intracranial lesions.[1,2] The internal surface of the skull is rough and irregular. When energy forces are applied to the head, the brain can move across these rough inner surfaces, resulting in contusions, lacerations, and shearing injuries. The facial bones also help to protect the brain and underlying structures from injury by absorbing some of the injury force.

Contents Within the Cranial Vault

Meninges

The meninges consist of three layers of protective coverings to **PAD** the brain and spinal cord (**Figure 6-2**). These three layers are the **P**ia mater, **A**rachnoid membrane, and **D**ura mater. The innermost layer, the pia mater, is firmly attached to the brain and spinal cord. The arachnoid is a thin transparent membrane. Cerebrospinal fluid (CSF) is produced in the ventricles of the brain and circulates around the brain beneath the arachnoid membrane (subarachnoid space) and through the central canal of the spinal cord. The CSF further cushions the brain and spinal cord. The outermost layer, the dura mater, is a tough, fibrous membrane that adheres to the internal surface of the skull. There are potential spaces both above (the epidural space) and below (the subdural space) the dura mater. Arteries, including the middle meningeal artery, are located within the epidural space. Small bridging veins traverse the subdural space. It is worthwhile to note that as individuals age, normal atrophy of the brain parenchyma results in a widening of the subdural space and greater susceptibility of these bridging veins to traumatic injury.

Tentorium

Part of the dura mater extends from the occipital bone to near the center of the cranium, forming the tentorium cerebelli. The tentorium divides the cranial

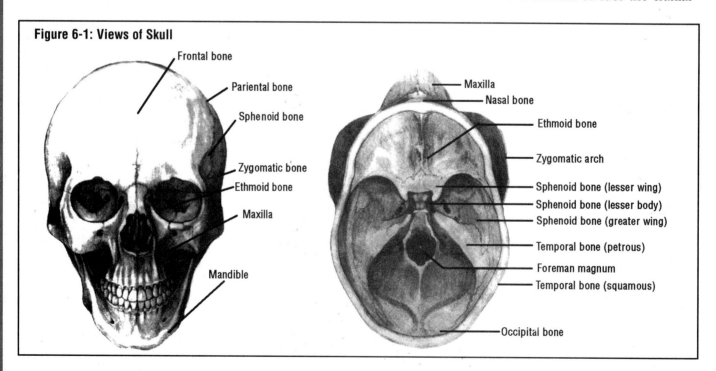

Figure 6-1: Views of Skull

Frontal bone
Pariental bone
Sphenoid bone
Zygomatic bone
Ethmoid bone
Maxilla
Mandible

Maxilla
Nasal bone
Ethmoid bone
Zygomatic arch
Sphenoid bone (lesser wing)
Sphenoid bone (lesser body)
Sphenoid bone (greater wing)
Temporal bone (petrous)
Foreman magnum
Temporal bone (squamous)
Occipital bone

vault into supratentorial and infratentorial compartments. The supratentorial compartment contains the cerebral hemispheres in the anterior and middle fossae. The infratentorial compartment contains the medulla, pons, and cerebellum in the posterior fossae. The midbrain, the upper portion of the brain stem, and the oculomotor nerve (cranial nerve III) pass through an elongated gap in the tentorium. Injury within the cranial cavity and resulting edema may cause shift and compression of brain stem structures and the oculomotor nerve against the tentorium.

Brain (Figure 6-3)

The two cerebral hemispheres are each divided into frontal, parietal, temporal, and occipital lobes. These lobes are responsible for judgment, behavior, and voluntary motor functions (frontal); sensory functions and spatial orientation (parietal); speech, auditory, and memory functions (temporal); and vision (occipital).

The diencephalon, connecting the cerebral hemispheres with the midbrain, includes the thalamus, hypothalamus, subthalamus, and epithalamus. The hypothalamus has numerous key roles in hormonal regulation and metabolic functions, including temperature regulation; release of hormones from the pituitary gland and adrenal cortex; emotional behaviors such as fear, rage, and pleasure; and activation of the sympathetic and parasympathetic functions of the autonomic nervous system.[2-4]

The three divisions of the brainstem are the midbrain, pons, and medulla. The reticular activating system, which originates in the midbrain and pons, is primarily responsible for vital reflexes, such as cardiovascular function and respirations, and consciousness or wakefulness. Stimulation of the reticular activating system, along with intact cerebral hemispheres, results in consciousness or an alert state. Conversely, a decrease in reticular activating system stimulation results in a decreased level of consciousness. Along

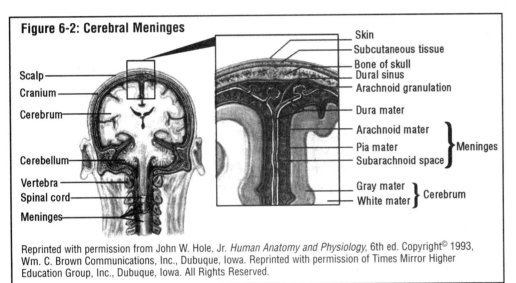

Figure 6-2: Cerebral Meninges

Scalp
Cranium
Cerebrum
Cerebellum
Vertebra
Spinal cord
Meninges
Skin
Subcutaneous tissue
Bone of skull
Dural sinus
Arachnoid granulation
Dura mater
Arachnoid mater
Pia mater
Subarachnoid space
Meninges
Gray mater
White mater
Cerebrum

Reprinted with permission from John W. Hole, Jr. *Human Anatomy and Physiology,* 6th ed. Copyright© 1993, Wm. C. Brown Communications, Inc., Dubuque, Iowa. Reprinted with permission of Times Mirror Higher Education Group, Inc., Dubuque, Iowa. All Rights Reserved.

Figure 6-3: Brain Structures

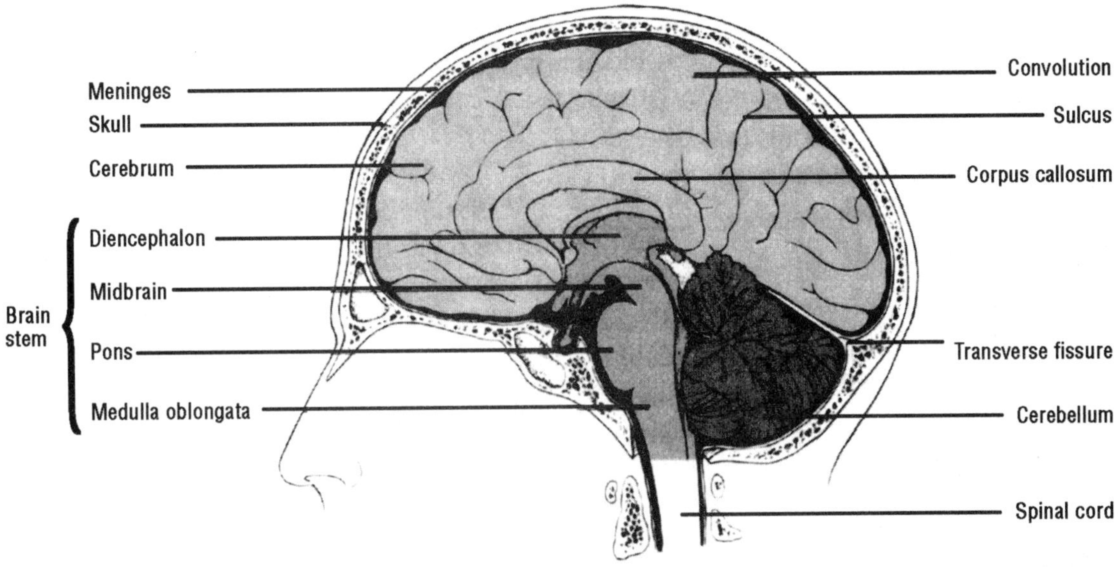

Meninges
Skull
Cerebrum
Diencephalon
Midbrain
Brain stem
Pons
Medulla oblongata
Convolution
Sulcus
Corpus callosum
Transverse fissure
Cerebellum
Spinal cord

with the reticular activating system, the medulla and pons have control over vital cardiorespiratory centers that regulate respirations, blood pressure, and heart rate.

The cerebellum, located in the posterior fossae, lies behind the brainstem and beneath the cerebral hemispheres. The cerebellum has extensive neural connections with the spinal cord, the midbrain, and the cerebral hemispheres.[2,4] Major functions of the cerebellum include conscious and unconscious muscle coordination, movement, balance, and posture.

Cranial Nerves

There are 12 pairs of cranial nerves; nine (cranial nerves III through X and XII) have their origins in the brainstem. The olfactory nerve (cranial nerve I) is actually a group of nerves within a fiber tract that connects the nasal mucosa to the olfactory bulb. The pair of optic nerves (cranial nerve II) originates in the retina and is considered a fiber tract once it leaves the optic chiasm. Millions of optic fibers travel to the occipital and temporal lobes of the cerebrum. The accessory nerve (cranial nerve XI) has both a cranial and spinal component. The spinal component is derived from the first five or six cervical spinal nerves. For further discussion on the anatomy of cranial nerves, refer to Chapter 7.

Blood Supply

Blood is supplied to the brain through the internal carotids and vertebral arteries. Branches of the internal and external carotid arteries provide the blood supply to the face. The external maxillary artery branches off the external carotid artery and supplies blood to the nasal area. Uncontrolled hemorrhage from any of these arteries can be life-threatening.[3,4] Venous outflow from the brain is through vessels that drain to large dural sinuses located between the dural layers and empty into the jugular veins.

Physiology

Cerebral Blood Flow (CBF)

The brain stores neither oxygen nor glucose; therefore, it requires a continuous supply of both nutrients. It uses approximately 20% of the body's total oxygen supply and metabolizes glucose at a rate of 60 mg/minute. These nutrients are delivered to the brain via a steady flow of blood from the internal carotid and vertebral arteries. CBF is regulated through sensitive autoregulatory mechanisms located in the cerebral arterioles or resistance vessels. These mechanisms cause the arterioles to constrict and dilate with changes in carbon dioxide levels, changes in arterial pressure, and in response to the cellular

nutritional needs of the brain tissue. Carbon dioxide is a primary regulator of blood flow to the brain.[4-6] Increased levels of carbon dioxide, a potent vasodilator, or decreased levels of oxygen result in dilation of cerebral vessels, increased blood flow, and increased blood volume. Decreased carbon dioxide levels result in vasoconstriction, decreased blood flow, and decreased volume.

Along with carbon dioxide and oxygen concentrations, cerebral vessels dilate and constrict in response to changes in systemic pressure. Cerebral autoregulation maintains a constant CBF and functions well as long as the systemic mean arterial pressure is within the range of 60 to 150 mm Hg.[2,6] Autoregulation is often severely compromised in the brain-injured patient.

Intracranial Pressure (ICP)

The brain parenchyma occupies approximately 80% of the cranial vault; blood, approximately 10%; and CSF, approximately 10%. These volumes are relatively fixed, and together they create a normal ICP of approximately 10 mm Hg. Small changes in the individual volumes can occur without adversely changing the constant total volume or affecting ICP. Pressures greater than 20 mm Hg are generally considered abnormal.[4,7,8] According to the Monro-Kellie doctrine, as one volume expands, one or both of the other two volumes must decrease to maintain a constant ICP.[4,9] Increased ICP is defined as a pressure greater than 15 mm Hg. The intracranial compensation is limited because the cranial vault is nonexpansive. Once this limit is reached, there may be a significant increase in ICP, even with a small additional increase in volume. Elevation in ICP may result in a decrease in CBF and a subsequent decrease in cerebral perfusion.

Cerebral Perfusion Pressure (CPP)

Adequate perfusion of oxygen and nutrients to the brain is dependent on the cerebral perfusion pressure (CPP). CPP is the pressure gradient across the brain or difference between the pressures of the cerebral arterial and venous vessels and a primary determinant of cerebral blood flow.[3,4,10] CPP is calculated by the following formula (with MAP standing for mean arterial pressure):

$$CPP = MAP - ICP$$

A close relationship exists between CBF and CPP, and thus there is an increased importance to maintaining an adequate blood pressure. CPP should be maintained at a minimum of 60 mm Hg in the absence of cerebral ischemia.[11] Cerebral perfusion pressure less than 70 mm Hg may cause increased risk of ischemia to areas of the brain.[11] Traumatic brain injury is associated with lowered CBF, particularly in areas near contusions and subdural hematomas. Therefore, augmenting systemic blood pressure may be necessary to bring CPP to normal levels and maintain CPP at a minimum of 60 mm Hg.[4,11,12] Moderate increases in blood pressure to maintain adequate CPP do not cause an increase in ICP.[1,4,11,12]

The physiologic characteristics of autoregulation are disrupted after severe brain injury. Once compensatory mechanisms are exhausted, there is an increase in ICP, and CPP is compromised. Cerebral perfusion pressure of less than 60 mm Hg is associated with poor outcomes after injury to the brain. Loss of autoregulation results in cerebral and brainstem ischemia. This ischemia initiates a central nervous system ischemic response, termed the Cushing response. The Cushing response stimulates an increase in systolic blood pressure, a widening pulse pressure, a reflex bradycardia, and a diminished respitory effort. The response is an attempt to increase the CBF because of an increase in arterial blood pressure.[4]

Epidemiology

Traumatic brain injury is an important public health problem in the United States and across the world. An estimated 1.4 million people sustain a traumatic brain injury annually, with approximately 50,000 deaths.[13,14] Additionally, 80% of traumatic brain injuries are treated in emergency departments, and almost 17% require hospitalization.[13] Traumatic brain injury results in varying degrees of permanent disability for more than 80,000 individuals, and more than 2% of our total population live with a disability related to traumatic brain injury.[7,13,14]

Our society remains highly mobile and dependent on a variety of vehicles for transportation and recreation. Because one of the primary mechanisms associated with brain injury is a motor vehicle crash, most of the population is at risk for injury during their life span. However, certain behaviors increase the risk of sustaining a brain injury. These behaviors include

- Acute or chronic alcohol ingestion
- Abuse of drugs (prescribed and illicit substances)
- Current use of anticoagulation medications
- Incorrect use or nonuse of automobile safety restraint systems[15]
- Nonuse of approved protective helmets when riding motorcycles, all-terrain vehicles, or bicycles[13,15-17]
- Participation in team sports without protective equipment[18-20]

Mechanisms of Injury

Motor vehicle/traffic-related incidents and falls remain the leading causes of traumatic brain injury for all ages.[7,13,14] Other mechanisms include sports, recreation and recreational vehicles, and unintentional injuries. Firearm-related brain injuries, although less common, are associated with a high mortality rate.[13]

The energy forces responsible for trauma to the head frequently result in injury to the cranial contents. When these forces are applied, shearing tensile and compressive stresses may lead to hemorrhage, hematomas, and contusions. As the force is applied, the brain may also be injured as it moves across the rough base of the skull.

When the head strikes a solid object, the sudden deceleration force may result in bony deformity and injury to cranial contents. A pressure wave is generated at the point of impact, travels across the cranial contents, and eventually dissipates. The initial impact and pressure wave may tear tissue and result in injury on the side of the impact and the side opposite the point

of impact. The injury on the same side of the impact is termed coup injury, and the injury on the opposite side is termed contrecoup injury.[21] (**Figure 6-4**)

Types of Injuries

Injuries can occur to the skull, the brain, soft tissues, vascular structures, and cranial nerves. Blunt brain and cranial injuries are associated with deformation, acceleration forces, deceleration forces, or a combination of acceleration/deceleration forces.

Penetrating brain injuries, particularly those that cross the midline and damage both cerebral hemispheres or affect the brainstem, carry a high mortality rate. Missile-type wounds may occur from rifles, handguns, semiautomatic weapons, or exploding objects (e.g., fireworks).

Scalp injuries bleed profusely because of their highly vascular nature and lack of blood vessel retraction. Bleeding from scalp lacerations should be promptly controlled during the primary assessment. Blood loss associated with these wounds can compound the effects of the patient's total blood loss and further compromise circulating blood volume.[3,4]

Usual Concurrent Injuries

Patients who have sustained brain or cranial injuries are at risk for concomitant injury to the cervical spine, with or without neurologic deficits; therefore, **all** patients with a brain or cranial injury should be assessed for cervical spine injury.[1]

Five percent of patients who have sustained a major brain or cranial injury have at least one additional significant injury to another system.[1] Injury to certain cranial nerves may alter the patient's facial expression or appearance. Injuries to the face may be associated with severe hemorrhage as a result of

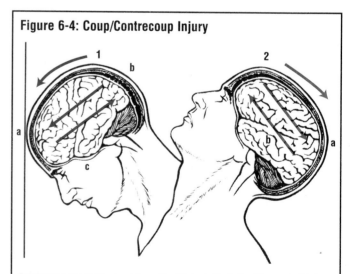

Figure 6-4: Coup/Contrecoup Injury

Reprinted from *Pathophysiology. The Biologic Basis for Disease in Adults and Children*, 4th edition, page 489, Alteration of Neurologic Function, Copyright 2002, with permission from Elsevier.

insult to the internal and external carotid arteries as well as the external maxillary artery that supplies blood flow to the nasal area. Further discussion of maxillofacial injuries can be found in Chapter 7, Ocular, Maxillofacial, and Neck Trauma.

Pathophysiology as a Basis for Signs and Symptoms

Injury to the brain may be classified as a primary or secondary injury. Primary injury involves the direct insult and inertial forces resulting in injuries such as a fractured skull or epidural hematoma. There is damage to neural tissue and a vascular response. Secondary brain injuries are produced by the many complex pathophysiologic changes and may be manifested hours to days after the initial injury. These secondary insults include hypotension, hypoxemia, hypercarbia, and cerebral edema resulting in increased ICP, decreased cerebral perfusion, and cerebral ischemia.[3,7,12,14,22,23] Secondary injuries compound the initial damage and diminish the effectiveness of autoregulatory and compensatory mechanisms of the brain. As previously mentioned, hypoxemia and hypotension are two secondary insults that have been highly correlated with an increase in morbidity and mortality after brain injury. Studies indicate that a single hypoxic episode in the prehospital setting as defined by a $PaO_2 < 60$ or a single hypotensive episode in the prehospital setting as defined by systolic pressure < 90 mm Hg were detrimental to outcomes.[4,11,12,14] Therefore, there has been an increased recognition of the importance of maintaining adequate oxygenation and cerebral perfusion.

Increased Intracranial Pressure

Intracranial pressure is a reflection of three volumes: brain, CSF, and blood within the nonexpansible cranial vault. As the volume of any one of these components increases, the volume of another must decrease to maintain ICP within a normal range. Normal compensatory mechanisms include displacement of CSF, decreased CSF production, and vasoconstriction to reduce cerebral blood volume. After brain injury, the normal compensatory mechanisms may be disrupted. These mechanisms also contribute to the development of cerebral edema. Once compensatory mechanisms are exhausted, ICP will rapidly increase.

As ICP rises, CPP decreases, leading to cerebral ischemia and the potential for hypoxia and lethal secondary insult.[3,12,14] In a hypotensive patient, even a marginally elevated ICP can be harmful. A slightly elevated blood pressure could protect against brain ischemia in a patient with a high ICP. Cerebral ischemia can lead to an increased concentration of carbon dioxide and decreased concentration of oxygen in cerebral vessels. Carbon dioxide dilates cerebral blood vessels, leading to an increase in blood volume and contributing to the further increase in ICP. Increased ICP produces observable signs and symptoms, depending on the stage of increased pressure.

Early signs and symptoms are

- Headache
- Nausea and vomiting
- Amnesia regarding events surrounding the injury
- Altered level of consciousness
- Restlessness, drowsiness, changes in speech, or loss of judgment

Late signs are

- Dilated, nonreactive pupil
- Unresponsiveness to verbal or painful stimuli
- Abnormal motor posturing patterns (e.g., flexion, extension, or flaccidity)
- Widening pulse pressure
- Increased systolic blood pressure
- Changes in respiratory rate and pattern
- Bradycardia

The triad of progressive hypertension, bradycardia, and diminished respiratory effort is known as Cushing's phenomenon or the Cushing reflex.[1,3,21]

Herniation Syndromes

Herniation occurs as a result of uncontrolled increases in ICP. Significant symptoms include[3,10]

- Unilateral or bilateral pupillary dilation
- Asymmetric pupillary reactivity
- Abnormal motor posturing
- Other evidence of neurologic deterioration

Two types of supratentorial herniation are classified by the site of herniation (**Figure 6-5**).

- Uncal herniation—The uncus (medial aspect of the temporal lobe) is displaced over the tentorium into the posterior fossa. This herniation is the more common of the two types of herniation syndromes.
- Central or transtentorial herniation—A downward movement of the cerebral hemispheres with herniation of the diencephalon and midbrain through the elongated gap of the tentorium.

Pressure on the pons and medulla results in blood pressure changes, cardiac deceleration, and asystole. If medullary brainstem function has been altered as a result of severe brain injury, hypotension can occur as an event signifying imminent death.

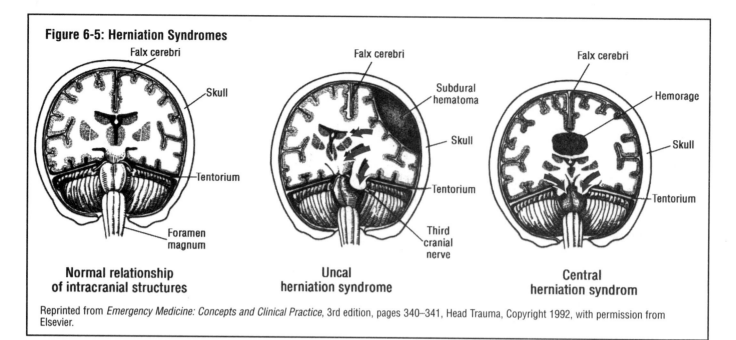

Figure 6-5: Herniation Syndromes

Normal relationship
of intracranial structures

Uncal
herniation syndrome

Central
herniation syndrom

Reprinted from *Emergency Medicine: Concepts and Clinical Practice*, 3rd edition, pages 340–341, Head Trauma, Copyright 1992, with permission from Elsevier.

Cerebrospinal Fluid Leakage

Disruption of the bony structures of the skull can result in either displaced or nondisplaced fractures. Fractures of the basilar skull or craniofacial structures may lacerate the dura mater, creating a passage for discharge of CSF either from the nose (rhinorrhea) or ear (otorrhea). A potential entrance for invading bacteria is also produced. Infections such as meningitis, encephalitis, or a brain abscess may occur as a result of these fractures.

Selected Brain and Cranial Injuries

Minor Head Trauma

Minor head trauma is usually defined as a head injury that produces a Glasgow Coma Scale (GCS) score of 13 to 15. Patients with minor head injuries may be further separated into two groups based on clinical presentation, the risk for significant intracranial pathology, and potential for deterioration[3] (**Table 6.1**).

Moderate Head Trauma

Moderate head trauma is defined as a head injury that produces a postresuscitative GCS score of 9 to 13. Patients may present to the emergency department with a wide variety of symptoms, including changes in level of consciousness, confusion, amnesia, and focal neurologic deficits.[3] Patients who initially sustain moderate head injuries may deteriorate to a condition of severe head injury over 48 hours and should be fully evaluated and closely mon-

itored to avoid hypoxia, hypotension, and other secondary insults.

Severe Head Trauma

Severe head trauma is defined as a head injury that produces a postresuscitative GCS score of 8 or less. Patients with severe head trauma may present in coma or with significant alterations in consciousness, abnormal pupil response, and abnormal motor posturing.[3]

Diffuse Brain Injuries

Concussion

A concussion is a temporary change in neurologic function that may occur as a result of minor head trauma. Concussions are typically the result of rapid acceleration/deceleration mechanisms or a direct blow to the head. Acute abnormalities on computed tomography (CT) scan or magnetic resonance imaging (MRI) are not usually found after concussions, but it is theo-

Table 6-1: Minor Head Injury Categories

High-Risk Patients	Low-Risk Patients
• Asymmetric pupils	• Currently asymptomatic
• Loss of consciousness lasting more than 2 minutes	• Normal pupils
• Vomiting	• No change in mentation/consciousness
• Seizure activity after injury	• Memory intact
• Headache	• No other injuries
• Skull fracture	• Accurate history
• Recent history of alcohol ingestion	• Trivial mechanism
• Anticoagulant therapy	• Reliable home observers

rized that there is some disruption of neuronal tissue and levels of neurotransmitters. Although there are several grading scales for concussion, the most common classifications are mild and classic.[3,4,20,21] A mild concussion produces cortical dysfunction and temporary, subtle neurologic deficits without loss of consciousness. A classic cerebral concussion involves a temporary loss of consciousness, usually lasting less than 6 hours, focal neurologic dysfunction, and retrograde amnesia.[1,4,21] Patients who sustain a concussion may manifest varying degrees of symptoms that last from several minutes to several hours.

Signs and Symptoms

- Transient loss of consciousness
- Headache
- Confusion and disorientation
- Dizziness
- Nausea and vomiting
- Loss of memory
- Difficulty with concentration
- Irritability
- Fatigue

Postconcussive Syndrome

Many patients who sustain a concussion will have postconcussive syndrome. Postconcussive syndrome may manifest immediately after the injury or may not occur until several days or months after head trauma. Symptoms typically resolve over several weeks but may persist for extended periods of time. Patients who experience postconcussive syndrome should be evaluated and may require treatment and rehabilitation.[3,7]

Signs and Symptoms

Symptoms are often vague, but may include

- Persistent headache
- Dizziness
- Nausea
- Memory impairment
- Attention deficit
- Irritability
- Insomnia
- Impaired judgment
- Loss of libido
- Anxiety
- Depression

Diffuse Axonal Injury

Diffuse axonal injury (DAI) is widespread, rather than localized, through the brain. Diffuse shearing, tearing, and compressive stresses from rotational or acceleration/deceleration forces result in microscopic damage primarily to axons within the brain.[4,21] Diffuse injury can also be caused by hypoxic insults to the brain caused by prolonged shock or apnea after the initial trauma.[1] It is manifested by diffuse, microscopic, hemorrhagic lesions and evidence of cerebral edema. The deeper white matter structures, the brainstem, and reticular activating system are particularly at risk, which leads to prolonged coma. The severity of injury may be graded as mild, moderate, or severe and is determined more by the patient's clinical signs and symptoms than the extent of radiographic findings.[1,4,7,21] Severe DAI is associated with significant morbidity and mortality.

Signs and Symptoms

- Immediate unconsciousness

  In mild DAI, coma may last from 6 to 24 hours. With severe injury, coma may persist for weeks or months, or the person may remain in a persistent vegetative state.

- Elevated intracranial pressure
- Abnormal posturing (flexion or extension)
- Hypertension with systolic blood pressure between 140 and 160 mm Hg, which can occur when there is damage to the diencephalon
- Hyperthermia with temperatures between 104 °F and 105 °F (40 °C and 40.5 °C)

  This symptom may not be observed initially in the emergency department.

- Excessive sweating because of autonomic dysfunction
- Mild to severe memory impairment, cognitive, behavioral, and intellectual deficits

Focal Brain Injury

Focal brain injury occurs in a localized area with grossly observable brain lesions. The injury may eventually expand, causing elevated intracranial pressure, compression and shift of intracranial contents, and damage to other areas of the brain, or there may be associated regions of the brain with more diffuse injury.[1,4,14,21] Common focal brain injuries include contusions and hematomas.

Cerebral Contusion

A contusion is a common focal brain injury in which brain tissue is bruised and damaged in a local area. Although contusions can occur in any area of the brain, most are located in the frontal and temporal lobes. Contusions may also develop in the brain tissue that underlies a depressed skull fracture. Contusions develop as the blood vessels within the brain parenchyma are damaged, resulting in hemorrhage, infarction, necrosis, and edema. If the contused area and subsequent swelling are significant, a shift of the injured cerebral hemisphere to the opposite side can be visualized on CT scan. The maximum effects of bleeding and edema formation peak 18 to 36 hours after injury.[1,4,21] Delayed hemorrhage or formation of an intracerebral hematoma may occur. Therefore, close observation and serial neurologic assessment are warranted to detect signs of increasing ICP.

Signs and Symptoms

- Alteration in level of consciousness
- Behavior, motor, or speech deficits
- Abnormal motor posturing (flexion, extension, or flaccidity)
- Signs of increasing ICP

Epidural Hematoma

An epidural hematoma results when a collection of blood forms between the skull and the dura mater. It is frequently associated (up to 90%) with fractures of the temporal or parietal skull that lacerate the middle meningeal artery.[3,21] Because the bleeding is usually arterial, blood accumulates rapidly. The expanding hematoma causes compression of the underlying brain, a rapid increase in ICP, decreased CBF, and secondary brain injury. Epidural hematomas of significant size require immediate surgical intervention, and the outcome is directly related to the neurologic status before surgery.

Signs and Symptoms

Classic signs of an epidural hematoma are[3,7]

- Transient loss of consciousness
- Lucid period lasting a few minutes to several hours
- Rapid deterioration in neurologic status

Other signs and symptoms may include

- Severe headache
- Sleepiness
- Dizziness
- Nausea and vomiting
- Hemiparesis or hemiplegia on the opposite side of the hematoma, which may rapidly progress to abnormal motor posturing
- Unilateral fixed and dilated pupil on the same side as the hematoma

Subdural Hematoma

A subdural hematoma is a focal brain injury beneath the dura mater that results from acceleration, deceleration, or combination forces. Subdural hematomas are usually venous in origin because the bridging veins are ruptured with the acceleration/deceleration forces. Cerebral contusions and diffuse axonal injury often accompany subdural hematomas. These hematomas, unlike epidural hematomas, are not necessarily associated with a skull fracture. There is, in addition to the hematoma formation, an associated incidence of direct injury to the underlying brain tissue.

The formation of a subdural hematoma may be acute or chronic. Patients with acute subdural hematomas manifest symptoms within 48 hours of the injury event. Patients with chronic subdural hematomas manifest symptoms as long as 2 weeks after the injury event. Chronic subdural hematomas are frequently associated with minor injury in older adults, patients taking anticoagulation medications, and chronic alcohol users because of the atrophy of the brain tissue, fragility of the bridging veins, and coagulation defects.

Signs and Symptoms

The onset of signs and symptoms and effect on neurologic function vary depending on the rapidity of hematoma formation. Signs and symptoms of acute subdural hematomas include

- Altered level of consciousness or steady decline in level of consciousness
- Signs of increased ICP
- Hemiparesis or hemiplegia on the opposite side of the hematoma
- Unilateral fixed and dilated pupil on the same side as the hematoma

Chronic subdural hematomas have similar symptoms, but these symptoms may manifest more slowly. Other signs and symptoms of chronic subdural hematomas include[4,7]

- Headache
- Progressive decrease in level of consciousness
- Ataxia
- Incontinence
- Seizures

Intracerebral Hematomas

Intracerebral hematomas occur deep within the brain tissue, may be single or multiple, and are commonly associated with contusions.[3,4,21] As with contusions, the most common sites are the frontal and temporal lobes. Intracerebral hematomas can result in significant mass effect, leading to increased ICP and neurologic deterioration.

Signs and Symptoms

- Progressive and often rapid decline in level of consciousness
- Headache
- Signs of increasing ICP
- Pupil abnormalities
- Contralateral hemiplegia

Skull Fractures

Because considerable force is required to fracture the skull, concurrent injury to the brain and cervical spine should always be considered. The three types of skull fractures are linear, depressed, and basilar. A linear skull fracture is a nondisplaced fracture of the cranium. It is of minor consequence unless the fracture site crosses an area where underlying vessels may be lacerated (e.g., temporal bone). A depressed skull fracture extends below the surface of the skull and can cause brain tissue compression and dural laceration. Basilar skull fractures are fractures of one or more of the five bones of the base of the skull. These fractures may accompany injury to other intracranial structures, such as the brain, dura mater, or cranial nerves, as well as significant facial trauma.

Linear Skull Fracture

Signs and Symptoms

- Headache
- Possible decreased level of consciousness

Depressed Skull Fracture

Signs and Symptoms

- Headache
- Possible decreased level of consciousness
- Possible open fracture
- Palpable depression of skull over the fracture site

Basilar Skull Fracture

Signs and Symptoms

- Headache
- Altered level of consciousness
- Periorbital ecchymosis (raccoon eyes), mastoid ecchymosis (Battle's sign), or blood behind the tympanic membrane (hemotympanum)
- Facial nerve (cranial nerve VII) palsy
- CSF rhinorrhea or otorrhea

Assessment

History

Refer to Chapter 3, Initial Assessment, for a description of general information that should be collected regarding every trauma patient. Only pertinent questions specific to patients with brain and cranial injuries are described following.

- If conscious, what are the patient's complaints?
  - Headache, nausea and vomiting, or memory deficits are important early signs of increasing ICP.
- If the patient has altered consciousness, does the history suggest brain or cranial trauma (or both)?
  - Impact to the head
  - Previous lucid interval
  - Witnessed vomiting or other associated signs or symptoms
- Was there any loss of consciousness after the injury, and if so, for how long?
- Does the patient have any amnesia from the injury event?
- Have drugs or alcohol been used that may affect the level of consciousness?
- Does the patient have any previous neurologic deficits or seizure history?

Physical Assessment

Refer to Chapter 3, Initial Assessment, for a description of the assessment of the patient's airway, breathing, circulation, and disability. Refer to **Appendix 6-A, *Initial Resuscitation of the Patient with a Severe Head Injury: Brain Trauma Foundation Guidelines* for an algorithm that depicts the initial resuscitation of the patient with a severe head injury.**

Inspection

- Assess the airway for obstruction, secretions, and foreign debris. The airway can be compromised as a result of decreased level of consciousness.
- Observe respiratory rate, pattern, and effort.
- Assess pupillary size and response to light.
  - A unilaterally fixed and dilated pupil may indicate oculomotor nerve compression from increased ICP and herniation syndrome.

- Bilateral fixed and pinpoint pupils may indicate a pontine lesion or effects of drugs (opiates).
  - A mildly dilated pupil with sluggish response may be an early sign of herniation syndrome.
  - A widely dilated pupil occasionally occurs with direct trauma to the globe of the eye.
  - Determine if the patient uses any eye medications.
- Observe for abnormal motor posturing patterns (e.g., abnormal flexion, abnormal extension, or flaccidity).
- Inspect the craniofacial area for ecchymosis or contusions. Basilar skull fractures can be accompanied by bleeding into the three fossae, producing ecchymosis. The ecchymosis may not be present until several hours after the injury.
  - Periorbital ecchymosis (raccoon eyes) indicates an anterior fossa fracture.
  - Mastoid process ecchymosis (Battle's sign) indicates a posterior fossa fracture.
  - Blood behind the tympanic membrane may indicate a middle fossa fracture.
- Inspect the nose and ears for drainage.
  - If drainage is present and not mixed with blood, test drainage with a chemical reagent strip. The presence of glucose indicates the drainage is CSF.
  - If drainage is present and mixed with blood (pink-tinged or red), test drainage by placing a drop of the fluid on linen or gauze. If a light outer ring forms around the dark inner ring (positive halo sign), the drainage contains CSF.

- Assess extraocular eye movements to test the function of cranial nerves III, IV, and VI (**Figure 6-6**).
  - The ability to perform extraocular eye movements indicates a functioning brainstem.
  - Limitation in range of ocular motion may indicate an orbital rim fracture with entrapment or paralysis of either a cranial nerve or ocular muscle.
- Determine the level of consciousness using the Glasgow Coma Scale (GCS) score (**Table 6-2**).

Palpation

- Palpate the cranial area for
  - Point tenderness
  - Depressions or deformities
  - Hematomas
- Assess all four extremities for
  - Motor function, muscle strength, and abnormal motor posturing
  - Sensory function

Glasgow Coma Scale

The Glasgow Coma Scale score ranges from 3 to 15 and is a measure of the patient's level of consciousness as well as a predictor of morbidity and mortality after brain injury.[3] It is not a measure of total neurologic function. The patient's total score results from a summative score of three aspects of behavior that are independently measured: **BEST** eye opening, **BEST** verbal response, and **BEST** motor response.[24] The motor component of the GCS score is the most sensitive subscore for identifying patients at risk for death and those with severe brain injury.[1,4,25] The initial GCS score provides a baseline score, and

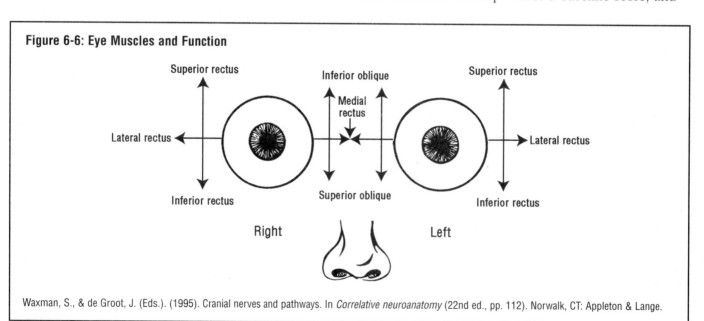

Figure 6-6: Eye Muscles and Function

Waxman, S., & de Groot, J. (Eds.). (1995). Cranial nerves and pathways. In *Correlative neuroanatomy* (22nd ed., pp. 112). Norwalk, CT: Appleton & Lange.

repeated assessments determine whether the patient's neurologic status is improving or deteriorating. Generally, a GCS score of 9 to 15 indicates mild to moderate head injury; a GCS score of 3 to 8 indicates severe head injury.

- **BEST** eye opening response is measured by observing whether the patient opens his or her eyes (**Table 6-3**).
- **BEST** verbal response is measured by the patient's response to questions. The response is characterized as ranging from oriented to no verbal response (**Table 6-4**).
- **BEST** motor response is measured by the patient's response to verbal or painful stimuli (**Table 6-5**).

Sometimes one or more limbs may be immobilized because of effects of sedation, pharmacologic paralysis, fractures, brain or spinal cord injury, or other circumstances. Take care not to misinterpret a grasp reflex or postural adjustments as a response to a command. Remember that the **BEST** response is to be measured. This is particularly important when one limb response is better than the other, or the patient moves his or her eyelids purposefully yet has paralysis from the neck down.

Diagnostic Procedures

Refer to Chapter 3, Initial Assessment, for frequently ordered radiographic and laboratory studies. Additional studies for patients with brain and cranial trauma are listed following.

Radiographic Studies

- CT scans[3,4]
  - Patient movement may produce artifacts and lead to an inaccurate CT reading.
  - Patients who are sedated or have received paralytic medications must be closely monitored during a CT procedure
- Skull series
  - This is not routinely ordered, especially if CT scan is available. If CT scan is unavailable, skull radiographs may be utilized to evaluate penetrating wounds to the head or suspected depressed skull fractures.
- Angiography
  - This may be indicated if vascular injury is suspected.

Table 6-2: Glasgow Coma Scale Score

Areas of Response	Points
Best Eye Opening:	
Eyes open spontaneously	4
Eyes open in response to voice	3
Eyes open in response to pain	2
No eye opening response	1
Best Verbal Response:	
Oriented (e.g., to person, place, time)	5
Confused, speaks but is disoriented	4
Inappropriate, but comprehensible words	3
Incomprehensible sounds but no words are spoken	2
None	1
Best Motor Response:	
Obeys command to move	6
Localizes painful stimulus	5
Withdraws from painful stimulus	4
Flexion, abnormal posturing of extremities	3
Extension, abnormal posturing of extremities	2
No movement or posturing	1
Total Possible Points:	**3–15**
Severe Head Injury	≤ 8
Moderate Head Injury	9–12
Minor Head Injury	13–15

Table 6-3: BEST Eye Opening Response from Glasgow Coma Scale

Score	Response	Comment/Description
4	Spontaneous eye opening	No stimulation is needed and the patient keeps eyes open spontaneously.
3	Responds to voice	There is no spontaneous eye opening, but the eyes open to the stimulus of speech. A response to voice does not need to be specifically to a command to open the eyes.
2	Responds to pain	There is no eye opening to voice, but the eyes open to a painful stimulus to the limbs (pinching of sternocleidomastoid muscle).
1	No response	There is no eye opening response to voice or painful stimulus. Eye opening may be precluded because of eye swelling or other physical reasons. In these circumstances, the best response should be measured or the score should be "1" with a comment as to the reason.

- MRI
  - This is typically not used in the acute resuscitation phase of care but may be indicated in the critical care or subacute phases to provide better delineation of a patient's injury and prognosis.

Laboratory Studies

- Arterial blood gases
- Coagulation studies
  - These studies may be beneficial in directing management for patients who have been previously treated with anticoagulants or for timing of insertion of ICP monitoring devices.
- Blood alcohol and urine toxicology screens may be beneficial to determine if changes in a patient's level of consciousness are related to substance abuse.

Planning and Implementation

Refer to Chapter 3, Initial Assessment, for a description of the specific nursing interventions for patients with compromises to airway, breathing, circulation, or disability.

- Open and clear the airway. Minimize or avoid stimulation of the gag reflex, which can produce a transient increase in ICP or may cause vomiting and subsequent aspiration.
- Administer oxygen via a nonrebreather mask at a flow rate sufficient to keep the reservoir bag inflated; this usually requires 12 to 15 liters/minute. The presence of hypoxia in patients with severe head trauma is associated with significant mortality.[12,14,23]
- Assist with early endotracheal intubation.

Table 6-4: BEST Verbal Response from Glasgow Coma Scale

Score	Response	Comment/Description
5	Oriented	Upon questioning, the patient is oriented to person, time, and place.
4	Confused/disoriented	The patient converses but is not fully oriented.
3	Inappropriate, comprehensible words	The patient articulates understandable words, but no comprehensible sustained conversation is possible.
2	Incomprehensible words	There are no recognizable words, but the patient is making noises (i.e., moaning).
1	No verbal response	There is no verbal response. Sometimes, speech may be precluded because of effects of sedation, intubation, or oral trauma. In these circumstances, the best response should be measured or the score should be 1 with a comment made as to the reason.

Table 6-5: BEST Motor Response from Glasgow Coma Scale

Score	Response	Comment/Description
6	Obeys commands	The patient purposefully moves in response to a verbal command.
5	Localizes painful stimuli	There is no response to a command, but there is purposeful movement (moves to attempt to remove stimulus) in response to a painful stimulus (pinching of the sternocleidomastoid muscle on each side) Maintain the stimulus until the maximal response is obtained.
4	Withdrawal from stimuli	There is no localization to pain, but there is a purposeful movement (i.e., flexion) in response to a painful stimulus (pinching of sternocleidomastoid muscle).
3	Abnormal flexion posturing	There is nonpurposeful movement (rapid withdrawal with abduction of shoulder, or slower adduction of shoulder response to a painful stimulus (pinching of sternocleidomastoid muscle on each side).
2	Abnormal extension posturing	There is nonpurposeful movement (abduction, internal rotation of shoulder, and pronation of forearm in response to a painful stimulus).
1	No movement	There is no movement in response to a painful stimulus to the limbs. If there is no motor response due to the effect of chemical paralysis, the patient should be scored 1 and a comment made as to the reason.

- This is done especially if the GCS score is less than 8 or the level of consciousness acutely decreases.[1,3,12,22]
  - Administer sedative and neuromuscular blocking agents, as prescribed, to assist with intubation (see Chapter 4).
- Consider hyperventilation in cases in which increased ICP is clinically evident and other methods to decrease it are unsuccessful (e.g., sedation, paralysis, CSF drainage, and osmotic diuretics).[12]
- A $PaCO_2$ above 45 mm Hg (6.0 KPa) may cause increased cerebral vasodilation, increased CBF, and ultimately increased ICP.
- Prolonged hyperventilation ($PaCO_2 \leq 25$ mm Hg or 3.7 KPa) is **not** recommended. Prophylactic hyperventilation ($PaCO_2 < 35$ mm Hg or 4.7 KPa) must be utilized judiciously.[12]
  - Hypocarbia that occurs as a result of hyperventilation causes cerebral vasoconstriction, decreased CBF, and ultimately decreased ICP. It is important to note that hyperventilation may cause ischemia secondary to severe vasoconstriction.
  - Hyperoxygenate the patient with 100% oxygen via a bag-mask device with an attached oxygen reservoir.
- Apply direct pressure to bleeding sites except over depressed skull fractures.
- Cannulate two veins with large-caliber intravenous catheters, and initiate infusions of an isotonic crystalloid solution with flow rate to be determined by the patient's hemodynamic status.
  - Hypotension in patients with severe head injury is associated with more than double the mortality as compared with patients with no hypotension.[11,12,14,23,26]
  - In certain situations, vasopressors may be indicated to maintain CPP. The goal of fluid support is to maintain hemodynamic stability while avoiding fluid overload. It is important to avoid even one episode of hypotension due to the resulting effect of decreased cerebral perfusion and subsequent secondary brain injury.
  - Research has been done to investigate the use of hypertonic saline solution (3% to 5%) in maintaining normovolemia and normotension without infusing large volumes of fluid.[22,27,28] Study results have been controversial as to whether or not hypertonic saline infusion contributes to better outcomes than infusion of large volumes of isotonic crystalloid solution. However, no research indicated that this treat-

ment modality is associated with negative patient outcomes.
- Insert an orogastric or nasogastric tube. An orogastric tube should be inserted if a basilar skull fracture or severe midface fractures are suspected.[1]
- Position the patient as guided by institutional protocols. Elevation of the patient's head to decrease ICP is controversial. An elevated head position may reduce ICP; however, it may also reduce CPP.[4,12,14,26]
  - Position the head midline to facilitate venous drainage. Rotation of the head can compress the veins in the neck and result in both venous engorgement and decreased drainage from the brain.[4]
- Prepare for insertion of an ICP monitoring device and then monitor the ICP, according to institutional protocols. Indications for ICP monitoring include[12]
  - Severe head injury (GCS score of 3 to 8) with an abnormal CT scan on admission
  - Severe head injury, but normal CT scan and two or more of the following:
    - Age older than 40 years
    - Unilateral or bilateral abnormal posturing
    - Systolic blood pressure < 90 mm Hg
- Administer mannitol, as prescribed. Administration via intermittent boluses (1 g/kg) may be more effective than a continuous infusion.[1,12,14,28,29]
  - Mannitol, a hyperosmolar, volume-depleting diuretic, decreases cerebral edema and ICP by pulling interstitial fluid into the intravascular space for eventual excretion by the kidneys. It is not recommended for prophylactic use because large doses can aggravate hypovolemia. It is generally indicated if the patient has signs of herniation or progressive neurologic deterioration. Although controversial, a loop diuretic (e.g., furosemide) may be an additional type of diuretic used in conjunction with mannitol.
- Administer anticonvulsant medication, as prescribed.
  - Prophylactic anticonvulsant medication is an option for early posttrauma seizures.[3,4,12] Seizure activity should be avoided because it increases both the cerebral metabolic rate and the ICP. Indications for seizure prophylaxis include
    - Depressed skull fracture
    - Seizure at the time of injury
    - Seizure on arrival to the emergency department

- History of seizures
- Penetrating brain injury
- Severe head injury
- Acute subdural hematoma
- Acute epidural hematoma

- Administer antipyretic medication, as prescribed, to treat hyperthermia. A cooling blanket may also be used.

  - Hyperthermia may increase the cerebral metabolic rate and ICP. Avoid causing shivering during the cooling process; shivering increases the cerebral metabolic rate and may precipitate a rise in ICP.

- Do not pack the ears or nose if a CSF leak is suspected.

- Administer tetanus prophylaxis, as appropriate.

- Assist with wound repair for facial and scalp lacerations.

- Administer other medications, as prescribed.

  - These may include analgesics, sedatives, naloxone (Narcan) if opiate use is suspected, and flumazenil (Romazicon) if benzodiazepine use is suspected.

- Administer antibiotics, as prescribed.

  - Patients with a basilar skull fracture may be given prophylactic antibiotics to prevent the development of meningitis. It is important to note that some organizations recommend monitoring the patient closely as opposed to administering prophylactic antibiotics.

- Prepare the patient for operative intervention, hospital admission, or transfer, as indicated.

Evaluation and Ongoing Assessment

Refer to Chapter 3, Initial Assessment, for a description of the ongoing evaluation of the patient's airway, breathing, circulation, and disability. Additional evaluations include the following.

- Changes in level of consciousness, using the GCS score for trend analysis
- Pupillary changes
- Trends in blood pressure, pulse, SpO$_2$, respiratory rate, and patterns for signs of increasing ICP, hypotension, or hypoxia
- Increasing edema
- Development of nausea, vomiting, seizure, or severe headache
- Changes in motor and sensory function
- Response to fluid administration and diuretic therapy by frequently monitoring urinary output

Summary

Head injury is the leading cause of trauma-related deaths. Appropriate and early intervention can prevent or minimize the development of irreversible brain injury. Secondary brain injury may result from cerebral hypoxemia, ischemia, cerebral edema, hypercarbia, hypotension, or increased ICP.

The priorities in treating patients with head injuries include facilitating oxygenation, ventilation, and adequate circulatory status; optimizing CPP; and controlling ICP. Maintaining adequate ventilation and CBF are essential to preserve neurologic function and prevent secondary injury. To maintain CPP, stabilize the patient's blood pressure and treat any increase in ICP through a collaborative team approach.

References

1. American College of Surgeons Committee on Trauma. (2004). Head Trauma. In *Advanced trauma life support® for doctors: Instructor course manual* (6th ed., pp. 151–176). Chicago: Author.

2. Sugerman, R. A. (2002). Structure and function of the neurologic system. In K. L. McCance & S. E. Huether (Eds.), *Pathophysiology: The biologic basis for disease in adults & children* (4th ed., pp. 363–400). St. Louis, MO: Mosby.

3. Biros, M. H., & Heegard, W. (2002). Head. In J. A. Marx, R. S. Hockberger, & R. M. Walls, (Eds.), *Rosen's emergency medicine: Concepts and clinical practice* (5th ed., pp. 286–314). St. Louis, MO: Mosby.

4. McQuillan, K. A., & Mitchell, P. H. (2002). Traumatic brain injuries. In K. A. McQuillan, K. T. Von Rueden, R. L. Hartsock, E. Whalen, & M. B. Flynn, (Eds.), *Trauma nursing: From resuscitation through rehabilitation* (3rd ed., pp. 394–461). Philadelphia: W. B. Saunders.

5. Guyton, A. C., & Hall, J. E. (2006). Cerebral blood flow, cerebrospinal fluid, and brain metabolism. In *Textbook of medical physiology* (11th ed., pp. 761–768). St. Louis, MO: W. B. Saunders.

6. Zauner, A., Daughtery, W. P., Bullock, M. R., & Warner, D. S. (2002). Brain oxygenation and energy metabolism: Part I biological function and pathophysiology. *Neurosurgery, 59*(2), 289–302.

7. Nolan, S. (2005). Traumatic brain injury: A review. *Critical Care Nursing Quarterly, 28*(2), 188–194.

8. Yanko, J. R., & Mitcho, K. (2001). Acute care management of severe traumatic brain injuries. *Critical Care Nursing Quarterly, 23*(4), 1–23.

9. Bader, M. K., Arbour, R., & Palmer, S. (2005). Refractory increased intracranial pressure in severe traumatic brain injury: Barbiturate coma and bispectral index monitoring. *American Association of Critical Care Nurses Clinical Issues, 16*(4), 526–541.

10. Boss, B. J. (2002). Alterations of neurologic function. In K. L. McCance & S. E. Huether (Eds.), *Pathophysiology: The biologic basis for disease in adults & children* (4th ed., pp. 438–486). St. Louis, MO: Mosby.

11. Brain Trauma Foundation, American Association of Neurological Surgeons. (2006). The joint section on neurotrauma and critical care. Guidelines for the management of severe traumatic brain injury: Cerebral perfusion pressure. Retrieved April 2, 2006, from http://www.braintrauma.org

12. Brain Trauma Foundation, American Association of Neurological Surgeons. (2000). The joint section on neurotrauma and critical care. Guidelines for the management of severe traumatic brain injury: Cerebral perfusion pressure. *Journal of Neurotrauma, 17*(6/7), 451–553.

13. Langlois, J. A., Rutland-Brown, W., & Thomas, K. E. (2004). *Traumatic brain injury in the United States: Emergency department visits, hospitalizations, and deaths*. Atlanta, GA: Centers for Disease Control and Prevention, National Center for Injury Prevention and Control.

14. Ghajar, J. (2000). Traumatic brain injury. *Lancet, 356*(9233), 923–929.

15. National Household Travel Survey. (2005). *Traffic safety facts 2004*. Washington, DC: Author.

16. Bledsoe, G. H., Schexnayder, S. M., Carey, M. J., Dobbins, W. N., Gibson, W. D., Hindman, J. W., et al. (2002). The negative impact of the repeal of the Arkansas motorcycle helmet law. *Journal of Trauma, 53,* 1078–1087.

17. Keenan, H. T., & Bratton, S. L. (2004). All-terrain vehicle legislation for children: A comparison of a state with and a state without a helmet law. *Pediatrics, 113*(4), 330–334.

18. Brown, G. J., Lam, L. T., & Parker, R. (2004). The nature and characteristics of sports and recreation-related concussive head injuries in children of young age. *Medicine and Science in Sports and Exercise, 36*(5), 275.

19. Delaney, J. S. (2004). Head injuries presenting to emergency departments in the United States from 1990 to 1999 for ice hockey, soccer, and football. *Clinical Journal of Sports Medicine, 14*(2), 80–87.

20. Terrell, T. R. (2004). Concussion in athletes. *Southern Medical Journal, 97*(9), 837–842.

21. Boss, B. J. (2002). Alterations of neurologic function. In K. L. McCance & S. E. Huether (Eds.), *Pathophysiology: The biologic basis for disease in adults & children* (4th ed., pp. 487–549). St. Louis, MO: Mosby.

22. Littlejohns, L. R., & Bader, M. K. (2001). Guidelines for the management of severe head injury: Clinical application and changes in practice. *Critical Care Nurse, 21*(6), 48–65.

23. Littlejohns, L. R., & Bader, M. K. (2005). Prevention of secondary brain injury: Targeting technology. *American Association of Critical Care Nurses Clinical Issues, 16*(4), 501–514.

24. Teasdale, G., & Jennent, B. (1974). Assessment of coma and impaired consciousness. *Lancet, 2,* 81–84.

25. Ross, S. E., Leipold, C., Terregino, C., & O'Malley, K. F. (1998). Efficacy of the motor component of the Glasgow Coma Scale in trauma triage. *Journal of Trauma, 45,* 42–44.

26. Robertson, C. S. (2001). Management of cerebral perfusion pressure after traumatic brain injury. *Anesthesiology, 95*(6), 1513–1517.

27. Bayir, H., Clark, R. S., & Kochanek, P. M. (2003). Promising strategies to minimize secondary brain injury after head trauma. *Critical Care Medicine, 31*(1), S112–S117.

28. Knapp, J. M. (2005). Hyperosmolar therapy in the treatment of severe head injury in children: Mannitol and hypertonic saline. *American Association of Critical Care Nurses Clinical Issues, 16*(2), 199–211.

29. Wakai, A., Roberts, I., & Schierhout, G. (2005). Mannitol for acute traumatic brain injury: The Cochrane collaboration. *The Cochrane Database of Systematic Reviews.* Hoboken, NJ: John Wiley and Sons.

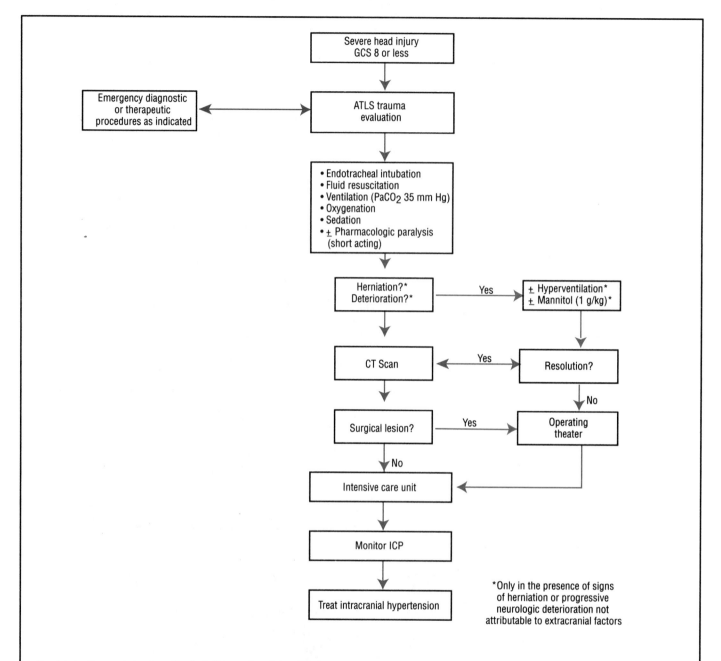

Reprinted with permission from The Brain Trauma Foundation. The American Association of Neurological Surgeons. The Joint Section on Neurotrauma and Critical Care. Initial management. (2000). Initial Management. *Journal of Neurotrauma*, 17, 465.

Original Source: Bullock, M. R., Chesnut, R. M., Clifton, G. L., Ghajar, J., Marion, D. W., Narayan, R. K. et al. (2000). Initial management. In Brain Trauma Foundation (Eds.), *Management and prognosis of traumatic brain injury.* (p. 26)

In addition to the nursing diagnoses outlined in Chapter 3, Initial Assessment, the following nursing diagnoses are potential problems for the patient with brain or cranial injuries or both. Once a patient has been assessed, diagnoses can be defined as either actual or risk. An actual nursing diagnosis is derived from a decision based on the patient's presenting signs and symptoms. A risk nursing diagnosis is a judgment that the nurse makes based on a particular patient's risk and potential for developing certain problems.

Nursing Diagnoses	Interventions	Expected Outcomes
Airway clearance, ineffective, related to: • Pain • Altered level of consciousness • Secretions and debris in airway • Soft tissue edema • Edema of the airway, vocal cords, epiglottis, and upper airway • Direct trauma • Presence of an artificial airway • Aspiration of foreign matter • Inhalation of toxic fumes or substances	• Stabilize cervical spine • Position patient • Open and clear airway • Insert oropharyngeal or nasopharyngeal airway • Avoid stimulation of gag reflex • Assist with early intubation	The patient will maintain a patent airway, as evidenced by: • Clear bilateral breath sounds • Regular rate, depth, and pattern of breathing • Effective cough • Absence of pain with coughing • Appropriate use of splinting techniques while coughing

Aspiration, risk, related to:
• Reduced level of consciousness secondary to injury, concomitant substance abuse
• Impaired cough and gag reflex
• Trauma to head, face, or neck
• Facial and/or neck soft tissue edema
• Secretions and debris in airway
• Increased intragastric pressure
• Impaired swallowing
	• Stabilize cervical spine
	• Position patient
	• Open and clear airway
	• Insert an oropharyngeal or nasopharyngeal airway
	• Avoid stimulation of gag reflex
	• Assist with early intubation
	• Insert an orogastric or nasogastric tube and evacuate stomach contents
		The patient will not experience aspiration, as evidenced by:
		• A patent airway
		• Clear and equal bilateral breath sounds
		• Regular rate, depth, and pattern of breathing
		• ABG values within normal limits:
		  ▪ PaO_2 80 to 100 mm Hg (10.0 to 13.3 KPa)
		  ▪ SaO_2 > 95%
		  ▪ $PaCO_2$ 35 to 45 mm Hg (4.7 to 6.0 KPa)
		  ▪ pH 7.35 to 7.45
		• Clear chest radiograph without evidence of infiltrates
		• Ability to handle secretions independently

Nursing Diagnoses	Interventions	Expected Outcomes
Gas exchange, Gas exchange, impaired, related to: • Deterioration of ventilatory efforts secondary to acute brain injury • Aspiration • Altered blood flow, oxygen-carrying capacity of the blood, oxygen supply • Ineffective airway clearance • Aspiration of foreign matter • Hypo- or hyperventilation • Inhalation of toxic fumes or substances	• Administer oxygen via nonrebreather mask • Ventilate, if needed, with 100% oxygen via a bag-mask device • Assist with early intubation • Monitor oxygen saturation with pulse oximeter • Administer blood, as indicated	The patient will experience adequate gas exchange, as evidenced by: • ABG values within normal limits: ▪ PaO$_2$ 80 to 100 mm Hg (10.0 to 13.3 KPa) ▪ SaO$_2$ > 95% ▪ PaCO$_2$ 35 to 45 mm Hg (4.7 to 6.0 KPa) ▪ pH 7.35 to 7.45 • SpO$_2$ 95% to 100% • Skin normal color, warm, and dry • Level of consciousness, awake and alert, age appropriate • Regular rate, depth, and pattern of breathing
Tissue perfusion, altered renal and cerebral, related to: • Cerebral edema, swelling, and expanding hematomas secondary to acute head injury • Decreased cerebral perfusion secondary to hypoxemia, hypercarbia, and hypotension • Hypovolemia	• Apply direct pressure to sites of active bleeding, except over depressed skull fractures • Cannulate two veins with large-caliber intravenous catheters and initiate infusion of isotonic crystalloid solution (flow rate to be determined by patient's hemodynamic status) • Position the patient as guided by institutional protocols (head midline) • Prepare for insertion of ICP monitoring device • Administer mannitol, as prescribed (not recommended for prophylactic use) • Hyperventilate only if signs of impending herniation • Obtain blood sample for ABGs, as indicated	The patient will have optimal cerebral tissue perfusion, as evidenced by: • GCS Score 14 to 15 (spontaneous eye opening, obeys verbal commands, oriented to person, place, and time) • Vital signs within normal limits for age: absence of vital sign abnormalities, including hypertension, bradycardia, respiratory irregularities or increase in pulse pressure • Normal pupil size, shape, and reactivity to light • Absence of signs and symptoms of increased intracranial pressure: headache, vomiting, lethargy, restlessness, change in orientation or consciousness • ABG values within normal limits: ▪ PaO$_2$ 80 to 100 mm Hg (10.0 to 13.3 KPa) ▪ SaO$_2$ > 95% ▪ PaCO$_2$ 35 to 45 mm Hg (4.7 to 6.0 KPa) ▪ pH 7.35 to 7.45 • Ability to maintain neck in proper neutral alignment • Absence of, or quickly controlled, seizure activity • Urine output 1ml/kg/hr

Nursing Diagnoses	Interventions	Expected Outcomes
Injury, risk, related to: • Increased intracranial pressure • Uncontrolled tonic/clonic movement • Altered sensorium secondary to head/facial injury • Visual field, motor, or perception deficits	• Administer anticonvulsant, as prescribed • Reorient patient as needed • Facilitate family presence	**The patient will be free from injury, as evidenced by:** • Patient will be seizure-free or seizures will be controlled rapidly once seizure activity evident • Absence of signs of injury such as bruises, broken teeth, or mucosal tears • Airway patency is maintained • Identifies safety measures to prevent injury • Requests assistance when needed
Hyperthermia, risk, related to: • Brain injury • Ambient temperature	• Administer antipyretic medication, as prescribed • Place hypothermia blanket, but avoid shivering • Keep ambient temperature of the room above 72 °F (22.4 °C)	**The patient will maintain a normal core body temperature, as evidenced by:** • Core temperature measurement of 98 to 99.5 °F (36 to 37.5 °C) • Skin normal color, warm, and dry
Infection, risk, related to: • Contamination of wounds from injury event or instrumentation • Prolonged immobility • Stress • Invasive procedures and devices	• Administer tetanus prophylaxis, as prescribed • Administer antibiotics, as prescribed • Assist with wound care • Maintain aseptic technique	**The patient will be free from infection, as evidenced by:** • Core temperature measurement of 98 to 99.5 °F (36 to 37.5 °C) • Absence of systemic signs of infection: fever, tachypnea, tachycardia • Wounds free from redness, swelling, purulent drainage, or odor • Urine output 1 ml/kg/hr • White blood cell count within normal limits • Level of consciousness, awake and alert, age appropriate

Chapter 7

Ocular, Maxillofacial, and Neck Trauma

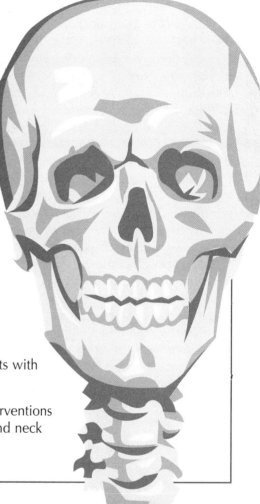

Objectives

On completion of this chapter/lecture, the learner should be able to:

1. Identify the common mechanisms of injury in ocular, maxillofacial, and neck trauma.

2. Describe the pathophysiologic changes as a basis for signs and symptoms of ocular, maxillofacial, and neck injuries.

3. Discuss the nursing assessment of the patient with ocular, maxillofacial, and neck injuries.

4. Plan appropriate interventions for patients with ocular, maxillofacial, and neck injuries.

5. Evaluate the effectiveness of nursing interventions for patients with ocular, maxillofacial, and neck injuries.

Preface

Lecture begins on page 119.

Knowledge of normal anatomy serves as the foundation for understanding the anatomic derangements and pathophysiologic compromises that may result from trauma. Before reading this chapter, it is strongly suggested that the learner read the following review material. Reading about the specific anatomic and physiologic concepts presented in this section will enhance the learner's ability to correlate such concepts with specific injuries. This material related to anatomy and physiology will not be covered during lectures, nor will it be evaluated by testing.

Globe

The globe (eyeball) is composed of three concentric layers. The outermost layer is formed by the sclera and cornea (**Figure 7-1**). The sclera is a white, opaque, fibrous coat that covers most of the globe. Its posterior portion is continuous with the outer sheath of the optic nerve[1,2] and is the attachment surface for the extraocular muscles and tendons responsible for normal movement of the globe in the orbit. The sclera's anterior portion is continuous with the cornea. The cornea is a multilayered, convex, transparent structure covering the anterior segment of the globe.[1] The circular margin where the cornea and sclera are contiguous is called the limbus. The outermost corneal layer, the anterior corneal epithelium, is continuous with the bulbar conjunctiva.

The uvea is the middle layer of the globe. It is composed of the iris, ciliary body, and choroid. The choroid is a thin, pigmented vascular sheath that underlies the optic portion of the retina. The innermost layer of the globe is the retina, which is continuous with the optic nerve (II) and lines the entire uveal layer of the globe.

The segments of the retina that line the ciliary body and the posterior aspect of the iris are not involved in visual perception.

Segments and Chambers

The eye is divided into the anterior and posterior segments. The posterior segment includes the retina, choroid, and vitreous humor. The vitreous humor is a transparent, colloidal gel. The anterior segment includes the cornea, iris, ciliary body, lens, and zonular fibers (suspensory ligaments of the lens). The anterior segment encloses the aqueous compartment and contains aqueous humor. The aqueous compartment is further subdivided (by the plane of the iris) into anterior and posterior chambers. The posterior chamber is bounded anteriorly by the posterior aspect of the iris, laterally by the ciliary body, and posteriorly by the lens and zonular fibers. The anterior chamber is bounded anteriorly by the endothelial layer (posterior aspect) of the cornea and posteriorly by the anterior aspect of the iris. Aqueous humor is secreted continuously by special cells in the ciliary body (i.e., in the posterior chamber of the aqueous compartment). The aqueous humor flows through the pupil and drains from the angle of the anterior chamber. The angle of the anterior chamber is the junction of the posterior surface of the cornea and outer margin of the iris.[3] Obstruction of the drainage of aqueous humor at this junction leads to an increase in intraocular pressure known as narrow-angle, or angle-closure, glaucoma.

Lens and Pupil

The lens is a transparent disc. The function of the lens is to "accommodate," or make adjustments for, viewing near objects and objects at a distance. The lens must be highly elastic so that its shape can be changed to more or less convex. It refracts and focuses light on the optic retina. The lens is supported by circumferentially radiating ligamentous fibers that attach to the ciliary body. Contractions of the muscles of the ciliary body alter how light is focused on the retina by altering the thickness of the lens. The pupil is not a structure; it is the aperture in the center of the iris. The pupillary sphincter muscle is a muscular ring in the iris that constricts the pupil in response to parasympathetic stimulation.[1] Pupil dilation occurs with sympathetic stimulation.

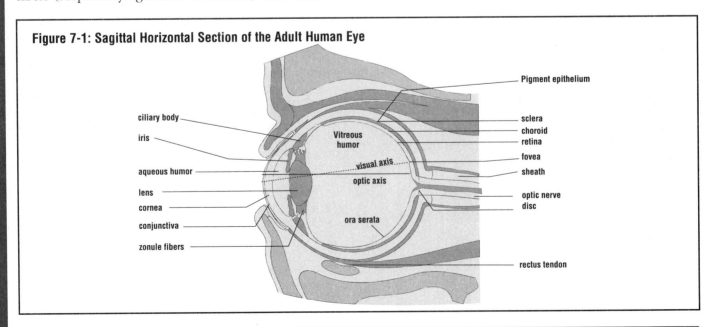

Figure 7-1: Sagittal Horizontal Section of the Adult Human Eye

ciliary body
iris
aqueous humor
lens
cornea
conjunctiva
zonule fibers

Vitreous humor
visual axis
optic axis
ora serata

Pigment epithelium
sclera
choroid
retina
fovea
sheath
optic nerve
disc

rectus tendon

Eyelids

The anterior surface of the globe is protected by the eyelids (palpebra). Each lid contains a tarsal plate and a band of cartilaginous connective tissue that gives the lids their shape. The eyelids have a rich blood supply and can accommodate significant edema or hematoma when injured. The palpebral conjunctiva lines the eyelids and is continuous with the bulbar conjunctiva of each eye. The conjunctiva is a vascularized, transparent membrane that takes on the color of the underlying tissue. Therefore, the palpebral conjunctiva appears to be pink and the bulbar conjunctiva white. The conjunctiva serves as a protective barrier to the surface of the globe and tarsal surface of the eyelids. Either or both conjunctival surfaces may be injured or inflamed, causing bloodshot eyes or subconjunctival hemorrhage. Conjunctival edema (chemosis) frequently accompanies eye injuries. The eyelashes (cilia) have a protective function in helping to screen the globe from small foreign bodies.

Lacrimal Glands

The lacrimal glands are in the upper lid, near the lateral canthus. Tears drain from the medial canthal region, via the small openings (puncta) of the canaliculi (lacrimal ducts). Therefore, injury to either canthal region may disrupt normal lacrimal lubrication.

Face

The face is divided into functional thirds. The upper third includes the lower portion of the frontal bone, supraorbital ridge, nasal glabellar region, and frontal sinuses. The middle third (midface) includes the orbits, maxillary sinuses, nasal bone, zygomatic bones, temporal bones, and basal bone of the maxilla. The basal bone of the mandible and the teeth-bearing bones of the maxilla and mandible compose the lower third of the face. The facial muscles covering the bones are responsible for facial movements. Mandibular muscles assist with the opening and closing of the jaw and mastication (**Figure 7-2**).

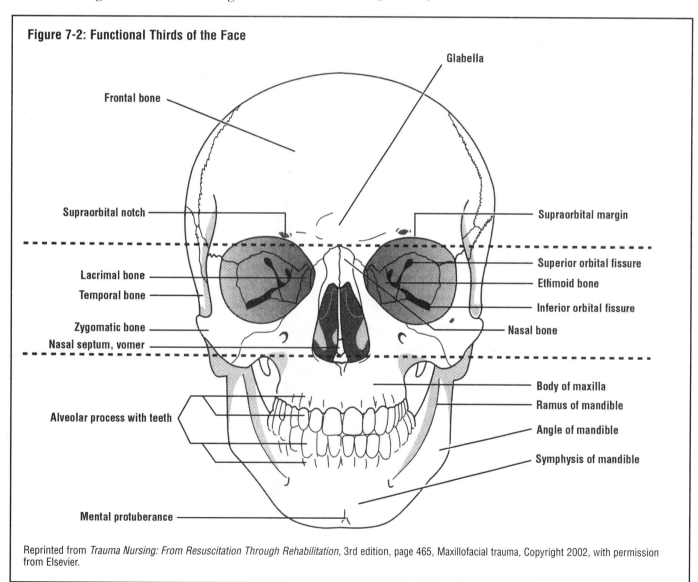

Figure 7-2: Functional Thirds of the Face

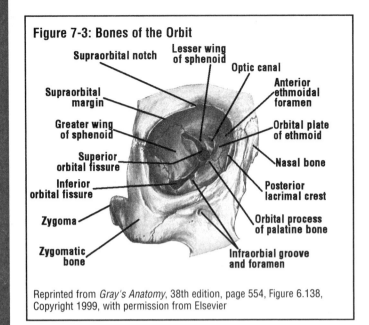

Figure 7-3: Bones of the Orbit

Supraorbital notch
Lesser wing of sphenoid
Optic canal
Supraorbital margin
Anterior ethmoidal foramen
Greater wing of sphenoid
Orbital plate of ethmoid
Superior orbital fissure
Nasal bone
Inferior orbital fissure
Posterior lacrimal crest
Zygoma
Orbital process of palatine bone
Zygomatic bone
Infraorbial groove and foramen

Reprinted from *Gray's Anatomy*, 38th edition, page 554, Figure 6.138, Copyright 1999, with permission from Elsevier

Orbit

The orbit, which is a bony socket formed by the junction of seven facial bones, protects the globe (Figure 7-3). The orbital rim is formed by the zygoma (laterally), maxilla (inferiorly and medially), and the frontal bone (superiorly). The orbital surfaces of these three bones form, respectively, parts of the lateral wall, floor, and ceiling of the orbit. The more posterior surfaces of the orbit are formed by portions of the sphenoid, ethmoid, and lacrimal bones and the orbital process of the palatine bone.

Neck

The neck contains a large concentration of anatomic structures relative to its size. The structures contained within the neck are the airway, common and internal carotid arteries, internal and external jugular veins, vertebral arteries, vagus nerves, thoracic

Figure 7-4: Vascular Supply to the Brain and Brain Stem

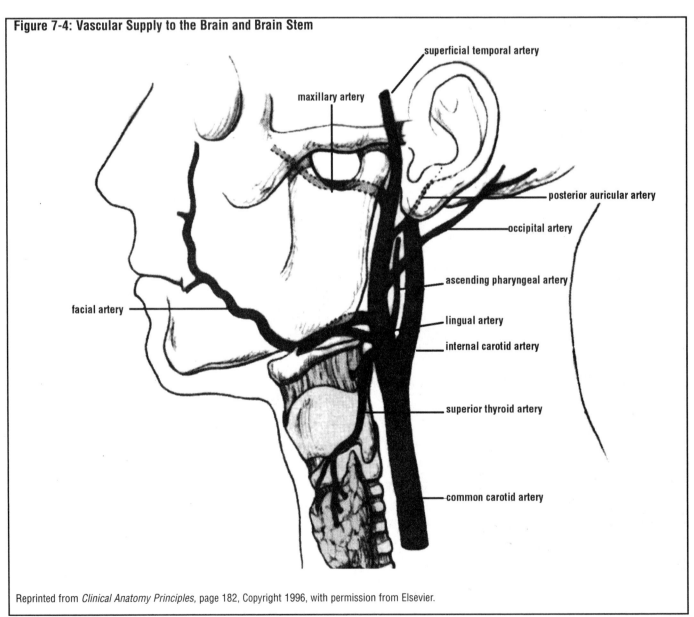

superficial temporal artery
maxillary artery
posterior auricular artery
occipital artery
ascending pharyngeal artery
facial artery
lingual artery
internal carotid artery
superior thyroid artery
common carotid artery

Reprinted from *Clinical Anatomy Principles*, page 182, Copyright 1996, with permission from Elsevier.

duct, trachea, pharynx, esophagus, spinal cord, cervical vertebral column, thyroid gland, parathyroid glands, lower cranial nerves, brachial plexus, muscle, and soft tissue.

The neck is commonly divided into three anatomic regions referred to as zones. The zones are based on bony and superficial landmarks. They are important in defining the potential structures injured, the diagnostic evaluation needed, and the surgical management approach. Zone I extends from the sternal notch and clavicle to the cricothyroid cartilage. Zone II extends upward to the angle of the mandible. Zone III extends from the angle of the mandible to the base of the skull.

Two fascial layers enclose the structures within the neck. The superficial fascia encompasses the platysma muscle, and the deep cervical fascia supports the muscles, vessels, and organs of the neck. The compartments formed by the fascia limit external bleeding, but bleeding within the closed spaces may compromise the airway with hematoma formation. The platysma muscle protects the underlying struc-

tures within the neck. If the platysma has been damaged, underlying injury may be suspected.

The vascular supply for the brain and brain stem (**Figure 7-4**) arises from the vertebral arteries and the internal carotids. Abrupt interruption in the blood flow through these structures will result in cerebral hypoxia and neurologic deficits.

The brachial plexus is a network of nerve fibers that incorporates the nerve roots of C-5 through T-1. These nerves subdivide to form the axillary, musculocutaneous, median, ulnar, and radial nerves. These nerves are responsible for arm and hand function (**Figure 7-5**).

Cranial Nerves

Certain cranial nerves are of particular importance in ocular, maxillofacial, and neck trauma (**Table 7-1**). Injuries to the eye and face may affect cranial nerves II to VII. Injuries to the neck may affect cranial nerves IX to XI.[4] Any of the cranial nerve functions can be altered by injury.

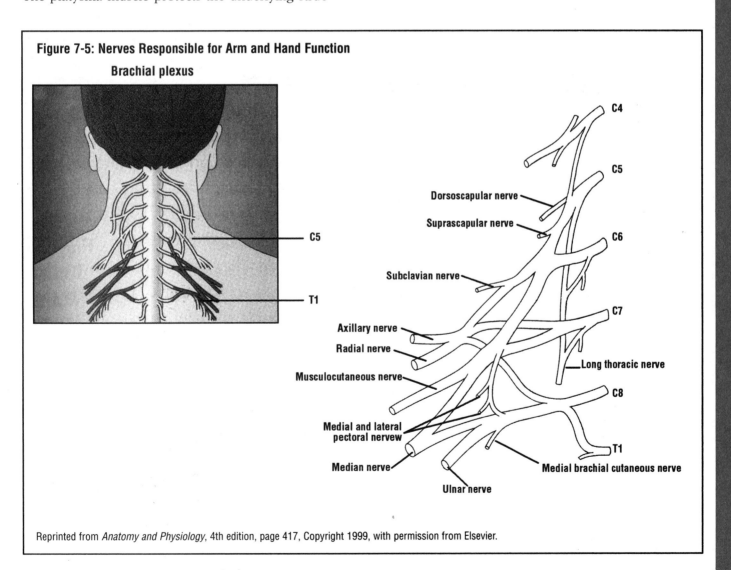

Figure 7-5: Nerves Responsible for Arm and Hand Function

Brachial plexus

Reprinted from *Anatomy and Physiology*, 4th edition, page 417, Copyright 1999, with permission from Elsevier.

Table 7-1: Results of Injury to Cranial Nerves

Cranial Nerve	Function	Results of Injury
Optic (II)	• Vision	• Visual loss • Alteration in visual fields
Oculomotor (III)	• Movement of the eyelid and eyeball • Dilation and constriction of the pupil	• Ptosis • Alteration in size, shape, and equality of pupil
Trochlear (IV)	• Movement of eyeball	• Double vision • Outward rotation of affected eye • Difficulty with downward gaze
Trigeminal (V)	• Chewing • Sensation face, upper teeth, gums, lip, and jaw	• Inability to open or close mouth • Misalignment of teeth • Numbness or pain of face, teeth, gums, lip, and jaw
Abducens (VI)	• Movement of eyeball	• Medially directed eye • Strabismus • Double vision
Facial (VII)	• Facial expression • Sensation to ear and tympanic membrane • Taste anterior tongue	• Facial asymmetry • Inability to close eye • Uncontrolled tearing • Drooling
Glossopharyngeal (IX)	• Sensation and taste posterior tongue • Swallowing • Muscle movement for speech	• Difficulty swallowing or speaking
Vagus (X)	• Muscle movement and sensory of pharynx and larynx • Parasympathetic nerve	• Hoarseness • Difficulty swallowing • Bradycardia
Spinal Accessory (XI)	• Movement of trapezius and sternocleidomastoid muscles	• Shoulder drooping • Difficulty turning head against resistance

Introduction

Epidemiology

In the United States in 2001, nearly 2 million individuals experienced an eye injury which required treatment in an emergency department (50.7%), private physician's office (38.7%), or outpatient (8.1%) and inpatient (2.5%) facilities. Eye injury rates were highest among individuals in their 20s, particularly for males and whites. Injury rates were highest for superficial injuries, foreign bodies, contusions, and open wounds.[5] Intraorbital foreign bodies are a relatively uncommon occurrence.[6] However, the military databases of combat casualties reveal many intraocular foreign bodies and an alarming increase in the incidence of all eye injuries.[7]

Maxillofacial injuries occur primarily in males aged 0 to 41 years, as a result of motor vehicle collisions and assaults, with the largest number of fractures occurring in the bones of the mandible and orbits.[8-11] Between 14% and 50% of all facial fractures involve the nose,[12-14] and between 5% and 30% involve the frontal sinus.[15] In the pediatric population, injuries during sports or play are the leading causes of orbital fractures in both boys and girls.[16] The use of seat belts and air bags has significantly decreased the incidence of maxillofacial fractures in motor vehicle crashes.[17,18] Blunt tracheobronchial, vertebral artery, and carotid artery injuries are rare.[19-21]

Penetrating injuries to the neck have been a significant cause of injury and death for centuries. In the United States, personal assaults from firearms and stabbings are the most common cause. Most cases of penetrating neck trauma in children, such as falls on sharp objects or motor vehicle crashes, are unintentional.[22]

Mechanism of Injury

Blunt or penetrating trauma, blast injuries, or chemical, thermal, and ultraviolet (actinic) radiation can all result in injury to the eyes, face, or neck. Blunt trauma occurs as a result of falls, motor vehicle crashes, assaults, and sports and recreational activities. Penetrating injuries are most commonly caused by guns, knives, fireworks, broken glass, shrapnel from bombs or blast injuries, and metal shards from machines or tools in the workplace. Blast forces can result in both blunt and penetrating injuries.

Chemicals may cause ocular injuries ranging from minor (superficial inflammation) to severe (permanent blindness). Caustic chemicals (i.e., strong acids and bases) are the most devastating. For further discussion of burns, refer to Chapter 12, Surface and Burn Trauma.

Usual Concurrent Injuries

Ocular, maxillofacial, and neck trauma may be an isolated injury or may be associated with head, cervical spine, or upper thoracic injuries. Therefore, **all** patients with a facial injury should be assessed for cervical spine injury. Intraocular hemorrhage is a common finding in pediatric head trauma patients with shaken baby syndrome. Intracranial injury, basal skull fractures, or both may accompany severe facial trauma. Brain injury may occur directly, because of comminuted fragments of orbital fractures, or indirectly, because of acceleration or deceleration forces. Optic nerve injury may occur with an anterior fossa basilar skull fracture. Injury to structures of the neck may occlude the airway, interrupt vascular flow to the brain, or cause cervical spine or spinal cord injury.

Pathophysiology as a Basis for Signs and Symptoms

Trauma to the ocular, maxillofacial, and neck areas may result in primary injuries such as fractures. Secondary injuries (which may occur as a result of primary injuries) include airway obstruction, hemorrhage, and neurologic deficits.

Airway Obstruction Causing Ineffective Ventilation

Trauma to the face or neck may compromise or occlude the airway. Facial injuries may cause edema of the oropharynx or nasopharynx and the entry of blood, vomit, unsupported soft tissue, bone, and teeth into the airway. Edema and hematomas from disrupted blood vessels following a neck injury can narrow or occlude the trachea. Tears or lacerations in the tracheobronchial tree may interrupt the integrity of the lower airway. Patients with these injuries manifest dramatic symptoms early in the resuscitative process as a result of massive air leaks into the subcutaneous tissue.

Bleeding

Facial injuries bleed profusely because of their highly vascular nature and lack of blood vessel retraction. This bleeding is usually venous, but insult to the temporal artery can occur, causing an arterial bleed. Disruption of nasal bones can result in active bleeding and epistaxis. There can be enough blood loss from maxillofacial injuries to result in hypovolemic shock, particularly when the patient has concurrent blood loss from fractured long bones or the pelvis or intra-abdominal injuries.[23] Penetrating traumatic injuries to certain vascular structures in the neck (carotid arteries or vertebral, brachiocephalic, and jugular veins) can cause rapid exsanguination. Carotid injuries may include tears that may progress to ischemia or a cerebrovascular accident on the ipsilateral side of the brain.

Neurologic Deficits

Injuries to cranial nerves in the ocular, face, and neck region may cause facial paresthesias, facial motor deficits, alteration in pupillary light responses, alteration in extraocular muscle movements, visual or olfactory disturbances, or spinal cord or brachial plexus injuries impairing motor or sensory function. Injury to carotid or vertebral arteries may also produce cerebral ischemia or cerebral infarction, resulting in cognitive, motor, or sensory impairment.[24]

Signs of Serious Eye Injury

Severe eye injury may occur concomitantly with periorbital or midface fractures. Signs include sudden decrease in vision, loss of field of vision, photophobia, diplopia, and abnormal pupillary reaction. Other signs include visual acuity of greater than 20/40 (corrected) and head injury resulting in amnesia.

Visual Disturbances

Loss of vision may occur as a result of direct injury to the globe or by the application of acceleration or deceleration forces to the eye region or to the brain. Causes of immediate or early-onset blindness include

- Posterior segment (vitreous) hemorrhage
- Prolapse or extrusion of globe contents
- A large intraocular foreign body
- Optic nerve laceration or avulsion
- Intracerebral hemorrhage, particularly in the occipital lobe

Causes of late-onset blindness or diminished acuity include

- Retinal detachment
- Hemorrhage
- Cataract formation
- Glaucoma associated with a hyphema

Blurred vision may result from injuries to the lens or posterior segment or from tearing or photophobia associated with a more superficial injury. Diplopia can be unilateral or bilateral. Unilateral diplopia may result from subluxation of the lens, orbital edema or hematoma, macular edema, or injury to the extraocular muscles. Bilateral diplopia may result from orbital fractures with extraocular muscle entrapment or from direct injury to the extraocular muscles or cranial nerves III, IV, or VI.

Pain

Eye pain varies depending on the depth of injury. Corneal injuries tend to be associated with intense, sharp, burning, or searing pain. Corneal foreign bodies are immediately painful and provoke considerable tearing.[25] Pain from the uveal structures, as in iritis or hyphema, is a deep aching or boring pain and may be accompanied by profuse tearing. Photophobia is a painful response to bright light. Photophobia may represent pain from a corneal injury, ciliary spasm, or posterior segment injury.[26]

Redness and Ecchymosis of the Eye

Many eye injuries are associated with different patterns of redness, from corneal or conjunctival inflammation or injury to uveal inflammation or deeper injury. The redness from a superficial foreign body tends to be diffuse, but with localized intensity in the area of the foreign body or resulting abrasion(s). Redness from actinic or noncorrosive chemical injury is very diffuse. Redness from subconjunctival hemorrhage is bright to deep red and opaque, and it may range from being localized to obscuring most of the sclera. Despite its appearance, the subconjunctival hemorrhage does not threaten the patient's vision, although it may exist concomitantly with other more serious injuries.

Periorbital Ecchymosis

Periorbital ecchymosis, or "black eye," is an accumulation of blood in the eyelids. Facial injuries (e.g., nasal fractures) may lead to unilateral periorbital ecchymosis. Bilateral periorbital ecchymosis may be seen with maxillofacial injuries or basal skull fracture.

Increased Intraocular Pressure

The eye is filled with intraocular fluid, which maintains sufficient pressure in the eyeball to keep it distended. The average normal intraocular pressure is about 15 mm Hg, with a range of 10 to 22 mm Hg. Patients with high intraocular pressure (> 30 mm Hg) may have glaucoma or retrobulbar hemorrhage. Urgent treatment is needed to lower elevated pressures and prevent permanent loss of vision caused by optic nerve damage. Patients with low (< 10 mm Hg) pressures may have a perforated globe or severe intraocular trauma and may require immediate evaluation by an ophthalmologist.[27]

Hyphema

Hyphema is an accumulation of blood, mainly red blood cells that disperse and layer within the anterior chamber.[28] It is generally caused by a direct blow to the globe. Initially blunt trauma indents and stretches the globe, which ultimately causes tearing and disruption of the well-vascularized ciliary body and iris. The degree of visual impairment that results from a hyphema is proportional to the degree of hemorrhage. A severe hyphema obscures the entire anterior chamber (eight-ball hemorrhage) and will diminish visual acuity severely or completely. Hyphema injuries are graded on the amount of blood in the anterior chamber (Table 7-2). Increased intraocular pressures may occur with hyphemas of any size. Outpatient management for patients with hyphemas should be considered only if the patient is compliant, does not have any blood dyscrasias or bleeding diathesis, has less than a grade 2+ hyphema, and has an intraocular pressure less than or equal to 35 mm Hg.[25]

Signs and Symptoms

- Blood in the anterior chamber
- Deep, aching pain
- Mild to severe diminished visual acuity
- Increased intraocular pressure

Chemical Burns to the Eye

Chemical injuries require immediate intervention if sight is to be preserved. Alkali combines with lipids in the cell membrane, disrupting the membrane and allowing rapid penetration of the caustic agent and extensive tissue destruction. Acids precipitate protein in the tissue, limiting extensive tissue penetration and causing corneal injury. For a more detailed discussion on chemical injuries, refer to Chapter 12, Surface and Burn Trauma.

Signs and Symptoms

- Pain
- Corneal opacification
- Coexisting chemical burn and swelling of lids

Penetrating Trauma/Open or Ruptured Globe

Penetrating ocular injury may result from projectiles, missiles, foreign bodies, impalement, or stab wounds and may leave foreign bodies in the eye. Intraocular foreign bodies may not be immediately obvious. The entry wound to the globe may be occult or very small. Suspect a globe injury if an eye-injured patient presents with substantial, acute, unilateral reduction in visual acuity.

An open globe injury also may result from forces that cause a sudden rise in intraocular pressure. Acceleration and deceleration of ocular tissues can lead to rupture, especially where the globe is fragile. Fragments from orbital fractures may lead to lacerations of the globe, extraocular muscles, or nerves or vascular structures. On occasion, severe orbital fractures may communicate with the anterior cranial fossa, giving rise to direct brain injury, internal carotid injury, or intracranial infection. Globe rupture is a serious ocular emergency and must always be considered when evaluating the condition of a patient who has sustained blunt trauma or lacerating injury to the head, face, or eye.[25] Rupture as a result of blunt trauma has a poor prognosis.

Signs and Symptoms

- Marked visual impairment
- Extrusion of intraocular contents
- Flattened or shallow anterior chamber
- Subconjunctival hemorrhage, hyphema
- Decreased intraocular pressure
- Restriction of extraocular movements

Orbital Fracture (Orbital Blowout Fracture)

The orbit is composed of multiple bones including the frontal bone, zygoma, maxilla, sphenoid, and ethmoid bones. An orbital blowout fracture is almost always secondary to a blunt blow from a relatively large object, such as a fist, elbow, or baseball bat.[29] With impact to the orbit, there is an increase in intra-orbital pressure, and energy is dissipated through the area of least resistance, usually the medial wall or orbital floor. Entrapment of cranial nerves and muscles may produce the signs associated with this injury. Visual disturbances may result from hematoma formation, from compression on the globe, optic nerve, or retinal artery, or all of these.

Table 7-2: Classification of Hyphemas

Grade	Classification
Grade I	Less than one-third filling of the anterior chamber
Grade II	One-third to one-half filling of the anterior chamber
Grade III	One-half to near total filling of the anterior chamber
Grade IV	Complete, total hyphema ("eight-ball")

Signs and Symptoms

- Diplopia (double vision)
- Loss of vision
- Altered extraocular eye movements
- Enophthalmos (displacement of the eye backward into the socket)
- Subconjunctival hemorrhage or ecchymosis of the eyelid
- Infraorbital pain or loss of sensation
- Orbital bony deformity

Maxillary Fracture

Maxillary fractures are commonly classified according to the LeFort classification system (**Figure 7-6**).

LeFort I Fractures

A LeFort I fracture is a transverse maxillary fracture that occurs above the level of the teeth and results in a separation of the teeth from the rest of the maxilla.

Signs and Symptoms

- Slight swelling of the maxillary area
- Possible lip lacerations or fractured teeth
- Independent movement of the maxilla from the rest of the face
- Malocclusion

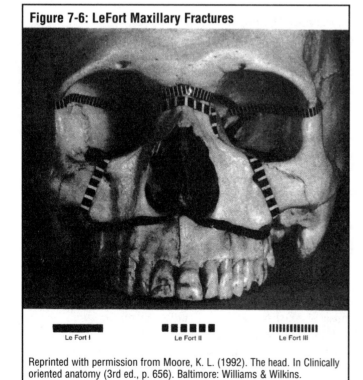

Figure 7-6: LeFort Maxillary Fractures

Le Fort I   Le Fort II   Le Fort III

Reprinted with permission from Moore, K. L. (1992). The head. In Clinically oriented anatomy (3rd ed., p. 656). Baltimore: Williams & Wilkins.

LeFort II Fractures

A LeFort II fracture is a pyramidal maxillary fracture involving the middle facial area. The apex of the fracture transverses the bridge of the nose. The two lateral fractures of the pyramid extend through the lacrimal bone of the face and ethmoid bone of the skull into the median portion of both orbits. The base of the fracture extends above the level of the upper teeth into the maxilla. A cerebrospinal fluid leak is possible.

Signs and Symptoms

- Massive facial edema
- Nasal swelling with obvious fracture of nasal bones
- Malocclusion
- Cerebrospinal fluid rhinorrhea

LeFort III Fractures

A LeFort III fracture is a complete craniofacial separation involving the maxilla, zygoma, orbits, and bones of the cranial base. This fracture is frequently associated with leakage of cerebrospinal fluid and a fractured mandible.

Signs and Symptoms

- Massive facial edema
- Mobility and depression of zygomatic bones
- Ecchymosis
- Anesthesia of the cheek
- Diplopia
- Open bite or malocclusion
- Cerebrospinal fluid rhinorrhea

Mandibular Fracture

The mandible, or lower jaw, is a horseshoe-shaped bone attached to the cranium at the temporomandibular joints. The common fracture sites are the canine and third molar tooth area, the angle of the mandible, and the condyles.

Signs and Symptoms

- Malocclusion
- Inability to open the mouth (trismus)
- Pain, especially on movement
- Facial asymmetry and a palpable step-off deformity
- Edema or hematoma formation at the fracture site
- Blood behind, or ruptured, tympanic membrane
- Anesthesia of the lower lip

Neck Injury

Neck trauma may result in injuries to airway structures (trachea or larynx), blood vessels (subclavian, jugular, carotid, and vertebrals), esophagus, endocrine structures (thyroid and parathyroid gland), thoracic duct, and brachial plexus.

Blunt ruptures or tears of the lower trachea, mainstem bronchus, neck vessels, or esophagus may be caused by such mechanisms of injury as striking the dashboard or steering wheel, karate-type blows, or "clothesline-type" injuries.

The evaluation and treatment of blunt neck injuries includes an evaluation of the integrity of the cervical vertebrae and the spinal cord. Penetrating injuries to the neck have the potential for injuring several organ systems. Wounds that extend through the platysma should not be explored manually or probed with instruments in the emergency department.[24]

Signs and Symptoms

- Dyspnea, tachypnea
- Hemoptysis (coughing up blood)
- Subcutaneous emphysema in the neck, face, or suprasternal area
- Decreased or absent breath sounds
- Penetrating wounds or impaled objects
- Pulsatile or expanding hematoma
- Loss of normal anatomic prominence of the laryngeal region
- Bruits
- Active external bleeding
- Neurologic deficit, such as aphasia or hemiplegia
- Cranial nerve deficits
- Facial sensory or motor nerve deficits
- Dysphonia (hoarseness)
- Dysphagia (difficulty swallowing)

Nursing Care of the Patient with Ocular, Maxillofacial, and Neck Trauma

Assessment

History

Refer to Chapter 3, Initial Assessment, for a description of general information that should be collected regarding every trauma patient. Only pertinent questions specific to patients with ocular, maxillofacial, and neck injuries are described following.

- What was the mechanism of injury?
- Was there major acceleration or deceleration injury?
- Was the injury caused by a missile, shrapnel, or foreign body? Was the projectile metal, wood, glass, plastic, or mineral? Was the velocity of the projectile such that intraocular penetration might have occurred? Is there a periorbital entry wound with no obvious exit? Is a foreign body still present, either superficially or intraocularly?
- Was the patient restrained? Did the air bag deploy? Was the helmet on? Was protective eyewear used?
- What are the patient's complaints?
  - Dyspnea (difficulty breathing)
  - Dysphagia (difficulty swallowing)
  - Dysphonia (hoarseness)
  - Numbness or tingling
  - Diminished visual acuity
  - Blurred or double vision in one or both eyes
  - Photophobia
  - Blepharospasm (prolonged, uncontrolled eye blinking)
  - Pain
- Does the patient normally wear glasses or contact lenses? Was the patient wearing them at the time of injury? If the patient was wearing glasses, did they shatter? If the patient wears contact lenses, what type are they, and are they still in place?
- Does the patient have a history of eye problems or prior eye injuries?
- Has the patient ever had eye surgery such as cataract surgery, lens implants, or corneal surgery?
- Does the patient have visual or ocular changes associated with a chronic illness (e.g., hypertension, congestive heart failure, diabetes mellitus, or glaucoma)?

Physical Assessment

Refer to Chapter 3, Initial Assessment, for a description of the assessment of the patient's airway, breathing, circulation, and disability.

Because of the potential for permanent impairment, and the consequences in terms of self-concept, work, and functional disability, eye, facial, and neck injuries have a high priority for intervention. In terms of triage, life-threatening injuries must be addressed initially. Once these issues are resolved, care of the serious eye injury takes priority over everything except life- or limb-threatening injuries. Deferred assessment of a badly swollen eye or failure to remove contact lenses can lead to serious eye injury and can contribute to serious, permanent impairment.

Inspection

- Inspect the eye, periorbital tissues, facial architecture, and neck.
- Observe for symmetry, edema, ecchymosis, ptosis, lacerations, and hematomas.
  - Periorbital ecchymosis (raccoon eyes) may indicate an anterior fossa fracture.
  - Mastoid process ecchymosis (Battle's sign) may indicate a posterior fossa fracture.
  - It is important to note that ecchymotic signs may take hours to develop and may not be visible on initial presentation.
- Inspect the globe for lacerations, large corneal abrasions, hyphema, and extrusion or prolapse of intraocular contents.
- Determine whether a lid laceration transects the lid margin or involves the lateral or medial canthus.
- Assess pupils for size, shape (roundness), equality, and reactivity to light.
  - A unilaterally fixed and dilated pupil may indicate oculomotor nerve compression as a result of increased intracranial pressure and herniation syndrome.
  - Bilateral fixed and pinpoint pupils may indicate pontine lesion or effects of drugs.
  - A mildly dilated pupil with sluggish response may be an early sign of herniation syndrome.
  - A widely dilated pupil occasionally occurs with direct trauma to the globe of the eye.
- Assess for consensual response.
- Assess for redness, eye watering, and blepharospasm.
- Assess for extraocular eye movements, except when an open globe injury is known or suspected.
  - Limitation in range of ocular motion may indicate an orbital rim fracture with entrapment or paralysis of a cranial nerve or ocular muscle.
- Perform a visual acuity examination.
  - Use a Snellen or handheld eye chart. Assess the uninjured eye first. Note visual acuity in each eye separately and then in both eyes together. If the patient has corrective lenses and can wear them, it is best to measure visual acuity as corrected. If the patient is unable to participate in the examination because of the extent of injury, developmental stage, cognitive

impairment, or intoxication, an assessment of finger-counting, hand-motion, and light perception should still be attempted.[3]

- Assess for blurred or double vision in the injured eye with the uninjured eye closed. Then, test with both eyes open.
- Inspect for rhinorrhea or otorrhea.
  - If drainage is present, it may indicate a cerebrospinal fluid leak.
- Observe for impaled objects.
- Assess occlusion of the mandible and maxilla.
  - Malocclusion or an inability to open and close the mouth is highly indicative of a maxillary or mandibular fracture.
- Observe for uncontrolled bleeding

Palpation

- Palpate the periorbital area, face, and neck for:
  - Tenderness
  - Edema
  - Step-off defects or depressions
  - Subcutaneous emphysema (esophageal or tracheobronchial tear)
- Palpate the trachea above the suprasternal notch.
  - Tracheal deviation may be a late indication of tension pneumothorax or massive hemothorax.
- Assess sensory function of the periorbital areas, face, and neck.
  - Facial fractures can impinge on the infraorbital nerve, causing numbness of the inferior eyelid, lateral nose, cheek, or upper lip on the affected side.
- Check the position of the trachea.

Diagnostic Procedures

Refer to Chapter 3, Initial Assessment, for frequently ordered radiographic and laboratory studies. Additional studies for ocular, maxillofacial, and neck trauma patients are listed following.

Radiographic Studies

- Eye radiographs to identify intraocular foreign bodies
- Computed tomography scan (CT) of head and face
- Magnetic resonance imaging (MRI) to ascertain the presence of wood or vegetable foreign bodies
- CT angiography or intravenous (IV) angiography if vascular injury is suspected

Other Diagnostic Studies

- Fluorescein staining

  Fluorescein staining and examination under cobalt blue lamp (Wood's light) or slit-lamp is conducted to identify surface defects (e.g., corneal abrasions, small conjunctival tears). The abraded areas absorb more dye and appear as punctate or larger areas of increased dye (green) intensity under fluorescent illumination. Single-use fluorescein strips should be stocked. Fluorescein drops are associated with increased infection rates.

- Slit-lamp examination

  Slit-lamp examination is used to identify a hyphema, or injury and inflammation of the cornea or anterior chamber. Removal of embedded corneal foreign bodies is generally performed under direct visualization with a slit-lamp.

- Tonometry (measures intraocular pressure)

- Bronchoscopy or esophagoscopy

Planning and Implementation

Refer to Chapter 3, Initial Assessment, for a description of the specific nursing interventions for patients with compromises to airway, breathing, circulation, and disability.

Nursing Interventions for the Patient with an Ocular Injury

Begin immediate copious, continuous irrigation with isotonic crystalloid solution for all chemical injuries. Do not attempt to neutralize the causative agent.

- Assess visual acuity as indicated; reassess at discharge, transfer, or admission.
- Elevate the head of the bed to minimize increases in intraocular pressure. If elevation is contraindicated, position the entire stretcher so that the patient's head is higher than the feet.
- Instruct the patient not to bend forward, cough, or perform a Valsalva maneuver because these actions may raise intraocular pressure.
- Assist with removal of foreign bodies as indicated; stabilize impaled objects.
- Apply cool packs to decrease pain and periorbital swelling, as indicated.
- Administer medications, as prescribed.
  - Instill prescribed topical anesthetic drops (ophthalmic tetracaine, proparacaine) for pain

control and to facilitate eye examination except in open globe injuries.

  - Instill normal saline drops or artificial tears to keep the corneas moist, as indicated. Use a solution without preservatives. Cover the eyelids with a sterile, moist saline dressing to prevent corneal drying and ulceration.
  - Antibiotics may be administered topically or systemically.
  - Administer tetanus prophylaxis, as prescribed.
- Use an eye patch to the affected eye, as prescribed.
  - Patch or shield both eyes to reduce movement and photophobia in patients with retinal injuries.
  - Patch, shield, or cover with a cool pack any injured eye that has been anesthetized, to protect it from further injury.
  - Do not patch the injured eye of a patient with a suspected open or ruptured globe. Patch the unaffected eye. Use a metal or plastic eye shield. Do not put pressure on the globe.
- Stabilize any impaled objects without placing pressure on the globe, and then patch the unaffected eye of a patient with an impaled object.
- Provide psychosocial support.
- Obtain an ophthalmology consultation.
- Provide discharge instructions:
  - Discuss the importance of protective eyewear.
  - Instruct the patient not to drive while wearing eye patches.
  - Advise the patient to wear sunglasses to reduce photophobia and tearing, especially if eye patches are not indicated or pupil-dilating medications have been instilled.
- Prepare for hospital admission, operative intervention, or transfer, as indicated.

Nursing Interventions for the Patient with a Maxillofacial or Neck Injury

- Administer oxygen via a nonrebreather mask at a flow rate sufficient to keep the reservoir bag inflated; this usually requires 12 to 15 liters/minute.
- For facial trauma, place the patient in a high-Fowler's position if no spinal injury is present. Conscious patients instinctively seek their optimal position for airway maintenance. If at all possible, do not force a patient with severe facial trauma into a supine, flat position. Monitor for the development of airway obstruction. Placing the patient

in a high-Fowler's position may also decrease facial edema.

- Insert an orogastric or nasogastric tube. An orogastric tube should be inserted if a basilar skull fracture or severe midface fractures are suspected.
- Monitor for progressive airway edema.
  - Prepare for endotracheal intubation, if necessary. Copious bleeding or secretions uncontrolled by suction may necessitate intubation to establish a patent airway. If intubation is unsuccessful, anticipate the need for a surgical airway.
- Cannulate two veins with large-caliber catheters and initiate infusions of an isotonic crystalloid solution.
- Control external bleeding with direct pressure.
- Monitor for continued bleeding and expanding hematomas.
- Apply cold compresses to the face to minimize edema.
- Assist with repair of oral lacerations, as indicated.
- Administer antibiotics, as prescribed. Patients with open or penetrating wounds of the face or sinus or oral areas may be given prophylactic antibiotics.
- Stabilize impaled objects.
- Administer analgesic medication, as prescribed.

Evaluation and Ongoing Assessment

Refer to Chapter 3, Initial Assessment, for a description of the ongoing evaluation of the patient's airway, breathing, circulation, and disability. Additional evaluations include the following.

- Reassessing visual acuity at reasonable intervals
- Reassessing pain, including the response to non-pharmacologic and pharmacologic interventions
- Monitoring the appearance, position, and movements of the globe, and pupillary responses
- Monitoring airway patency, respiratory effort, and arterial blood gases

Summary

The spectrum of ocular, maxillofacial, and neck injuries ranges from minor to severe. Having knowledge of the potential complications, frequently assessing for signs and symptoms of these complications, and applying the appropriate interventions will prevent morbidity and potential mortality in this patient group. Providing pain relief and addressing the patient's and family's specific concerns will help to alleviate fear and anxiety. The goals of emergency care include prevention or limitation of further injury; prevention of infection and other complications; reduction of pain, fear, and anxiety; and facilitation of appropriate follow-up. Because most eye injuries are preventable, the trauma nurse should discuss prevention strategies with the patient.

References

1. *Dorland's Illustrated Medical Dictionary* (30th ed.). (2003). Philadelphia: W. B. Saunders.
2. Netter, F. H. (2003). *Atlas of human anatomy* (3rd ed.). Teterboro, NJ: Icon Learning Systems.
3. Ganong, W. F. (1999). *Review of medical physiology* (19th ed.). Norwalk, CT: Appleton & Lange.
4. Cranial nerves summary. (n.d.). Retrieved December 19, 2005, from http://www.meddean. luc.edu/lumen/MedEd/GrossAnatomy/h_n/cn/ cn1/table1.htm
5. McGwin, G., Xie, A., & Owsley, C. (2005). Rate of eye injury in the United States. *Archives of Ophthalmology, 123*, 970–976.
6. Ho, V. H., Wilson, M. W., Fleming, J. C., & Haik, B. G. (2004). Retained intraorbital metallic foreign bodies. *Ophthalmic Plastic and Reconstructive Surgery, 20*(3), 232–236.
7. Nguyen, Q. D., Kruger, E. F., Kim, A. J., Lashkari, M. H., & Lashkari, K. (2002). Combat eye trauma: Intraocular foreign body injuries during the Iran–Iraq War (1980–1988). *International Ophthalmology Clinics, 42*(3), 167–177.
8. Hogg, N. J., Stewart, T. C., Armstrong, J. E., & Girotti, M. J. (2000). Epidemiology of maxillofacial injuries at trauma hospitals in Ontario, Canada, between 1992 and 1997. *Journal of Trauma: Injury, Infection, and Critical Care, 49*(3), 425–432.
9. Aksoy, E., Unlu, E., & Sensoz, O. (2002). A retrospective study on epidemiology and treatment of maxillofacial fractures. *Journal of Craniofacial Surgery, 13*(6), 772–775.
10. Erol, B., Tanrikulu, R., & Gorgun, B. (2004). Maxillofacial fractures. Analysis of demographic distribution and treatment in 2901 patients (25-year experience). *Journal of Cranio-Maxillo-Facial Surgery, 32*(5), 308–313.
11. Ferreira, P. C., Amarante, J. M., Silva, P. N., Rodrigues, J. M., Choupina, M. P., Silva, A. C., et al. (2005). Retrospective study of 1251 maxillofacial fractures in children and adolescents. *Plastic and Reconstructive Surgery, 115*, 1500–1508.

12. Thomas, G. R., Sandeep, D., Furze, A., Lehman, D., Ruiz, J., Checcone, M., et al. (2005). Managing common otolaryngologic emergencies. *Emergency Medicine, 37*(6), 39–48.

13. Fernandes, S. V. (2004). Nasal fractures: The taming of the shrewd. *Laryngoscope, 114,* 587–592.

14. Kulcik, C. J., Clenney, T., & Phelan, J. (2004). Management of acute nasal fractures. *American Family Physician, 70,* 1315–1320.

15. Rice, D. H. (2004). Management of frontal sinus fractures. *Current Opinion in Otolaryngology & Head and Neck Surgery, 12,* 46–48.

16. Jatla, K. K., & Enzenauer, R. W. (2004). Orbital fractures: A review of current literature. *Current Surgery, 61,* 25–29.

17. Simoni, P., Ostendorf, R., & Artemus, J., (2003). Effect of airbags and restraining devices on the pattern of facial fractures in motor vehicle crashes. *Archives of Facial Plastic Surgery, 5*(1), 113–115.

18. Murphy, R. X., Birmingham, K. L., & Okunski, W. J. (2000). The influence of airbag and restraining devices on the patterns of facial trauma in motor vehicle collisions. *Plastic and Reconstructive Surgery, 105,* 516–520.

19. Norwood, S. H., McAuley, C. E., Vallina, V. L., Berne, J. D., & Moore, W. L. (2001). Complete cervical transection from blunt trauma. *Journal of Trauma: Injury, Infection, and Critical Care, 51*(3), 568–571.

20. Rogers, F. B., Baker, E., Osler, T. M., Shackford, S. R., & Wald, S. L. (1998). A new diagnostic modality to screen for blunt cervical arterial injuries. *Journal of Trauma: Injury, Infection, and Critical Care, 44*(2), 432.

21. Mayberry, J. C., Brown, C. V., Mullins, R. J., & Velmahos, G. C. (2004). Blunt carotid artery injury: The futility of aggressive screening and diagnosis. *Archives of Surgery, 139,* 609–613.

22. Murphy, M. C., Lydiatt, W. M., & Lydiatt, D. D. (2003). Penetrating injuries of the neck. Retrieved December 19, 2005, from http://www.emedicine.com/ent/topic489.htm

23. Bynoe, R. P., Kerwin, A. J., Parker, H. H., Nottingham, J. M., Bell, R. M., Yost, M. J., et al. (2003). Maxillofacial injuries and life-threatening hemorrhage: Treatment with transcatheter embolization. *Journal of Trauma: Injury, Infection, and Critical Care, 55,* 74–79.

24. American College of Surgeons Committee on Trauma. (2005). *Advanced trauma life support® for doctors (Student course manual)* (7th ed., p. 24). Chicago: Author.

25. Hoyt, K. S., & Haley, R. J. (2005). Assessment and management of eye emergencies. *Topics in Emergency Medicine, 27*(2), 101–117.

26. Hitchings, R. (1994). Eye pain. In P. D. Wall & R. Melzack (Eds.), *Textbook of pain* (3rd ed., pp. 555–562). Edinburgh, Scotland: Churchill Livingstone.

27. Smith, S. C. (2002). Ocular injuries. In K. A. McQuillan, K. T. Von Rueden, R. L. Hartsock, M. B. Flynn, & E. Whalen, *Trauma nursing: From resuscitation through rehabilitation* (3rd ed., pp. 484–506). Philadelphia: W. B. Saunders.

28. Sankar, P. S., Chen, T. C., Grosskreutz, C. L., & Pasquale, L. R. (2002). Traumatic hyphema. *International Ophthalmology Clinics, 42*(3), 57–68.

29. Orbital blowout fracture. (2001). Retrieved December 19, 2005, from http://www.eyemdlink.com/Condition.asp?ConditionID=317

In addition to the nursing diagnoses outlined in Chapter 3, Initial Assessment, the following nursing diagnoses are potential problems for the patient with injuries to the eyes, face, or neck. Once a patient has been assessed, diagnoses can be defined as either actual or risk. An actual nursing diagnosis is derived from a decision based on the patient's presenting signs and symptoms. A risk diagnosis is a judgment that the nurse makes based on a particular patient's risk and potential for developing certain problems.

Nursing Diagnoses	Interventions	Expected Outcomes
Airway clearance, ineffective, related to: • Pain • Altered level of consciousness • Secretions and debris in airway • Soft tissue edema • Edema of the airway, vocal cords, epiglottis, and upper airway • Direct trauma • Presence of an artificial airway • Aspiration of foreign matter • Inhalation of toxic fumes or substances	• Immobilize the cervical spine • Position the patient • Open and clear the airway • Insert an oropharyngeal or nasopharyngeal airway • Avoid stimulation of a gag reflex • Assist with early intubation	**The patient will maintain a patent airway, as evidenced by:** • Clear bilateral breath sounds • Regular rate, depth, and pattern of breathing • Effective cough • Absence of pain with coughing • Appropriate use of splinting techniques while coughing

Aspiration, risk, related to:
 	
• Impaired cough and gag reflex
• Trauma to face or neck
• Facial and/or neck soft tissue edema
• Secretions and debris in airway
• Increased intragastric pressure
• Impaired swallowing
	• Immobilize the cervical spine
	• Position the patient
	• Open and clear the airway
	• Insert an oropharyngeal or nasopharyngeal airway
	• Avoid stimulation of a gag reflex
	• Assist with early intubation
	• Insert an orogastric or nasogastric tube and evacuate stomach contents
		The patient will not experience aspiration, as evidenced by:
		
		• A patent airway
		• Clear and equal bilateral breath sounds
		• Regular rate, depth, and pattern of breathing
		• Arterial blood gas (ABG) values within normal limits:
		  ▪ PaO_2 80 to 100 mm Hg (10.0 to 13.3 KPa)
		  ▪ SaO_2 > 95%
		  ▪ $PaCO_2$ 35 to 45 mm Hg (4.7 to 6.0 KPa)
		  ▪ pH 7.35 to 7.45
		• Clear chest radiograph without evidence of infiltrates
		• Ability to handle secretions independently

Nursing Diagnoses	Interventions	Expected Outcomes

Gas exchange, impaired, related to:
 	
• Aspiration
• Altered blood flow, oxygen-carrying capacity of the blood, oxygen supply
• Ineffective airway clearance
• Aspiration of foreign matter
• Hypo- or hyperventilation
• Inhalation of toxic fumes or substances
	• Administer oxygen via nonrebreather mask
	• Ventilate, if needed, with 100% oxygen via a bag-mask device
	• Assist with early intubation
	• Monitor oxygen saturation with pulse oximeter
	• Administer blood, as indicated
		The patient will experience adequate gas exchange, as evidenced by:
		
		• ABG values within normal limits:
		  ▪ PaO_2 80 to 100 mm Hg (10.0 to 13.3 KPa)
		  ▪ SaO_2 > 95%
		  ▪ $PaCO_2$ 35 to 45 mm Hg (4.7 to 6.0 KPa)
		  ▪ pH 7.35 to 7.45
		• SpO_2 > 95%
		• Skin normal color, warm, and dry
		• Level of consciousness, awake and alert, age appropriate
		• Regular rate, depth, and pattern of breathing

Tissue perfusion, altered renal and cerebral, related to:
 	
• Hypovolemia
• Interruption of flow: arterial and/or venous
	• Apply direct pressure to sites of active bleeding
	• Cannulate two veins with large-caliber catheters and initiate infusion of an isotonic crystalloid solution (flow rate to be determined by patient's hemodynamic status)
	• Position the patient as guided by institutional protocols (head midline)
	• Obtain blood sample for ABGs, as indicated
		The patient will maintain adequate tissue perfusion, as evidenced by:
		
		• Vital signs within normal limits for age: absence of vital sign abnormalities, including hypotension, bradycardia, respiratory irregularities, or increase in pulse pressure
		• Normal pupil size, shape, and reactivity to light
		• ABG values within normal limits:
		  ▪ PaO_2 80 to 100 mm Hg (10.0 to 13.3 KPa)
		  ▪ SaO_2 > 95%
		  ▪ $PaCO_2$ 35 to 45 mm Hg (4.7 to 6.0 KPa)
		  ▪ pH 7.35 to 7.45
		• Urine output 1ml/kg/hr

Sensory/perception, altered visual, related to: • Visual impairment • Involvement of sensory receptors, CNS function • Direct trauma to the eye	• Check visual acuity • Protect the patient from injury	The patient will experience normal vision, as evidenced by: • Normal responses to visual acuity examination

Nursing Diagnoses	Interventions	Expected Outcomes
Pain, related to: • Direct trauma to eye • Irritation and inflammation • Visible foreign body or substance • Chemical injury • Fractures • Soft tissue injury	• Administer topical analgesics as prescribed unless contraindicated • Administer systemic analgesics, as prescribed • Administer cycloplegic agents, as prescribed • Patch the affected eye, if indicated • Stabilize impaled objects • Assist with foreign body removal, as indicated • Irrigate the eyes with normal saline, as indicated • Use touch, positioning, or relaxation techniques to give comfort	**The patient will experience relief of pain, as evidenced by:** • Diminishing or absent level of pain through patient's self-report • Absence of physiologic indicators of pain, which include tachycardia, tachypnea, pallor, diaphoretic skin, increasing blood pressure, and restlessness • Absence of nonverbal cues of pain: crying, grimacing, inability to assume position of comfort • Ability to cooperate with care, as appropriate

Infection, risk, related to:
 	
• Loss of skin or structural integrity secondary to direct trauma
• Foreign bodies
• Contamination of wound from injury event or instrumentation
	• Monitor temperature
	• Maintain aseptic technique
	• Administer antibiotics, as prescribed
	• Check wounds for drainage
	• Monitor urinary output
	• Obtain blood samples as indicated for:
	  ▪ Blood cultures
	  ▪ Complete blood count
	• Administer tetanus prophylaxis, as prescribed
		The patient will be free from infection, as evidenced by:
		
		• Core temperature measurement of 98 °F to 99.5 °F (36 °C to 37.5 °C)
		• Absence of systemic signs of infection: fever, tachypnea, and tachycardia
		• Wounds free from redness, swelling, purulent drainage, or odor
		• Level of consciousness, awake and alert, age appropriate
		• White blood cell count within normal limits

Injury, risk, related to: • Visual field defect • Impaired depth perception secondary to patching • Disruption of orbit architecture • Concomitant brain injury	• Protect eye(s) with eye diaphragm/patch as indicated • Shield **(do not patch)** an eye with a suspected open or ruptured globe • Patch the unaffected eye • Stabilize impaled objects with patch/diaphragm; patch the unaffected eye • Shield (do not patch) the eye of a patient who has a hyphema, infection (corneal ulceration), or other anterior chamber injury (traumatic iritis) • Occasionally double-patch (2 patches) the injured eye for a patient with a superficial corneal injury • Explain to the patient the purpose of eye patching	**The patient will have minimal complications of the injury, as evidenced by:** • No iatrogenic extension of the injury • Movement of the eye is minimized with patching • Verbalization of an understanding of the need for patching of the eye • Absence of increase in extent of original injury • Identification of safety measures to prevent injury • Maintenance of airway patency

Nursing Diagnoses	Interventions	Expected Outcomes
Fear (patient and family), related to: • Actual or perceived threat of vision loss • Unfamiliar environment • Invasive procedures and therapeutic treatment • Separation from support systems • Pain	• Communicate with the patient • Establish a trusting relationship • Describe all procedures • Orient the patient to his or her surroundings • Administer topical analgesics, as prescribed unless contraindicated	**The patient and family will experience decreasing fear, as evidenced by:** • Absence of fear-related behavior: crying, shouting, agitated behavior, noncommunicative behavior, blank stare; facial expressions, voice tone, and body posture are within normal parameters for the patient • Acknowledgment of fear and stating that there is decreasing fear • Absence of physiologic indicators of fear: palpitations, increased blood pressure, diaphoresis, and tachycardia • Decreased level of pain • Orientation to surroundings • Participation in decision making regarding care when appropriate

Chapter 8

Thoracic Trauma

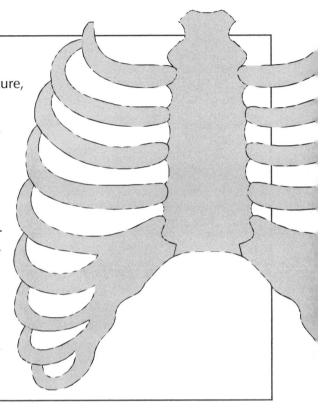

Objectives

On completion of this chapter/lecture, the learner should be able to:

1. Identify the common mechanisms of injury associated with thoracic trauma.

2. Describe the pathophysiologic changes as a basis for the signs and symptoms of thoracic trauma.

3. Discuss the nursing assessment of patients with thoracic trauma.

4. Plan appropriate interventions for patients with thoracic trauma.

5. Evaluate the effectiveness of nursing interventions for patients with thoracic trauma.

Preface

Lecture begins on page 136.

Knowledge of normal anatomy serves as the foundation for understanding the anatomic derangements and pathophysiologic compromises that may result from trauma. Before reading this chapter, it is strongly suggested that the learner read the following review material. Reading about the specific anatomic and physiologic concepts presented in this section will enhance the learner's ability to correlate such concepts with specific injuries. This material related to anatomy and physiology will not be covered during lectures, nor will it be evaluated by testing.

Refer to Chapter 4, Airway and Ventilation, for a detailed description of the physiology of ventilation.

Respiratory System

The respiratory system's primary function is the transport of oxygen to, and the removal of carbon dioxide from, the cells. This is achieved by the following processes: pulmonary ventilation, the movement of air between the atmosphere and alveoli; diffusion, the movement of oxygen and carbon dioxide between the alveoli and the blood; transport of oxygen to the peripheral tissues, exchange of carbon dioxide at the cellular level, and return of carbon dioxide to the lungs; and regulation of ventilation.[1]

The anatomy of the respiratory system is divided into those structures considered the upper airways, such as the nose, oropharynx, larynx, and trachea. These structures filter, warm, and humidify inhaled air. The bronchi and bronchioles are lower airway structures and conduct atmospheric air to the alveoli, where gas exchange takes place. The alveoli and pulmonary capillaries are responsible for gas exchange.[1]

The thoracic cavity extends from the top of the sternum to the diaphragm. Key structures within the thoracic cavity include the lungs and the space between the lungs, termed the mediastinum. The mediastinum is bound anteriorly by the sternum, posteriorly by the 12 thoracic vertebrae, and inferiorly by the diaphragm. The contents of the mediastinal space include the heart and pericardium, thoracic aorta, esophagus, trachea, inferior and superior vena cavae, vagus nerves, phrenic nerves, and other vascular structures. Correlation of anatomical structures and surface landmarks can be important in physical assessment of the chest (**Figure 8-1**).

Heart and Thoracic Great Vessels

The heart is situated in the mediastinum, with the most anterior chamber, the right ventricle, located beneath the sternum. The left ventricle is anterior to the thoracic spine. The heart is enclosed by the pericardium (pericardial sac). The double-layered pericardium is composed of a tough, outer fibrous layer and a thinner, serous layer, referred to as the epicardium. Between the two layers is approximately 30 to 50 ml of lubricating fluid that allows frictionless motion during systole and diastole.

Cardiac function and cardiac output are affected by:

- Preload, which refers to the volume in the left and right ventricles at the end of diastole[1]
- Afterload, which refers to the resistance or pressure in the arteries against which the ventricles must contract
- Myocardial contractility
- Heart rate

Factors affecting preload are blood volume, right atrial pressure, and intrathoracic pressure. Afterload is affected by the arterial pressure in the aorta and pulmonary arteries. Cardiac contractility can be affected by hypoxemia, ventricular diastolic volume, stimulation of the sympathetic nervous system, blunt cardiac injury, and myocardial infarction.

The thoracic aorta, the main vessel carrying oxygenated blood out of the left ventricle, is located in the mediastinum. It is divided into three portions: the ascending aorta, the aortic arch, and the descending thoracic aorta. The portion of the aorta immediately

Figure 8-1 Chest and anatomical landmarks

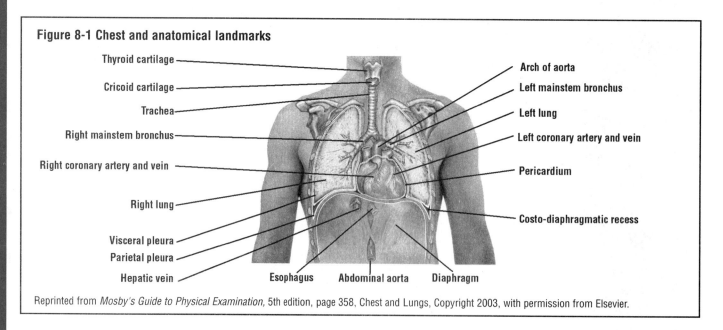

Thyroid cartilage
Cricoid cartilage
Trachea
Right mainstem bronchus
Right coronary artery and vein
Right lung
Visceral pleura
Parietal pleura
Hepatic vein
Esophagus
Abdominal aorta
Diaphragm
Arch of aorta
Left mainstem bronchus
Left lung
Left coronary artery and vein
Pericardium
Costo-diaphragmatic recess

Reprinted from *Mosby's Guide to Physical Examination*, 5th edition, page 358, Chest and Lungs, Copyright 2003, with permission from Elsevier.

proximal to the heart is referred to as the ascending aorta. The aortic arch is attached to the pulmonary artery by the fetal remnant of the ductus arteriosus, termed the ligamentum arteriosum. The aortic isthmus is that portion of the aorta near the ligamentum where the left subclavian artery originates. This portion of the aorta is part of the descending aorta, which is tethered in position and, therefore, has less ability to tolerate acceleration and/or deceleration forces.

Segmental arteries arise from the descending aorta. The segmental arteries branch into the intercostal and radicular arteries. The radicular arteries, which supply the anterior and posterior spinal arteries, are the primary vascular supply for the spinal cord.[2]

Epidemiology

Patients with trauma to the chest present with some of the most life-threatening conditions in emergency care. Thoracic injuries are second only to brain and spinal cord injuries as the leading causes of traumatic death.[3] The increase in interpersonal violence has had an impact on the pattern of injuries to the chest.[3]

Mechanisms of Injury and Biomechanics

Mechanical energy is the most common energy source associated with chest injuries. Acceleration and deceleration forces may be responsible for injuries to intrathoracic contents. The first and second ribs and the sternum tend to resist energy loads better than other bones of the body; therefore, if these bones are fractured, suspect significant injury to underlying structures. Mechanical energy applied to the chest can lead to fractures, blunt cardiac injury, and pulmonary contusions. Because of the relative fixation of the descending aorta distal to the ligamentum arteriosum, this structure is more susceptible to injury produced by deceleration forces. Structural cardiac injuries, such as chamber rupture or perforation, carry a high mortality rate.[4] Forces that cause penetrating cardiac injury most often injure the right ventricle.

Motor vehicle crashes account for an estimated two-thirds of all chest trauma-related deaths. Additional mechanisms of injury commonly associated with thoracic injuries are falls, crush injuries, assaults, use of firearms, stabbings, and motor vehicle versus pedestrian incidents.

Types of Injuries

The most common type of injury associated with chest trauma is blunt; the most common cause of blunt chest trauma are motor vehicle crashes, accounting for approximately 70%.[5] Penetrating injuries to the chest are usually the result of firearm injuries or stabbings.

Usual Concurrent Injuries

Injuries to the chest are frequently associated with immediate life-threatening conditions. Chest trauma may disrupt the airway, impair breathing, or result in serious alterations in circulation.

Isolated blunt thoracic injury is uncommon.[5] Head, extremity, and abdominal injuries frequently occur concurrently. Penetrating trauma to the thorax, particularly gunshot or shotgun injuries, are frequently associated with abdominal trauma because of the anatomical proximity of the chest and abdomen. Patients with penetrating injuries to the lower thoracic region should be assumed to have both chest and abdominal injuries until proven otherwise.

Table 8-1 lists organs that may be injured when the sternum or ribs are fractured.

Pathophysiology as a Basis for Signs and Symptoms

Ineffective Ventilation

Ineffective ventilation can be a result of thoracic trauma. The pathophysiology is related to the loss of integrity of anatomical structures, as well as compromises to the normal physiologic process of respiration. Tears or lacerations in the tracheobronchial tree interrupt the integrity of the lower airway.[3] Patients with these injuries manifest dramatic symptoms early during resuscitation with massive air leaks into the subcutaneous tissue of the chest, neck, and face.

Ineffective ventilation may also result from rib fractures or sternal fractures. Pain resulting from these fractures may impair the patient's ability to adequately ventilate.

When the ribs or sternum are fractured, there is often injury to underlying organs. Interstitial and alveolar edema may occur, in addition to hemorrhage and laceration, when the lung is contused or punctured. The interstitial and alveolar edema results in impaired diffusion of gases across the alveolar membrane. Damaged alveoli and capillary injuries produce abnormalities in the ventilation to perfusion ratio.[1]

Penetrating injury of the chest wall and laceration of lung tissue affects the patient's ability to maintain negative intrapleural pressure. Air or blood leaking into the intrapleural space collapses the lung. The degree of lung collapse is dependent on the severity of the underlying lung injury.

Table 8-1: Thoracic Skeletal Fractures

Injury	Associated Injury
Sternal fractures	• Blunt cardiac injury
First and second rib fractures	• Great vessel injuries • Brachial plexus injuries • Head and spinal cord injuries
Rib fractures and flail chest	• Pulmonary contusions • Pneumothorax • Hemothorax
Fractures of lower ribs (7th to 12th)	• Liver and spleen injuries

Ineffective Circulation

Injury to the heart or thoracic great vessels results in internal and external hemorrhage leading to hypovolemia and shock. Direct trauma to the heart may lead to a reduction in cardiac output because of reduced myocardial contractility.

Air or blood that continues to accumulate in the thoracic cavity will increase the intrapleural pressure. If the pressure rises to an abnormally high level, the heart and great vessels may shift, causing compression of the vena cava, obstruction of venous return, and collapse of the lung. Compression of the vena cava with obstruction of venous return will result in decreased cardiac output. The primary symptoms the patient will exhibit are respiratory distress, tachycardia, hypotension, and unilateral absence of breath sounds. Neck vein distention because of increased intrathoracic pressure and tracheal deviation are late signs that may not be clinically appreciated.

Rapid accumulation of even small amounts of blood in the pericardial sac (pericardial tamponade) may result in compression of the heart and inability of the heart to fill during diastole. This injury results in decreased cardiac output. The patient may exhibit hypotension, tachycardia, muffled heart sounds, and neck vein distention.

Neurologic Deficits

Paraplegia associated with aortic injuries is related to ischemia or infarction of the spinal cord because of hematoma formation or occlusion of the blood flow from the aorta to the spinal arteries.[2,6]

Selected Thoracic Injuries

Rib and Sternal Fractures

Rib fractures are the most common type of blunt chest injury.[5,7] The injured area of lung underlying the fracture is usually of more clinical significance than the fracture. Fracture of the sternum or the first or second rib requires significant force and, therefore, may be associated with serious injuries of underlying structures. Left lower rib fractures may be associated with splenic injury, right lower rib fractures with hepatic injury, and sternal fractures with heart or great vessel injury.[7] Sternal fracture is associated with a blunt injury (e.g., the chest colliding with the steering wheel). The most common fracture site is the junction of the manubrium and the body of the sternum (angle of Louis), which is adjacent to the 2nd intercostal space.

Signs and Symptoms

- Dyspnea
- Localized pain on movement, palpation, or inspiration
- Patient assumes a position intended to splint the chest wall to reduce pain
- Chest wall ecchymosis or sternal contusion
- Bony crepitus or deformity

Flail Chest

Flail chest is defined as a fracture of two or more sites on two or more adjacent ribs, or when rib fractures produce a free-floating sternum (Figure 8-2). The unsupported chest wall or flail segment moves paradoxically or opposite from the rest of the chest wall during inspiration and expiration. Flail segments may not be clinically evident in the first several hours after injury because of muscle spasms that cause splinting.[7] After positive pressure is initiated, paradoxical chest wall movement ceases. A flail chest may be associated with the following

- Ineffective ventilation
- Pulmonary contusion
- Lacerated lung parenchyma

Signs and Symptoms

- Dyspnea
- Chest wall pain
- Paradoxical chest wall movement—the flail segment moves in during inspiration and out during expiration

Pneumothorax

A simple pneumothorax results when an injury to the lung leads to accumulation of air in the pleural space with a subsequent loss of the negative intrapleural pressure. Partial or total collapse of the lung may ensue.[8]

An open pneumothorax results from a wound through the chest wall. Air enters the pleural space both through the wound and the trachea.

Signs and Symptoms

- Dyspnea, tachypnea
- Tachycardia
- Hyperresonance (increased echo produced by percussion over the lung field) on the injured side
- Decreased or absent breath sounds on the injured side
- Chest pain
- Open, sucking wound on inspiration (open pneumothorax)

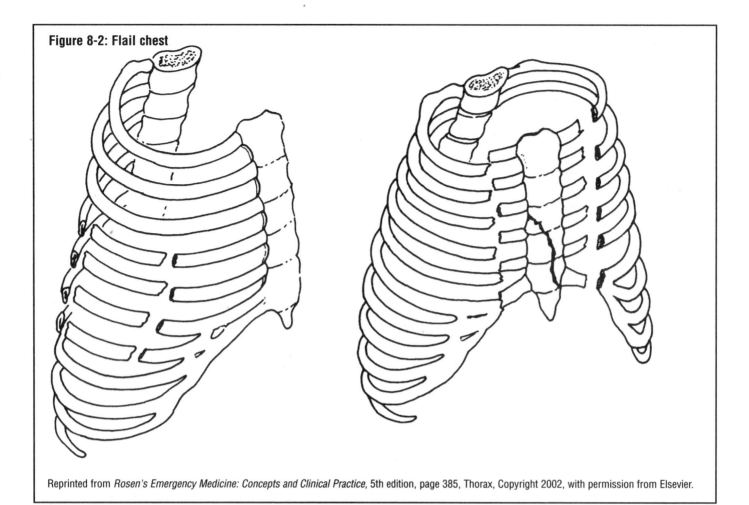

Figure 8-2: Flail chest

A tension pneumothorax is a life-threatening injury. Air enters the pleural space on inspiration, but the air cannot escape on expiration. Rising intrathoracic pressure collapses the lung on the side of the injury causing a mediastinal shift that compresses the heart, great vessels, trachea, and ultimately, the uninjured lung. Venous return is impeded, cardiac output falls, and hypotension results.[8]

Tension pneumothorax is a clinical diagnosis and immediate decompression should be performed. Treatment should not be delayed to obtain more definitive diagnostic tests when a tension pneumothorax is suspected.[8]

Signs and Symptoms

- Severe respiratory distress
- Markedly diminished or absent breath sounds on the affected side
- Hypotension
- Distended neck, head, and upper extremity veins—may not be clinically appreciated if significant blood loss present
- Tracheal deviation—shift toward uninjured side (late sign; may not be clinically appreciated)
- Cyanosis (late sign)

Hemothorax

A hemothorax is an accumulation of blood in the pleural space. A massive hemothorax is a rapid accumulation of 1,500 ml or more in the intrapleural space.[8] Massive, intrapleural hemorrhage may result in a mediastinal shift, decreased venous return, and hypotension.

Signs and Symptoms

- Dyspnea, tachypnea
- Chest pain
- Signs of shock
- Decreased breath sounds on the injured side
- Dullness to percussion on the injured side

Pulmonary Contusion

Pulmonary contusions may occur as a result of direct impact, deceleration, or high-velocity bullet wounds.[9] A contusion develops when blood leaks into the lung parenchyma, causing edema and hemorrhage. The contusion may be localized or diffuse. The degree of respiratory insufficiency is related to the size of the contusion, the severity of injury to the alveolar-capillary membrane, and the development of atelectasis. The subtle signs and symptoms of respiratory insufficiency associated with pulmonary contusion usually develop over time rather than manifesting immediately.[8]

Signs and Symptoms

- Dyspnea
- Ineffective cough
- Hemoptysis
- Hypoxia
- Chest pain
- Chest wall contusion or abrasions

Ruptured Diaphragm

A ruptured diaphragm is a potentially life-threatening injury that may result from forces that penetrate the body, such as gunshot wounds, or from acceleration or deceleration forces, such as motor vehicle crashes. Blunt injuries are more likely to injure the left hemidiaphragm because the right hemidiaphragm is somewhat protected by the liver.[10] A rupture or tear of the diaphragm may allow herniation of abdominal contents, such as the stomach, small bowel, or spleen, into the thorax. Herniation may result in respiratory compromise because of impairment of lung capacity and displacement of normal lung tissue. Mediastinal structures may shift to the opposite side of the injury.[10]

Penetrating injuries below the nipple line should be evaluated for the potential of diaphragmatic injury and concurrent abdominal injury. Stab wounds to the lateral chest walls and flanks can be associated with diaphragmatic lacerations because of the close proximity, steep slope, and large surface area of the diaphragm.

Signs and Symptoms

- Dyspnea or orthopnea
- Dysphagia (difficulty swallowing)
- Abdominal pain
- Sharp epigastric or chest pain radiating to the left shoulder (Kehr's sign)
- Bowel sounds heard in the lower to the middle chest
- Decreased breath sounds on the injured side

Tracheobronchial Injury

Tracheobronchial injury can be a result of blunt trauma; however, it is more likely caused by penetrating mechanisms. Blunt ruptures of the lower trachea or mainstem bronchus should be suspected in karate-type blows, "clothesline-type" injuries, or when the neck strikes the steering wheel. It has been reported

that the majority of tracheobronchial ruptures (> 80%) occur within 2.5 cm of the carina. The majority of penetrating injuries to the trachea and bronchi (75%) occur in the proximal trachea.[3] Patients with suspected bronchial injury should undergo bronchoscopy as part of the diagnostic evaluation. Patients with injuries causing large defects in the trachea or bronchial tree will require urgent surgical intervention.

Signs and Symptoms

- Dyspnea, tachypnea
- Hoarseness
- Hemoptysis
- Subcutaneous emphysema in the neck, face, or suprasternal area
- Decreased or absent breath sounds
- Signs and symptoms of airway obstruction

Blunt Cardiac Injury

Formally called "cardiac contusion" or "concussion," the phrase *blunt cardiac injury* has become preferred to describe the spectrum of potential blunt injuries to the heart, including more specific descriptions of associated structures and cardiac injury involved[11] (e.g., blunt cardiac injury with septal rupture). Blunt cardiac injury should be suspected following an associated mechanism of injury or in patients that exhibit an abnormally poor cardiovascular response to their injury. It is most commonly associated with motor vehicle crashes,[11] especially with direct impact of the chest with the steering wheel, or falls from heights.

Signs and Symptoms

- ECG abnormalities, the most common of which are sinus tachycardia, premature ventricular contractions (PVCs), and atrioventricular (AV) blocks[8]
- Chest pain
- Chest wall ecchymosis

Pericardial Tamponade

Pericardial tamponade is a collection of blood in the pericardial sac. This life-threatening cardiac injury occurs most often with penetrating injury, although blunt trauma may also result in pericardial tamponade.[8] As blood accumulates in the noncompliant pericardial sac, it exerts pressure on the heart, inhibiting or compromising ventricular filling. A subsequent decrease in stroke volume leads to a decrease in cardiac output. Impairment in cardiac function is related to both the rate and amount of fluid accumulation.

Signs and Symptoms

- Hypotension
- Tachycardia or pulseless electrical activity (PEA)
- Dyspnea
- Cyanosis
- Beck's triad

   The classic findings of hypotension, distended neck veins, and muffled heart sounds are defined as Beck's triad. However, these symptoms occur in only 10% to 40% of patients. If there are other sources of blood loss, the central venous pressure (CVP) will be low, and neck vein distention will be absent.[3] Additionally, it may be difficult to appreciate muffled heart sounds in the resuscitative setting.

- Progressive decreased voltage of conduction complexes on an electrocardiogram (ECG)[3]

Aortic Injuries

Injuries to the thoracic aorta may be the result of penetrating or, more commonly, blunt trauma. The descending thoracic aorta is susceptible to rupture from rapid deceleration forces. The mechanism of injury is associated with a combination of shearing forces, compression of the aorta on the vertebral column, and an increase in pressure inside the vessel during the episode of the trauma.[12] The usual site of damage to the descending aorta is at the aortic isthmus distal to the ligamentum arteriosum and the takeoff of the left subclavian artery where the aorta is relatively fixed. Ascending aortic injuries are immediately fatal in most cases.[13] Patients with descending aortic injury have an 85% mortality prior to arrival at a hospital. There is a 10% to 30% mortality in those patients who are admitted and receive surgical intervention.[12,13]

Signs and Symptoms

- Hypotension
- Decreased level of consciousness
- Hypertension in upper extremities[12]
- Decreased quality (amplitude) of femoral pulses compared to upper extremity pulses
- Loud systolic murmur in parascapular region
- Chest pain
- Chest wall ecchymosis
- Widened mediastinum on chest radiograph
- Paraplegia

Assessment

History

Refer to Chapter 3, Initial Assessment, for a description of general information that should be collected regarding every trauma victim. Only pertinent questions specific to patients with thoracic injuries are described following.

- What was the mechanism of injury?
   - What was the type of motor vehicle crash?
      - Head-on collision or impact with a stationary object, such as a tree or cement wall, will result in deceleration forces that may be associated with chest injuries, such as a traumatic aortic rupture (**Table 8-2**).
   - What was the damage to the exterior and interior of the vehicle?
      - A bent steering wheel or steering column imprint on the patient's chest may be associated with sternal fractures, blunt cardiac injury, or a transected aorta. The amount of structural intrusion into the passenger compartment may be useful to identify patterns of injury, such as lateral rib fractures.
- What are the patient's complaints?
   - Dyspnea
   - Dysphagia
   - Dysphonia
   - Pain

Table 8-2: Type of Impact and Associated Thoracic Injuries

Mechanism	Associated Thoracic Injuries
Frontal impact	• Anterior flail chest • Blunt cardiac injury • Pneumothorax • Transection of aorta (decelerating injury)
Side impact	• Lateral flail chest • Pneumothorax • Traumatic aortic rupture • Diaphragmatic rupture
Motor vehicle–pedestrian	• Transection of the aorta • Abdominal visceral injuries

American College of Surgeons. (2004). Initial assessment and management. In *Advanced Trauma Life Support® for doctors* (Student Course Manual). (7th ed., p. 22). Chicago: Author.

- What were the patient's vital signs prior to admission?
  - Were vital signs or signs of life observed by prehospital care personnel or another reliable source? If cardiopulmonary resuscitation is being performed, when was it started? When did the patient lose signs of life? This information is important in determining the indications for performing a thoracotomy in the emergency department.

Physical Assessment

Refer to Chapter 3, Initial Assessment, for a description of the assessment of the patient's airway, breathing, circulation, and disability.

Inspection

Observe the chest wall for injuries that may severely impair the adequacy of breathing, such as open chest wounds or flail segments. This may require the removal of debris or blood to avoid overlooking any wounds.

- Assess breathing effectiveness and rate of respiration.
- Observe the chest wall for symmetrical movement.

  The presence of a flail segment may produce paradoxical movement.
- Inspect the jugular veins.

  Distended neck veins may indicate increased intrathoracic pressure as a result of a tension pneumothorax or pericardial tamponade. Flat external jugular veins may reflect hypovolemia.
- Inspect the upper abdominal region for evidence of blunt or penetrating injury.

Percussion

- Percuss the chest.

  Dullness is associated with hemothorax, and hyperresonance suggests a pneumothorax.

Palpation

- Palpate the chest wall, clavicles, and neck for:
  - Tenderness
  - Swelling or hematoma
  - Subcutaneous emphysema
- Note the presence of bony crepitus (possible fractured ribs or sternum).
- Palpate central and peripheral pulses and compare quality between:
  - Right and left extremities
  - Upper and lower extremities

- Palpate the trachea.

  Palpate the trachea above the suprasternal notch. Tracheal shift may indicate a tension pneumothorax or massive hemothorax. (This is a late sign and may not be clinically appreciated.)
- Palpate extremities for motor and sensory function.

  Lower extremity paresis or paralysis may indicate aortic injury.[12]

Auscultation

- Auscultate and compare blood pressure in both upper and lower extremities.
- Auscultate breath sounds.

  Decreased or absent breath sounds may indicate the presence of a pneumothorax or hemothorax. Diminished sounds may result from splinting. Shallow respirations may be exhibited because of pain.
- Auscultate the chest for the presence of bowel sounds.

  Bowel sounds heard in the middle to lower lung fields may occur with diaphragmatic rupture.
- Auscultate heart sounds.

  Muffled heart sounds may be associated with pericardial tamponade.
- Auscultate the neck vessels for bruits, which may indicate vascular injury.

Diagnostic Procedures

Refer to Chapter 3, Initial Assessment, for frequently ordered radiographic and laboratory studies. Additional studies for patients with thoracic injuries are listed following.

Radiographic Studies

- Chest

  After the potential for spinal cord injury has been ruled out, an upright chest radiograph may be necessary to evaluate the presence of a hemothorax, especially if blood accumulation is less than 300 ml.[14] Chest radiograph is the primary diagnostic screening tool for diagnosis of blunt aortic injuries, with loss of the aortic knob contour as the most reliable marker.[12,15]
- Arteriography

  Arteriography may be used to evaluate suspected vascular injuries in the chest. Aortography may be done if there is a mechanism of injury, or physical or radiographic signs that result in a high index of suspicion for aortic injury.[16]
- Bronchoscopy and laryngoscopy

- Computed tomography (CT) scan

  A thoracic CT scan evaluates pulmonary parenchymal injuries, pulmonary contusions, and aortic injuries. Transesophageal echocardiography and the use of spiral CT are used as diagnostic tools for patients with normal chest radiography and a history of significant deceleration injury. Although thoracic CT does not replace aortography in the definitive evaluation of aortic injury, patients who are having CT scanning performed for other reasons (e.g., head or abdominal trauma) may have a CT performed as a screening exam prior to more invasive tests (e.g., aortography).[12,14,16]

- Focused Assessment Sonography for Trauma (FAST)

  A FAST exam may be indicated to detect the presence of pericardial blood or effusions. The FAST exam is a screening ultrasound study that is noninvasive, rapid and portable, accurate, inexpensive, and can be repeated. Many regional trauma centers use FAST, appreciating the fact that it has limited comprehensiveness and accuracy of the results are operator dependent.[17] For further discussion about the FAST exam, refer to Chapter 9, Abdominal Trauma.

Laboratory Studies

- Cardiac enzymes

  Cardiac enzymes may be useful in diagnosing myocardial infarction. Their usefulness in diagnosing blunt cardiac injury, however, is inconclusive. Therefore, they should not be used in the evaluation and treatment of a patient with blunt cardiac injury.[8]

Other

- Electrocardiogram

  Sinus tachycardia, PVCs, and AV blocks are most frequently observed following blunt chest injury.[8]

- Central venous pressure (CVP)

  Patients with cardiac tamponade or tension pneumothorax may have an elevated CVP. Patients with hypovolemia may have a decreased CVP. Normal CVP is between 5 and 10 cm H_2O (2 and 5 mm Hg).

- Echocardiography

Planning and Implementation

Refer to Chapter 3, Initial Assessment, for a description of the specific nursing interventions for patients with compromises to airway, breathing, circulation, and disability.

- Ensure patent airway.
  - Suction airway to maintain patency, as needed.
  - Prepare for endotracheal intubation or surgical airway with cervical spine stabilization if the patient has severe chest trauma. Consider using rapid sequence intubation.
  - Intubation of the patient with a tracheobronchial injury in the emergency department is controversial. Attempts at intubation may cause further injury. The use of a flexible bronchoscope may be helpful in guiding the endotracheal tube distal to the injury.
- Administer oxygen via a nonrebreather mask at a flow rate sufficient to keep the reservoir bag inflated (12 to 15 liters/minute).
- Prepare for ventilatory support, as necessary. Administer 100% oxygen using either a bag-mask device with an attached reservoir system or a mechanical ventilator.
  - Sandbags, strapping, or rib belts are not used in patients with rib fractures or a flail chest because therapy is aimed at correcting abnormalities in gas exchange rather than providing chest wall stability.[7]
- Cover open wound with sterile, nonporous dressing (e.g., petroleum-impregnated dressing), and tape securely on three sides.
  - If signs or symptoms of a tension pneumothorax develop after application of the dressing, remove the dressing and re-evaluate the patient.
- If a tension pneumothorax is suspected, **immediately** prepare for a needle thoracentesis. A 14-gauge needle is inserted into the 2nd intercostal space in the midclavicular line on the affected side. Prepare for subsequent chest tube insertion (see **Figure 8-3**).
- Prepare for chest tube insertion (thoracostomy).
  - A chest tube is inserted to decompress a pneumothorax or hemothorax. Chest tubes may be placed prophylactically in patients with blunt or penetrating chest trauma who require positive pressure ventilation. If the pneumothorax is small, the physician may decide to defer chest tube placement.
  - Contraindications: The only absolute contraindication is the need for an immediate open thoracotomy.
  - Chest drainage systems: If air or blood accumulates in the pleural cavity, negative pressure is lost and the lung collapses. The therapeutic

goal of drainage devices is restoration of negative pressure.

- Chest tube placement: The insertion site is the 4th or 5th intercostal space, at the anterior or midaxillary line (**Figure 8-3**). After the chest tube is inserted, the tube is connected to drainage tubing of a chest drainage system and the suction chamber tubing is connected to a suction source.

- Management of a patient with a chest drainage system

    - For the safety of the patient, all tubing connections between the patient and underwater seal or chest drainage unit should be taped or banded to prevent inadvertent disconnection. The chest tube insertion site should be covered with 4 × 4 gauze dressings and the tube secured to the chest wall with heavy tape. Follow institutional protocols for specific dressing procedures. A chest radiograph is needed to document correct tube placement.

    - Maintain the chest drainage unit below the level of the chest to facilitate the flow of drainage and prevent reflux into the chest cavity. With water seal chest drainage units, keep the unit upright to prevent the loss of the water seal.

    - The tubing should be gently coiled without dependent loops or kinks.

    - Assess and document **fluctuation** in the water seal chamber, **output**, **color** of drainage, and **air leak** (FOCA).

    - Troubleshooting for problems with chest tube drainage should follow the D.O.P.E. mnemonic —Dislodgement, Obstruction, Pneumothorax, and Equipment.

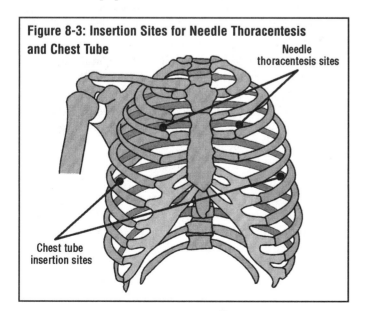

Figure 8-3: Insertion Sites for Needle Thoracentesis and Chest Tube

Needle thoracentesis sites

Chest tube insertion sites

- Notify the physician if initial chest drainage output is greater than 1,000 ml or if there is continued blood loss of greater than 200 ml/ hour for 3 to 4 hours. Prepare for transport to the operating room for emergency thoracotomy if either of these situations occurs.[8]

- During patient transport, clamping of chest tubes is NOT necessary and is contraindicated. Clamping of chest tubes before the patient's lung is fully reexpanded may lead to the development of a tension pneumothorax.

- Prepare for aggressive ventilatory support if a major bronchial air leak exists after chest tube insertion.

    - A tracheobronchial laceration can result in persistent bubbling in the chest drainage unit and failure of the involved lung to reexpand despite suction. Prepare for surgical intervention if tracheobronchial injury is suspected.

- Prepare for autotransfusion, as indicated.

    - Consider autotransfusion if a large blood loss is anticipated or greater than 500 ml of blood is collected.

    - Indications: To transfuse patients with their own blood. In the emergency department, autotransfusion is usually limited to blood drained from a hemothorax. In significant chest trauma, autotransfusion should be anticipated and the collection device prepared prior to chest tube insertion, if possible.

    - Precautions/contraindications: Blood contaminated with bowel contents or infection at the site of blood retrieval. Blood salvaged from a bacteria-contaminated cavity is considered in dire emergencies or when no alternative source of blood is available.

        - Blood potentially contaminated with malignant cells

        - Injuries greater than six hours old

        - Autotransfusion greater than 50% of patient's estimated blood loss

        - Careful consideration should be given when autotransfusing patients with hepatic or renal dysfunction.

- Stabilize impaled objects.

- Cannulate two veins with large-caliber intravenous catheters and initiate infusions of isotonic crystalloid solution.

- Prepare for massive transfusion of blood and blood products, as indicated.

- If pulmonary contusion is suspected and no signs of hypovolemic shock are present, restrict fluid administration to prevent pulmonary complications.

- Prepare for pericardiocentesis, as indicated.

  Pericardiocentesis is an emergency procedure performed by a physician to relieve cardiac tamponade. The patient is placed with head and torso elevated at a 45-degree angle. A 16- or 18-gauge, 6-inch (15 cm) or longer, over-the-needle catheter is attached to a 60-ml syringe. The needle is inserted at a 45-degree angle, lateral to the left side of the xiphoid, 1 to 2 cm inferior to the xiphochondral junction. Blood is aspirated during introduction of the needle until as much blood as possible is withdrawn from the pericardial sac.[8,11]

  Blood removed from the pericardial sac will generally not clot (because blood is defibrinated from agitation during systole), and the hematocrit will be lower than venous blood.[3] Blood clots may be present in the pericardial sac and require operative removal.

- Assist with an emergency resuscitative thoracotomy.

  The indications for this procedure have been subject to considerable review. Resuscitative thoracotomy in the emergency department for patients with no documented vital signs or signs of life (e.g., pupillary reflexes, spontaneous movement, organized ECG activity) and/or with blunt injuries has been demonstrated to have doubtful benefit. The best results are obtained in patients with a single penetrating injury of the anterior or precordial thoracic area and in patients who had a witnessed cardiac arrest in the emergency department. In such patients, especially those with stab wounds, a timely resuscitative thoracotomy may lead to complete recovery.[18,19,20] This procedure is recommended only in situations where physicians are experienced in the technique and surgical resources are available for continuing surgical therapy.[8]

- Monitor and treat cardiac dysrhythmias or dysfunction if significant blunt cardiac injury is suspected.

- Administer analgesic medication, as prescribed.

  Pain control helps to prevent hypoventilation. Prepare to assist with an intercostal nerve block, if ordered.

Evaluation and Ongoing Assessment

Refer to Chapter 3, Initial Assessment, for a description of the ongoing evaluation of the patient's airway, breathing, circulation, and disability. Additional evaluations include

- Monitoring airway patency, respiratory effort, and arterial blood gases
- Monitoring respiratory effort after covering a wound because this may lead to the development of a tension pneumothorax
- Monitoring vital signs
- Monitoring chest tube drainage to determine the amount and any change in drainage characteristics

Summary

Trauma to the chest may result in life-threatening injuries because of catastrophic compromises in breathing and circulation. Knowledge of anatomy, mechanism and pattern of injury, and the physiologic consequences of any disruption of the pulmonary and cardiovascular systems are the foundations of the trauma nursing process for patients with an injury to the chest.

Early identification of all injuries requires a collaborative team approach to conduct the necessary diagnostic and therapeutic interventions. Determining the patient's need for operative management and/or transfer to a comprehensive trauma center is a major consideration for members of the trauma team.

References

1. Guyton, A. C., & Hall, J. E. (2005). *Textbook of medical physiology* (11th ed.). Philadelphia: W. B. Saunders.

2. Gabella, G. (Ed.). (1999). Thorax: Aorta. In P. L. Williams, L. H. Bannister, M. M. Berry, P. Collins, M. Dyson, J. E. Dussek, et al. (Eds.), *Gray's anatomy: The anatomical basis of medicine and surgery* (38th ed., pp. 1504–1513). Edinburgh: Churchill Livingstone.

3. Sherwood, S. F., & Harstock, R. L. Thoracic injuries. (2002). In K. A. McQuillan, K. T. Von Rueden, R. L. Hartsock, M. B. Flynn, & E. Whalen (Eds.), *Trauma nursing: From resuscitation through rehabilitation* (3rd ed., pp. 543–590). Philadelphia: W. B. Saunders.

4. Fitzgerald, M., Spencer, J., Johnson, F., Marasco, S., Atkin, C., & Kossmann, T. (2005). Definitive management of acute cardiac tamponade secondary to blunt trauma. *Emergency Medicine Australasia, 17,* 494–499.

5. American College of Surgeons Committee on Trauma. (2002). *National trauma data bank report 2002®.* Chicago: Author.

6. Mattox, K. L., Wall, M. J., & LeMaire, S. A. (2004). Injury to the thoracic great vessels. In E. E. Moore, D. V. Feliciano, & K. L. Mattox (Eds.), *Trauma* (5th ed., pp. 576–578). New York: McGraw-Hill.

7. Livingston, D. H. & Hauser, C. J. (2004). Trauma to the chest wall and lung. In E. E. Moore, D. V. Feliciano, & K. L. Mattox (Eds.), *Trauma* (5th ed., pp. 507–537). New York: McGraw-Hill.

8. American College of Surgeons. (2004). Thoracic trauma. In *Advanced trauma life support for doctors® (Instructor course manual)* (7th ed., pp. 103–130). Chicago: Author.

9. Vignesh, T., Arun Kumar, A. S., & Kamat, V. (2004). Outcome in patients with blunt chest trauma and pulmonary contusions. *Indian Journal of Critical Care Medicine, 8*(2), 73–77.

10. Asensio, J. A., Petrone, P., & Demetriades, D. (2004). Injury to the diaphragm. In E. E. Moore, D. V. Feliciano, & K. L. Mattox (Eds.), *Trauma* (5th ed., pp. 613–635). New York: McGraw-Hill.

11. Ivatury, R. R. (2004). The injured heart. In E. E. Moore, D. V. Feliciano, & K. L. Mattox (Eds.), *Trauma* (5th ed., pp. 555–568). New York: McGraw-Hill.

12. Mattox, K. L., Wall, M. J., & LeMaire, S. A. (2004). Injury to the thoracic great vessels. In E. E. Moore, D. V. Feliciano, & K. L. Mattox (Eds.), *Trauma* (5th ed., pp. 571–590). New York: McGraw-Hill.

13. Nzewi, O., Slight, R. D., Zamvar, V. (2006). Management of blunt thoracic aortic injury. *European Journal of Vascular and Endovascular Surgery, 1,* 18–27.

14. Livingston, D. H., & Hauser, C. J. (2004). Injury to the chest wall and lung. In E. E. Moore, D. V. Feliciano, & K. L. Mattox (Eds.), *Trauma* (5th ed., pp. 522–523). New York: McGraw-Hill.

15. Fabian, T. (1997). Prospective study of blunt aortic injury: Multicenter trial of the American Association for the Surgery of Trauma. *The Journal of Trauma, 42,* 374–383.

16. Exadaktylos, A. K., Duwe, J., Eckstein, F., Stoupis, C., Schoenfeld, H., Zimmermann, H., et al. (2005). The role of contrast-enhanced spiral CT imaging versus chest x-rays in surgical therapeutic concepts and thoracic aortic injuries. *Cardiovascular Journal of South Africa, 16,* 162–165.

17. Catalano, O., & Siani, A. (2004). Focused assessment with sonography for trauma (FAST): What it is, how it is carried out, and why we disagree. *La Radiologia Medica, 108,* 443–453.

18. Cothren, C. C., & Moore, E. E. (2006). Emergency department thoracotomy for the critically injured patient: Objectives, indications, and outcomes. *World Journal of Emergency Surgery, 1*(4), 1–13.

19. Grove, C. A., Lemmon, G., Anderson, G., & McCarthy, M. (2002). Emergency thoracotomy: Appropriate use in the resuscitation of trauma patients. *The American Surgeon, 68*(4), 313–316.

20. Aihara, R., Millham, F. H., Blansfield, J., & Hirsch, E. F. (2001). Emergency room thoracotomy for penetrating chest injury: Effect of an institutional protocol. *The Journal of Trauma, 50*(6), 1027–1030.

In addition to the nursing diagnoses outlined in Chapter 3, Initial Assessment, the following nursing diagnoses are potential problems for the patient with thoracic injury. Once a patient has been assessed, diagnoses can be defined as either actual or risk. An actual nursing diagnosis is one derived from a decision based on the patient's presenting signs and symptoms. A risk nursing diagnosis is a judgment the nurse makes based on a particular patient's risk and potential for developing certain problems.

Nursing Diagnoses	Interventions	Expected Outcomes
Airway clearance, ineffective, related to: • Presence of an artificial airway • Edema of the airway, vocal cords, epiglottis, and upper airway • Direct trauma • Irritation of the respiratory tract • Altered level of consciousness • Tracheobronchial secretions or obstruction • Aspiration of foreign matter • Inhalation of toxic fumes or substances	• Stabilize cervical spine • Position the patient • Open and clear the airway • Insert oro- or nasopharyngeal airway • Assist with endotracheal intubation or surgical airway	**The patient will maintain a patent airway, as evidenced by:** • Effective cough and gag reflex • Absence of signs and symptoms of airway obstruction: stridor, dyspnea, hoarse voice • Clear sputum of normal amount without abnormal color or odor • Absence of signs and symptoms of retained secretions: fever, tachycardia, tachypnea

Breathing pattern, ineffective, related to:
 	
• Pain
• Musculoskeletal impairment
• Unstable chest wall segment
• Lack of intact thoracic cavity wall
• Lung collapse
	• Administer oxygen via a nonrebreather mask
	• Prepare for ventilatory support with either bag-mask device or endotracheal intubation and mechanical ventilation
	• Obtain blood sample for ABGs as indicated
	• Cover open wounds with sterile, nonporous dressing
	• If signs and symptoms of a tension pneumothorax develop:
	  ▪ After application of the dressing, remove the dressing and re-evaluate the patient
	  ▪ Immediately prepare for a needle thoracentesis
		The patient will have an effective breathing pattern, as evidenced by:
		
		• Normal rate, depth, and pattern of breathing
		• Symmetrical chest wall expansion
		• Absence of stridor, dyspnea, or cyanosis
		• Clear and equal bilateral breath sounds
		• ABG values within normal limits:
		  ▪ PaO_2 80–100 mm Hg (10.0–13.3 KPa)
		  ▪ SaO_2 > 95%
		  ▪ $PaCO_2$ 35–45 mm Hg (4.7–6.0 KPa)
		  ▪ pH between 7.35–7.45
		• Trachea midline

Gas exchange, impaired, related to:
 	
• Ineffective breathing pattern: loss of integrity of thoracic cage, impaired chest wall movement, loss of negative intrathoracic pressure
• Retained secretions
• Accumulation of blood in thoracic cavity
• Decrease in inspired air
• Pulmonary contusion
• Altered blood flow, oxygen-carrying capacity of the blood, oxygen supply
• Aspiration of foreign matter
• Hypo- or hyperventilation
• Inhalation of toxic fumes or substances
	• Administer analgesic medication, as prescribed
	• Prepare for ventilatory support, as necessary
	• Prepare for/assist with chest tube insertion
	• Administer analgesic medication, as prescribed
	• Administer high flow oxygen
	• Monitor oxygen saturation with continuous pulse oximetry
	• Administer blood, as indicated
		The patient will experience adequate gas exchange, as evidenced by:
		
		• ABG values within normal limits:
		  ▪ PaO_2 80–100 mm Hg (10.0–13.3 KPa)
		  ▪ SaO_2 > 95%
		  ▪ $PaCO_2$ 35–45 mm Hg (4.7–6.0 KPa)
		  ▪ pH between 7.35–7.45
		• Skin normal color, warm, and dry
		• Level of consciousness, awake and alert, age appropriate
		• Regular rate, depth, and pattern of breathing

Nursing Diagnoses	Interventions	Expected Outcomes
Fluid volume deficit, related to: • Hemorrhage • Impaired cardiac filling and ejection • Mechanical compression of heart and great vessels • Alteration in capillary permeability	• Control any uncontrolled external bleeding • Cannulate two veins with large-caliber catheters and initiate infusion of lactated Ringer's solution or normal saline • Stabilize impaled objects • Prepare for definitive care if control of internal bleeding is indicated • Consider autotransfusion for a patient with a hemothorax • Position patient with legs elevated • Administer blood, as indicated	**The patient will have an effective circulating volume, as evidenced by:** • Stable vital signs appropriate for age • Urine output 1 ml/kg/hr • Strong, palpable peripheral pulses • Level of consciousness, awake and alert, age appropriate • Skin normal color, warm, and dry • Maintains hematocrit of 30 ml/dl or hemoglobin of 12 to 14g/dl or greater • Control of external hemorrhage
Cardiac output, decreased, related to: • Hypovolemic shock secondary to acute blood loss • Compression of heart and great vessels • Impairment of cardiac filling and ejection	• **Immediately** prepare for a needle thoracentesis if a tension pneumothorax is suspected • Prepare for pericardiocentesis or surgical intervention (pericardial window), as indicated • Monitor and treat cardiac dysrhythmias • Assist with emergency resuscitative thoracotomy, as indicated	**The patient will maintain adequate circulatory function, as evidenced by:** • Strong, palpable peripheral pulses • Apical pulse rate age appropriate • Normal heart sounds • ECG with normal sinus rhythm • Absence of jugular vein distension, deviated trachea • Skin normal color, warm, and dry • Level of consciousness, awake and alert, age appropriate
Tissue perfusion, altered renal, cardiopulmonary, cerebral, gastrointestinal, peripheral (specify type), related to: • Hypovolemia • Interruption of flow: arterial and/or venous	• Control any uncontrolled bleeding • Cannulate two veins with large-caliber intravenous catheters and initiate infusion of lactated Ringer's solution or normal saline • Administer blood, as indicated • Prepare for definitive care	**The patient will maintain adequate tissue perfusion, as evidenced by:** • Vital signs within normal limits for age • Level of consciousness, awake and alert, age appropriate • Skin normal color, warm, and dry • Strong and equal peripheral pulses • Urine output of 1 ml/kg/hr
Pain, related to: • Effects of trauma • Pleural irritation • Experience during invasive procedures/diagnostic tests	• Administer analgesic medication, as prescribed • Stabilize impaled objects • Use touch, positioning, or relaxation techniques to give comfort	**The patient will experience relief of pain, as evidenced by:** • Diminishing or absent level of pain through patient's self-report • Absence of physiologic indicators of pain that include: tachycardia, tachypnea, pallor, diaphoretic skin, increasing blood pressure • Absence of nonverbal cues of pain: crying, grimacing, inability to assume position of comfort • Ability to cooperate with care, as appropriate

Chapter 9

Abdominal Trauma

Objectives

On completion of this chapter/lecture, the learner should be able to:

1. Identify the common mechanisms of injury associated with abdominal trauma.

2. Describe the pathophysiologic changes as a basis for signs and symptoms.

3. Discuss the nursing assessment of patients with abdominal trauma.

4. Plan appropriate interventions for patients with abdominal trauma.

5. Evaluate the effectiveness of nursing interventions for patients with specific types of abdominal injuries.

Preface

Lecture begins on page 152.

Knowledge of normal anatomy serves as the foundation for understanding the anatomic derangements and pathophysiologic compromises that may result from trauma. Before reading this chapter, it is strongly suggested that the learner read the following review material. Reading about the specific anatomic and physiologic concepts presented in this section will enhance the learner's ability to correlate such concepts with specific injuries. This material related to anatomy and physiology will not be covered during lectures, nor will it be evaluated by testing.

The abdominal cavity extends from the diaphragm to the pelvis and is bounded anteriorly by the abdominal wall and posteriorly by the vertebral column. The left side of the diaphragm is slightly lower than the right and may extend to the level of the 5th rib in the mammary line. The abdominal contents are located in the peritoneal cavity, retroperitoneal space, or pelvic cavity.

For the purposes of abdominal evaluation, the abdomen can be divided into four quadrants (**Figure 9-1**).

A serous, smooth membrane called the peritoneum covers the abdominal structures. The parietal peritoneum lines the abdominal wall. The visceral layer surrounds organs of the abdomen. Because the peritoneum is a smooth, lubricated layer of tissue, the viscera can move within the abdomen without friction. Mesenteries are double layers of peritoneum. Their function is to surround and attach organs (e.g., large and small bowels) to the abdominal wall. Additionally, the mesenteries contain blood vessels that supply blood to the large and small bowels. Other organs are only partially covered by the peritoneum. These organs are in the retroperitoneal space (e.g., kidneys, pancreas, aorta, vena cava, and a portion of the duodenum). In men, the peritoneum is a closed sac. In women, the peritoneum is open where the distal ends of the fallopian tubes enter the peritoneal cavity.

Solid Organs

Liver

The liver, spleen, kidneys, and pancreas are solid organs. The liver is an extremely vascular organ located in the upper right quadrant and extends transversely across the midline. It has a solid consistency, but is friable enough to be lacerated, ruptured, or fragmented. The liver substance, hepatic parenchyma, forms lobules that are surrounded by a capsule. The diaphragmatic surface of the liver is smooth and convex, lying at the level of the 6th to 10th ribs on the right side, and at the 7th to 8th ribs on the left side. Circulation through the liver is via the hepatic artery and portal vein. Blood flow to the liver is approximately 30% of the total cardiac output.

Besides its role in metabolism, the liver has two other major functions. The first is as a secretory gland releasing bile. Bile salts help emulsify fat particles in food and absorb fatty acids. The second major function is to filter and store blood. The liver has a large vascular capacity and can store as much as 500 ml of blood at one time.

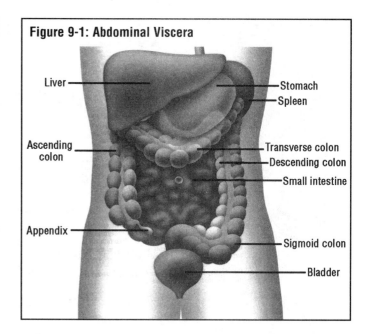

Figure 9-1: Abdominal Viscera

Liver — Stomach — Spleen — Ascending colon — Transverse colon — Descending colon — Small intestine — Appendix — Sigmoid colon — Bladder

Spleen

The spleen is located in the upper left quadrant under the diaphragm and lateral to the stomach. The vascular, friable spleen has a diaphragmatic surface at the level of the 9th through 11th ribs. It is covered by peritoneum, which forms the external layer of the spleen's capsule. The spleen plays an important role in our body's immune function by clearing blood-borne bacteria. The spleen also acts as a blood filter and reservoir for up to 200 ml of blood.

Kidneys

The kidneys are located in the retroperitoneal space at the level of T-12 to L-3. The right kidney is slightly lower than the left because of the position of the liver. The kidneys are behind the stomach, spleen, colonic flexure, and small bowel. Because they are not fixed to the abdominal wall, they move with inspiration and exhalation. A capsule of fatty tissue and a layer of renal fascia surround the kidneys. This fascia, along with the renal vessels, maintains the position of the kidneys. The ureters serve as a conduit for urine from the kidneys to the bladder.

Pancreas

The pancreas is a gland that lies along the abdomen's posterior wall in the retroperitoneum. The head of the pancreas is close to the duodenum and the transverse colon, whereas the upper border is near the hepatic and splenic arteries. As an exocrine organ, it produces fluid which contains enzymes, electrolytes, and bicarbonate to aid in digestion and nutrient absorption. Its endocrine function includes the secretion of insulin and glucagon, the hormones involved in carbohydrate metabolism.

Hollow Organs

Stomach

The stomach, small bowel, large bowel, and bladder are hollow organs. The stomach is located in the left upper quadrant of the abdomen between the liver and spleen at the level of the 7th to 9th ribs. The stomach contains acidic gastric secretions.

Small Bowel

The small bowel is approximately 7 meters long and is comprised of three sections. In descending order from the stomach, the sections are the duodenum, jejunum, and ileum. The first portion of the duodenum, part of the second portion of the duodenum, the jejunum, and the ileum are located in the peritoneal cavity. The rest of the duodenum is retroperitoneal. The small bowel is held in position by the adjacent viscera, the peritoneal membrane attachments to the posterior abdominal wall, and ligaments. Enzymes are secreted into the small bowel to aid in digestion and absorption.

Large Bowel

The large bowel is approximately 1.5 meters long and is comprised of four sections: the cecum, colon, rectum, and anal canal. The colon is further divided into four sections. The first section, the ascending colon, travels past the right lobe of the liver. The second section, the transverse colon, crosses the abdomen from the upper right quadrant to the upper left quadrant. As it crosses the end of the spleen, it curves to become the descending colon located in the left quadrants. The last section, the sigmoid colon, is S-shaped and ends at the level of S-3. The rectum continues for approximately 13 cm, where it dilates and forms the anal canal. The anal canal has both an internal and an external sphincter.

Bladder

The bladder is a membranous sac that stores urine. When it is empty, the bladder is located in the pelvic cavity. When full, it can expand into the abdomen. In women, the bladder is anterior to the uterus and behind the symphysis pubis. The urethra is a membranous canal that conducts urine from the bladder to the exterior of the body at the urinary meatus. The urethra in females is shorter than in males. The prostate is a gland in the male surrounding the neck of the bladder and part of the urethra.

Epidemiology

Abdominal injuries are a significant source of morbidity and mortality in patients who sustain both blunt and penetrating trauma. Abdominal injuries, with a mortality rate of 13% to 15%, rank third as a cause of traumatic death preceded only by head and chest injuries.[1] Patients with multiple abdominal organ injuries (with or without an injury to another body system) have significantly higher mortality rates than those with an isolated abdominal injury. Despite the trend toward nonoperative management of traumatic abdominal injuries, nearly one-fifth of all patients requiring operative intervention have sustained trauma to the abdomen. A frequent cause of preventable death is the unrecognized or missed abdominal injury.[2-4] The initial physical examination is often unreliable due to an altered level of consciousness from head injury, sedation, alcohol, or other illicit drugs. Historical data may be incomplete or presumptive. Therefore, the assessment and management of a patient with suspected abdominal injures should be approached in an organized and collaborative manner relying on both clinical examination and diagnostic procedures.

Mechanisms of Injury

Understanding the mechanism of injury, as well as the forces involved, helps the nurse and health care team focus their assessment and raises the suspicion of specific organ involvement. Blunt and penetrating abdominal injuries may be associated with extensive damage to the viscera resulting in massive blood loss, spillage of intestinal contents into the peritoneal space, and peritonitis. The extent of the injury is related to the

- Type of force applied
- Tissue density of the structure injured (e.g., solid organ, encapsulated, gas-filled organ, hollow organ)

Blunt Trauma

Blunt trauma is the leading cause of intra-abdominal injury, with motor vehicle crashes being the leading mode of injury.[2] Other blunt trauma mechanisms include motor vehicle–pedestrian incidents, assaults, falls, and contact sports. Blunt abdominal injuries result from compression, shearing, or deceleration forces. For example, in frontal impact crashes, the driver may sustain compression injury to the abdominal viscera as the steering wheel comes in direct contact with the abdominal and chest wall. These crushing forces can rupture the capsule sur-

rounding solid organs and injure organ parenchyma. Hollow organs may rupture due to a sudden increase in intraluminal pressure. Rapid deceleration injuries occur when a person falls from a height or when a moving vehicle stops suddenly during a crash. Rapid deceleration produces shearing and stretching forces. Some abdominal organs are semifixed by ligaments, such as the mesenteric attachments of the intestines. During energy transfer, the longitudinal shearing forces may cause rupture of these organs at their attachment points or where the blood vessels enter the organ.[3]

Safety restraint devices, particularly three-point safety belts, provide significant protection; however, improper positioning of these devices may result in shearing injuries to the lower abdomen.[3] Crashes with a bent steering wheel are associated with more significant abdominal injuries to both the driver and front-seat passengers of the vehicle.[5] Riders of bicycles and motorcycles are also at risk for significant blunt abdominal injury as the handlebars impact the abdominal wall.[6]

Penetrating Trauma

Although gunshots and stabbings are the most common causes of penetrating abdominal trauma, other less-common instruments of penetrating injury include flying glass, scissors, arrows, horned animals, and picket fences.[3,4] Stab wounds occur nearly three times more often than gunshot wounds, are generally less destructive, and have a very low mortality rate (1% to 2%).[4] The most commonly injured organs from stab wounds include the liver, small bowel, diaphragm, and colon; however, many stab wounds do not ever violate the peritoneum. Gunshot wounds have greater kinetic energy, produce fragmentation and cavitation, and the bullet has the potential to ricochet off bony structures making the trajectory difficult to determine. The extent of internal injury should never be based on the external appearance of the wound. Gunshot wounds are responsible for almost 90% of the mortality associated with penetrating trauma.[4] Abdominal injury should be suspected not only when the penetrating wound is in the anterior abdomen, but also when there is penetrating injury to the back, flank, or buttocks. The most commonly injured organs from gunshot wounds include the small bowel, colon, liver, and abdominal vascular structures.[2,3]

Usual Concurrent Injuries

As previously mentioned, abdominal trauma is rarely a single-system injury. Patients with abdominal trauma may have thoracic injuries including pulmonary and cardiac injury. Because of their anatomical location, patients with liver or spleen injuries frequently have fractures of the lower rib cage. In high-energy blunt trauma, such as high-speed motor vehicle crashes or significant crush injuries to the lower torso, patients may sustain pelvic and lower extremity fractures in addition to intra-abdominal injuries. With penetrating trauma, any wounds between the nipple line and the inguinal crease anteriorly are considered to have the potential for both thoracic and abdominal injury. Diaphragm injuries, although relatively uncommon, are more frequently associated with penetrating mechanisms of injury.[1] Left-sided diaphragmatic rupture is more common, as the liver acts as a protective barrier to the right diaphragm.

Pathophysiology as a Basis for Signs and Symptoms

Patient manifestations of abdominal trauma are frequently subtle. The abdomen may sequester large amounts of fluid without apparent distention. Signs and symptoms associated with abdominal injury are blood loss, abdominal tenderness, specific pain patterns, and absent bowel sounds.

Blood Loss

Injuries to organs or abdominal blood vessels may lead to extensive hemorrhage. The spleen and liver are extremely vascular and serve as reservoirs for

blood. Injury to these organs may result in rapid blood loss. Because they are encapsulated, compression of the abdomen may rapidly increase pressure within the capsule, resulting in rupture and hemorrhage. In addition, the consistency of the tissues makes hemostasis difficult. Bleeding from organs in the anterior abdomen is usually confined to that cavity. Bleeding from structures in the retroperitoneum is often confined to the retroperitoneal space, making evaluation and diagnosis more difficult (**Figure 9-2**).

Pain

Pain, rigidity, guarding, or spasms of the abdominal musculature are classic signs of intra-abdominal pathology. Sudden movement of irritated peritoneal membranes against the abdominal wall causes rebound tenderness and guarding of the abdominal muscles. Irritation may be because of the presence of free blood or gastric contents in the peritoneal cavity. Manifestations of pancreatic and duodenal injury are related to hemorrhage in the area and the effect of active enzymes on their surrounding tissues. The resultant "chemical peritonitis" from the enzymes released into the retroperitoneum and the significant tissue swelling may not appear as signs and symptoms until several hours after injury.[4,7] The patient with pancreatic and duodenal injury may also complain of diffuse abdominal tenderness and pain radiating from the epigastric area to the back.

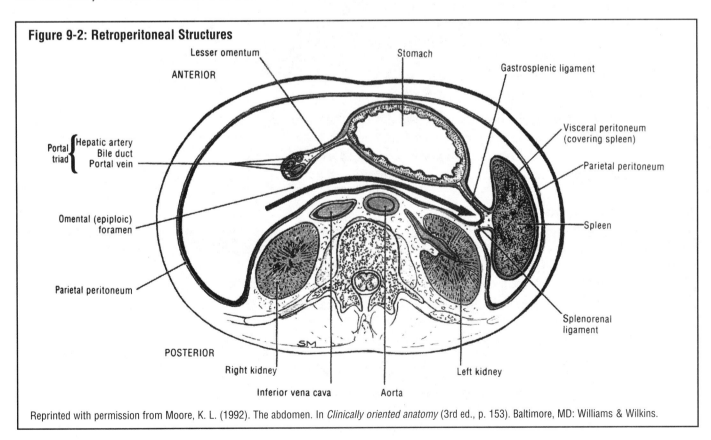

Figure 9-2: Retroperitoneal Structures

Reprinted with permission from Moore, K. L. (1992). The abdomen. In *Clinically oriented anatomy* (3rd ed., p. 153). Baltimore, MD: Williams & Wilkins.

Pain can be referred to other areas of the body. An example is the referred shoulder pain known as Kehr's sign associated with splenic rupture. The blood that collects under the diaphragm causes irritation of the phrenic nerve, which innervates the diaphragm. The pain is perceived along the course of the nerve and is commonly referred to the left subscapular region. Pain referred to the testicles may be indicative of duodenal injury.

Selected Abdominal Injuries

Hepatic Injuries

The severity of hepatic injuries ranges from a controlled subcapsular hematoma and lacerations of the parenchyma to a severe vascular injury of the hepatic veins, retrohepatic cava, or hepatic avulsion (**Table 9-1**).[8] The friability of liver tissue, the extensive blood supply, and the blood storage capacity cause hepatic injury to result in profuse hemorrhage. Patients with less severe injures (Grades I to III) are often successfully managed nonoperatively. More severe injuries often require surgical control of bleeding. The success of nonoperative management for hepatic injuries is predicted based on adherence to rigid criteria for patient selection. These criteria include hemodynamic stability, the absence of peritoneal signs, neurologic integrity, and precise CT scan delineation of the injury, as indicated by the degree of free intraperitoneal blood and absence of associated intra-abdominal injuries.[7,9]

Signs and Symptoms

- Upper right quadrant pain
- Abdominal wall muscle rigidity, spasm, or involuntary guarding
- Rebound tenderness
- Hypoactive or absent bowel sounds
- Signs of hemorrhage or hypovolemic shock

Splenic Injuries

Injury to the spleen is usually associated with blunt trauma, but may also be associated with penetrating trauma. Fractures of the left 10th to 12th ribs are associated with underlying damage to the spleen.

Table 9-1: Liver Injury Scale

Grade	Injury Description
I	• Hematomas: subcapsular & nonexpanding; affect < 10% of surface area • Lacerations: < 1 cm parenchymal depth and nonbleeding
II	• Hematomas: 10%–50% of subcapsular surface and < 1 cm intraparenchymal hematoma • Lacerations: Capsular tear with active bleeding; 1–3 cm in length
III	• Hematomas: > 50% surface area or actively bleeding; ruptured subcapsular or parenchymal hematoma. Intraparenchymal hematoma > 10 cm or expanding • Lacerations: > 3 cm deep into parenchyma
IV	• Ruptured parenchymal hematomas with active bleeding or parenchymal disruption involving 25%–75% of a hepatic lobe
V	• Parenchymal disruption involving > 75% of hepatic lobe. • Vascular injury involves retrohepatic cava or juxtahepatic venous injury
VI	• Hepatic avulsion with avulsion from vascular structures

Table 9-2: Spleen Injury Scale

Grade	Injury Description
I	• Hematomas: Subcapsular involving < 10% surface area and nonexpanding • Laceration: Capsular tears < 1 cm into parenchymal depth and non-bleeding
II	• Hematomas: Subcapsular involving 10%–50% of the surface area or are < 5 cm in diameter • Lacerations: Capsular tear 1–3 cm into parenchymal depth with active bleeding
III	• Hematomas: Greater than 50% surface area and expanding, or a ruptured subcapsular or parenchymal hematoma with active bleeding • Lacerations: > 3 cm into parenchyma with active bleeding or involving the trabecular vessels
IV	• Lacerations involving hilar vessels producing major devascularization (> 25% spleen)
V	• Completely shattered spleen; hilar vascular injury with total devascularization

Injuries to the spleen range from laceration of the capsule or a nonexpanding hematoma to ruptured subcapsular hematomas or parenchymal laceration (**Table 9-2**).[8] The most serious splenic injury is a severely fractured spleen or vascular tear, producing splenic ischemia and massive blood loss (**Figure 9-3**).

In cases of minor blunt trauma, the treatment approach is generally less invasive and dependent on the patient's age and other clinical factors. Nonoperative management of the patient with an isolated splenic injury mandates that the patient be hemodynamically stable.[9-11] This may involve bed rest and possibly blood transfusions (Classes I and II shock only); however, observation, selective embolization, or surgical management should be directed at eliminating the need for transfusion.

Signs and Symptoms

- Signs of hemorrhage or hypovolemic shock
- Pain in the left shoulder (Kehr's sign) when lying supine or Trendelenburg
- Tenderness in the upper left quadrant
- Abdominal wall muscle rigidity, spasm, or involuntary guarding

Large and Small Bowel Injuries

Blunt hollow viscus injuries occur in less than 1% of trauma patients.[2] The small bowel is the hollow organ most frequently injured. It is most commonly injured by a direct blow to the abdominal wall, causing the small intestine to be crushed between the external force and the vertebral column. Deceleration may lead to shearing, which causes avulsion or tearing of the small bowel. The areas of the small bowel most commonly affected are the areas relatively fixed or looped.

Lap seat belts causing compression have resulted in rupture of the small bowel or colon. Clinical signs and symptoms may develop slowly and be overshadowed by other injuries. Delays in diagnosis and management result in significant morbidity and mortality. Patients presenting with ecchymosis over the lower abdominal wall (seat belt sign) should heighten the suspicion of intestinal injury.[3,4]

Large bowel injuries carry a high morbidity and mortality rate due to fecal contamination and the probability of sepsis. The majority of injuries to the colon and rectum are related to penetrating trauma.[1]

Signs and Symptoms

- Peritoneal irritation manifested by abdominal wall muscle rigidity, spasm, involuntary guarding, rebound tenderness, or pain
- Evisceration of the small bowel or stomach

- Hypovolemic shock
- Diagnostic peritoneal lavage (DPL) may show presence of bile, feces, or food fibers
- Gross blood from the rectum

Gastric and Esophageal Injuries

Gastric and esophageal injuries are both quite rare, occur more with multiorgan and multisystem injuries, and are most commonly associated with penetrating trauma.[1,2] Blunt gastric trauma may be more common in children due to the elasticity of the anterior abdominal wall. The cervical region of the esophagus is the most frequently injured. The bacterial content of stomach contents is very low; therefore, signs and symptoms of gastric injury are related to the chemical irritation of nearby tissues by the highly acidic gastric contents.

Signs and Symptoms

Gastric Injury

- Abdominal pain
- Peritoneal irritation
- Evisceration of stomach
- Gross blood in gastric aspirate (nonspecific sign)

Esophageal Injury

- Subcutaneous emphysema
- Peritoneal irritation
- Pain radiating to the neck, chest, shoulders, or throughout the abdomen
- Gross blood in gastric aspirate (nonspecific sign)

Figure 9-3: Grade I Splenic Laceration

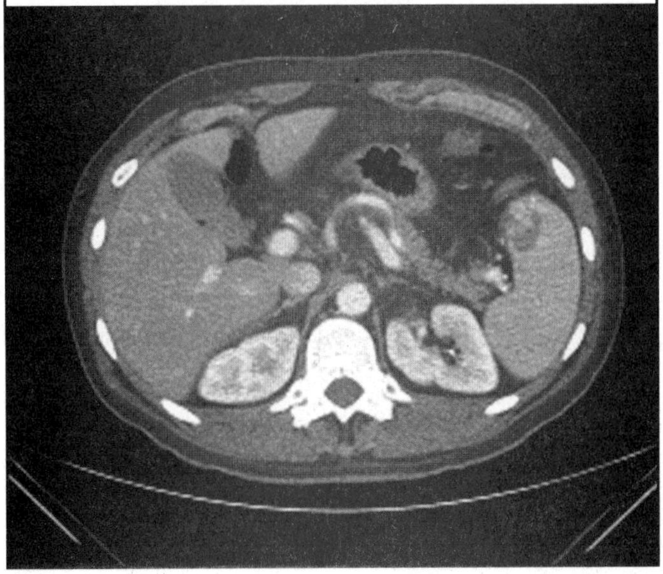

Renal Injuries

Renal injuries are the most frequent urologic trauma and occur in up to 10% of patients. Blunt mechanisms account for more than 80% of all renal injuries.[12] The most common injury to the kidney is a blunt contusion. Severe injuries involve the vascular pedicle and often result in a devascularized kidney. Renal injury should be suspected if there are fractures of the posterior ribs or lumbar vertebrae. Renal parenchyma can be damaged by shearing or compression forces, causing lacerations or contusions. The bleeding will become more serious as the depth of the laceration increases. Rupture of the kidney is not usually associated with hypovolemia unless laceration of a renal artery has occurred. Deceleration forces may cause vascular damage to the renal artery. Because there is little collateral circulation in the area of the renal artery, any ischemia is serious and may lead to acute tubular necrosis. Injury to the kidney is graded by the degree of injury to the collecting system or vascular structures (**Table 9-3**),[13] and diagnosis is best accomplished via CT scan.

Signs and Symptoms

- Hematuria: gross or microscopic. Almost 95% of significant renal injuries are associated with hematuria,[12] although its absence does not rule out injury.
- Flank or abdominal tenderness elicited during palpation
- Ecchymosis over the flank (Grey Turner's sign) may occur, but normally develops 6 to 12 hours after injury.

Bladder and Urethral Injuries

The majority of bladder injuries are a result of blunt mechanisms. The mechanism of injury causing bladder trauma is usually severe and usually associated with other nonurologic injuries that must be treated first. Normally, the bladder lies below the level of the symphysis pubis, but when full, it rises above the pubis into the abdominal cavity. If the bladder is not full when the rupture occurs, urine may leak into the surrounding pelvic tissues, vulva, or scrotum. If a distended bladder ruptures or is perforated, urine is likely to extravasate into the abdomen. Most ruptures of the bladder occur in association with pelvic fractures. Bladder injuries are classified into three categories: [14]

- Partial-thickness bladder wall contusions
- Extraperitoneal rupture (involves lacerations below the pelvic peritoneum)
- Intraperitoneal rupture (pelvic peritoneum is violated)

Classification is made based on retrograde cystography or CT cystography findings. Because treatment modalities are different, proper classification is essential.

Urethral trauma is more common in males than females because the male urethra is longer and less protected. The presence of an anterior pelvic fracture should raise the index of suspicion for a concomitant urethral injury. Urethral injury in females is almost always associated with pelvic fractures. Injury to the penile portion of the urethra in males is most commonly caused by straddle trauma. Prostatic (posterior) urethral injury is usually caused by pelvic fractures and frequently leads to incontinence and impotence.

Signs and Symptoms

- Suprapubic pain
- Urge, but inability, to urinate
- Hematuria (may be microscopic)
- Blood at the urethral meatus
- Blood in scrotum

Table 9-3: Renal Injury Scale

Grade	Injury Description
I	• Contusion: Microscopic or gross hematuria may be present, but urologic studies normal • Hematoma: Subcapsular, nonexpanding without parenchymal laceration
II	• Hematoma: Nonexpanding perirenal hematoma confined to the renal retroperitoneum • Laceration: > 1 cm depth of renal cortex without urinary extravasation
III	• Laceration > 1 cm in parenchymal depth of renal cortex without collecting system rupture or urinary extravasation
IV	• Lacerations extending through the cortex, medulla, and collecting system. • Vascular injuries involving the main renal artery or vein with contained hemorrhage
V	• Completely shattered kidney • Vascular injury includes avulsion of renal hilum, which devascularizes the kidney

- Rebound tenderness
- Abdominal wall muscle rigidity, spasm, or involuntary guarding
- Displacement of prostate gland

Nursing Care of the Patient with Abdominal Trauma

Assessment

History

Refer to Chapter 3, Initial Assessment, for a description of general information that should be collected regarding every trauma victim. Only pertinent questions specific to patients with abdominal injuries are described following.

Blunt mechanisms

- Type of crash
  - Was the patient wearing any restraints or protective devices, or was the patient ejected?
    - Inappropriately positioned lap belts may injure lower abdominal structures.
- Speed of the vehicle
  - The speed of the vehicle on impact influences the severity of the injury.
- Extent of vehicular damage
- Patient's location within the vehicle
- Extrication time
- Height of the fall

Penetrating mechanisms

- Type of weapon or wounding agent
- Distance from the assailant
- Suspected number of shots
- Blood loss at the scene
- What is the location, intensity, and quality of pain?
- Is nausea or vomiting present?
- Does the patient feel an urge to defecate or urinate?

Physical Assessment

Refer to Chapter 3, Initial Assessment, for a description of the assessment of the patient's airway, breathing, circulation, and disability.

Inspection

- Observe the lower chest for asymmetric chest wall movement. Chest wall asymmetry may indi-

cate lower rib fractures, and liver, spleen, or diaphragm injury should be suspected.

- Observe the contour of the abdomen (i.e., flat or distended). Distention may be an indication of massive bleeding or gastric distention.
- Inspect the lower chest, abdomen, flanks, and back for seat belt abrasions or other soft tissue injuries.
  - Ecchymosis over the upper left quadrant suggests soft tissue trauma or splenic injury.
  - Ecchymosis or abrasions across the abdomen (lap belt marks or steering wheel-shaped contusions) suggests a significant mechanism of injury, and small bowel and other intra-abdominal injuries should be suspected.
  - Ecchymosis around the umbilicus (Cullen's sign) and ecchymosis of the flank (Grey Turner's sign) suggest retroperitoneal bleeding.[4] These ecchymotic signs may take hours or days to develop and may not be noted on initial presentation.
- Inspect gunshot and stab wounds. Wounds should be described by size, appearance, and location. Wounds should NOT be labeled as entrance and exit, but clearly identified and numbered.
- Inspect the pelvic area for soft tissue bruising.
- Inspect the perineum for hematomas, bloody drainage from the urethral meatus, and vaginal or rectal bleeding.

Auscultation

- Auscultate the chest. If bowel sounds are heard in the chest, it is an indication of diaphragmatic rupture with herniation of the stomach or small bowel into the thoracic cavity.
- Auscultate all four quadrants of the abdomen for bowel sounds. Absence of bowel sounds, in combination with abdominal distention and guarding, are highly indicative of visceral injury.

Percussion

- Percuss the abdomen for hyperresonance or dullness. Hyperresonance indicates air, whereas dullness indicates fluid accumulation. Percussion tenderness constitutes a peritoneal sign and mandates further evaluation.

Palpation

- Begin palpation of the abdomen in an area where the patient has not complained of pain. Gently palpate each of the four quadrants separately for involuntary guarding, rigidity, spasm, and localized pain. Press on the abdomen and quickly release to determine the presence of rebound tenderness. Any positive findings of involuntary guarding, rigidity, pain, or spasm during palpation indicate peritoneal irritation. These signs may be absent if the patient has any of the following

- Distracting pain from another injury
- Retroperitoneal hematoma
- Spinal cord injury
- Ingestion of alcohol or narcotics
- Decreased level of consciousness

- Palpate the pelvis for bony instability, asymmetry, or pain, which indicate possible dislocations or fractures.
- Palpate the flanks for tenderness.
- Palpate the anal sphincter for presence or absence of tone.

Diagnostic Procedures

*Refer to Chapter 3, Initial Assessment, for frequently ordered radiographic and laboratory studies. Additional studies for patients with abdominal trauma are listed below. See **Table 9-4** for a comparison of DPL, FAST, and CT scans in blunt abdominal trauma.*

Radiographic Studies

- Computed tomography (CT) scan
  - Abdominal CT scan has become the primary diagnostic modality for the diagnosis of intra-abdominal injuries. CT scan may be performed

to identify and grade solid organ injuries and hematomas or to estimate the amount of free fluid or air in the abdominal cavity.[3,15,16] It is also useful in diagnosing retroperitoneal and pelvic injuries. The utility of CT scan in the patient with a penetrating injury is questionable. Patients with penetrating injuries and obvious peritoneal violation or hemodynamic compromise require emergent operative exploration. CT scan is being used as an adjunct to local wound exploration and clinical examination in patients with abdominal stab wounds or other low-velocity penetrating injury, with no signs of peritoneal violation or irritation, and hemodynamic stability.

- CT scan of the abdomen is most commonly and appropriately used in the patient who is deemed hemodynamically stable and does not have other injuries requiring immediate diagnostic or therapeutic intervention that would be delayed by CT examination of the abdomen.
- Controversy exists over the need for oral contrast when using CT scan to diagnose abdominal injury. The current opinion is that oral contrast provides no significant benefit in the initial diagnosis of solid organ or hollow viscus injury, but may prove beneficial in follow-up CT scans for pancreatic or intestinal injury.[15]
- Use of intravenous (IV) contrast aids in the diagnosis of active bleeding from the vascular structures. A blush on the scan is an indication

Table 9-4: Indications, Advantages, Disadvantages of DPL, FAST, and CT Scan for Patients With Blunt Abdominal Trauma

Diagnostic Peritoneal Lavage (DPL)	Focused Assessment Sonography for Trauma (FAST)	Computed tomography (CT) Scan
Indications Document bleeding if hypotensive	Document fluid if hypotensive	• Document organ injury if blood pressure is normal
Advantages • Early diagnosis • All patients • Performed rapidly • 98% sensitive • Detects bowel injury • Transport: No	• Early diagnosis • All patients • Noninvasive • Performed rapidly • Repeatable • 86% to 97% accurate • Transport: No	• Most specific for injury • Sensitive: 92% to 98% accurate
Disadvantages • Invasive • Specificity: Low • Misses injury to diaphragm and retroperitoneum	• Operator dependent • Bowel gas and subcutaneous air distortion • Misses diaphragm, bowel, and pancreatic injuries	• Increased cost and time • Misses diaphragm, bowel, and some pancreatic injuries • Transport: Required

of active bleeding and possible need for embolization of the vascular supply to the liver, spleen, or kidney.

- Focused assessment sonography for trauma (FAST)
  - FAST is a portable (bedside), rapid, accurate, and inexpensive diagnostic modality that is used to detect the presence of hemoperitoneum in patients primarily with blunt abdominal trauma.[3,15,16] Four areas of the abdomen are examined: the hepatorenal fossa, the splenorenal fossa, the pericardial sac, and the pelvis (**Figure 9-4**). FAST is considered to be extremely sensitive, with the ability to detect as little as 100 ml of fluid. However, FAST is typically not considered positive until at least 200 to 500 ml of fluid is detected in the abdomen.[4] The primary disadvantage of FAST is its inability to diagnose hollow visceral and retroperitoneal injuries or intraperitoneal injuries not associated with hemoperitoneum. Additionally, the sensitivity of FAST is influenced by operator experience and the amount of free fluid in the peritoneal cavity.

- Intravenous pyelogram (IVP)
  - IVP should only be used as an alternative when CT scan is unavailable.
  - Extravasation of the contrast media into surrounding tissues indicates a disruption in the integrity of the kidney, ureters, or bladder.

- Flat plate, lateral, or upright abdominal radiographic studies should not be routinely used unless CT scan is unavailable. Plain films may be used to
  - Visualize foreign bodies and associated visceral damage
  - Visualize free air in the abdomen indicating disruption of the gastrointestinal tract
  - Diagnose diaphragmatic rupture on upright or chest x-ray

- Cystogram and urethrogram
  - Cystogram and urethrogram should be used in conjunction with CT scan to diagnose urethral or bladder injury. These tests are typically reserved for use after the initial evaluation and resuscitation have been completed.

- Angiography
  - There is increasing awareness and utilization of angiography and embolization in the acute evaluation and nonoperative management of patients with abdominal injuries. Once CT scan has identified a blush or ongoing bleeding, angiography and embolization of bleeding vascular structures may be indicated.[11,17,18]

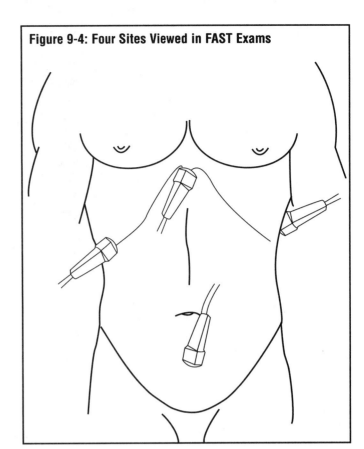

Figure 9-4: Four Sites Viewed in FAST Exams

Angiography may be an adjunct in both the hemodynamically stable and unstable patient.

Laboratory Studies

- Hematocrit
- Base deficit
- Serum lactate
- Coagulation studies
- Analysis of urine, stool, or gastric contents for blood
- Pregnancy testing for females of childbearing age

Other Studies

- Diagnostic peritoneal lavage (DPL)
  - DPL is one method used to detect intra-abdominal bleeding after blunt abdominal trauma. The popularity of DPL as a diagnostic tool has decreased with the introduction of high-speed, helical CT scanners. However, in the hemodynamically unstable patient, DPL may afford rapid diagnosis of intra-abdominal hemorrhage when an ultrasound (FAST) is equivocal or unavailable.[16] DPL is not useful for identifying retroperitoneal bleeding.[3] After decompressing the bladder with an indwelling catheter and the stomach with a gastric tube to avoid inadvertent puncture, a peritoneal catheter is inserted into the abdomen (usually

below the umbilicus). The catheter is introduced via a puncture or a small incision. Withdrawal of gross blood from the catheter is considered a positive finding. If gross blood is not initially aspirated, a liter of warmed isotonic crystalloid solution is rapidly infused through the catheter. The lavage fluid is then allowed to drain out via gravity and analyzed for the presence of red or white blood cells, bile, amylase, food fiber, or feces. DPL has a 98% accuracy rate in the identification of intra-abdominal bleeding.[3,16] A positive DPL requires a surgical consult.

- The American College of Surgeons Committee on Trauma recommends that a DPL be performed early to evaluate the severely injured, hemodynamically unstable patient, especially if the abdominal examination is[3]
  - Suggestive of injury
  - Unreliable (e.g., patient is unresponsive, injury to spinal cord)
- Diagnostic peritoneal lavage is contraindicated when the decision has already been made to perform abdominal surgery. Relative contraindications include[3]
  - Previous abdominal surgery—there is increased potential for adhesions
  - Advanced cirrhosis of the liver
  - Morbid obesity, making technical performance of the procedure difficult
  - Pre-existing coagulopathy

Planning and Implementation

Refer to Chapter 3, Initial Assessment, for a description of the specific nursing interventions for patients with compromises to airway, breathing, circulation, and disability.

Interventions

- Cannulate two veins with large-caliber (14- or 16-gauge), intravenous (IV) catheters, and initiate infusions of warmed, isotonic crystalloid solution.
- Administer blood, as indicated, via fluid warming device.
  - After two liters of crystalloid solution have infused, consider packed red blood cell (RBC) transfusion.
- Consider insertion of an indwelling urinary catheter.
  - An indwelling urinary catheter is inserted to minimize urine leakage into the abdomen or

supporting tissues. Suspected injury to the urethra (i.e., gross blood at the urethral meatus) is a contraindication to catheterization through the urethra. Consider catheterizing the bladder through a suprapubic approach.

- Frequently observe for, and quantify the degree of, hematuria with an indwelling urinary catheter. The initial urine obtained may have been in the bladder prior to the traumatic event. If hematuria is noted, this may be due to the placement of the urinary catheter. Measure and discard the initial urine specimen and test the subsequent urine specimen for the presence of blood.

- Consider insertion of a gastric tube and aspirate gastric contents to
  - Decompress the stomach and prevent aspiration
  - Prevent vagal stimulation and resultant bradycardia
  - Minimize gastric content leakage and subsequent contamination of the abdominal cavity
  - Test the gastric aspirate for the presence of blood
- Cover open abdominal wounds with a sterile dressing. If evisceration of abdominal contents has occurred, place a sterile, moist dressing over the injury. Do not attempt to push the contents back into the abdominal cavity.
- Stabilize impaled objects.
- Administer antibiotics, as prescribed. Leakage of gastric and bowel contents will result in peritonitis and possibly sepsis.
- Administer analgesics, as prescribed.
- Prepare the patient for operative intervention including local wound exploration, hospital admission, or transfer, as indicated.
- Provide psychosocial support.

Evaluation and Ongoing Assessment

Refer to Chapter 3, Initial Assessment, for a description of the ongoing evaluation of the patient's airway, breathing, circulation, and disability. Additional evaluations include the following:

- Monitor cardiovascular status for changes suggestive of hypovolemic shock. These changes include tachycardia and hypotension. If the patient requires continuous assessment of arterial perfusion of a more aggressive nature, consider preparing for insertion of invasive monitoring devices (e.g., arterial line, pulmonary artery catheter).

- Reassess the abdomen frequently and thoroughly to detect subtle changes in pain, tenderness, guarding, or rigidity.
- Reassess pain level and need for additional analgesics or other adjuncts for pain control.
- Monitor urinary output for changes suggestive of hypovolemic shock or insult to renal structures.

Nonoperative management of blunt hepatic, splenic, and most renal injuries is the treatment of choice in the hemodynamically stable patient. Patients with conditions including altered neurologic status or multisystem injury do not preclude the decision for nonoperative management. Nonoperative management has been particularly successful in patients with a lower grade of solid organ injury, but it also has relatively high success rates in patients with higher grades of injury.[4,9,19]

Nonoperative management focuses on serial vital signs, abdominal physical examinations, and laboratory values.[2,9] However, no Class I data is available to support the frequency for serial evaluations.[9] Once the decision has been made to manage the patient nonoperatively, collaborative management is vital to ensure that subtle changes in the patient's condition are recognized, which may indicate the need for urgent exploratory laparotomy. Serial examinations include

- Monitoring cardiovascular changes, primarily tachycardia, indicating ongoing bleeding
- Abdominal physical exams for increasing peritoneal signs
- Hemoglobin and hematocrit (typically every 4 to 6 hours) following institutional guidelines
- Although no Class I evidence supports the performance of repeat or serial CT scans, in select patients, a repeat abdominal CT scan may be ordered to evaluate ongoing bleeding, the development of pseudoaneurysms, or stabilization of the injury.[9]

Nonoperative management of patients with certain types of penetrating abdominal trauma is now an accepted, though controversial, standard of care. However, studies have established the low incidence of intraperitoneal injuries based on the specificity of certain diagnostic tests. This has resulted in a significant reduction in the number of unnecessary laparotomies.[4] Management is based on the following criteria:

- Hemodynamic stability of the patient
- Wound location
- Organ involvement (typically liver or spleen)
- Diagnosis based on CT scan

Hemodynamically stable patients who present with stab wounds that have not violated the anterior fascia or peritoneum typically are candidates for this type of management.[3] Management is based on the results of serial physical evaluations, local wound exploration, DPL, and laparoscopy.[4]

Summary

Abdominal trauma is frequently associated with injuries to other body regions, including the chest. Because of the high vascularity of the solid organs and the presence of major vessels, abdominal trauma has the potential to produce hemorrhage and hypovolemic shock. Patients with abdominal injuries may not present with obvious signs and symptoms. Frequent reassessment is an essential component of the trauma nursing process to detect changes in the patient's condition. Unrecognized abdominal trauma is a frequent cause of preventable death.

The trauma nurse is part of a team who recognizes the nature of multisystem trauma and the need for an organized, standardized approach to the assessment, diagnosis, and interventions for the management of the patient. The nurse who is familiar with the anatomy of the abdomen, mechanisms and patterns of injury, and the pathophysiologic consequences of injury as a basis for signs and symptoms contributes significantly to the collaborative efforts of the trauma team.

References

1. Montonye, J. M. (2002). Abdominal injuries. In K. A. McQuillan, K. T. VonRueden, R. L. Hartsock, M. B. Flynn, & E. Whalen (Eds.), *Trauma nursing: From resuscitation through rehabilitation* (3rd ed., pp. 591–619). Philadelphia: W. B. Saunders.
2. Todd, S. R. (2004). Critical concepts in abdominal injury. *Critical Care Clinics, 20,* 119–134.
3. American College of Surgeons. (2004). Abdominal trauma. In *Advanced Trauma Life Support for Doctors® (Instructor Course Manual)* (7th ed., pp. 131–150). Chicago: Author.
4. Marx, J. A. (2002). Abdominal trauma. In J. A. Marx, R. S. Hockberger, & R. M. Walls (Eds.), *Rosen's emergency medicine: Concepts and clinical practice* (5th ed., pp. 415–436). St. Louis, MO: Mosby.
5. Newgard, C. D., Lewis, R. J., & Kraus, J. F. (2005). Steering wheel deformity and serious thoracic or abdominal injury among drivers and passengers involved in motor vehicle crashes. *Annals of Emergency Medicine, 45,* 43–50.

6. Nadler, E. P., Potoka, D. A., Shultz, B. L., Morrison, K. E., Ford, H. R., & Gaines, B. A. (2005). The high morbidity associated with handlebar injuries in children. *Journal of Trauma, 58,* 1171–1174.

7. Fabian, T. C., & Croce, M. A. (2000). Abdominal trauma, including indications for celiotomy. In K. L. Mattox, D. V. Feliciano, & E. E. Moore (Eds.), *Trauma* (4th ed., pp. 583–602). New York: McGraw-Hill.

8. Moore, E. E., Cogbill, T. H., Jurkovich, G. J., Shackford, S. R., Malangoni, M. A., & Champion, H. R. (1994). Organ injury scaling: Spleen and liver. *Journal of Trauma, 38,* 323–324.

9. Alonso, M., Brathwaite, C., Garcia, V., Patterson, L., Scherer, T., Stafford, P., et al. (2003). *Practice management guidelines for the nonoperative management of blunt injury to the liver and spleen.* Chicago: Eastern Association for the Surgery of Trauma.

10. Haan, J. M., Bochicchio, G. V., Kramer, N., & Scalea, T. M. (2005). Nonoperative management of blunt splenic injury: A 5-year experience. *Journal of Trauma, 58,* 492–498.

11. Harbrecht, B. G. (2005). Is anything new in adult blunt splenic trauma? *American Journal of Surgery, 190,* 273–278.

12. Smith, J. K., & Kenney, P. J. (2003). Imaging of renal trauma. *Radiologic Clinics of North America, 41,* 1019–1035.

13. Moore, E. E., Shackford, S. R., Pachter, H. L., McAninch, J. W., Browner, B. D., Champion, H. R., et al. (1989). Organ injury scaling: Spleen, liver, and kidney. *Journal of Trauma, 29,* 1664–1666.

14. Gibbs, M., & Schnieder, R. (2001). Genitourinary tract and renovascular trauma. In P. C. Ferrera, S. A. Coluccciello, J. A. Marx, V. P. Verdile, & M. A. Gibbs (Eds.), *Trauma management: An emergency medicine approach* (pp. 317–329). St. Louis, MO: Mosby.

15. American College of Emergency Physicians. (2004). Clinical policy: Critical issues in the evaluation of adult patients presenting to the emergency department with acute blunt abdominal trauma. *Annals of Emergency Medicine, 43,* 278–290.

16. Hoff, W. S., Holevar, M., Nagy, K. K., Patterson, L., Young, J., Arrillaga, A., et al. (2001). *Practice management guidelines for the evaluation of blunt abdominal trauma.* Chicago: Eastern Association for the Surgery of Trauma.

17. Haan, J. M., Biffl, W., Knudson, M. M., Davis, K. A., Oka, T., Majercik, S., et al. (2004). Splenic embolization revisited: A multicenter review. *Journal of Trauma, 56,* 542–547.

18. Pryor, J. P., Braslow, B., Reilly, P. M., Guillamondegi, O., Hedrick, J. H., & Schwab, C. W. (2005). The evolving role of interventional radiology in trauma care. *Journal of Trauma, 59,* 102–104.

19. Sharma, O. P., Oswanski, M. F., & Singer, D. (2005). Role of repeat computed tomography in nonoperative management of solid organ trauma. *The American Surgeon, 71,* 244–249.

In addition to the nursing diagnoses outlined in Chapter 3, Initial Assessment, the following nursing diagnoses are potential problems for the patient with abdominal injuries. Once a patient has been assessed, diagnoses can be defined as either actual or risk. An actual nursing diagnosis is derived from a decision based on the patient's presenting signs and symptoms. A risk nursing diagnosis is a judgment that the nurse makes based on a particular patient's risk and potential for developing certain problems.

Nursing Diagnoses	Interventions	Expected Outcomes
Fluid volume deficit, related to: • Hemorrhage secondary to evisceration, disruption in integrity of intra-abdominal organs, drainage	• Elevate extremities • For evisceration of abdominal contents, place a sterile moist dressing over the injury • Stabilize impaled objects • Cannulate two veins with large-caliber intravenous catheters and initiate infusion of crystalloid solution—rate to be determined by patient's condition • Administer blood, as indicated • Prepare for definitive care	**The patient will have an effective circulating volume, as evidenced by:** • Stable vital signs appropriate for age • Urine output of 1 ml/kg/hr • Strong, palpable peripheral pulses • Level of consciousness, awake and alert, age appropriate • Skin normal color, warm, and dry • Maintains hematocrit of 30 ml/dl or hemoglobin of 12 to 16 g/dl or greater • External hemorrhage is controlled
Cardiac output, decreased, related to: • Decreased venous return secondary to acute blood loss	• Elevate extremities • For evisceration of abdominal contents, place a sterile moist dressing over the injury • Stabilize impaled objects • Cannulate two veins with large-caliber intravenous catheters and initiate infusion of crystalloid solution—rate to be determined by patient's condition • Initiate CPR and ALS measures, if indicated • Administer blood, as indicated • Prepare for definitive care	**The patient will maintain adequate circulatory function, as evidenced by:** • Strong, palpable peripheral pulses • Normal heart sounds • ECG with normal sinus rhythm, absence of dysrhythmias • Absence of jugular vein distension, deviated trachea • Skin normal color, warm, and dry • Level of consciousness, awake and alert, age appropriate • Urine output of 1 ml/kg/hr • Vital signs within normal limits for age
Tissue perfusion, altered renal, cardiopulmonary, cerebral, gastrointestinal, peripheral (specify type), related to: • Hypovolemia • Interruption of flow: arterial and/or venous	Control any uncontrolled bleeding • Cannulate two veins with large-caliber intravenous catheters and initiate infusion of crystalloid solution—rate to be determined by patient's condition • Administer blood, as indicated • Prepare for definitive care	**The patient will maintain adequate tissue perfusion, as evidenced by:** • Vital signs within normal limits for age • Level of consciousness, awake and alert, age appropriate • Skin normal color, warm, and dry • Strong and equal peripheral pulses • Urine output of 1 ml/kg/hr

Nursing Diagnoses	Interventions	Expected Outcomes
Infection, risk, related to: • Presence of invasive lines and procedures • Contamination of peritoneal cavity by blood, urine, feces, gastric contents, bile	• Maintain aseptic technique • Cover open wounds with sterile dressings • Stabilize impaled objects • Administer antibiotics, as prescribed • Monitor temperature • Check wounds for drainage • Obtain blood cultures and laboratory studies • Prepare for definitive care	**The patient will be free from infection, as evidenced by:** • Core temperature measurement of 98 to 99.5 °F (36 to 37.5 °C) • Urine output 1 ml/kg/hr • White blood cell count within normal limits • Level of consciousness, awake and alert, age appropriate • Abdomen nontender, nondistended, with bowel sounds present
Urinary elimination, altered, related to: • Urethral or renal trauma	• Insert urinary catheter unless contraindicated • Monitor urinary output	**The patient will have normal patterns of urinary elimination, as evidenced by:** • Urine output of 1 ml/kg/hr • Absence of or decreasing hematuria • Adequate bladder emptying
Pain, related to: • Blunt or penetrating injury • Stimulation of nerve fibers, secondary to abdominal distension • Experience during invasive procedures/diagnostic tests	• Administer analgesics, as prescribed • Use touch, positioning, or relaxation techniques to give comfort	**The patient will experience relief of pain, as evidenced by:** • Diminishing or absent level of pain through patient's self-report • Absence of physiologic indicators of pain, including: tachycardia, tachypnea, pallor, moist skin, increasing blood pressure • Absence of nonverbal cues of pain: crying, grimacing, inability to assume position of comfort • Ability to cooperate with care, as appropriate

Chapter 10

Spinal Cord and Vertebral Column Trauma

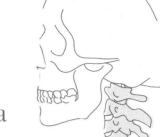

Objectives

On completion of this chapter/lecture, the learner should be able to:

1. Identify the common mechanisms of injury associated with spinal cord and vertebral column trauma.

2. Describe the pathophysiologic changes as a basis for signs and symptoms.

3. Discuss the nursing assessment of patients with spinal cord or vertebral column trauma or both.

4. Plan appropriate interventions for patients with spinal cord or vertebral column trauma or both.

5. Evaluate the effectiveness of nursing interventions for patients with spinal cord or vertebral column injuries or both.

Preface

Lecture begins on page 172.

Knowledge of normal anatomy serves as the foundation for understanding the anatomic derangements and patho-physiologic compromises that may result from trauma. Before reading this chapter, it is strongly suggested that the learner read the following review material. Reading about the specific anatomic and physiologic concepts presented in this section will enhance the learner's ability to correlate such concepts with specific injuries. This material related to anatomy and physiology will not be covered during lectures, nor will it be evaluated by testing.

Vertebral Column

The vertebral column is a series of stacked bones that support the head and trunk and provide the bony encasement for the spinal cord. The vertebral column is composed of 26 vertebrae divided into four regions. The first seven vertebrae are the cervical vertebrae. There are 12 thoracic vertebrae, 5 lumbar vertebrae, 1 sacral bone (composed of 5 vertebrae fused into one), and 1 coccygeal bone formed by the fusion of the final 4 vertebrae (**Figure 10-1**). The typical vertebra is composed of a weight-bearing body and a vertebral arch. The arch is made of 2 pedicles (right and left), 2 laminae, 4 articular processes (facets), 2 transverse processes, and 1 spinous process (**Figure 10-2**). The spinous process can be felt by an examiner when palpating the back. Together, the arch and the body form an enclosure called the vertebral foramen that encircles and protects the spinal cord.[1,2]

Cervical Vertebrae

The cervical vertebrae are the smallest and most mobile. The first cervical vertebra, the atlas, supports the weight of the head and articulates with the occipital condyles of the skull. The atlas is different from the other vertebrae because it has no spinous process or vertebral body. In addition, the foramen opening for the spinal cord is larger than in the rest of the vertebrae. The axis, C-2, has a perpendicular projection called the odontoid process, or dens. The atlas articulates with the axis on the odontoid process.[2] The cervical spine is the most common site for injury.[1]

Thoracic Vertebrae

The thoracic vertebrae, T-1 through T-12, articulate with the ribs. The attachment to the ribs limits flexion and extension but permits more rotation than the lumbar region and less than the cervical region. The vertebrae in this region are strong, and additional support is provided by the ribs. Extreme forces are required to produce fractures and dislocations in this region of the vertebral column; therefore, vertebral fractures in the thoracic region can be frequently accompanied by spinal cord injury.[3]

Lumbar, Sacral, and Coccygeal Vertebrae

The five lumbar vertebrae (L-1 to L-5) are the largest and strongest in the vertebral column.[2] This area of the spine has some freedom of movement and rotation, but not as much as the cervical region. The five sacral vertebrae (S-1 to S-5) are fused to

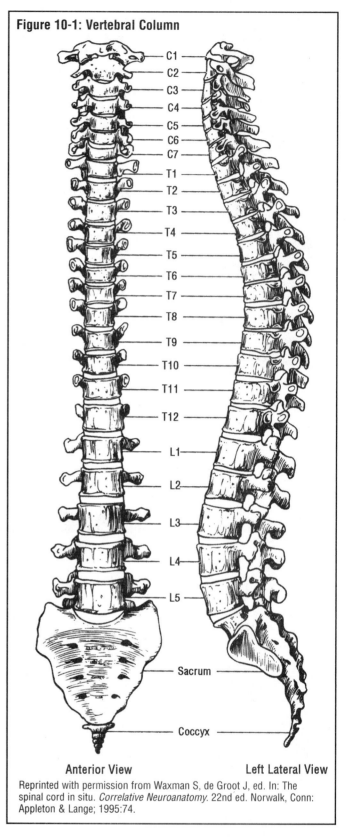

Figure 10-1: Vertebral Column

C1
C2
C3
C4
C5
C6
C7
T1
T2
T3
T4
T5
T6
T7
T8
T9
T10
T11
T12
L1
L2
L3
L4
L5
Sacrum
Coccyx

Anterior View   **Left Lateral View**

Reprinted with permission from Waxman S, de Groot J, ed. In: The spinal cord in situ. *Correlative Neuroanatomy*. 22nd ed. Norwalk, Conn: Appleton & Lange; 1995:74.

form the sacrum in the adult, and the final four coccygeal vertebrae are fused to form the coccyx.[1,4]

Ligaments and Intravertebral Discs

The vertebral bodies are connected by a series of ligaments that provide support and stability for the

Figure 10-2: Structure of Vertebrae

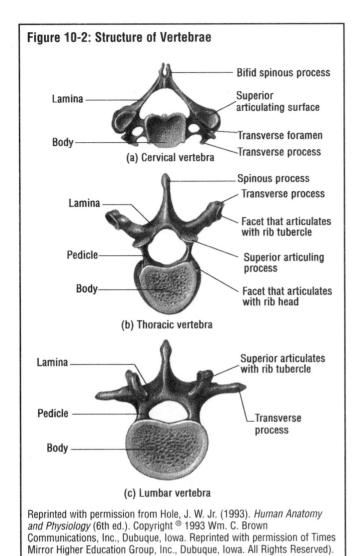

(a) Cervical vertebra

Labels: Lamina, Body, Bifid spinous process, Superior articulating surface, Transverse foramen, Transverse process

(b) Thoracic vertebra

Labels: Lamina, Pedicle, Body, Spinous process, Transverse process, Facet that articulates with rib tubercle, Superior articuling process, Facet that articulates with rib head

(c) Lumbar vertebra

Labels: Lamina, Pedicle, Body, Superior articulates with rib tubercle, Transverse process

Reprinted with permission from Hole, J. W. Jr. (1993). *Human Anatomy and Physiology* (6th ed.). Copyright ® 1993 Wm. C. Brown Communications, Inc., Dubuque, Iowa. Reprinted with permission of Times Mirror Higher Education Group, Inc., Dubuque, Iowa. All Rights Reserved).

Figure 10-3: Section of Vertebral Column

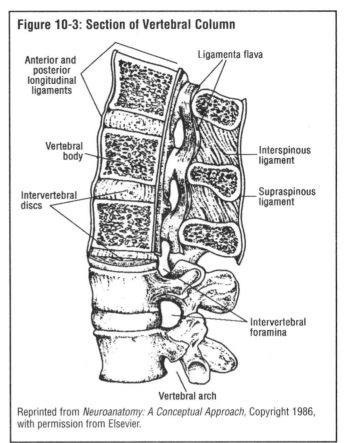

Labels: Anterior and posterior longitudinal ligaments, Vertebral body, Intervertebral discs, Ligamenta flava, Interspinous ligament, Supraspinous ligament, Intervertebral foramina, Vertebral arch

Reprinted from *Neuroanatomy: A Conceptual Approach,* Copyright 1986, with permission from Elsevier.

vertebral column. The anterior and posterior longitudinal ligaments are major ligaments that run the length of the vertebral column and hold the discs and vertebral bodies in position. The ligaments prevent the vertebral column from experiencing excessive flexion and extension. The spinous and transverse processes serve as attachment points for muscles and other ligaments (**Figure 10-3**). Located between the vertebral bodies are fibrocartilaginous discs, which act as shock absorbers during weight bearing and as articulating surfaces for the subsequent vertebral bodies. The more flexible cervical and lumbar regions contain thicker intervertebral discs.[2,4]

Vascular Supply

The spinal cord receives its blood supply from branches off the vertebral arteries and the aorta. Primarily, the cord is fed from the anterior and posterior spinal arteries, which branch off the vertebral artery at the cranial base.[5,6] Injuries to the cord or surrounding area can lacerate these arteries, resulting in hematoma formation that may compress the cord.

Injury to the vessels can be devastating because collateral circulation does not develop in this area.

Spinal Cord

The spinal cord is an elongated mass of nerve tissue. The spinal cord extends from the foramen magnum to the level of L-2. The spinal cord varies in diameter; the thickest point is at its origin in the superior end and the narrowest at the inferior end. Cervical and lumbar area enlargements of cord diameter are also seen at areas where nerves supplying the upper and lower limbs enter and exit the cord.[1] Just below the lumbar enlargement, the cord tapers and terminates into a cone-shaped structure called the conus medullaris. Spinal nerve roots continue to exit below the conus medullaris and are collectively referred to as the cauda equine.[1]

The spinal cord, when viewed in a cross section, has an H-shaped core (**Figure 10-4**). The core is made up of gray matter, which consists of nerve cell bodies. The gray matter is surrounded by white matter, which forms ascending and descending tracts. The descending pathways are termed the corticospinal (pyramidal) tracts and are motor tracts, and the ascending pathways, termed spinothalamic and posterior column, are sensory tracts.[1,5,6] Most voluntary motor movement impulses originate in the motor cortex in the frontal lobe of the brain. The impulses

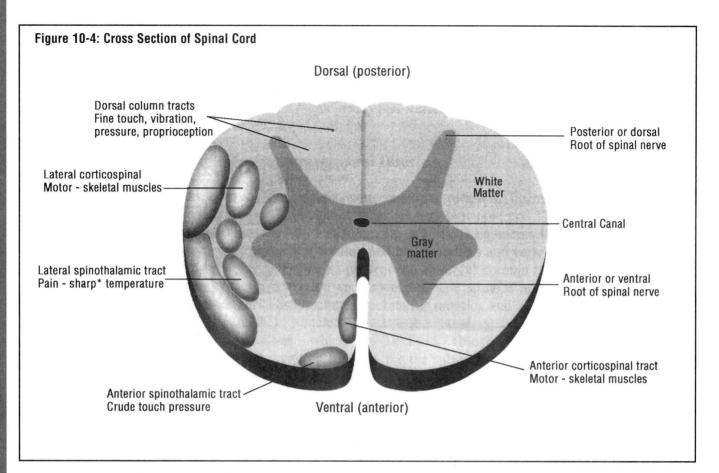

Figure 10-4: Cross Section of Spinal Cord

Dorsal (posterior)

Dorsal column tracts
Fine touch, vibration,
pressure, proprioception

Lateral corticospinal
Motor - skeletal muscles

Lateral spinothalamic tract
Pain - sharp* temperature

Anterior spinothalamic tract
Crude touch pressure

Posterior or dorsal
Root of spinal nerve

White
Matter

Central Canal

Gray
matter

Anterior or ventral
Root of spinal nerve

Anterior corticospinal tract
Motor - skeletal muscles

Ventral (anterior)

travel down specific motor tracts to muscle groups. Most of the descending fibers cross in the medulla. This is the basis for a patient experiencing contralateral loss of movement. There are, however, some fibers that descend through the white matter on the same side and cross at specific spinal cord segments, resulting in ipsilateral loss of movement.[5,6]

Motor

Voluntary motor movement originates from cells in the frontal lobe of the cerebral cortex (upper motor neurons). Upper motor neurons cross to the opposite side in the medulla of the brain stem and then descend in the corticospinal (pyramidal) tract. Upper motor neurons synapse with cell bodies of lower motor neurons on the anterior horn of the gray matter in the spinal cord. The lower motor neurons innervate skeletal muscle. The cervical nerve fibers of the corticospinal tract, which innervate the upper extremities, are located in the central portion of the anterior horn or gray column of the spinal cord. The sacral fibers of the corticospinal tract, which innervate the lower extremities, are located in the peripheral portion of the anterior horn or gray column of the spinal cord.[1,2]

Sensory

Sensory input can be integrated into spinal reflexes or relayed to higher centers in the brain for interpre-

tation. Sensation is classified as superficial, deep, or combined. Superficial sensation is related to touch, pain, and temperature. Deep sensation is muscle or joint position sense (proprioception), vibration sensation, and deep muscle pain.[4] The afferent (ascending) impulses transmit sensory information from specific segments of skin referred to as dermatomes (Figure 10-5). Afferent impulses enter the spinal cord via the posterior (dorsal) roots and ascend in a tract of the spinal cord, depending on the type of sensation. Proprioception and vibration fibers ascend via the posterior column and cross in the medulla. Pain and temperature fibers cross immediately on entering the spinal cord, or within one to two spinal segments, before ascending in the spinothalamic tract. Touch sensation fibers cross immediately on entering the spinal cord and then ascend in the spinothalamic tract[1,2,4] (Table 10-1).

The Reflex Arc

The reflex arc is a stimulus-response mechanism that does not require ascending or descending spinal cord pathways to the cerebral cortex to function. The essential structures of the reflex are:[1]

- Receptor (sense organ, cutaneous end-organ, or neuromuscular spindle)
- Afferent (sensory) neuron
- Association (interneuron) neuron

Figure 10-5: Dermatomes

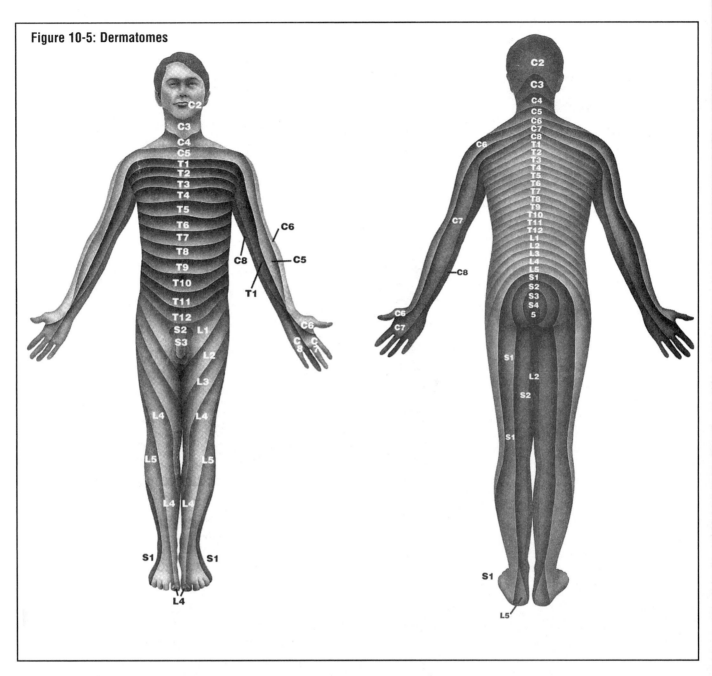

Table 10-1: Motor and Sensory Spinal Nerve Tracts

Nerve Tracts	Origin	Cross Over	Function	Location in Spinal Cord
Descending Tracts • Corticospinal (pyramidal)	Cerebral cortex	Medulla oblongata	• Voluntary motor	Anterolateral
Ascending Tracts • Spinothalamic	Sensory receptors located throughout body	Level they enter spinal cord	• Pain • Temperature • Crude touch	Anterolateral
Posterior tracts (dorsal)	Sensory receptors located throughout body	Medulla oblongata	• Proprioception • Fine touch • 2-point discrimination	Posterior (dorsal)

- Efferent (motor) neuron
- Effector (muscle, tendon, or gland that produces response)

An anatomically and physiologically intact reflex arc will function even if there is disruption of spinal cord function above the level of the reflex.[1,2]

Spinal Nerves

There are 31 pairs of spinal nerves, which include 8 cervical, 12 thoracic, 5 lumbar, 5 sacral, and 1 coccygeal (**Figure 10-6**). Each pair of spinal nerves exits the spinal cord bilaterally, and each has a posterior (dorsal) root and anterior (ventral) root. The posterior (dorsal) root transmits sensory impulses. The anterior (ventral) roots transmit motor impulses. The dorsal

Figure 10-6: Spinal Nerves and Plexuses

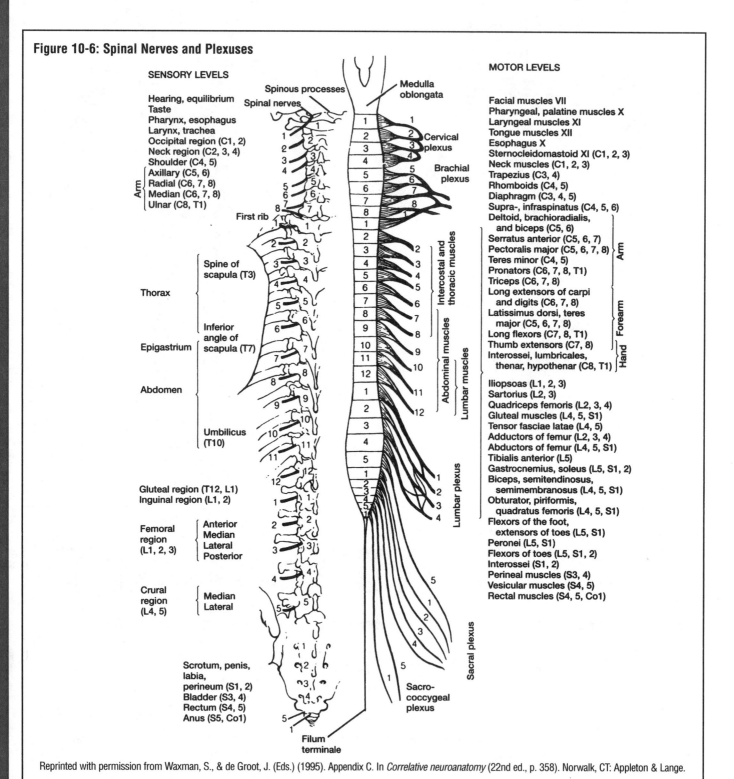

Reprinted with permission from Waxman, S., & de Groot, J. (Eds.) (1995). Appendix C. In *Correlative neuroanatomy* (22nd ed., p. 358). Norwalk, CT: Appleton & Lange.

TNCC Sixth Edition

root of each nerve innervates particular regions of the body referred to as dermatomes.

The thoracic nerves innervate the thorax, abdomen, buttocks (skin), and portions of the upper arm. The intercostal muscles are innervated by spinal nerves T-2 through T-8. The lumbar nerves innervate the groin region and lower extremities. The sacral nerves S-3 to S-5 supply the perianal muscles, which control voluntary contraction of the external bladder sphincter and the external anal sphincter.[1,2]

Plexes

A plexus is an interlacing network of nerve fibers. There are four major nerve plexes: cervical, brachial, lumbar, and sacral. The cervical plexus is formed by the first four cervical nerves, which innervate the muscles of the neck and shoulders. In addition, C-4 of the cervical plexus, with additional origins from the 3rd and 5th cervical nerve, gives rise to the phrenic nerve, which innervates the diaphragm. Spinal nerves C-5 to C-8, along with T-1, form the brachial plexus, which supplies motor control and sensation to the arm, wrist, and hand.[5,6] The brachial plexus branches include the ulnar and radial nerves. The femoral nerve arises from the lumbar plexus, formed by spinal nerves L-1 to L-4 (**Figure 10-6**), and innervates the anterior portion of the lower body.

The sciatic nerve arises from the sacral plexus, formed by L-5 to S-4. The sacral plexus innervates the posterior portion of the lower body.[1,2]

Autonomic Nervous System

The autonomic nervous system fibers innervate smooth muscle, cardiac muscle, and glands. The autonomic nervous system controls involuntary vital functions such as blood pressure, heart rate, body temperature, appetite, fluid balance, gastrointestinal motility, and sexual function.[5,6]

The autonomic nervous system has two subdivisions. The parasympathetic originates from nerves in the craniosacral regions of the central nervous system, and the sympathetic originates from the thoracolumbar region of the spinal cord. The parasympathetic division regulates bodily function under normal body conditions. Sympathetic system activity increases during physiologic and psychological stress. Specific responses from autonomic stimulation are dependent on the type and number of receptors located within a tissue, organ, or system. The generalized responses resulting from stimulation of each of these systems are listed in **Table 10-2**.[1,2]

Table 10-2: Effects of Sympathetic and Parasympathetic Stimulation[1,2]

Target Tissue, Organ, or System	Result of Sympathetic Stimulation	Result of Parasympathetic Stimulation
Skin	• ↑ Secretions from sweat glands • Piloerection	—
Cardiac	• ↑ Heart rate, conduction and contractility • Coronary artery dilation	• ↓ Heart rate, conduction, and contractility • Coronary artery constriction
Vascular	• Peripheral vasoconstriction	—
Respiratory	• ↑ Respiratory rate • Bronchial dilation • Pulmonary vascular constriction	• Bronchial constriction
Hepatic	• ↑ Glycogen breakdown and synthesis of new glucose	• Promotes glycogen synthesis
Stomach and Intestines	• ↓ Motility and tone • Sphincter contraction • ↓ Gastric secretions and mesenteric blood flow	• ↑ Motility and tone • Sphincter relaxation • ↑ Gastric secretions
Renal	• ↑ Renin secretion • Vascular constriction causes ↓ urinary output	—
Adrenal medulla	• Catecholamines, norepinephrine, and epinephrine released from adrenal glands	—

Epidemiology

Since the year 2000, approximately 11,000 Americans have sustained spinal cord injuries annually.[7] From 2000 to 2004, 79% of spinal cord injured victims were males.[7] Most men injured (41%) are between 16 and 30 years of age. Across all age groups, motor vehicle crashes account for the largest number of spinal cord and vertebral column injuries (45.6%). Falls (19.6%), violence (17.8%), and sports injuries (10.7%) are also frequent causes. More than 60% of the spinal cord injuries in people older than 75 years of age are associated with falls.[7]

Mechanisms of Injury and Biomechanics

Rapid acceleration or deceleration forces may cause the spine to move beyond its usual range of motion during a vehicular crash. Four distinct categories of injuries to the vertebral column may result from hyperextension, hyperflexion, rotation, or axial loading forces sustained in vehicular crashes. **Table 10-3** summarizes common mechanisms and their associated injuries.

The proper use of safety restraint systems minimizes the possibility of ejection. Incorrectly applied seat belts may be associated with concurrent injuries. Serious injury to the anterior neck may be associated with the use of diagonal torso belts only. Lumbar vertebral frac-

tures or dislocations may result from the use of a lap belt only.[8,9]

Types of Injuries

Most injuries to the spinal cord or vertebral column are blunt injuries from acceleration or deceleration forces on the spinal cord or vertebral column (or both). Most penetrating injuries result from gunshots that often disrupt the integrity of the vertebral column. Stab wounds do not often cause instability of the vertebral column; however, the wounding object may lacerate the spinal cord, nerve roots, or both.

Usual Concurrent Injuries

Usual concurrent injuries include closed head injuries, long-bone fractures, thoracic injuries, and abdominal injuries. Thoracic vertebral injuries may be associated with rib fractures or chest injury.[3] Pelvic fractures are frequently associated with injuries to the lumbar spine. A fall from a height, resulting in calcaneus fracture, is an additional pattern of injury associated with compression fractures of the lumbar vertebrae.[8] Because of the patient's inability to feel pain, potentially serious injuries elsewhere in the body (such as abdominal injuries) may be difficult to identify.

Associated Conditions and Special Situations

Spinal cord injuries should be suspected in near drowning victims when the events leading up to the injury are unclear. Contributing risk factors include a history of epilepsy, intoxicant use, and miscalculation of water depth. A definite association has been identi-

Table 10-3: Mechanisms of Injury to the Vertebral Column[5,6]

Mechanism of injury	Etiology of Injury (Cause)	Result of Injury (Effect)	Example	Location of Injury
Hyperextension	Backward thrust of the head beyond the anatomical capacity of the cervical vertebral column	Damage to anterior ligaments ranging from stretching to ligament tears and bony dislocations	Rear-end MVC resulting in "whiplash"	Cervical spine
Hyperflexion	Forceful forward flexion of the cervical spine with the head striking an immovable object	Wedge fractures; facet dislocations; subluxation (due to ligament rupture); teardrop, odontoid or transverse process fractures	Head-on MVC with head striking windshield creating a "star burst" effect	Cervical spine
Rotational	A combination of forceful forward flexion with lateral displacement of the cervical spine[7]	Rupture of the posterior ligament and/or anterior fracture or dislocation of the vertebral body	MVC to front or rear lateral area of vehicle resulting in conversion of forward motion to a spinning-type motion[7]	Cervical spine
Axial loading	Direct force transmitted along the length of the vertebral column	Deformity of the vertebral column; secondary edema of the spinal cord, resulting in neurologic deficits	Diver striking head on bottom of pool	T-12 to L-2

MVC = motor vehicle crash.

fied between diving and cervical spine injuries, most commonly at the C-5 or C-6 levels (or both) and particularly in the pediatric population.[10] In adult submersion victims, most cervical spine injuries result from high-impact injury such as diving, water skiing, or surfing.[11]

Patients with signs or symptoms of other "distracting injuries" (i.e., large blood loss, open fractures) and those with obvious intoxication or altered mental status of unknown etiology must be presumed to have sustained a vertebral injury until proven otherwise.[3,12] Additionally, for patients with suspected cervical spine injury, the nurse must also anticipate a closed head injury (refer to Chapter 6, Brain and Cranial Trauma).

Pathophysiology as a Basis for Signs and Symptoms

Neurologic Deficits

Whenever excessive force is applied to the spinal cord, hemorrhage, cellular damage, structural changes, biochemical responses to the injury, or all of these cause damage to the cord. The spinal cord is rarely actually severed or transected; it is usually bruised or compressed initially, resulting in hemorrhage into the tissue and edema formation. Within a few minutes after the injury, microscopic hemorrhages develop in the central gray matter. Edema also develops in the white matter, impairing cord circulation and leading to the development of ischemic areas. These changes are most prominent at the level of the injury and in the two cord segments above and below it.[5,6]

Secondary damage to the spinal cord can occur from:

- Hypovolemic shock and resulting hypoperfusion[12,13]
- Hypoxia[5,6]
- Neurogenic shock, resulting in bradycardia, peripheral vasodilation, and hypotension[5,6,9]
- Injury due to inadequate spinal immobilization
- Endogenous biochemical responses causing edema and cellular necrosis[13]

Because spinal cord neurons do not regenerate, severe injury with cellular death results in permanent loss of function. Injury to the spinal cord may result in loss of all motor and sensory functions below the level of the lesion. Loss of function may be temporary if only cellular ischemia and not cellular death has occurred.

Spinal Cord Pathology

Spinal cord injuries result from concussion, contusion, transection, or disruption of the blood supply to the cord.

- Cord concussion is a temporary loss of function lasting 24 to 48 hours. This injury may be observed in patients with preexisting degenerative disease, with resultant narrowing of the vertebral foramen.[5,6,14]
- Cord contusion is bruising of the neural tissue causing edema and possible necrosis of tissue from cord compression. The amount of neurologic deficit is dependent on the physiologic changes and the presence of necrosis.[5,6]
- A cord transection is the complete or incomplete disruption of the spinal tracts. With complete transections, all cord-mediated functions below the level of the injury are permanently lost. With incomplete transections, all function is lost temporarily; however, the potential for recovery remains based on the location and severity of injury to individual tracts. A laceration of the cord may produce permanent deficits.[5,6]
- Interruption in the vascular supply to the spinal cord may result in cord ischemia or necrosis. Temporary deficits may be caused by episodes of ischemia, whereas prolonged ischemia will result in necrosis of the spinal cord with permanent neurologic deficits.

Inadequate Ventilation

Injuries to the upper cervical region of the spinal cord are most critical because this region supports respiratory function. The most likely cause of death when a spinal cord injury occurs above C-3 is respiratory arrest due to loss of phrenic nerve function and resultant paralysis of the diaphragm. Because diaphragmatic innervation occurs at C-3 to C-5, cord injuries at this level often lead to respiratory insufficiency. Injuries between C-6 and T-8 may result in a loss of function of the intercostals and abdominal muscles, which can result in disruption of the mechanics of ventilation.[15]

Manifestations of Spinal Injury

Spinal Shock

Spinal shock results in the temporary loss of motor, sensory, and reflex functions below the level of the lesion (**Table 10-4**). The onset is usually immediate, but it can occur several days after the initial injury. The intensity and duration of spinal shock varies with the level of the lesion. Spinal shock may last for days or weeks. The patient may present with flaccid paralysis, areflexia, and bowel and bladder dysfunction. The return of sacral reflexes, bladder tone, and the presence of hyperreflexia indicates the resolution of spinal shock.[5,6,9] The presence of rectal tone and intact perineal sensation indicates sacral sparing.

Neurogenic Shock

Neurogenic shock, a form of distributive shock, is associated with spinal cord injuries at the level of T-6 or above. Impairment of the descending sympathetic pathways in the spinal cord results in loss of vasomotor tone and sympathetic innervation to the heart.[5,6] When these pathways are interrupted, loss of sympathetic activity leads to massive vasodilation and a maldistribution of blood volume, resulting in decreased preload, decreased cardiac filling, decreased stroke volume, bradycardia, and hypotension. It is important to understand that even though the patient experiences hypotension, the blood volume is normal.[12]

Vertebral Column Fractures and Dislocations

Vertebral fractures most often occur in the vertebral body or in combination with another part. Because of the mobility of the cervical and lumbar regions, they are more frequently injured.[5,6,9] Greater force is required to fracture the thoracic vertebrae because they are supported by the ribs.[15] Vertebral fractures are classified into four major categories (**Table 10-5**).

- Simple fractures
- Compression or wedge fractures
- Comminuted or burst fractures
- Teardrop fractures

Injuries to the anterior and posterior ligaments may produce unilateral or bilateral facet dislocation, resulting in malalignment (dislocation) of the vertebrae. If

Table 10-4: Neurogenic and Spinal Shock[5,6,12]

Neurogenic Shock	Spinal Shock
Precipitating injury • Spinal cord injury at T-6 or above	• Spinal cord injury at any level
Pathophysiology • Temporary loss of sympathetic tone	• Loss of reflex function below the level of injury
Duration • Temporary, often less than 72 hours[8]	• Variable (hours to weeks)
Signs/symptoms • Hypotension • Bradycardia • Loss of ability to sweat below level of injury	• Flaccidity • Loss of reflexes

Table 10-5: Vertebral Column Fractures

Fracture/Dislocation	Mechanism of Injury	Description
Simple	• Acceleration or deceleration forces	• Linear fracture of the spinous or transverse process, facets, or pedicles • Compression of spinal cord is rare • Vertebral column remains aligned
Compression (Wedge)	• Compression of vertebral body • Anterior or lateral flexion • Hyperflexion	• Fracture of vertebral body • Compression of the spinal cord may or may not be present
Comminuted (Burst)	• Axial loading	• Comminuted fracture of vertebral body • May result in spinal cord injury
Teardrop	• Hyperflexion • Axial compression	• Small fracture of anterior edge of vertebra • Fragment may impinge on cord • May have associated posterior dislocation

Reprinted from *Atlas of Emergency Radiology*, Copyright 2001, with permission from Elsevier.

the vertebrae are not completely dislocated, the injury is termed a subluxation. Dislocations and subluxations may occur simultaneously with a fracture.

Atlas and Axis Fractures

The first two vertebrae, C-1 and C-2, because of their articulation, have a wide range of motion. **Table 10-6** describes four fractures or dislocations of this region.

Vertebral Fracture Stability

Vertebral fractures are frequently classified as stable or unstable. Spinal stability is defined as:[14]

- No potential for progressive impingement or injury to the spinal cord.
- No potential for displacement of injured bony area during the healing process.
- No displacement or angulation from normal physiologic loading after healing has occurred.

Stability of the vertebral column depends on the integrity of ligamentous and bony structures. The loss of ligamentous integrity results in an unstable spinal injury. During resuscitation, assume an unstable injury exists and maintain spinal immobilization.

Spinal Cord Injury

The initial evaluation and treatment of a spinal cord injury includes distinguishing between complete and incomplete lesions.

Incomplete Spinal Cord Lesions

A patient with an incomplete lesion may have preservation of some motor or sensory function below the level of the injury. Sacral sparing (represented by intact perianal sensation, anal sphincter tone, and great toe flexor function) represents some structural integrity of the ascending and descending tracts. It is important to recognize that a patient with an incomplete lesion may not exhibit sacral sparing if spinal shock is present. As spinal shock resolves, sacral sparing becomes evident.

Patients with incomplete lesions demonstrate different signs and symptoms (**Table 10-7**). Selected incomplete lesions are referred to as specific syndromes, such as central cord syndrome, anterior cord syndrome, posterior cord syndrome, and Brown-Séquard syndrome. Comparison of bilateral upper to lower extremity motor and sensory function is important to discern the exact cord syndrome.

Complete Spinal Cord Lesion

Patients with a complete spinal cord syndrome lose all motor and sensory function below the level of the lesion. Spinal shock is frequently the initial response, resulting in loss of motor, sensory, and reflex function below the level of the injury.[5,6] The patient may also develop neurogenic shock, which results in loss of sympathetic function.

Signs and Symptoms[5,6]

- Loss of motor function below the level of the injury; flaccid paralysis of musculature
- Loss of sensory function below the level of the injury; loss of pain, touch, temperature, pressure, vibration, and proprioception
- Loss of all reflexes below the level of the injury
- Bilateral external rotation of the legs at the hips
- Loss of autonomic nervous system function (neurogenic shock)

Table 10-6: C-1 and C-2 Fractures and Dislocations

Fracture/Dislocation	Mechanism of Injury	Description
(C-1) Atlanto-occipital dislocation	• Hyperextension and extreme force	• Dislocation of atlas from the occipital bone • Usually fatal
(C-1) Atlas fracture (Jefferson fracture)	• Axial loading forces transmitted from occiput to C-1	• Varies; may be a burst fracture, comminuted, arch fracture, or transverse process fracture • Compression of spinal cord is rare
(C-2) Hangman's fracture	• Axial loading • Lateral bending forces • Hyperflexion with rapid deceleration	• Fracture(s) of C-2 may be associated with dislocation of one or both facets • Unstable fracture, but uncommon to have neurological deficit
(C-2) Odontoid fracture	• Hyperextension • Hyperflexion	• Relatively common disruption of the odontoid process projection of C-2

Reprinted from *Atlas of Emergency Radiology*, Copyright 2001, with permission from Elsevier.

- Hypotension because of loss of autonomic function, resulting in venous pooling in the extremities
  - Bradycardia and loss of thermoregulation, which are related to the loss of autonomic function. The patient may become poikilothermic, which means the patient assumes the environmental temperature. This is primarily because of the absence of vasoconstriction, but it is also related to the inability of the patient to shiver or sweat to regulate body temperature.
- Loss of voluntary bowel and bladder function, because of loss of autonomic function
- Paralytic ileus with abdominal distention
- Priapism (continuous erection of the penis) and respiratory depression may be present

Nursing Care of the Patient with a Spinal Cord and Vertebral Column Trauma

Assessment

History

Refer to Chapter 3, Initial Assessment, for a description of general information that should be collected regarding every trauma patient. Only pertinent questions specific to patients with spinal cord or vertebral column injuries are described following.

- Does the patient complain of neck or back pain?
- Was there spontaneous movement or altered sensation of the extremities?
- Was there a loss of bowel or bladder control?

The absence of these symptoms initially with subsequent development later may indicate expansion of a hematoma or additional edema formation.

Physical Assessment

Refer to Chapter 3, Initial Assessment, for a description of the assessment of the patient's airway, breathing, circulation, and disability.

Inspection

- Assess breathing effectiveness and rate of respirations.

  Assess for increased work of breathing or use of abdominal muscles and the potential for rapid deterioration in patients with cervical or upper thoracic level lesions.
- Assess motor functions.
  - Ask the patient to wiggle his or her toes and fingers; gently lift an arm and a leg.
  - The inability to perform gross extremity movement indicates a lesion above the level of injury. **Table 10-8** lists movements with their associated levels of nervous innervation.
- Logroll the patient and examine the vertebral column for deformity or open wounds.

Table 10-7: Incomplete Cord Syndromes

Syndrome	Mechanism/Etiology	Symptoms
Central cord	• Hyperextension injuries or interrupted blood supply • Swelling in the center of the cord • Bony abnormality may be absent • Most common	• Loss of motor and sensory function below the level of the lesion • Greater loss in arms than in legs • Varied degrees of bladder dysfunction
Anterior cord	• Acute anterior cord compression • Disruption of anterior spinal artery	• Loss of motor function, pain and temperature below level of injury • Crude touch, pressure, proprioception, and vibration are intact
Posterior cord	• Acute posterior cord compression or hyperextension • Rare	• Loss of proprioception, vibration, fine touch, and fine pressure below injury • Intact motor function, pain, temperature, crude touch, and crude pressure
Brown-Séquard	• Transverse hemisection of cord • Usually because of penetrating injury • Uncommon	• Loss of motor function, proprioception, and vibration sense below injury on same side • Loss of pain and temperature below injury level on opposite side of injury • Paralysis or paresis below injury level on same side

- Observe for priapism.
  - Continued erection (priapism) may be present due to the parasympathetic nervous system stimulation and loss of sympathetic nervous system control.[1,5,6]

Palpation

- Palpate pulse rate and quality.
  - Pulse is slow and strong in neurogenic shock, as opposed to rapid and weak in hypovolemic shock.
- Palpate skin temperature.
  - Skin is warm and dry in neurogenic shock, as opposed to cool and moist in hypovolemic shock. The patient may assume the temperature of the environment (poikilothermy).
- Assess all four extremities for muscle strength.
- Assess sensory function.
  - The use of a tactile stimulus such as a pinprick or cotton swab to determine levels of sensory function should begin at the area of no feeling and proceed toward the area of feeling. This will aid in localizing the level of injury to the affected dermatome (Figure 10-5). Commonly referenced dermatomes are listed in Table 10-9.
  - Proprioception is the ability of the patient to sense the position of a particular body part. Move the patient's great toe up, down, or leave it neutral. Ask the patient to describe the various positions.
- Gently palpate the entire vertebral column for pain, tenderness, crepitus, or step deformities between vertebrae.
- Palpate the anal sphincter for presence or absence of tone.
- Assess for sacral sparing.
  - The presence of perianal sensation and anal sphincter tone when seen in conjunction with other focal deficits represents an incomplete spinal cord injury.[16]

Test Reflexes

Assist with the examination of deep tendon reflexes and for presence of Babinski's reflex. In the presence of spinal shock, the patient will present with areflexia. A Babinski's reflex is a pathologic response because of dysfunction of upper motor neurons of the corticospinal tract. A positive Babinski's reflex is dorsiflexion of the great toe and fanning of the other toes when the sole of the relaxed foot is stroked.[2]

Table 10-8: Innervation Levels

Movement	Innervation
Extend and flex arms	C-5 to C-7
Extend and flex legs	L-2 to L-4
Flexion of foot; extension of toes	L-4 to L-5
Tighten anus	S-3 to S-5

Table 10-9: Dermatomal Landmarks

Anatomical Landmark	Dermatome
Top of shoulders	C-5
Nipple line	T-4
Umbilicus	T-10
Great toe	L-4

Diagnostic Procedures

Refer to Chapter 3, Initial Assessment, for frequently ordered radiographic and laboratory studies. Additional studies for patients with spinal cord or vertebral trauma or both are listed following.

Radiographic Studies

- Vertebral column radiographs
  - Obtain an initial cross-table lateral view of the cervical spine. Additional views can determine the exact site and nature of the bony injury. These views may include anterior/posterior, odontoid, and obliques. Cervical spine films should visualize all seven cervical vertebrae and T-1.
  - Radiographic studies of the thoracic and lumbar spine, as indicated. Complete radiographic evaluation is indicated if the patient has an altered mental status.
- Computed tomography scan
  - If C-7 to T-1 cannot be visualized on x-ray, consider computed tomography scan of the cervical spine.[3]
- Magnetic resonance imaging (MRI)
  - MRI is most frequently used to evaluate suspected or confirmed ligamentous and cord injuries[3] but is unable to be performed if the patient has any attached or implanted metal devices.

Planning and Implementation

Refer to Chapter 3, Initial Assessment, for a description of the specific nursing interventions for patients with compromises to airway, breathing, circulation, and disability.

- Protect the cervical spine by manual in-line stabilization until more definitive treatment is available. Manual hand stabilization of the cervical spine may be initiated without any additional equipment until a rigid cervical collar or other cervical stabilization device is available. Full spinal immobilization includes not only the use of a rigid cervical collar with secured head blocks or rolled towels but also a long spine board with a minimum of three secure straps to restrict spinal motion at all levels of the vertebral column.

- Follow individual facility protocols for "clearing" the cervical spine. Clearance of the cervical spine involves both radiographic and clinical assessments.

- Suction the airway, as needed.

  Use caution because vigorous suctioning can lead to bradycardia. Bradycardia can be caused by stimulation of the vagus nerve in combination with a loss of sympathetic function.[3]

- Administer intravenous fluids judiciously.

  Hypotension because of hypovolemia may result from occult injuries (e.g., hemothorax, splenic lacerations); therefore, fluid resuscitation to treat hypovolemia should be considered[3,12] before initiation of vasopressor therapy.

- Administer vasopressors, as prescribed.

  Hypotension may also be a symptom of neurogenic shock. Neurogenic shock results from loss of cardiac sympathetic tone and vasomotor paralysis below the level of the lesion. Hypotension and bradycardia occur when blood vessels below the level of the injury vasodilate and blood pools in the lower extremities. If neurogenic shock is present, blood pressure will not usually be restored with fluid infusion; judicious use of vasopressors may be indicated. Attempts to restore blood pressure with more than 2 liters of fluid may lead to volume overload and pulmonary edema.[3,12]

- Administer steroids, as prescribed, for nonpenetrating injuries.

  Much debate exists regarding steroid use in patients with spinal cord injuries. High-dose steroid (methylprednisolone) administration has been reported to minimize the effects of certain biochemical responses to spinal cord injury if administered within 8 hours of injury, but more recent studies have called the routine use of steroids into question based on risk-benefit ratios.[17] The primary benefit appears to be limitation of cord edema, ischemia, and the prevention of cellular death. Studies have demonstrated higher wound infections and even higher overall mortality rates in patients receiving the high-dose

steroids. If given, the recommended regimen for administration is a 30 mg/kg intravenous loading dose over 15 minutes. Wait 45 minutes; then initiate a 5.4 mg/kg/hr intravenous infusion over the next 23 hours. For maximum effect, the initial dose must be administered within the first 8 hours of injury.[12,17]

- Keep the patient warm. This may be accomplished by increasing the room temperature, infusing warmed intravenous fluids, using a commercial warming device/blanket, covering the patient with a warm blanket to prevent loss of body heat, or all of these.

- Insert a gastric tube to prevent gastric distention due to decreased peristalsis, ileus, or both.[3]

- Provide psychosocial support.

- Initiate skin care early.

  Identify and document high-risk areas of abrasions or loss of skin integrity. Because prolonged immobilization can lead to ischemic pressure ulcers, remove or pad the backboard as soon as possible.[3] Keep clean, dry linen beneath the patient and protect all bony prominences from pressure with padding.

- Assist with the application of skeletal tongs or halo device.

  Skeletal tongs with traction or halo devices or both are frequently applied in the emergency department to obtain and maintain spinal alignment and reduce patient discomfort because of muscle spasm. Once traction is applied, ensure that weights are hanging freely at all times. If a halo device is applied, make sure that the wrench for removing the chest piece is taped to the halo vest.[9]

- Prepare for interfacility transfer.

  Consider transferring the patient with a spinal cord injury (either suspected or confirmed) to a specialized facility. Consult the receiving facility regarding stabilization techniques during transfer.

Evaluation and Ongoing Assessment

Refer to Chapter 3, Initial Assessment, for a description of the ongoing evaluation of the patient's airway, breathing, circulation, and disability. Additional evaluations include:

- Monitoring breathing effectiveness

  Patients with disruption of innervation to the intercostal muscles develop respiratory fatigue

- Monitoring changes in sensory or motor function or both

- Monitoring temperature to avoid hypothermia
- Maintaining spinal protection

Summary

Blunt and penetrating injuries to the bony vertebral column may result in fractures, subluxations, or dislocations. Injury to the spinal cord may result in incomplete or complete spinal cord injuries. Anatomic transection of the cord is rare; however, physiologic cord damage may be demonstrated by motor, sensory, and sympathetic nervous system deficits.

Knowledge of the pattern of injury, including the type of forces applied to the vertebral column and the resulting flexion, extension, rotation, or all of these, is important in the assessment phase of the trauma nursing process. The patient with spinal cord or vertebral column injury needs collaborative team intervention to ensure adequate ventilation and circulation.

References

1. Seeley, R. R., Stephens, T. D., & Tate, P. (2003). *Anatomy & physiology* (6th ed.). Boston: McGraw-Hill.

2. Tortora, G. J., & Grabowski, S. R. (1996). *Principles of anatomy & physiology* (8th ed.). New York: HarperCollins.

3. Lee, T. T., & Green, B. A. (2002). Advances in the management of acute spinal cord injury. *Orthopedic Clinics of North America, 33*, 311–315.

4. Waxman, S. G., & deGroot, J. (1995). *Correlative neuroanatomy*. Norwalk, CT: Appleton & Lange.

5. Boss, B. J. (2002). Concepts of neurologic dysfunction. In K. L. McCance & S. E. Huether (Eds.), *Pathophysiology: The biologic basis for disease in adults & children* (4th ed., pp. 438–486). St. Louis, MO: Mosby.

6. Boss, B. J. (2002). Alterations of neurologic function. In K. L. McCance & S. E. Huether (Eds.), *Pathophysiology: The biologic basis for disease in adults & children* (4th ed., pp. 487–549). St. Louis, MO: Mosby.

7. Jackson, A. B., Dijker, S. M., Deviv, O. M., & Poczatek, R. B. (2004). A demographic profile of new traumatic spinal cord injuries: Change & stability over 30 years. *Archives of Physical Medicine and Rehabilitation, 85*, 1740–1748.

8. Campbell, J. E. (Ed.). (2004). *Basic trauma life support for paramedics and other advanced providers*. Upper Saddle River, NJ: Pearson Education.

9. Newberry, L. (Ed.). (2003). *Sheehy's emergency nursing principles and practice* (5th ed.). St. Louis, MO: Mosby.

10. Hwang, V., Shofer, F. S., Durbin, D. R., & Baren, J. M. (2003). Prevalence of traumatic injuries in drowning and near drowning in children and adolescents. *Archives of Pediatrics and Adolescent Medicine, 157*, 50–53.

11. Watson, R. S., Cummings, P., Quan, L., Bratton, S., & Weiss, N. S. (2001). Cervical spine injuries among submersion victims. *Journal of Trauma, 51*, 658–662.

12. Chestnut, R. M. (2004). Management of brain and spine injuries. *Critical Care Clinics, 20*, 24–55.

13. Okonkwo, D. O., & Stone, J. R. (2003). Basic science of closed head injuries and spinal cord injuries. *Clinics in Sports Medicine, 22*, 467–481.

14. Lindsey, R. W., & Gugala, Z. (2004). Injury to the vertebrae and spinal cord. In E. E. Moore, D. V. Feliciano, & K. L. Mattox (Eds.), *Trauma* (5th ed., pp. 459–492). New York: McGraw-Hill.

15. Johnson, G. A., Cohen, H., Wojtowycz, A. R., & McCabe, J. (2001). *Atlas of emergency radiology*. Philadelphia: W. B. Saunders.

16. Mermelstein, L. E., Keenen, T. L., & Benson, D. R. (1998). Initial evaluation and emergency treatment of the spine-injured patient. In B. D. Browner, J. B. Jupiter, A. M. Levine, & P. G. Trafton (Eds.), *Skeletal trauma: Fractures, dislocations, ligamentous injuries* (pp. 745–768). Philadelphia: W. B. Saunders.

17. Gomes, J. A., Stevens, R. D., Lewin J. J. III,, Mirski, M. A., & Bhardwaj, A. (2005). Glucocorticoid therapy in neurologic critical care. *Critical Care Medicine, 33*(6), 1214–1224.

In addition to the nursing diagnoses outlined in Chapter 3, Initial Assessment, the following nursing diagnoses are potential problems for the patient with spinal cord or vertebral column injuries or both. Once a patient has been assessed, diagnoses can be defined as either actual or risk. An actual nursing diagnosis is derived from a decision based on the patient's presenting signs and symptoms. A risk nursing diagnosis is a judgment that the nurse makes based on a particular patient's risk and potential for developing certain problems.

Nursing Diagnoses	Interventions	Expected Outcomes
Airway clearance, ineffective, related to: • Decreased strength of cough secondary to paralysis of chest and abdominal muscles • Presence of an artificial airway • Direct trauma • Tracheobronchial secretions or obstruction • Aspiration of foreign matter	• Open the airway with jaw thrust or chin lift while maintaining cervical spine immobilization • Suction the airway • Obtain a blood sample for arterial blood gases (ABGs) as indicated • Assist with endotracheal intubation	**The patient will maintain a patent airway, as evidenced by:** • Clear and equal bilateral breath sounds • Clear sputum of normal amount without color or odor • Absence of signs and symptoms of retained secretions: fever, tachycardia, tachypnea • Absence of signs and symptoms of airway obstruction: stridor, dyspnea, hoarse voice • Effective cough when assisted

Aspiration, risk, related to:
 	
• Impaired cough and gag reflex secondary to spinal cord injury
• Spinal immobilization devices
• Gastric distension secondary to paralytic ileus
• Reduced level of consciousness secondary to injury or concomitant substance abuse
• Trauma to head, face, and/or neck
• Increased intragastric pressure
• Impaired swallowing
• Secretions and debris in airway
	• Maintain spinal precautions
	• Position the patient
	• Open and clear the airway
	• Consider and assist with endotracheal intubation, as indicated
	• Insert gastric tube and evacuate stomach contents
	• Administer antiemetics as ordered
		The patient will not experience aspiration, as evidenced by:
		
		• Patent airway
		• Clear and equal bilateral breath sounds
		• Regular rate, depth, and pattern of breathing
		• ABG values within normal limits:
		  ▪ PaO_2 80 to 100 mm Hg (10.0 to 13.3 KPa)
		  ▪ SaO_2 > 95%
		  ▪ $PaCO_2$ 35 to 45 mm Hg (4.7 to 6.0 KPa)
		  ▪ pH 7.35 to 7.45
		• Clear chest radiograph without evidence of infiltrates
		• Ability to handle secretions independently

Nursing Diagnoses	Interventions	Expected Outcomes

Gas exchange, impaired, related to:
 	
• Altered and/or maldistributed blood flow
• Decreased oxygen-carrying capacity secondary to blood loss
• Aspiration of foreign matter
	• Administer oxygen via a nonrebreather mask
	• Ventilate with 100% oxygen via a bag-mask device, if indicated
	• Monitor oxygen saturation with continuous pulse oximetry
	• Assist with intubation and ventilatory support if diaphragm is paralyzed or if respiratory effort does not provide adequate gas exchange
	• Administer blood, as indicated
		The patient will experience adequate gas exchange, as evidenced by:
		
		• Patent airway
		• Vital signs within normal limits for age
		• Clear and equal bilateral breath sounds
		• Regular rate, depth, and pattern of breathing
		• ABG values within normal limits:
		  ▪ PaO_2 80 to 100 mm Hg (10.0 to 13.3 KPa)
		  ▪ $SaO_2 > 95\%$
		  ▪ $PaCO_2$ 35 to 45 mm Hg (4.7 to 6.0 KPa)
		  ▪ pH 7.35 to 7.45
		• $SpO_2 > 95\%$
		• Skin normal color, warm, and dry
		• Level of consciousness, awake and alert,

Fluid volume deficit, related to: • Alteration in vascular tone secondary to spinal cord injury • Maldistribution of blood volume secondary to neurogenic shock	• Cannulate two veins with large-caliber catheters and initiate infusion of isotonic crystalloid solution; monitor rate carefully • Consider vasopressors as needed • Insert urinary catheter to monitor output • Monitor hemodynamic status of patient	**The patient will have an effective circulating volume, as evidenced by:** • Stable vital signs appropriate for age • Urine output of 1 ml/kg/hr • Strong, palpable peripheral pulses • Level of consciousness, awake and alert, age appropriate • Skin normal color, warm, and dry
Tissue perfusion, altered renal, cardiopulmonary, cerebral, gastrointestinal, peripheral (specific type), related to: • Hypovolemia • Interruption of flow: arterial and/or venous • Vasoconstriction secondary to hypotension and shock	• Control any uncontrolled bleeding • Cannulate two veins with large-caliber catheters and initiate infusion of isotonic crystalloid solution • Administer blood, as indicated • Provide supplemental oxygen as needed • Prepare for definitive care	**The patient will maintain adequate tissue perfusion, as evidenced by:** • Vital signs within normal limits for age • Level of consciousness, awake and alert, age appropriate • Skin normal color, warm, and dry • Strong and equal peripheral pulses • Urine output of 1 ml/kg/hr
Thermoregulation, ineffective, related to: • Loss of hypothalamic control secondary to spinal cord injury	• Provide warm environment, warm blankets or warming lights to prevent body heat loss • Warm all intravenous fluids administered • Consider warmed oxygen	**The patient will maintain a normal core body temperature, as evidenced by:** • Core temperature measurement of 98 °F to 99.5 °F (36 °C to 37.5 °C) • Skin normal color, warm, and dry

Nursing Diagnoses	Interventions	Expected Outcomes
Injury, risk, related to: • Instability of vertebral column fracture • Altered level of consciousness • Lack of knowledge regarding spinal precautions • Increasing edema of spinal cord with ascending paralysis	• Establish and maintain immobilization • Consider a sedative or short-acting paralytic agent to maintain adequate immobilization of the restless, agitated, or violent patient • Administer methylprednisolone, as prescribed, for nonpenetrating injuries within the first 8 hours	**The patient will be free from increase in injury, as evidenced by:** • No iatrogenic extension of the injury • Movement of spine is minimized due to proper alignment and immobilization of the spinal column • Verbalizes and demonstrates understanding of need for no movement of neck • Absence of increase in extent of original injury
Ineffective coping, risk, related to: • Impact of injury on lifestyle • State of shock and denial • Loss of control over body and bodily functions • Knowledge deficit	• Provide support to the patient and family • Provide information and answer questions • Make appropriate referrals for support	**The patient will demonstrate absence or resolution of ineffective coping, as evidenced by:** • Utilizing coping strategies
Impaired skin integrity, risk, related to: • Pressure, shear, friction forces on skin and tissue • Mechanical irritants: fixation devices • Impaired mobility • Urinary and bowel incontinence • Sensory and motor deficits	• Remove patient from backboard as soon as possible • Avoid allowing a paralyzed patient to lie on backboard for more than 2 hours • Consider placement on special bed	**The patient will demonstrate absence or resolution of impaired skin integrity, as evidenced by:** • Absence of signs of irritation: redness, ulceration, blanching, itching • Verbalizes understanding of immobilization devices

Chapter 11

Musculoskeletal Trauma

Objectives

On completion of this chapter/lecture,
the learner should be able to:

1. Identify the common mechanisms
   of injury associated with musculoskeletal trauma.

2. Describe the pathophysiologic changes
   as a basis for signs and symptoms.

3. Discuss the nursing assessment
   of the patient with musculoskeletal trauma.

4. Plan appropriate interventions for
   patients with musculoskeletal trauma.

5. Evaluate the effectiveness of nursing interventions for patients with specific types of
   musculoskeletal trauma.

Preface

Lecture begins on page 186.

*Knowledge of normal anatomy and physiology serves as
the foundation for understanding the anatomic
derangements and pathophysiologic compromises that may
result from trauma. Before reading this chapter, it is strongly suggested that the
learner read the following review material. Reading about the specific anatomic
and physiologic concepts in this section will enhance the learner's ability to correlate such concepts with specific injuries. This material related to anatomy and
physiology will not be covered during lectures, nor will it be evaluated by testing.*

The musculoskeletal system and associated neurovascular structures are composed of bones, joints, tendons, ligaments, muscles, vessels, and nerves. This system provides support, strength, movement, and protection to the human body. Additionally, bones store calcium.

Types of Bone

Bone is composed of 60% mineral and 40% organic material, of which the majority is collagen. The two types of bone are compact and spongy (cancellous).[1] Compact bone is dense and more rigid than spongy bone; it forms the shaft of long bones and the exterior surface of other bones (e.g., short bones). Spongy bone is located in the interior of the bone and is constructed in a lattice-like pattern. Spongy bone contains red marrow, which is involved in the production of red blood cells. By adulthood most red marrow is converted to yellow marrow that contains adipose cells; however, the vertebrae, ribs, sternum, and ilium maintain their red bone marrow.

Classification of Bones

There are 206 bones classified into four different categories: long, short, flat, and irregular. Long bones include the femur, tibia, fibula, humerus, radius, and ulna. Short bones, such as the tarsals, are spongy bone with a compact bone surface. Flat bones provide protection and include the skull, scapula, ribs, and sternum. Flat bones are made of a layer of spongy bone and two layers of compact bone. The vertebrae and facial bones are examples of irregular bones.

Structure of Bone

The structural components of a long bone are as follows (**Figure 11-1**):

- Epiphyses—one located at each end of the bone.
- Epiphyseal plate—where longitudinal bone growth occurs (growth ceases between 18 and 25 years of age).
- Diaphysis—the compact bone that forms the shaft surrounding a medullary cavity.
- Medullary cavity—the canal located within the shaft. The medullary cavity contains yellow marrow consisting mostly of fat cells.
- Articular cartilage—a thin layer of cartilage that covers the epiphyses.
- Periosteum—the vascular layer that covers the bone except at articular surfaces. Tendons and ligaments are continuous with the periosteum.[1]

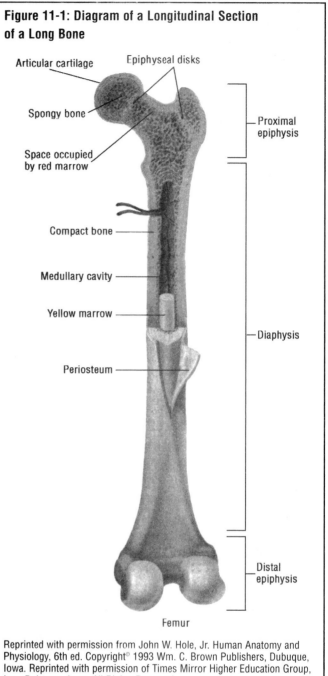

Figure 11-1: Diagram of a Longitudinal Section of a Long Bone

Articular cartilage

Epiphyseal disks

Spongy bone

Space occupied by red marrow

Proximal epiphysis

Compact bone

Medullary cavity

Yellow marrow

Periosteum

Diaphysis

Distal epiphysis

Femur

Joints, Tendons, and Ligaments

The human body has three structural types of joints: fibrous (synarthroses), cartilaginous (amphiarthroses), and synovial (diarthroses). Fibrous joints allow for little or no movement and are found between the bones of the cranium, teeth and jaw, and maxillary bones. Cartilaginous joints allow for slight movement and are found between the vertebrae and between the symphysis pubis bones. The most common and most complex types of joints are the synovial joints, which are freely movable. Examples include the knee, wrist, hip, and shoulder.

The musculoskeletal system is also supported by other structures, which include tendons and ligaments. Tendons are thick, white, fibrous materials that attach muscles to bones. The white color comes from collagen fibers, which give tendons their tensile strength. Tendons allow for movement of the extremity by extension or flexion of the muscle groups. As the muscle group moves, the tendon pulls the distal bone in the desired direction. Tendons are not elastic and contain a minimal blood supply.

Ligaments are bands of fibrous connective tissue that attach bones to bones. They have elastic fibers to provide the stretch necessary to move bones. These structures help stabilize joints and assist in movement.

Skeletal (striated) muscles are voluntary muscles whose fibers fuse with tendon fibers and insert into bones. Muscles are covered by fascia, a fibrous membrane that supports and separates muscles.

Blood and Nerve Supply

Small blood vessels permeate the bone and periosteum. Large vessels enter and exit through the articular ends and supply the open spaces of the spongy bone. A medullary artery that enters through the middle of the diaphysis usually supplies the medullary canal. Large and small vessels traverse the length of long bones, often curving around the bone and through surrounding muscle and soft tissue.

Nerves are distributed throughout the periosteum and usually accompany arteries. Nerves transmit impulses from the brain to the skeletal muscles along descending pathways to initiate fine and gross extremity movement.

Pelvis

The pelvis is a ring formed by the sacrum and two innominate bones (**Figure 11-2**). Each innominate bone is formed by the fusion of the ilium, ischium, and pubis.[2] The innominate bones are connected posteriorly to the sacrum at the sacroiliac joints and are joined anteriorly at the symphysis pubis. The stability of the pelvis is maintained by ligaments. Many blood vessels are located in the pelvic cavity and along the inner wall of the pelvis. Those veins in the pelvis form a large venous plexus. The pelvis is a weight-bearing structure and provides protection to the lower abdominal viscera.[1,2]

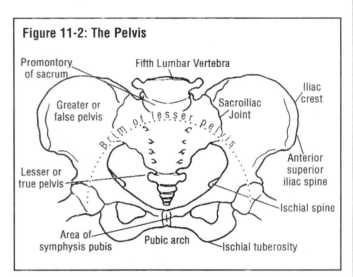

Figure 11-2: The Pelvis

Introduction

Epidemiology

More than half of all hospital admissions because of trauma are patients with some type of fracture, usually of the lower limb.[3] The National Center for Health Statistics reported an annual estimate of 54.9 million musculoskeletal injuries, with fractures accounting for 10.5 million of this total. Sprains and dislocations accounted for 22.9 million.[4] Older adults (those over 65 years of age) are at particularly high risk of being hospitalized for an extremity injury.

Mechanisms of Injury and Biomechanics

Musculoskeletal trauma can be sustained as a single-system injury or in combination with other systems. Injuries to the extremities are not usually considered the first priority unless the injury affects the hemodynamic status. Mechanisms of injury include motor vehicle crashes, assaults, falls, sports, or home activities. Close attention to the mechanism of injury can aid in the treatment and prognosis of the patient.

Musculoskeletal injuries can result from the application of both acceleration and deceleration forces. Injuries to the bone result from tension, compression, bending, and torsion-type forces.[5] When there is enough force to fracture the shaft of a bone, this force may be transmitted to the joints; for example, fractures of the shaft of the radius and ulna may be associated with fractures to the wrist, elbow, and shoulder.

Falls are a frequent mechanism of injury, especially for older adults. Older adults who fall often sustain pelvic or lower extremity injuries. These injuries, even if not life-threatening, can seriously alter an older person's lifestyle and reduce his or her functional independence. Underlying bone disease, such as osteoporosis or cancer metastases, may predispose the patient to an extremity injury.[5]

Calcaneus fractures may occur when people fall or jump and land on their feet. The force of the impact is transmitted upward, compressing the vertebral bodies. People then tend to fall forward and extend their arms to cushion the fall, which results in wrist fractures. Thus, patients with fractured calcaneus bones may have concurrent thoracolumbar vertebral fractures, bilateral wrist fractures, or both.

When the patella comes in contact with the dashboard during a motor vehicle crash, the impact often results in a femur fracture, posterior hip fracture/dislocation, popliteal artery damage, or all three.[6] A pedestrian hit by an automobile may have bilateral tibia and fibula fractures from contact with the front bumper of the car.

Differentiating between unintentional and intentional injury can be difficult. Suspicion of abuse should be raised if the type or degree of injury does not correspond to the history.

Types of Injuries

Musculoskeletal injuries may be blunt or penetrating. They may involve bone, soft tissue, muscles, nerves, blood vessels, or all of these. Injuries include fractures or dislocations of the bone or joint (or both), sprains, strains, ligamentous tears, tendon lacerations, and neurovascular compromises.

Usual Concurrent Injuries

Bony extremity injuries may be associated with concurrent injury to nerves, arteries, veins, or soft tissue. Neurovascular injury should be suspected with any injury to the bones of an extremity. Severe pelvic fractures can be associated with injuries to pelvic organs and large-volume blood loss. Genitourinary injuries, especially to the bladder or the urethra in males, can result from pelvic fractures. Depending on the mechanism of injury, bony injury of the extremities may be associated with vertebral column injuries.

Pathophysiology as a Basis for Signs and Symptoms

Blood Loss

Musculoskeletal trauma can be associated with large-volume blood loss because of disruption of arteries or veins in close proximity to bones. Up to 1,500 ml of blood can be lost from an isolated femur fracture. A tibial or humeral fracture can lead to a blood loss of up to 750 ml.[7] Multiple fractures may result in significant blood loss, which can potentiate shock from other injuries. Blood loss from pelvic fractures varies significantly based on the mechanism of injury, the type of fracture, the particular vessels injured, and whether there are other intra-abdominal injuries.

Capillaries and cellular membranes can be disrupted or torn with all types of musculoskeletal injuries. Blood from vascular disruption and intracellular fluid are released into the area surrounding the injury. Edema from fluid and blood accumulation can cause compression of surrounding structures. Normal physiologic mechanisms are activated to minimize damage caused by these structural disruptions:

- Initiation of the clotting system to decrease bleeding
- Restoration of cellular membrane integrity to enhance fluid reabsorption
- Increased collateral blood flow to promote healing

Bone or joint displacement can compress surrounding vessels and nerves, causing pathophysiologic changes distal to the injury. As arterial blood flow is obstructed, tissue oxygenation decreases, resulting in tissue ischemia and cellular death. During this process, pain increases; pulses become more difficult to palpate; the limb becomes pale, cyanotic, and cool; and capillary refill time increases.

Neurologic Deficits

If nerves are compressed or lacerated, conduction pathways are interrupted, and the relay of nerve impulses is blocked or diminished. Nerve injury can result in diminished pain sensation. Injury distal to a nerve may result in partial or complete loss of motor and sensory function.

Fractures

Fractures involve a disruption of bony continuity (Table 11-1).

Selected Musculoskeletal Injuries

Joint Injuries

A joint may become dislocated when the normal range of motion is exceeded. Joint dislocations may be complicated by neurovascular compromise and associated fractures. Delayed reduction of a hip dislocation can lead to avascular necrosis of the femoral head and permanent disability.[8] More recent research has shown that avascular necrosis may also result from the initial injury, therefore early reduction (6 to 24 hours after injury) is suggested.[8] Dislocation of the knee requires immediate intervention because per-

Table 11-1: Types of Fractures

Type of Fracture	Description
Open	Skin integrity over or near a fracture site is disrupted
Closed	Skin integrity over or near a fracture site is intact
Complete	Total interruption in bony continuity
Incomplete	Incomplete interruption in bony continuity
Comminuted	Splintering of bone into fragments
Greenstick	Bone buckles or bends; fracture does not go through the entire bone
Impacted	Distal and proximal fracture sites are wedged into each other
Displaced	Proximal and distal fracture sites are out of alignment

oneal nerve injury and compromises to the popliteal artery and vein may develop. Angiography is necessary to diagnose vascular trauma.

Signs and Symptoms

- Pain
- Joint deformity
- Edema
- Inability to move the affected joint
- Abnormal range of motion
- Neurovascular compromise: Distal pulses may be diminished or absent; sensory function may be affected

Femur Fractures

Femur fractures are a result of major trauma, such as falls, motor vehicle crashes, or missiles causing penetrating wounds. Fractures of the femoral neck are common after a fall in the older adult population. Certain types of femur fractures can result in a collection of 1,000 to 1,500 ml of blood in the thigh.[7]

Signs and Symptoms

- Pain and inability to bear weight
- Shortening of the affected leg
- Rotation internally or externally, depending on the location of the fracture site in the hip
- Edema of the thigh
- Deformity of the thigh
- Evidence of hypovolemic shock

Pelvic Fractures

Pelvic fractures are classified as either stable or unstable.[9] A stable fracture is defined as "one that can withstand normal physiologic forces without abnormal deformation."[9] An unstable fracture occurs when the pelvic ring is fractured in more than one place, resulting in two displacements on the ring; rotational displacement is always present. Pelvic fractures may be further classified by the type of force that caused the injury. The forces are external rotation (anteroposterior), lateral compression, external rotation (abduction), and shear.[9] Attention to both biomechanical and anatomic aspects of the injury is required.

These fractures can be life-threatening and are often accompanied by large-volume blood loss and injury to the genitourinary system.[9] Bleeding may originate from lacerated veins, arteries, or the fracture itself. Arterial injuries occur in 20% of patients, and posterior fractures are more likely than anterior fractures to cause bleeding. Anteroposterior compression may cause significant hemorrhage. Patients with lateral compression fractures may require two to four units of blood replacement.[10] The bleeding may be significant enough to cause hypovolemic shock.

Injuries to the pelvis may be open or closed. Open pelvic fractures may be associated with injuries to the perineum, genitourinary structures, or rectum and have a significantly higher mortality rate.[9]

Signs and Symptoms

- Pain
- Evidence of hypovolemic shock
- Shortening or abnormal rotation of the affected leg
- Genitourinary (look for blood at the meatus) or intra-abdominal injury

Open Fractures

All open fractures are considered contaminated because of the foreign materials and bacteria that can be introduced into the wound. Any open fracture may result in an infection, which may be manifested by poor wound healing, osteomyelitis, or sepsis. The risk of serious infection is greater with severe fractures. Open fractures are graded from I to III according to the degree of skin and soft tissue injury surrounding the fracture site. Grade I open fractures have minimal soft tissue damage. Grade II open fractures have wounds larger than 2 cm with the presence of slight crush injury. Grade III open fractures have extensive soft tissue damage and a high degree of contamination.[11] Grade III open fractures are further described by the amount of nonviable tissue and vascular trauma.[12]

Signs and Symptoms

- Evidence of skin disruption (e.g., laceration or puncture) near or over the fracture
- Protrusion of bone through open wounds
- Pain
- Neurovascular compromise
- Bleeding (may be minimal to severe)

Amputations

Amputations may be partial or complete and usually involve the digits, distal half of the foot, the lower leg, the hand, or the forearm. The axiom of saving "life over limb" is a reminder to the trauma team to fully resuscitate the patient before managing the amputation.

Guillotine-type amputations have a better chance of being successfully replanted than avulsive/tearing types of injuries. The decision to replant should be made by a surgeon or reimplantation team, if available.

The following have been identified as candidates for reimplantation[13]

- Multiple digits
- Thumb
- Wrist
- Forearm
- Pediatric patients (children typically have a more positive outcome from reimplantation procedures)[13,14]

Signs and Symptoms

- Obvious tissue loss
- Pain
- Bleeding (may be minimal to severe)

  Complete amputations will have less active bleeding than partial amputations because of retraction of the severed arteries. An exception is an avulsive type of complete amputation, which can result in extensive bleeding.

- Evidence of hypovolemic shock

Crush Injuries

Crush injuries can result from prolonged entrapment or a crushing blow. Certain crush injuries, depending on the location of the injury, may be life-threatening (e.g., pelvis and both lower extremities). Cellular destruction and damage to vessels and nerves make crush injuries difficult to treat. Hemorrhage from the damaged tissue, destruction of muscle and bone tissue, fluid loss resulting in hypovolemic shock, compartment syndrome, and infection are sequelae associated with crush injuries. The destruction of muscle tissue associated with release of myoglobin can result in renal dysfunction.[15]

Signs and Symptoms

- Massively crushed pelvis or extremity(ies) with soft tissue swelling
- Pain
- Evidence of hypovolemic shock
- Signs of compartment syndrome
- Loss of neurovascular function distal to the injury

Compartment Syndrome

Compartment syndrome occurs as pressure increases inside a fascial compartment (**Figure 11-3**). This pressure increase results in impaired capillary blood flow and cellular ischemia. Compartment syndrome occurs more frequently in the muscles of the lower leg or forearm, but it can involve any fascial compartment. The increased pressure may be because of an internal source, such as hemorrhage or edema caused by open or closed fractures, or crush injuries. It can also result from an external source, such as a cast,

Figure 11-3: Compartments of the Lower Leg

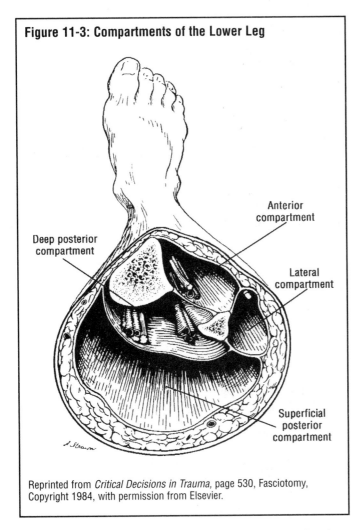

Deep posterior compartment

Anterior compartment

Lateral compartment

Superficial posterior compartment

Reprinted from *Critical Decisions in Trauma*, page 530, Fasciotomy, Copyright 1984, with permission from Elsevier.

excessive traction, air splint, or pneumatic antishock garment. Nerves, blood vessels, and muscles can be compressed.[13] If pressures are not released within the compartment, the muscle and nerve tissue can die within 6 hours. The muscle death can result in permanent loss of function or even require amputation. The degree of damage depends on the amount of pressure as well as the length of time blood flow in the compartment has been compromised. The nurse must remain vigilant for signs of compartment syndrome.

Signs and Symptoms

The six Ps associated with compartment syndrome are

- **Pain:** Pain out of proportion to the extent of the injury is suspicious for developing or having actual compartment syndrome. A hallmark sign of compartment syndrome is pain on passive range of motion of the affected compartment.
- **Pallor:** Poor skin color and cool temperature reflects poor perfusion to the area.
- **Pulses:** Vascular compromise can be associated with circumferential edema or direct injury to the vessels.

- **Paresthesia:** Sensory deficits, such as numbness, tingling, or loss of sensation may occur as nerves and blood vessels are compressed.
- **Paralysis:** Motor dysfunction reflects injury to the nervous system.
- **Pressure:** Involved compartment or limb will feel tense on palpation.[16]

Other signs and symptoms include

- Progressive muscle weakness
- Elevated muscle compartment pressures

Nursing Care of the Patient with Musculoskeletal Trauma

Assessment

History

Refer to Chapter 3, Initial Assessment, for a description of general information that should be collected regarding every trauma patient. Only pertinent questions specific to patients with musculoskeletal injuries are described following.

- What was the mechanism of injury?
- Was it a high-energy or low-energy incident?
- What position was the patient in when the incident occurred?
- What position was the patient found in?
- Where did the incident occur?

  Information regarding the specific injuring agents or points of contact with any extremity provides important clues in identifying the specific type and extent of injury as well as in anticipating and treating any potential sequelae resulting from the original injury.

- Was any previous treatment or splinting done before arrival?
- Is there a history of previous orthopedic problems?

Physical Assessment

Refer to Chapter 3, Initial Assessment, for a description of assessment of the patient's airway, breathing, circulation, and disability.

Inspection

- Observe the general appearance of the extremities. Note the color, position, and obvious differences of the injured extremity as compared to the uninjured extremity, such as shortening, rotation, displacement, or loss of function.

- Assess the integrity of the injured area.

  Note protrusion of bone, any break in the skin, or soft tissue abnormalities that may indicate fractures or dislocations beneath the skin.

- Assess for bleeding.

  Estimation of external blood loss is an essential aspect of the inspection phase because it provides important information about the patient's hemodynamic status.

- Assess for deformity or angulation of the extremity (or both).

- Assess for muscle spasm.

Palpation

- Extremity assessment is described by the six Ps: pain, pallor, pulses, paresthesia, paralysis, and pressure.[16] This assessment relates to the neurovascular status of the injured extremity. Assess the injured extremity and compare it with the opposite, uninjured extremity.

  - Pain

    Carefully palpate the entire length of each extremity for pain or tenderness. Determine the location and quality of pain. Ischemic pain is often described as burning or throbbing.

    Assess for full range of motion to all extremities.

  - Pallor

    Note the color and temperature of the injured extremity. Pallor, delayed capillary refill (greater than 2 seconds), and a cool extremity may indicate vascular compromise; however, consider the ambient temperature.

  - Pulses

    Palpate pulses proximal and distal to the injury for comparison. Then compare the quality of pulses with those of the opposite, uninjured extremity. Note: Maintaining a pulse does not rule out compartment syndrome, because loss of pulses is a late sign.

  - Paresthesia

    Determine the presence of abnormal sensations (e.g., burning, tingling, numbness).

  - Paralysis

    Assess motor function for both active and passive range of motion. The ability to move can be related to neurologic function.

    In extremities where there is an obvious injury, motor function or range of motion may be deferred because of the risk of exacerbating damage to the surrounding structures (muscles and nerves).

  - Pressure

    Palpate the extremity for firmness of compartments and muscle spasm.

- Palpate the pelvis for pain or bony instability.

  Apply gentle pressure on the iliac crests toward the midline, noting any instability or increased pain. Gently press downward on the symphysis pubis. If a fracture is suspected, carefully palpate the pelvis. Do not rock the pelvis.

- During palpation, note bony crepitus, which is a crackling sound produced by the grating of the ends of fractured bones.

Diagnostic Procedures

Refer to Chapter 3, Initial Assessment, for frequently ordered radiographic and laboratory studies. Additional studies for patients with musculoskeletal trauma are listed following.

Radiographic Studies

- Obtain at least two views at right angles of the injured extremity. These are usually anterior-posterior and lateral views. Consider also an oblique view.

  Some fractures can only be seen from one radiographic angle; therefore, an oblique view may be indicated. The film should include the joints immediately above and below the injury.

- Angiography

  Angiography may be indicated to identify tears or compressions in the arterial or venous network of the injured extremity.

Planning and Implementation

Refer to Chapter 3, Initial Assessment, for a description of the specific nursing interventions for patients with compromises to airway, breathing, circulation, and disability.

- Control bleeding.
- Splint and immobilize the affected extremity.
  - Splinting is indicated when there is evidence of the following:
    - Deformity
    - Pain
    - Bony crepitus
    - Edema
    - Ecchymosis
    - Circulatory compromise

- Open soft tissue injury
- Impaled object
- Paresthesia or paralysis

- Select an appropriate splint. Three types of splints are available:
  - Rigid splints, such as cardboard, plastic devices, or metal splints
  - Soft splints, such as pillows, slings, or air splints
  - Traction splints—applied for actual or suspected femur or proximal tibial fractures
- Remove jewelry or constricting items of clothing before immobilization.
- Do not reposition protruding bone ends.
- Immobilize the joints above and below the deformity.
- Modify the splint to fit the fracture, if necessary.
- Avoid excessive movement of the fractured bone fragments. Any manipulation can increase bleeding into the tissues, increase the risk of fat emboli, or convert a closed fracture to an open fracture.
- Assess neurovascular status before and after immobilization. If the neurovascular status is compromised, reassess, remove, adjust, or reapply the splint.

- Apply ice to reduce swelling and pain. Ice is not indicated if compartment syndrome is suspected.
- Elevate the extremity above the level of the heart to reduce swelling and pain. However, if compartment syndrome is suspected, maintain the extremity at the level of the heart.
- Administer analgesic medications, as prescribed.
- Consider regional analgesia, such as a nerve block.
- Prepare for definitive stabilization. Traction, casting, closed reduction, or internal or external fixation may be indicated.
- Prepare for procedural sedation, as prescribed.
- Provide psychosocial support.
- Prepare the patient for operative intervention or hospital admission or transfer, as indicated.

Nursing Interventions for the Patient with a Pelvic Fracture

- Stabilize pelvic fractures with one of the following options:
  - Wrap the pelvis in a folded sheet that is clamped or knotted at the front, or use a commercially prepared device for this purpose.

- Apply a pneumatic antishock garment to splint pelvic fractures.
- Prepare for application of an external fixator. Unstable pelvic fractures with severe blood loss may require immediate stabilization with an external fixator.[11] External fixation is a method of fracture immobilization in which percutaneous pins are connected to a rigid frame. It is the treatment of choice for a closed fracture that will not maintain position. This method is often used with open fractures, fractures with extensive soft tissue damage, or the unstable patient.[17]

- Assist with additional diagnostic radiographs, including cystogram, angiogram, or computed tomography (CT) scan of the pelvis, as ordered. Patients must be carefully monitored during angiography and related therapeutic embolization.

Nursing Interventions for the Patient with an Open Fracture

- Irrigate any wound with sterile saline, as indicated.
- Cover open wounds with dry, sterile dressings. Avoid frequent dressing changes to minimize the risk of bacterial contamination.
- Administer antibiotics, as prescribed.
- Inspect dressings frequently for continued bleeding.
- Administer tetanus prophylaxis, as indicated.

Nursing Interventions for the Patient with an Amputation

- Control any active bleeding with pressure dressings and elevation. Utilize tourniquets as a last resort when pressure and elevation do not control the bleeding.
- Elevate the stump.
- Splint the stump as needed.
- Remove gross dirt or debris.
- Keep the amputated part cool and wrap it in a saline-moistened gauze, then place in a sealed plastic bag, and finally place the bag in crushed ice and water. Do not allow the part to freeze.
- Prepare for radiographs of both the stump and the amputated part.
- Prepare the patient for hospital admission, operative intervention, or transfer to a facility with a reimplantation team, as indicated.
- Administer antibiotics, as prescribed.
- Administer tetanus prophylaxis, as indicated.

Nursing Interventions for the Patient with a Crush Injury

- Administer an intravenous isotonic crystalloid solution to increase urinary output and facilitate excretion of myoglobin.

- Elevate the injured extremity above the level of the heart to reduce swelling and pain unless compartment syndrome is suspected. For suspected compartment syndrome, maintain the injured extremity at the level of the heart.

- Gently clean open wounds.

- Prepare the patient for surgical debridement, fasciotomy, and/or amputation.

Nursing Interventions for the Patient with Possible Compartment Syndrome

- Elevate the limb to the level of the heart to promote venous outflow and prevent further swelling. Do not elevate the limb above the heart because this may decrease perfusion to a compromised extremity.

- Assist with measurement of fascial compartment pressure, as indicated. Normal pressure is 0 to 8 mm Hg. A reading of greater that 30 to 40 mm Hg is suggestive of possible anoxia to muscles and nerves. Measurement is performed by a physician inserting a large-caliber needle or catheter into the fascia of the involved muscle and attaching it to a manometer or pressure monitor.[18]

- Prepare for fasciotomy, as indicated. A fasciotomy may prevent muscle or neurovascular damage (or both) and loss of the limb.

- Reassess and document the neurovascular status on an ongoing basis. Communicate changes to the physician immediately.

Evaluation and Ongoing Assessment

Refer to Chapter 3, Initial Assessment, for a description of the ongoing evaluation of the patient's airway, breathing, circulation, and disability. Additional evaluations include

- Monitoring breathing effectiveness and rate of respiration.

  Tachypnea, rales, and wheezes may be indicators of fat embolus syndrome. Fat embolism is a potential complication of long-bone fractures that may present as acute respiratory insufficiency.[18]

- Reassessing and documenting the six Ps.

- Reassessing the following:
  - Urinary output
  - Presence of myoglobin in the urine
  - Motor and sensory function

Summary

Injuries of the extremities are usually not the first priority of care for the patient with multiple trauma. However, there is a high incidence of injuries to upper and lower extremities that, although usually not life-threatening, can result in functional disability, loss, or both, and long-term rehabilitation.

The proximity of vessels and nerves to musculoskeletal structures increases the risk of neurovascular damage ranging from motor, sensory, or vascular deficits to paralysis or hemorrhage (or both) and shock. Disruptions and fractures of the pelvis may result in significant blood loss because of concurrent injury to the blood vessels in the pelvic cavity. Nurses should collaborate with members of the trauma team to correct any life-threatening compromises to circulation.

During the secondary assessment, assess the extremities for indications of a fracture or dislocation. Intervene early to splint the suspected fracture and reassess neurovascular function both before and after the application of any splinting device.

Timely identification and management of suspected musculoskeletal injuries, including the use of pain control, splints, traction, external fixation, or all of these, contributes to improved functional patient outcomes.

References

1. Stendring, S. (2005). Functional anatomy of the musculoskeletal system. In *Gray's anatomy: The anatomical basis of clinical practice* (39th ed., pp. 83–112). Edinburgh: Elsevier Churchill Livingston.

2. Cwinn, A. A. (2002). Pelvis and hip. In P. Rosen & R. M. Barkin (Eds.), *Emergency medicine: Concepts and clinical practice* (5th ed., pp. 625–642). St. Louis, MO: Mosby.

3. Trafton, P. G. (2004). Lower extremity fractures and dislocations. In K. L. Mattox, D. V. Feliciano, & E. E. Moore (Eds.), *Trauma* (5th ed., pp. 939–969). New York: McGraw-Hill.

4. National Center for Health Statistics. (2001). *National hospital ambulatory medical care survey and national ambulatory medical care survey.* Retrieved January 25, 2006, from http://www.usbjd.org/healthcare_pro/resources/Facts_in_Brief_2004.doc

5. Hipp, J. A., & Hayes, W. C. (2003). Biomechanics of fractures. In B. D. Browner, J. B. Jupiter, A. M. Levine, & P. G. Trafton (Eds.), *Skeletal trauma fractures, dislocations, ligamentous injuries* (3rd ed., pp. 90–119). Philadelphia: W. B. Saunders.

6. American College of Surgeons Committee on Trauma. (2004). Biomechanics of trauma. In *Advanced trauma life support® course for doctors (Instructor course manual)* (6th ed., pp. 417–438). Chicago: Author.

7. American College of Surgeons Committee on Trauma. (2004). Musculoskeletal trauma. In *Advanced trauma life support® for doctors (Student course manual)* (7th ed., pp. 205–219). Chicago: Author.

8. Goulet, J., & Levin, P. (2003). Hip dislocations. In B. D. Browner, J. B. Jupiter, A. M. Levine, & P. G. Trafton (Eds.), *Skeletal trauma fractures, dislocations, ligamentous injuries* (3rd ed., pp. 1657–1690). Philadelphia: W. B. Saunders.

9. Mayo, K., Kellam, J. F., & Browner, B. D. (2003). Pelvic ring disruptions. In B. D. Browner, J. B. Jupiter, A. M. Levine, & P. G. Trafton (Eds.), *Skeletal trauma fractures, dislocations, ligamentous injuries* (3rd ed., pp. 1052–1108). Philadelphia: W. B. Saunders.

10. Scalea, T. M., & Burgess, A. R. (2004). Pelvic fractures. In K. L. Mattox, D. V. Feliciano, & E. E. Moore (Eds.), *Trauma* (5th ed., pp. 779–809). New York: McGraw-Hill.

11. Kunkler, C.E. (2002). Fractures. In A. B. Maher, S. W. Salmond, & T. A. Pellino (Eds.), *Orthopaedic nursing* (3rd ed., pp. 609–650). Philadelphia: W. B. Saunders.

12. Sirkin, M., & Behrens, F. F. (2003). Fractures with soft tissue injuries. In B. D. Browner, J. B. Jupiter, A. M. Levine, & P. G. Trafton (Eds.), *Skeletal trauma fractures, dislocations, ligamentous injuries* (3rd ed., pp. 293–319). Philadelphia: W. B. Saunders.

13. Antosia, R. E., & Lyn, E. (2002). The hand. In P. Rosen & R. Barkin (Eds.), *Emergency medicine: Concepts in clinical practice* (5th ed., pp. 493–534). St. Louis, MO: Mosby.

14. Meyer, F. (2004). Upper extremity and hand injuries. In K. L. Mattox, D. V. Feliciano, & E. E. Moore (Eds.), *Trauma* (5th ed., pp. 901–939). New York: McGraw-Hill.

15. Chandler, C. F., Blinman, T., & Cryer, H. G. (2004). Acute renal failure. In K. L. Mattox, D. V. Feliciano, & E. E. Moore (Eds.), *Trauma* (5th ed., pp. 1323–1351). New York: McGraw-Hill.

16. Harvey, C. (2001, May/June). Compartment syndrome: When it is least expected. *Orthopaedic Nursing, 20*(3), 15–25.

17. Redemann, S. (2003). Modalities for immobilization. In A. Maher, S. Salmond, & T. Pellino (Eds.), *Orthopedic nursing* (3rd ed., pp. 302–324). Philadelphia: W. B. Saunders.

18. Pellino, T., Preston, M., Bell, N., Newton, M., & Hansen, K. (2003). Complications of orthopedic disorders and orthopedic surgery. In A. Maher, S. Salmond, & T. Pellino (Eds.), *Orthopedic nursing* (3rd ed., pp. 230–269). Philadelphia: W. B. Saunders.

In addition to the nursing diagnoses outlined in Chapter 3, Initial Assessment, the following nursing diagnoses are potential problems for the patient with musculoskeletal injuries. Once a patient has been assessed, diagnoses can be defined as either actual or risk. An actual nursing diagnosis is derived from a decision based on the patient's presenting signs and symptoms. A risk nursing diagnosis is a judgment the nurse makes based on a particular patient's risk and potential for developing certain problems.

Nursing Diagnoses	Interventions	Expected Outcomes
Fluid volume deficit, related to: • Hemorrhage	• Control any uncontrolled bleeding by applying direct pressure over bleeding site; elevating extremity; applying pressure over arterial pressure sites • Cannulate two veins with large-caliber catheters and initiate infusion of isotonic crystalloid solution • Administer blood, as indicated	**The patient will have an effective circulating volume, as evidenced by:** • Stable vital signs appropriate for age • Urine output of 1 ml/kg/hr • Strong, palpable peripheral pulses • Level of consciousness, awake and alert, age appropriate • Skin normal color, warm, and dry • Maintenance of hematocrit of 30 ml/dl or hemoglobin of 12 to 14 g/dl or greater • Capillary refill time of < 2 seconds • Control of external hemorrhage
Physical mobility, impaired, related to: • Bone, soft tissue, and/or nerve injury of extremity • Pain • Edema • External immobilization devices • Limited range of motion of affected bone	• Splint injured extremity • Splint and immobilize affected extremity • Immobilize joints above and below the deformity • Administer analgesic medications, as prescribed • Use touch, positioning, or relaxation techniques to give comfort	**The patient will experience increased mobility, as evidenced by:** • Ability to tolerate movement and increased activity • Willingness to move affected part to degree allowed • Maintenance of proper body alignment
Infection, risk, related to: • Impaired skin integrity • Contamination of wound from initial injury or instrumentation • Invasive fixation devices • Interruption in perfusion • Suppressed inflammatory response	• Obtain blood/wound cultures • Monitor vital signs • Administer antibiotics, as prescribed • Keep wound clean and apply dressing using aseptic technique • Maintain aseptic technique • Cover open wounds with a sterile dressing • Do not reposition protruding bone fragments • Prepare for definitive care • Stabilize impaled objects	**The patient will be free from infection, as evidenced by:** • Core temperature measurement of 98 to 99.5 °F (36 to 37.5 °C) • White blood cell count within normal limits • Absence of signs of infection: redness, swelling, purulent drainage, odor, and tenderness
Impaired skin integrity, risk, related to: • Movement of fractured bones • Pressure, shear, friction on skin and tissue • Mechanical irritants: fixation devices, splints, and casting material • Impaired mobility • Effects of trauma/injury agents	• Assess skin integrity frequently • Keep skin dry • Maintain aseptic/clean technique, as appropriate • Splinting, as indicated	**The patient will experience absence or resolution of impaired skin integrity, as evidenced by:** • Maintenance of intact skin overlying fracture • Absence of signs of irritation: redness, blanching, and itching

Nursing Diagnoses	Interventions	Expected Outcomes
Pain, related to: • Soft tissue injury and pressure • Fractures • Tissue stretching and edema • Neurovascular compromise • Experience during invasive procedures/diagnostic tests	• Administer analgesic medication, as prescribed • Administer analgesia before invasive therapy • Use touch, positioning, or relaxation techniques to give comfort • Immobilize and elevate the injured extremity • Apply ice to reduce pain and swelling	**The patient will experience relief of pain, as evidenced by:** • Diminishing or absent level of pain through patient's self-report • Absence of physiologic indicators of pain, which include tachycardia, tachypnea, pallor, diaphoretic skin, and increasing blood pressure • Absence of nonverbal cues of pain: crying, grimacing, inability to assume position of comfort • Ability to cooperate with care, as appropriate • Relief of pain when injury is not manipulated • Proper alignment of extremity
Tissue perfusion, altered peripheral, related to: • Vessel compression secondary to edema • Vessel compression secondary to compartment syndrome • Loss of normal contour or alignment • Hypovolemia • Interruption of flow: arterial and/or venous	• Assess neurovascular status before and after application of a splint • Remove jewelry or constrictive clothing before splinting • Elevate to the level of the heart if compartment syndrome is suspected • Control any uncontrolled bleeding • Cannulate two veins with large-caliber catheters and initiate infusion of isotonic crystalloid solution • Administer blood, as indicated • Prepare for definitive care	**The patient will maintain adequate peripheral tissue perfusion, as evidenced by:** • Absence of ischemic pain and motor paralysis • Capillary refill time of < 2 seconds • Skin normal color, warm, and dry distal to injury • Strong and regular peripheral pulses • Absence of changes in mobility • Normal sensation
Injury, risk, related to: • Immobility • Instability of skeleton • Mechanical irritants	• Monitor the six Ps • Reposition, as indicated • Protect patient from environmental hazards • Monitor for the development/progression of pain, pressure, paresthesia, decreasing pulse, or paralysis in an injured extremity	**The patient will not experience a secondary injury or compromise, as indicated by:** • Absence of increasing pain, pressure, paresthesia, paralysis, or a decreasing pulse in an injured extremity • Awareness of limitations

Chapter 12

Surface and Burn Trauma

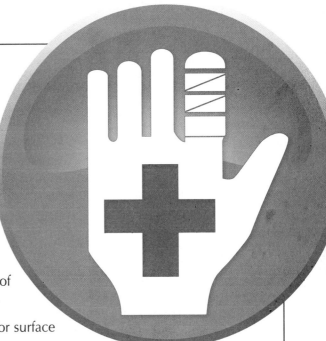

Objectives

On completion of this chapter/lecture, the learner should be able to:

1. Identify the common mechanisms of injury associated with surface trauma.

2. Describe the pathophysiologic changes as a basis for the signs and symptoms.

3. Discuss the nursing assessment of the patient with surface trauma.

4. Plan appropriate interventions for surface trauma patients.

5. Evaluate the effectiveness of nursing interventions for patients with specific types of surface trauma injuries.

Preface

Lecture begins on page 200.

Knowledge of normal anatomy serves as the foundation for understanding the anatomic derangements and pathophysiologic compromises that may result from trauma. Before reading this chapter, it is strongly suggested that the learner read the following review material. Reading about the specific anatomic and physiologic concepts presented in this section will enhance the learner's ability to correlate such concepts with specific injuries. This material related to anatomy and physiology will not be covered during lectures, nor will it be evaluated by testing.

The Skin

The skin is the elastic, self-generating, waterproof covering of the body. It functions as a protective barrier from injury and infection, provides tactile interaction with the environment, assists with fluid and electrolyte management, and is involved in the body's temperature-regulating mechanisms. The two layers of skin, the epidermis and the dermis, cover the subcutaneous tissue layer, or hypodermis (**Figure 12-1**).

The epidermis is the outermost layer. It is avascular, receiving nourishment from the dermis, and is composed of epithelial cells. The thickness of the epidermis varies—it is thickest over the palmar surfaces of the hands and the plantar surfaces of the feet and tends to be leanest over the face. The epidermis is composed of five layers, of which the deepest layer is a single layer of cells (basal cells) capable of producing new skin cells that move to the skin's surface to replace lost cells. If, after injury, a sufficient number of basal cells survive, regeneration is possible.

The dermis is formed by connective tissue and contains collagen and elastic fibers. The two-layered dermis contains blood vessels, nerve endings, sweat glands, sebaceous glands, lymph vessels, and hair follicles. The dermis supplies nutrition to the epidermis. Under the dermis is a layer of subcutaneous tissue composed of fat and connective tissues. The dermal layer cannot regenerate if the cells are destroyed.

The four major functions of the skin are sensory perception, thermoregulation, secretion, and protection. The sensations of pain, touch, temperature, and pressure are transmitted through the sensory nerve fibers to areas in the cerebral cortex. The sweat glands secrete sweat to maintain a normal body temperature. The skin also assists in the body's regulation of fluids and electrolytes. The sebaceous glands secrete sebum, an oily substance that contributes to lubrication of the skin, maintains the skin's texture, and contains antifungal and antibacterial properties. The skin protects the body against damage from heat, cold, bacteria, fungi, and chemicals. The integument houses the subcutaneous and fatty tissues that protect the underlying structures from external forces.

Surface trauma that disrupts the integrity of the skin may result in loss of some or all of the functions of the skin. The skin provides not only these physiologic and anatomic functions, but also secondary functions such as the storage of fat, production of vitamins, and the facilitation of motion. One of the skin's most important secondary functions is its contribution to appearance and individual identity; disruption of this individuality may pose major readjustment problems, most significantly in burn injury patients.

Capillary and Fluid Dynamics

The body's fluids are composed of water, electrolytes, proteins, and other substances contained in the intracellular and extracellular compartments. Because electrolytes and other molecular substances are dissolved in body water, the fluid compartments have both electrical and chemical properties. The size of all cells is controlled by the movement of water between the compartments. Because water is in motion, the pressure that is generated is termed osmotic pressure. The osmotic activity that results is because of the number, not the size, of nondiffusible particles.[1] Water molecules, separated by a semipermeable membrane, will move from the compartment with the lesser number of nondiffusible particles to the compartment with more.

Four forces contribute to the fluid movement across the capillary membrane (**Table 12-1**).

Because the hydrostatic pressure is higher at the arterial end of a capillary than at the venule end, fluid can move out at the arterial end. At the venule end of the capillary, the hydrostatic pressure is lower. The capillary colloid osmotic pressure is the dominant pressure that pulls fluid back into the capillary at the venule end. Proteins, the only dissolved particles in the plasma that do not pass through the pores of the cell's semipermeable membrane, are responsible for generating the capillary colloid osmotic pressure. Any disruption in the integrity of the capillary membrane will lead to a reduction in the capillary osmotic pressure and a loss of intracapillary water into the interstitium.

Refer to the Anatomy and Physiology section in Chapter 4, Airway and Ventilation, for a review of respiratory anatomy and physiology.

Figure 12-1: Layers of the Skin and Depth of Burn Wound

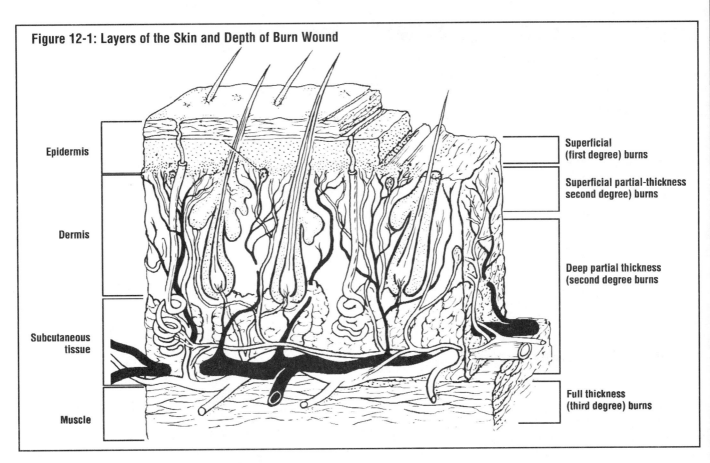

Epidermis

Dermis

Subcutaneous tissue

Muscle

Superficial (first degree) burns

Superficial partial-thickness second degree) burns

Deep partial thickness (second degree burns

Full thickness (third degree) burns

Table 12-1: Pressures Contributing to Capillary Flow

Pressure	Function
Hydrostatic or Capillary Pressure Arterial end = 30 mm Hg Venous end = 10 mm Hg	• Forces fluid out of the capillary at the arterial end
Plasma Colloid Osmotic Pressure 28 mm Hg	• Pulls fluid into the capillary at the venule end
Interstitial Free Fluid Pressure (IFFP) Usually slightly less than atmospheric, −3 to −5, but can be positive (e.g., in the brain)	• Pulls fluid out of the capillary (when the IFFP is negative) • Forces fluid into capillary (when the IFFP is positive)
Interstitial Fluid Osmotic Pressure 8 mm Hg	• Pulls fluid out of the capillary

Introduction

Surface trauma can be defined as any disruption in the integumentary system; it can be a skin or a soft-tissue injury. Surface trauma can be the primary injury or a concurrent injury. Burns, lacerations, abrasions, avulsions, contusions, punctures, hematomas, and degloving injuries are forms of skin trauma often encountered in the acutely injured patient. Soft-tissue injuries can involve muscles, tendons, cartilage, ligaments, vessels, and nerves. Because the resultant effects on the body are so different, this chapter will cover basic skin and soft tissue trauma followed by burn trauma. Basic injury to the skin and soft tissue is seen in most trauma events and tends to have responses that are more localized, whereas burn trauma of any significant size will result in systemic effects.

Basic Skin and Soft-Tissue Trauma

Epidemiology

Trauma patients are exposed to multiple forces of energy, which are transferred through the skin and may cause injury.

Emergency departments treat 12.2 million patients with surface trauma each year.[2] Most basic skin and soft-tissue injuries occur on the face and scalp (51%), the upper extremities (34%), and the lower extremities (13%).[2] Most patients (74%) are young men (average age, 23 years).[2] The Centers for Disease Control and Prevention (CDC) reports that the most frequently encountered primary diagnosis is contusions and that the fifth most common primary diagnosis is open wounds.[3] Infection is the most common complication of skin and soft-tissue injury. Infections are more likely to occur in human bite wounds, grossly contaminated wounds, wounds with retained foreign debris, and wounds in the lower extremities.

Mechanisms of Injury and Biomechanics

Surface trauma occurs under a variety of circumstances (e.g., self-inflicted wounds, assault, work-related accidents, home accidents, motor vehicle or motorcycle crashes, or falls). Surface trauma can be the primary injury or a concurrent injury. The mechanism of injury for primary skin or soft tissue trauma can be classified by the forces of shearing, tensile, compression, and burn (**Table 12-2**). Burns will be discussed later in the chapter.

Usual Concurrent Injuries

The mechanism of injury will give clues to the anticipated severity of the skin and soft-tissue injury as well as to suspected concurrent injuries. Musculoskeletal injuries are common concurrent injuries and often result in skin and soft-tissue trauma.

Pathophysiology as a Basis for Signs and Symptoms of Skin and Soft-Tissue Trauma

Wound healing is a complex process involving hemostasis, inflammation, fibroblast growth, angiogenesis, epithelialization, and tissue contraction (**Figure 12-2**).[4]

Complications can occur at any time in this process. The most common complication of wound care is infection. Approximately 3.5% to 6.3% of laceration wounds in adults treated in the emergency department become infected.[2] Infection can dramatically impede the healing process. Comorbid medical conditions such as diabetes and peripheral vascular disease can impede healing as well.

Injury to the skin and soft tissues predisposes an individual to secondary complications such as (1) localized and systemic infection, (2) hypoproteinemia, (3) hypothermia, and (4) sequelae related to tissue necrosis.[5]

Selected Skin and Soft Tissue Trauma

Abrasion

Abrasion is an injury caused by the friction of skin rubbing against a hard object or surface. Motorcycle and bicycle crashes often result in abrasion injuries. These wounds can be partial thickness or full thickness but are not deeper than the dermis. Abrasions vary in size of body surface area involved as well as in depth of injury. They can be impregnated with dirt, debris, and road surface debris. "Traumatic tattooing" occurs if debris become trapped in the epidermis or dermis and cause unsightly discoloration, which may eventually require surgical intervention.

Avulsion

An avulsion is a full-thickness injury caused by a tearing or ripping of the skin or soft tissue where the wound edges cannot be approximated. The treatment of an avulsion is dependent on the extent of injury and amount of tissue loss. Tissue grafting may be necessary with full-thickness avulsions extending greater than 2 cm².[6] A degloving injury is an avulsion where the skin is torn or pulled away from the soft tissue.

Contusion/Hematoma

A contusion/hematoma is a closed wound that results from the rupture of small blood vessels and the subsequent oozing of blood into the soft tissue. Contusions/hematomas are characterized by swelling and pain. There may be underlying tissue damage or fractures.

Laceration

A laceration is an open wound caused by the cut of a sharp object or the rupture of skin from the impact of a blunt object. It is classified as superficial if the laceration affects the epidermis and dermis. Lacerations may involve damage to underlying tissues. For example, a deep laceration extends beyond the dermis into the underlying soft tissue.

Puncture

A puncture is an open wound caused by a spearlike object penetrating the skin and soft tissue to varying depths. The outward appearance of a puncture wound may seem minor compared to the severity of the underlying tissue damage. Foreign debris may become embedded into the soft tissue as a result of the puncture. Animal and human bites are specific types of puncture wounds caused by the crush of teeth and jaws. These puncture wounds are grossly contaminated, and the risk of infection is apparent. Microorganisms in human saliva can cause both gram-negative and gram-positive infections.

Nursing Care of the Patient with Basic Skin and Soft-Tissue Trauma

Assessment

History

Refer to Chapter 3, Initial Assessment, for a description of general information that should be collected regarding every trauma patient. Only pertinent questions specific to patients with skin and soft tissue trauma are described following.

Table 12-2: Mechanism of Injury for Primary Skin or Soft-Tissue Trauma

Energy Source	Description	Complications
Shearing Sharp object (knife, glass)	Laceration Puncture	Minimal scarring Minimal risk infection Infection with embedded foreign debris
Friction	Abrasion	Minimal risk infection Traumatic tattooing
Tensile Blunt object impact Tearing or pulling of tissue	Hematoma Laceration Avulsions Degloving	Vascular disruption Moderate scarring Tissue ischemia Infection Scarring
Compression Blunt object impact Fall	Complex laceration Contusion	Devitalized tissue Infection Scarring Compartment syndrome
Burn Thermal Chemical Electrical Ultraviolet Ionizing radiation	Partial- to full-thickness burns	Scarring Infection Compartment syndrome Multisystem dysfunction per severity

Figure 12-2: Activity of Wound Healing Components

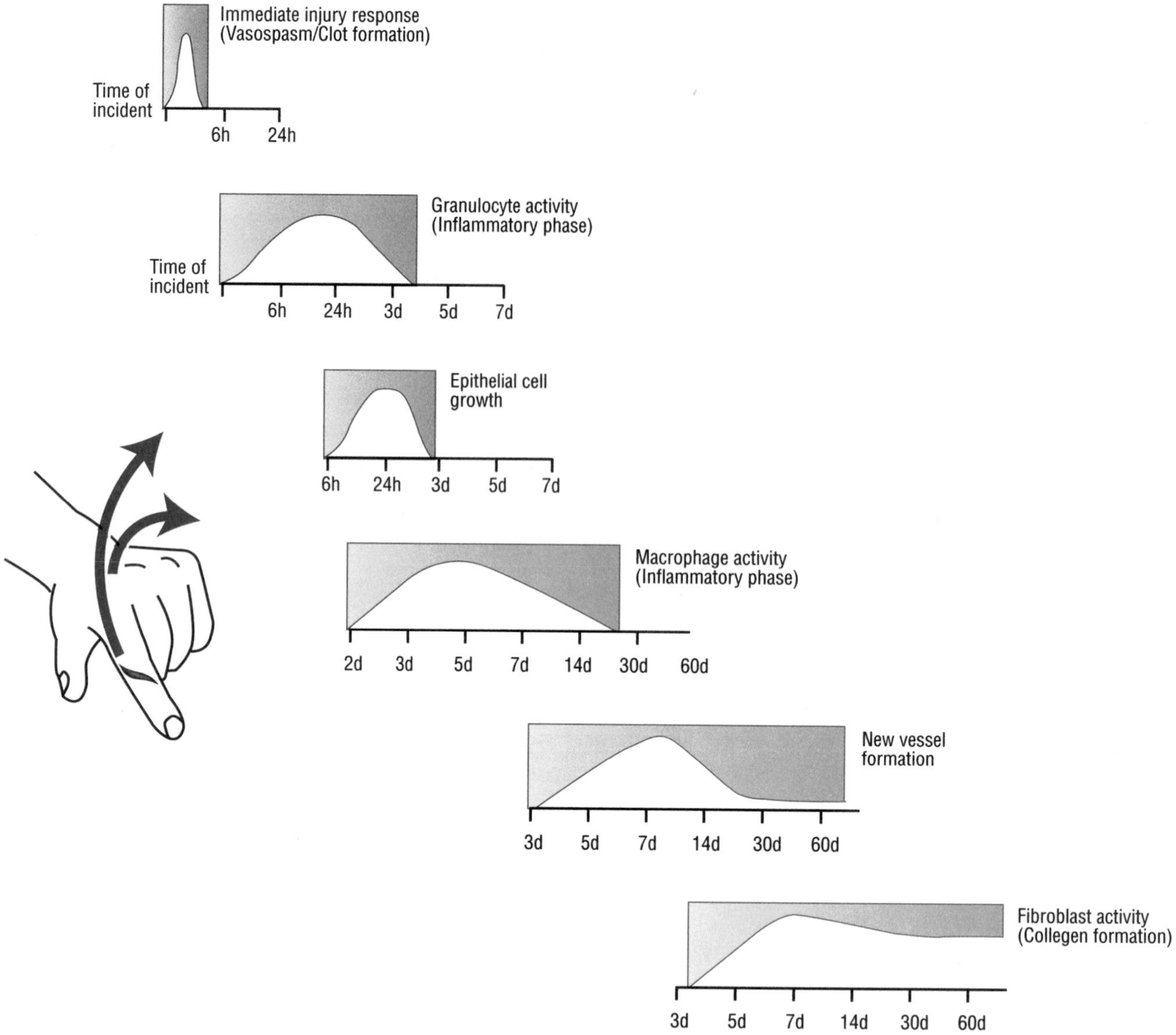

Immediate injury response
(Vasospasm/Clot formation)

Time of incident

6h   24h

Granulocyte activity
(Inflammatory phase)

Time of incident

6h   24h   3d   5d   7d

Epithelial cell growth

6h   24h   3d   5d   7d

Macrophage activity
(Inflammatory phase)

2d   3d   5d   7d   14d   30d   60d

New vessel formation

3d   5d   7d   14d   30d   60d

Fibroblast activity
(Collegen formation)

3d   5d   7d   14d   30d   60d

Reprinted from *Wounds and Lacerations: Emergency Care and Closure*, 3rd edition, page 23, Surface injury and wound healing, Copyright 2005, with permission from Elsevier.

- What was the mechanism of injury (motor vehicle crash, assault with sharp or blunt object, human or animal bite)?
- Where did the injury occur?
- What time did the injury occur? (Delay in treatment will change the treatment options.)
- Are there associated signs/symptoms (bleeding, pain, paresthesia, weakness, loss of function, swelling, deformity)?
- Are there comorbid diseases that would decrease healing of wounds (diabetes, peripheral vascular disease, bleeding disorders)?
- Is the patient taking medication that may affect bleeding time or the healing process?

- When did the patient receive his or her last tetanus shot?

Physical Assessment

Refer to Chapter 3, Initial Assessment, for a description of the assessment of the patient's airway, breathing, circulation, and disability.

Inspection

Identify soft-tissue damage, including edema, ecchymosis, contusions, abrasions, avulsions, and lacerations. Also assess patient wounds for the presence of crepitus. Assess the

- Location, length, depth, and shape of wound
- Swelling

- Exudate from wound
- Sensory and motor function
- Vascular integrity, tissue perfusion (capillary refill, pulses, skin color, skin temperature)
- Evidence of embedded foreign body or wound contamination
- Evidence of fracture

Auscultation

- Auscultate breath sounds

Palpation

- Assess the six Ps
  - **Pain:** Pain out of proportion to the extent of the injury is suspicious for developing or having actual compartment syndrome.
  - **Pallor:** Poor skin color and cool temperature reflect poor perfusion to the area.
  - **Pulses:** Palpate peripheral pulses to detect any vascular compromise associated with circumferential edema or direct injury to the vessels.
  - **Paresthesia:** Palpate the extremities to determine sensory function.
  - **Paralysis:** Motor dysfunction reflects injury to the nervous system. Palpate and assess for full range of motion for all extremities.
  - **Pressure:** Palpate the extremity for firmness of compartments and muscle spasm.

Diagnostic Procedures

Refer to Chapter 3, Initial Assessment, for frequently ordered radiographic and laboratory studies. Additional studies for patient's skin and soft-tissue trauma are listed following.

Radiographic Studies

- Specific local radiographic images are necessary when you:
  - Suspect a foreign body
  - Suspect underlying injury (fracture, joint penetration)

Laboratory Studies

- Check for evidence of excess bleeding (hematology, coagulation factors).
- Check serum creatine phosphokinase, which may indicate muscle necrosis as a result of compartment syndrome.

Refer to Chapter 3, Initial Assessment, for a description of the specific nursing interventions for patients with compromises to airway, breathing, circulation, and disability.

Interventions

The goals of wound care are to promote optimal healing, prevent complications, maintain function, and minimize scar formation. Appropriate interventions will serve to accomplish these four goals.

Interventions of wound care follow a four-step approach: hemostasis, wound preparation, wound closure decision, and aftercare/follow-up regimen.

1. **Hemostasis**
   - Apply direct pressure to the wound to control bleeding.
   - Anticipate electrocautery or suture ligation if bleeding cannot be controlled with direct pressure.
   - Consider using a tourniquet when severe bleeding continues with direct pressure.

2. **Wound Preparation**
   - Anticipation of anesthesia

     Effective local anesthesia will decrease or eliminate pain sensation so that more thorough wound preparation can be done. Lidocaine 0.5% to 2.0% is used most often because it has a rapid onset (1 to 2 minutes). Avoid vascular injection by aspirating before tissue infiltration.
   - Wound cleansing

     The main purpose for peripheral wound cleansing is to remove any visible contamination or dried blood.[7] Use a 4 × 4 sponge and cleansing agent (such as 10% povidone-iodine solution and saline, 1:10 to 1:20 mix ratio).
   - Hair clipping

     Clipping the hair near the wound site can be done to facilitate cleansing and possible closure. Never shave a patient's eyebrows.
   - Wound irrigation

     Irrigation is the most important step in reducing bacterial contamination and potential for wound infection. Copious wound irrigation with normal saline solution is recommended for open wounds. Low-pressure irrigation, such as with a bulb syringe, will remove large particles but not smaller contaminants and bacteria.[8] A 35-ml Luer-Lok™ syringe with an attached 19-g soft intravenous catheter (needle removed) or a 20- to 35-ml syringe with a splash shield in place will generate the appropriate amount of pressure necessary to thoroughly irrigate the wound.[7]

- Wound culture

  Obtain a wound culture as indicated from open sites.

- Antibiotic administration

  If you use antibiotics, they should be given as soon as possible after injury. The administration of prophylactic antibiotics is controversial, but is considered for high-risk, contaminated wounds. High-risk wounds include intraoral lacerations, complicated human or dog bites, cat bites, and foot puncture wounds.[9] In addition to high-risk wounds, the use of a single dose of a systemic antibiotic with activity against Staphylococcus aureus is logical at the time of wound debridement, irrigation, and primary closure.[10]

  - Anticipation of wound exploration in instances where there is suspicion of contamination with a foreign body

    Glass is the most commonly found foreign body. Road or surface debris can be embedded into the skin or soft tissue with certain mechanisms of injury (i.e., deep abrasions occurring as a person is ejected from a vehicle and then slides across the road surface).

  - Anticipation of debridement

    All nonviable, devitalized tissue should be excised with surgical scissors or a surgical scalpel blade.

- Tissue preservation

  No unnecessary tissue excision is done. All viable tissue is preserved.

3. Wound Closure

The principles of wound closure involve using the least invasive method with the best cosmetic outcome and the lowest risk of complication. The method of closure is dependent on the approximation of the skin or soft tissue, the amount of contamination, and the location of the wound.

- Primary intention
  This type of closure can be accomplished with sutures, staples, or skin tape. These wounds are usually well approximated and noncontaminated. Primary intention closure is ideally accomplished within the first 6 to 8 hours postinjury; however, facial or scalp wounds that are highly vascular can be sutured 24 hours after injury.[4]

  - Staples are useful to approximate wounds in which the cosmetic effect is not extremely

important. Tape is used in superficial wounds or for approximation after the staples have been removed.

- Delayed primary intention

  Bite wounds and lacerations can be considered for this technique.[2] Cleansing, irrigation, debridement, and antibiotic administration promote wound preparation for 3 to 5 days before delayed primary closure.[2]

- Secondary intention

  These wounds are not closed and are allowed to heal gradually by granulation and eventual re-epithelialization. Wounds that are best closed by secondary intention are ulcerations, human bite wounds, full- or partial-thickness abrasions, or punctures or other wounds with gross contamination. Large wounds may eventually need to be closed with skin grafts or muscle flaps.

4. Aftercare/Follow-Up Regimen

- Antibiotic ointment is thinly applied to closed wounds or superficial abrasions.

- Wounds heal best in a moist environment with a properly applied wound dressing. Basic wound covering consists of a nonadherent base dressing, absorbent gauze sponges, gauze wrap if needed, and tape to secure the dressing.

- Inspect dressings frequently for continued bleeding.

- Prepare for radiographs of the involved extremity if contamination by foreign bodies is suspected.

- Educate patients about wound care, signs/symptoms of infection, elevation, ice therapy if indicated, and pain management.

- Regarding follow-up, patients should make a timely return for wound assessment, suture removal, etc.

- Tetanus administration
  - Determine the need for tetanus prophylaxis following surface trauma. The decision will be based on the condition of the wound, the cause of the wound, the actual or possible contamination of the wound, and the patient's vaccination history (**Table 12-3**).
  - Patients without a clear history of at least three tetanus vaccinations who have any wound other than clean and minor require tetanus immune globulin (TIG), not just Td.[11]
  - Please check the CDC website at www.cdc.gov for the most current recommendations for tetanus administration.

Epidemiology

The incidence of serious burn injury, subsequent hospitalization, and burn death rates have all declined by at least 50% in the past four decades.[12,13] These data reflect societal changes such as an increase in educational programs related to fire and burn prevention, legislation, an increased presence of smoke alarms in all households, improved building codes, increased safety in industrial settings, and the use of safer appliances and heating devices.[13-15] Although its incidence has been reduced, burn injury remains the sixth leading cause of death in children younger than 14 years and the fifth leading cause of death in the 1- to 4-year age group.[16]

There are an estimated 1.25 million burn injuries each year. These injuries result in an estimated 700,000 emergency department (ED) visits, with 45,000 hospitalizations per year.[13,17] About half of these are admitted to 125 specialized, regional burn treatment centers across the United States. Advances in trauma systems and treatments have reduced mortality from over 6% of these patients dying from their injury or its complications to 4.7%.[13,17]

Overall, burns rank as the sixth leading cause of death because of unintentional injury.[16] Most burn deaths occur as a result of residential fires; more than three fourths of the deaths are related to inhalation of toxic substances.[13,18] Careless use of smoking materials and alcohol consumption are common factors in fatal house fires. More than 40% of the deaths in house fires are related to alcohol or drugs.[13]

The southeastern United States has the highest death rates (highest along coastal plains and along the Mississippi River) from house fires because of differences in construction, economic status, and heating devices. Improperly positioned or unattended cooking and heating devices are the leading cause of house fires resulting in death, with an increased incidence in the cold winter months.[13]

The cost of care for a hospitalized burn patient ranges from $30,000 to $118,000; a fire-related death, including lost years of estimated productivity, has been estimated to cost $250,000 to $1.5 million.[13]

Scald burns are more frequent for those younger than 5 years or older than 65 years. In these individuals, such burns are related to the thinness of the skin and the decreased reaction time to move away from the heated liquid. Burns caused by scalds from hot liquids frequently lead to hospital admissions but, fortunately, to few deaths (approximately 100 per year).[13] For children younger than 5 years old, hot water from taps, showers, and bathtubs is the leading source of scald burns. Water at 155 °F (68 °C) can cause a deep partial- or full-thickness burn in 1 second (**Table 12-4**).[13,19,20]

Careless smoking accounts for one of four residential fire deaths and is compounded by alcohol and drug intoxication, which impair mentation.[13] In residential fires, a significant number of clothing fires occur in the over-65 age group, principally from nightwear (e.g., robes, pajamas, or nightgowns). Of the clothing fire deaths reported, about three fourths occurred in those aged 65 years and older.[21] Most occurred while people were cooking (33%), smoking (23%), or burning trash or having contact with heaters (8% each).[22]

Electrical contact injuries cause approximately 1,000 deaths per year. Lightning accounts for about 100 deaths per year.[12] The incidence is greatest among those between ages 10 and 19; males have a death rate seven times greater than females. More lightning deaths occur during the summer months,

Table 12-3: CDC Guidelines for Tetanus and Diphtheria Toxoids (Td) or Tetanus and Diphtheria Toxoids and Pertussis Vaccine Adsorbed (Tdap) Administration

Vaccination History	Clean, Minor Wounds	All Other Wounds
Unknown or < 3 doses	Td or Tdap (Tdap preferred for ages 11 to 18)	Td or Tdap (Tdap preferred for ages 11 to 18) **plus** tetanus immune globulin (TIG)
3 or more doses and ≤ 5 years since last dose	Nothing else needed	Nothing else needed
3 or more doses and 6 to 10 years since last dose	Nothing else needed	Td or Tdap (Tdap preferred for ages 11 to 18)
3 or more doses and > 10 years since last dose	Td or Tdap (Tdap preferred for ages 11 to 18)	Td or Tdap (Tdap preferred for ages 11 to 18)

Adapted from *Total Burn Care*, 2nd edition, 455–460, Copyright 2002, with permission from Elsevier.

and close to one third of these deaths are in outdoor workers (e.g., farmers, construction workers). Although they can occur at any time, lightning strikes are most prevalent during thunderstorms, with the highest mortality rates in the southern and eastern states.[13,23,24]

Burn patients and their support networks experience devastating problems, beginning with the initial event and continuing through subsequent hospitalizations and lengthy periods of rehabilitation. In addition, the burn survivor must cope with changes in body image, altered self-esteem, long-term rehabilitation, and new financial burdens.

Caring for burn patients in an emergency setting is stressful for the entire trauma team. This patient population may not be often seen in some facilities and is very resource-intensive in its use of personnel, medical equipment, and social services.

Mechanisms of Injury and Biomechanics

The energy agents that can cause burns are

- Thermal
- Chemical
- Electrical
- Ultraviolet or ionizing radiation

The most common mechanisms of injury leading to thermal burns are events generating heat, flames, or both.[11] Such burns can be caused by flames, flashes,

Table 12-4: Temperature of Hot Substances and Length of Time until Skin Burns

Temperature	Length of Exposure
110 °F (43 °C)	up to 6 hours
118 °F (48 °C)	5 minutes to burn
124 °F (51 °C)	3 minutes to burn
126 °F (52 °C)	1 minute to burn
130 °F (54 °C)	30 seconds to burn
133 °F (56 °C)	15 seconds to burn
140 °F (60 °C)	5 seconds to burn
147 °F (64 °C)	2 seconds to burn
155 °F (68 °C)	1 second to burn
160 to 180 °F (71 to 82 °C)	Hot beverages
200 °F (93 °C)	Electric crock pot
212 °F (100 °C)	Water boils
298 °F (148 °C)	Frying
392 °F (200 °C)	Baking
392 to 500 °F (200 to 260 °C)	Deep frying

Reprinted from Am J Pathol 1947, 23: 695-720 with permission from the American Society from Investigative Pathology.

scalds, and contact with burning substances, objects, and chemicals. The mechanism of injury leading to pulmonary injury is related to the inhalation of heat, smoke, and toxic substances (both gases and particulate matter) released during the burning process. As natural and synthetic materials burn, byproducts of combustion, such as carbon monoxide, hydrogen cyanide, and other gases are released. Additionally, as the combustion process consumes oxygen, the atmospheric concentration of oxygen decreases, carbon dioxide levels increase, and the temperature in the environment rises.

Usual Concurrent Injuries

In the burn injury population, although the burn to the skin may be the first injury observed, the potential for injury to the pulmonary system requires immediate assessment and intervention. The primary focus must be on lifesaving measures. Inhalation injury as a single factor increases the mortality from burns by 20%.[25] Inhalation injury is more common when the fire has occurred in an enclosed space, particularly in residential fires. Direct thermal injury is usually limited to the upper airway with the inhalation of superheated air. Inhalation injury below the glottis is rarer and is usually limited to chemical exposure, as opposed to thermal. Superheated air often causes laryngospasm, thereby closing the glottis and decreasing the incidence of thermal damage to the lungs. Water conducts heat approximately 30 times as efficiently as air; in an incident involving large amounts of steam the risk of injury is far greater because water has a heat-carrying capacity 4,000 times greater than air.[26] Additional injuries may be a direct result of explosive forces that caused the initial fire or may result from falls or jumps to safety. Fractures, head injuries, abdominal injuries, or chest injuries may occur. Electrical injuries may cause fractures, particularly of the spine and long bone, from subsequent violent, tetanic skeletal muscle contraction; the cervical spine must be protected, and compression fractures of vertebral bodies should be ruled out.[26,27]

Pathophysiology as a Basis for Signs and Symptoms of Burn Trauma

Heat, or thermal energy, that exceeds the body's ability to dissipate can burn the layers of the skin and underlying structures. (Chemical and electrical injuries will be discussed later in the chapter.)

Severe burns on the skin present zones of injury (**Figure 12-3**).

Figure 12-3: Zones of the Burn Wound

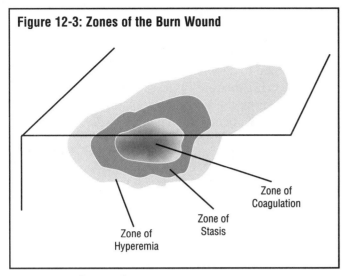

Zone of Coagulation

Zone of Stasis

Zone of Hyperemia

- Zone of coagulation

  The most seriously affected cells form an area of coagulation at the center, where the tissue is not viable. This tissue is necrotic and has lost the ability to regenerate.

- Zone of stasis

  Surrounding the zone of coagulation is the area where capillary occlusion, diminished perfusion, and edema occur in the first 24 to 48 hours after the burn. This area, if treated in a timely and appropriate manner, has the potential to be salvaged.

- Zone of hyperemia (increased blood flow)

  This is the area around the zone of stasis. The increased flow is just one of the consequences of the resulting inflammatory response through active and reactive hyperemia.

Several vasoactive chemicals are released from mast cells, white blood cells, and platelets as a result of the injury process. The seriousness of a thermal burn is related to the degree of systemic problems, such as hypovolemia or cardiovascular, respiratory, or renal failure. In the presence of severe injury of the skin (greater than 20% to 30% total burn surface area), systemic pathophysiologic changes can be anticipated.[28]

Plasma Loss and Other Vascular Responses

The burn patient may present in shock because of intravascular volume loss, diminished tissue perfusion, or associated traumatic injury. As a result of both the direct injury to capillaries and the release of vasoactive substances, the semipermeability of the capillary is lost, leading to movement of proteins and other dissolved substances out of the intravascular spaces into the interstitium. The active hyperemia (increased blood flow in response to tissue demand) increases the capil-

lary pressure at the arterial end of the capillary. The loss of proteins decreases the capillary colloid osmotic pressure. Both of these pressure changes contribute to hypovolemia and edema. Edema formation after a burn is caused by the hyperosmolar state of the interstitium from the presence of [1,19]

- Sodium and osmotically active cellular debris
- Protein leakage

The rate of fluid loss from intravascular spaces depends on the

- Patient's age
- Burn size and depth
- Intravascular pressures
- Time elapsed since the burn

Additionally, the body's inflammatory response leads to release of several substances that contribute to edema and cardiovascular consequences. They are[29]

- Histamine: Leads to arteriolar vasodilation and increased capillary permeability
- Prostaglandins: Lead to vasodilation and increased permeability of the microcirculation
- Thromboxane A_2 (a prostaglandin): Leads to platelet aggregation and may cause expansion of the zone of ischemia
- Leukotrienes and cytokines: Contribute to inflammatory response
- Bradykinin: Causes increased permeability of venules
- Oxygen-free radicals: May lead to damage of the endothelial cells of the microcirculation

The pathophysiologic response to the burn leads to the following changes in the vascular system:

- Hemoconcentration of the blood through the loss of plasma volume, as manifested by an elevated hematocrit.
- Increased blood viscosity. Because the percentage of red blood cells is higher, the friction between cells is greater. The friction of cells influences the ability of the cells to move; the more friction, the greater the viscosity and resistance to flow.
- Increased peripheral resistance because of the increased viscosity.
- Greater percentage of red blood cells. Although the percentage of red blood cells is greater, the actual number of red blood cells is diminished because of direct hemolysis and thrombi formation.[29]

Hypoxemia/Asphyxia

The process of combustion consumes oxygen; therefore, victims of fires who are in an enclosed space, such as a house or a car, inhale air that has a concentration of oxygen less than 21%. The reduction in the fraction of inspired oxygen (FiO_2) leads to arterial hypoxemia. Asphyxia occurs when the blood has a decreased amount of oxygen and there is an increase in carbon dioxide or toxic substances in the blood and tissues of the body.[25] Asphyxiation, or deprivation of oxygen, may result from the lack of oxygen in the environment or the inhalation of toxic substances. The inhalation of substances, most commonly carbon monoxide, has been cited as the leading cause of death resulting from house fires.[25,30]

Carbon Monoxide Poisoning

Carbon monoxide is a tasteless, odorless, and colorless gas that is present in the smoke of the combustion of organic materials, such as wood, coal, and gasoline. Carbon monoxide is also released when the available oxygen to support combustion is consumed and incomplete combustion occurs. Carbon monoxide, when inhaled, crosses the alveolar-capillary membrane and binds to the oxygen-binding sites on hemoglobin molecules. Because carbon monoxide has 200 to 300 times greater affinity and tenacity to stay bound to hemoglobin than does oxygen, the oxygen-carrying capacity of hemoglobin is reduced. Carbon monoxide can also affect cardiac muscle by binding with myoglobin (the oxygen-transporting pigment of muscle), leading to such changes as hemorrhage and necrosis of cardiac muscle. Treatment with 100% oxygen will decrease the half-life of carbon monoxide from 4 hours to 45 minutes.[25,28]

The oxygen remaining on the hemoglobin molecule is not readily released to the tissues. Thus, tissue hypoxia is even more serious for patients who have preexisting cardiac or pulmonary conditions (or both). The presence of carbon monoxide on hemoglobin does not affect the patient's partial pressure of oxygen (PaO_2), but does affect the oxygen content (oxygen content = oxygen combined with hemoglobin in physical solution).[25] The patient will have a below-normal oxygen saturation (SaO_2) as calculated from an arterial blood gas sample. The SpO_2 (arterial oxygen saturation) obtained by pulse oximetry may be inaccurate because the pulse oximeter cannot accurately discriminate between oxyhemoglobin and carboxyhemoglobin. Because the PaO_2 stays normal, the chemoreceptors are not stimulated to increase ventilation, and the patient sustains tissue hypoxia.[19,31] In fires, the inhalation of toxic substances is not limited to carbon monoxide.

Pulmonary Injury

Combustion and incomplete combustion of organic and inorganic materials produces byproducts, some of which can be toxic when inhaled (**Table 12-5**).

Smoke is the mixture of gases and particulate matter produced during the decomposition and combustion of natural or synthetic materials. The actual composition of the smoke depends on the

- Substance burning
- Temperature and rate at which it is being generated
- Amount of oxygen present in the burning environment

As a person inhales, smoke and soot particles will enter the respiratory tract. The size of the particles and the anatomic location of their deposit will be reflected in the severity of the lung injury. Larger particles may affect the upper airways but will be somewhat filtered and prevented from entering the lower airways. Some gases, when inhaled, produce harmful acids or alkalies, resulting in edema of the membranes with subsequent ulcer formation and necrosis. Other gases destroy the cellular membrane and interfere with the cell's ability to use oxygen. Steam, which has 4,000 times more heat-carrying capacity than dry air, can directly injure the airways by direct thermal (heat) damage when inhaled.

Airway obstruction, atelectasis, and impaired ciliary clearance occur because of the accumulation of debris and secretions. Smoke inhalation may extend to the alveoli, leading to edema and collapse. Additionally, there may be a loss of surfactant, which normally lines the interior surface of the alveoli and reduces surface tension. Without surfactant, the alveoli collapse, and pulmonary compliance is reduced.

Pulmonary edema may be seen in patients who have sustained severe thermal injury to the skin with or without inhalation injury. Pulmonary edema, decreased lung compliance, ventilation/perfusion mismatch, increased airway resistance, tracheobronchitis, and pneumonia are possible sequelae.[32] The inci-

Table 12-5: Toxic Chemicals from Combustion

Burning Source	Toxic Substance
• Organic materials	• Carbon monoxide
• Polyurethane	• Hydrogen cyanide, ammonia, halogen acids
• Polyvinyl chloride	• Phosgene
• Rubber	• Sulfur dioxide
• Upholstery	• Hydrogen chloride
• Wool, silk	• Hydrogen cyanide, hydrogen sulfide

dence of pneumonia independently increases the risk of death by up to 40%.[25]

Hypermetabolism

An increase in the metabolic rate after major trauma and burns is related to the autonomic nervous system response and subsequent hormonal release from the adrenal glands, hypothalamus, and pituitary gland. This metabolic change results in an increase in heart rate and heat production, with elevation of body temperature. The degree of increase in the metabolic rates of patients postburn is related to the severity of the burn, the percentage of the body surface area burned, and the degree of hyperemia.[26] Other influences on the body's response to the burn and rate of metabolism are[26]

- Age
- Ambient temperature
- Pain
- Anxiety
- Patient activity
- Infection (late complication)

Hypermetabolism is demonstrated in the burn patient by

- Tachypnea, due in part to increased oxygen consumption
- Tachycardia, due in part to increased sympathetic response
- Low-grade fever

Selected Burn Trauma

Electrical Burns

Burns from exposure to electrical sources, such as direct exposure to current or from a lightning strike, result in different types of injuries than burns from heat sources. Electrical burns are divided into categories based on exposure to low versus high voltage. High voltage, such as electrical power wires, is any exposure greater than 1,000 volts. Higher voltage results in higher temperatures, leading to greater direct thermal injury.

Electrical current can be either direct current (DC—continuous current flow in one direction) or alternating current (AC—periodic reversal in the current direction). Alternating current is the electricity supplied to homes and businesses. Many medical devices and most electronics use DC, electricity supplied by batteries or power supplies that convert AC supplied from an electric socket to DC. Alternating current is more dangerous than direct current; it may cause tetany, so that a person's grip on an electrical source tightens, which lengthens the exposure to the current. Direct current tends to pass in one direction straight through the body. The electrical current in the United States (and Canada) used in most dwellings is 60 cycle, 110 volt, AC, whereas in Europe and Australia, 50 Hz AC is used.[33]

During assessment of electrical burns, it is important to determine the

- Voltage
- Type of current
- Location of electrical source
- Duration of contact with the electrical source
- Loss of consciousness or required resuscitation

In electrical burns, it is difficult to assess the true extent of damage because electricity enters the body at the point of contact and travels the path of least resistance. The skin is not a good conductor of electrical current and is the most resistant organ of the body. In the body, less resistance is found in muscle tissue, and the largest mass of muscle is located along the bone; the result is twofold, because bones do not conduct electricity. Therefore, electrical injuries can be the most difficult to appreciate because the external damage does not reflect the potentially massive tissue damage or predict outcome.

The path of electricity may traverse internal structures and deeper tissues before eventually exiting the body. The skin may be intact except for the contact points, commonly referred to as entrance and exit wounds, whereas underlying tissues may be injured to the point of necrosis. The electricity may injure any type of tissue, and its effect depends on the tissue's resistance, the intensity (voltage divided by resistance), and the length of contact. Electrical current follows the path of certain tissues in the order of their ability to conduct the current; nerves are the first structures that current will pass through, followed by blood vessels, muscles, skin, tendons, fat, and finally bone. More important than tissue resistance is current density; the smaller the area that comes in contact with the electricity, the greater the tissue damage.

Electrical injuries cause significant damage to the extremities and less damage to the torso and viscera.[26] High-voltage electricity can pass violently through the body. The hollow organs must be evaluated for potential injury, particularly if there was prolonged contact. Cardiac muscle is very susceptible to the effects of electrical current because it has an intrinsic pacemaker ability. Electrical injury can cause immediate or delayed cardiac dysrhythmia, damage, or arrest, or all three. The patient should be observed for abnormalities, even if asymptomatic, when exposed to current greater than 1,000 volts.

The damage to vessels and muscles is an important aspect of electrical injury.[34] Vascular disruption, hemorrhage, or thrombi (or all three) may result from damage to blood vessels. Hemoglobin may be released and appear in the urine. If striated muscle fibers are destroyed (rhabdomyolysis), then myoglobin, the protein pigment in muscle that transports oxygen, may be released and excreted in the urine (myoglobinuria). Muscle damage may lead to edema formation and subsequent elevation of compartment pressures, as well as other complications such as acute renal failure.

Chemical Burns

Chemical burns occur when the patient comes in direct contact with caustic chemical agents, such as acids, alkalies, or petroleum-based products. Chemicals act to break down the cell wall and destroy intracellular proteins.[35] Alkaline chemicals (e.g., lime or sodium and potassium hydroxide present in many household cleaning products and wet cement) are generally responsible for more serious burns through ingestion or cutaneously because alkalies penetrate the contact area more deeply than acids. Damage to the skin in any type of chemical burn is influenced by the length of contact and the concentration and amount of the chemical. In most cases, damage is limited to the local area and does not involve a systemic response.

During the assessment phase of nursing care, it is imperative to identify the causative agent. Contact with a regional poison center may be needed to identify the characteristics of certain substances and neutralization methods. The extent of tissue damage from exposure to chemicals is not immediately apparent, and the extent of injury may progress after the initial exposure, depending on the type of chemical involved and the effectiveness of decontamination procedures.

Nursing Care of the Patient with Burn Trauma

Assessment

History

Refer to Chapter 3, Initial Assessment, for a description of general information that should be collected regarding every trauma patient. Only pertinent questions specific to patients with burn trauma are described here.

- What was the causative agent/mechanism of the burn (e.g., flash fire, direct contact with flame, scald from steam or hot liquid, or contact with a hot object, chemical, or electrical source)?
- Does the causative agent pose a threat to the health care team?
- Does the patient have any clothing or jewelry that must be immediately removed to stop the burning process and prevent constriction leading to edema formation?
- What are the patient's complaints?
- Is the patient hoarse or do they have stridor? Does the patient feel that his or her voice has changed?

  Patients with hoarseness or stridor have a partial airway obstruction and are at significant risk for complete obstruction.[36]
- Where was the patient located in the environment?
  - An inhalation injury should be suspected if the fire was in an enclosed space, in association with heated air, steam, or the burning of potentially toxic materials. An explosion increases the chances of other life-threatening injuries, including penetrating trauma.
  - A patient who has sustained facial burns in an enclosed space, with a carbon monoxide level greater than 15%, has a 90% probability of inhalation injury.[17]
- What was the patient's approximate weight before the burn?
- Has the patient recently consumed alcohol or other substances of abuse?
- Is the mechanism/pattern of the burn suspicious for abuse?
- Is the patient a smoker?

Physical Assessment

Refer to Chapter 3, Initial Assessment, for a description of the assessment of the patient's airway, breathing, circulation, and disability.

Inspection

- Determine airway patency and effectiveness of breathing.
- Inspect the nasopharynx and oropharynx.

  Look for evidence of soot, carbonaceous sputum, irritation of mucous membranes, increased secretions, or all three. Determine the presence or absence of cough, hoarseness, stridor, and gag reflex.
- Inspect for singed nasal, facial, and eyebrow hairs.

- Inspect for burns and edema, especially around the face and neck.
- Count respiratory rate, determine breathing pattern, and watch the expansion of the chest during inspiration.

  An increased respiratory rate may indicate hypercarbia, pulmonary injury, shock, anxiety, pain, hypermetabolism, or all of these. Circumferential burns of the thorax may prevent total inflation of the lungs and lead to respiratory compromise.

- In patients where electrical injury is suspected, inspect the patient for entrance and exit wounds.
- Also monitor the patient's cardiac rhythm because cardiac dysrhythmias (atrial fibrillation, ventricular fibrillation, and asystole) may occur after the incident.
- Determine the depth of the burn injury (**Table 12-6**).
  - Superficial (first-degree) burns are dry, erythematous areas with no bullae (blisters). The burned area blanches and is tender, and the epidermis is intact.
  - Partial-thickness (second-degree) burns usually appear hyperemic in color, are moist, and have blisters. The patient will complain of pain. The two classifications of partial-thickness burns are
    - Superficial partial-thickness burns involve the epidermis and the upper portion of the dermis. The skin is typically a mottled, red color. Blisters are formed, or the tissue is weeping serous fluid. These burns are very painful because the destruction of the epidermal layer has left nerve endings exposed. Often these burns can be covered with a synthetic dressing/skin substitute, and the patient can be treated on an outpatient basis after minimal observation. These burns will usually heal in 10 to 14 days without surgical intervention and leave minimal scarring.
    - Deep partial-thickness burns involve the entire epidermal layer and extend more deeply into the dermis. There is decreased moistness because the glands become damaged and lose the ability to secrete. The skin will be pale, with absent or greatly prolonged blanching. There will be some degree of healing in 21 to 28 days, but this will depend on the burn size and anatomic location. Deep partial-thickness burns of significant size will require surgical intervention.
- Distinguishing between deep partial-thickness burns and full-thickness burns may initially be difficult.
  - Full-thickness (third-degree) burns range in color from pale yellow to cherry red, brown, or carbon black. These burns have a dry, leathery appearance. The burned tissue is inelastic and lacks sensation. This depth of burn can be limb- or life-threatening (or both).
  - Fourth-degree burn is a less common term used to describe burns in which the destruction extends completely through the dermal layer and subcutaneous tissue into deep structures such as the underlying fat, fascia, muscle, tendon, or bone. Treatment will require elaborate debridement and, oftentimes, amputation.
  - Depth of burn injury may not be completely determined in the emergency department. Depth can only be determined after careful examination, debridement, and cooling of the heated area.
- Determine the extent of the burn injury.

  The extent of burn injury may progress over the first 48 hours.[37]
  - The extent of the burn is the percentage of total body surface area (TBSA) burned. Fluid amounts for intravenous infusion are calculated using the percentage of TBSA burned for patients with partial- (second-degree) and full-

Table 12-6: Depth and Degree of Burn

Depth	Degree	Characteristics
Superficial	First	• Dry, red, blanches, tender
Partial-thickness • Superficial partial-thickness • Deep partial-thickness	Second	• Hyperemic, moist, bullae, painful • Involves upper dermis • Involves deeper dermis
Full-thickness	Third	• Dry • May be leathery looking or translucent • Color varies from yellow to red to brown or black • Not painful (insensate)

thickness (third-degree) burns only. This is open tissue that will cause the patient to lose plasma and require fluid replacement. The tissue integrity of superficial (first-degree) burns remains intact.

- The rule of nines divides the TBSA into areas comprising 9% or multiples of 9%, except for the perineum, which is equal to 1% of the TBSA. The rule of nines is an estimate and is most useful for adults and children older than age 10 (**Figure 12-4**).

- In the hospital setting, the Lund and Browder chart provides a more accurate calculation of the TBSA burned because body proportions change during childhood growth. The percentages are related to the patient's age and represent a more accurate estimate of the proportions of specific body surfaces (**Table 12-7**).

- The rule of palms is used to measure the extent of small or scattered burns. The percentage of burned surface can be estimated by considering the palmar surface of the patient's hand (to include the fingers) as equal to 1% of the total body surface and then estimating the TBSA burned in reference to the palm.[28,38]

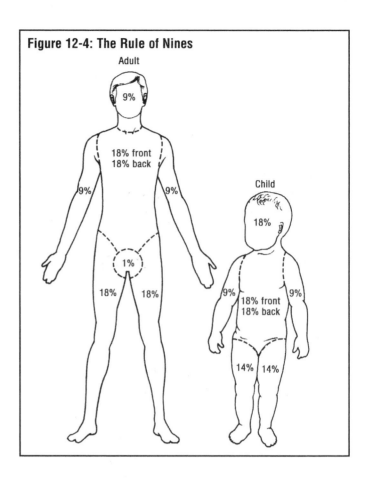

Figure 12-4: The Rule of Nines

Table 12-7: Modified Lund and Browder Chart

	Age (years)					
Burned Area	**1**	**1 to 4**	**5 to 9**	**10 to 14**	**15**	**Adult**
Total Body Surface (%)						
Head	19	17	13	11	9	7
Neck	2	2	2	2	2	3
Anterior trunk	13	13	13	13	13	13
Posterior trunk	13	13	13	13	13	13
Right buttock	2.5	2.5	2.5	2.5	2.5	2.5
Left buttock	2.5	2.5	2.5	2.5	2.5	2.5
Genitalia	1	11	11	1	1	1
Right upper arm	4	4	4	4	4	4
Left upper arm	4	4	4	4	4	4
Right lower arm	3	3	3	3	3	3
Left lower arm	3	3	3	3	3	3
Right hand	2.5	2.5	2.5	2.5	2.5	2.5
Left hand	2.5	2.5	2.5	2.5	2.5	2.5
Right thigh	5.5	6.5	8	8.5	9	9.5
Left thigh	5.5	6.5	8	8.5	9	9.5
Right leg	5	5	5.5	6	6.5	7
Left leg	5	5	5.5	6	6.5	7
Right foot	3.5	3.5	3.5	3.5	3.5	3.5
Left foot	3.5	3.5	3.5	3.5	3.5	3.5

- Determine the location of the burn injuries.
  - Circumferential burns of the chest or neck may lead to respiratory compromise.
  - Circumferential burns of the extremities may contribute to neurovascular compromise.
  - Certain locations of thermal burns present specific patient problems. Burns of the face and neck may cause respiratory problems if edema is present. Burns in this area may also interfere with the patient's ability to talk, swallow, eat, or drink. Burns of the hands inhibit the ability to perform many activities, including those of daily living. Burns of the feet interfere with ambulation. Patients with burns of the perineum are at increased risk of infection, difficulties with urinary and bowel elimination, and sexual activity.
- Determine the severity of the burn.
  - On the basis of the depth, extent, and location of the burn, the severity of the thermal injury can be determined.
  - Monitor the color of the patient's urine if myoglobinuria is suspected after injury. In the presence of myoglobinuria, urine may be pigmented.
  - Age, general preexisting health status, presence of other injuries, and mechanism of injury contribute to overall severity.

Auscultation

- Auscultate breath sounds.
  - Burn patients may have inhaled the byproducts of combustion. If the patient has a circumferential burn of the thorax, increased inspiratory pressure may be noted during mechanical ventilation as the chest is auscultated.
- Auscultate pulses in burned extremities (radial, ulnar, palmar arch, fingers, posterior tibial, dorsalis pedis, and toes) with a Doppler ultrasonic flow meter, if available.

Palpation

- Palpate the peripheral pulses to detect any vascular compromise associated with circumferential burns to the extremities and any direct injury to vessels.
- Palpate the extremities to determine sensory function and detect any neurologic compromise. Full-thickness burns, which destroy nerve endings, will not be painful. Areas around the full-thickness burn that are not as severely burned will still have sensation and be painful.

- Feel the temperature of the skin to determine peripheral perfusion status. Burn tissue feels cold because of decreased perfusion and fluid loss.

Diagnostic Procedures

Refer to Chapter 3, Initial Assessment, for frequently ordered radiographic and laboratory studies. Additional studies for patients with burn trauma are listed following.

Radiographic Studies

- A chest radiograph is performed to establish a baseline to evaluate evolving pulmonary injury.
- In the event of explosion, fall, or jump, obtain radiographic studies where indicated.
- There is a low index of suspicion for radiographic studies in any high-voltage electrical injury, with the primary focus placed on the cervical spine and long bones.

Laboratory Studies

- Electrolytes
- Arterial blood gases, pH, and SaO_2
  - An arterial blood sample can be used for extended testing of oxyhemoglobin, carboxyhemoglobin, and methemoglobin.
  - The normal level of carboxyhemoglobin is 0% to 13%, the toxic level is considered 25% to 35%, and the lethal level is over 60%.[39]
- A urinalysis and test for hemoglobin and myoglobin may be ordered; however, diagnosis is usually based on urine color. In the presence of myoglobinuria, the urine may take on a pink or red color.

Other Studies

- Pulse oximetry: Although it is important to measure SpO_2, caution must be used because pulse oximeters cannot differentiate between carboxyhemoglobin and oxyhemoglobin.[40]
- Fiberoptic, flexible bronchoscopy may be performed to determine the degree of inhalation injury.

Planning and Implementation

Refer to Chapter 3, Initial Assessment, for a description of the specific nursing interventions for patients with compromises to airway, breathing, circulation, and disability.

Interventions

- Stop the burning process, if still active.

- Ensure a patent airway.

  Prepare for early intubation as needed, especially if signs of inhalation injury are present. Intubation of the trachea may be difficult because of edema. Complete airway obstruction can occur rapidly. Summon someone skilled in difficult intubations and surgical airway techniques. It is important that a large tube be used to facilitate adequate ventilation and pulmonary clearing, especially in patients with inhalation injury. If facial burns are present, consider using umbilical tape to secure the endotracheal tube.

- Administer oxygen via a nonrebreather mask at a flow rate sufficient to keep the reservoir bag inflated; this usually requires 12 to 15 L/minute.

- Assist ventilation, if needed.

  Positive end expiratory pressure (PEEP) or continuous positive airway pressure (CPAP) may be used to maintain alveolar inflation and prevent respiratory distress. Ventilators should be equipped to administer oxygen that is warmed and humidified.

- Cannulate two veins with large-caliber intravenous catheters, and initiate infusion of a warmed intravenous solution. Avoid burned areas, if possible.

- Patients with more than 20% of their TBSA burned require fluid resuscitation.[40]

  - The primary goal of fluid resuscitation is to maintain adequate tissue perfusion and organ function while avoiding complications related to inadequate or excessive fluid therapy.

  - The latest guidelines established by the American Burn Association for fluid resuscitation follow[38]

    - Adults: 2 to 4 ml of a crystalloid solution (such as normal saline or lactated Ringer's solution) × body weight (kilograms) × percentage of TBSA burned

    - Children: 3 to 4 ml of a crystalloid solution (such as normal saline or lactated Ringer's solution) × body weight (kilograms) × percentage of TBSA burned

    - Infants and young children: Should receive fluid with 5% dextrose at a maintenance rate in addition to the resuscitation fluid noted above for children

  - One-half the amount calculated should be infused within the first 8 hours **from the time of the burn.** The remaining half is infused over the subsequent 16 hours postburn. The 24-hour time period begins from the time of the actual burn, not the time of arrival at the emergency department.

  - The following is an example:

    24-Hour Burn Fluid Calculation

    - 40% total body surface area burn

    - 70-kg patient

    - Burn occurred at 10:00 p.m.

    - Order reads: Give 2 ml per kg per % TBSA burned

      - 2 × 70 × 40 = 5,600 ml in first 24 hours postburn event

      - 2,800 ml infused by 6:00 a.m. (first 8 hours since burn event)

      - 2,800 ml or 175 ml/hour infused from 6:00 a.m. to 10:00 p.m. (subsequent 16 hours postburn)

- Ongoing fluid resuscitation is adjusted based on the individual patient's response to the injury, primarily evidenced by urinary output but taking into consideration all hemodynamic parameters such as heart rate, blood pressure, and level of consciousness.

- Patients who may require more fluid than predicted are those who have[28,41]

  - An inhalation injury

  - A high-voltage electrical injury

  - Consumed alcohol

  - Delayed fluid resuscitation since the time of injury

  - Preexisting medical conditions

- The use of additional maintenance fluids in children may be considered.[38,41]

- Insert an indwelling urinary catheter with a urimeter to monitor output of urine.

  - The urine output target is 30 to 50 ml/hour (or 0.5 ml/kg/hour). For children weighing less than 30 kg, the goal for urine output is 1 ml/kg/hour.[38] The cause of the burn; mentation; pulmonary, renal, and cardiovascular status; and size of the patient are all considerations.

- Monitor pediatric patients' blood glucose frequently because children have limited glycogen stores, which are rapidly exhausted in the early postburn stage.

- Remove all clothing and jewelry (e.g., rings, watches, necklaces) in anticipation of edema formation and to prevent heat transfer to the skin.

- Administer analgesic medications, as prescribed. Narcotics (e.g., morphine) should be administered intravenously. Absorption may be altered if the intramuscular or subcutaneous route is used. The intravenous route also allows a more accurate titration of medication to control the pain.

- Insert a gastric tube. Prevention of gastric ileus is necessary in patients with major burns.

- Do not use ice.

- Keep small burn areas cool (will help to relieve pain).

- Apply cool dressings within 10 minutes of the burn to reduce the heat content of the tissues and the depth of the burn injury.[26]

- Apply cool, saline-moistened, sterile dressings to burns less than 10% TBSA.

- Avoid using cool dressings for longer than 20 minutes to avoid further injury to tissue and hypothermia.[38]

- Cover burns greater than 10% TBSA with a clean, dry sheet.

- Keep the patient warm, especially during any transport.

- Because a burn patient cannot maintain body heat, keep the room warm to prevent hypothermia. Keeping the ambient temperature warm is also important because the patient may be in a hypermetabolic state. For patients with burns greater than 50% TBSA, increasing the ambient temperature above 86 °F (30 °C) can reduce their hypermetabolism.

- Assist with escharotomies of the chest wall, extremities, or both as needed to facilitate chest wall expansion or adequate blood flow. An escharotomy is an incision made into the eschar or burned tissue to relieve circumferential tension.

- Position extremities to prevent contractures.

- Elevate burned extremities, if not contraindicated, to facilitate venous return.

- Elevate the head of the bed to reduce airway edema and reduce the risk of pneumonia, especially ventilator-associated pneumonia in the intubated patient.

- Treat or assist with care of the burn wound.
  - If the patient is being transferred to a burn center within 24 hours of injury, wound care is deferred.
  - General care of a localized (less than 15% TBSA for the adult, less than 10% TBSA for the child) burn wound includes[26]
    - Administering an analgesic medicine before wound care.
    - Cleaning the wound gently with tepid water and a mild soap solution.

- Debriding nonviable epidermis.
- Unroofing of bullae (blisters) (often debated). Although some experts (Advanced Trauma Life Support®[40]) recommend leaving blisters intact, it is more widely agreed that wound-healing factors are lower than normal, and if in a facility of definitive treatment, debridement and proper dressing are indicated.[37]
- Clipping hair around the wound. Never shave eyebrows.
- Applying a topical antimicrobial agent, such as 1% mafenide acetate cream (Sulfamylon) or 1% silver sulfadiazine cream (Silvadene).

- Wound care is a low priority in the initial care of a severely burned patient. Direct wound care should not be attempted until well after the patient's airway, breathing, and circulatory status have been addressed.

- Provide psychosocial support to the patient and family, especially because burn wounds may be difficult for the patient and family to view.

- Prepare the patient for operative intervention, hospital admission, or transfer, as indicated. If the patient is to be transferred, consult with the receiving facility for instructions on wound care. If wound care is to be done before transfer, wash wounds, debride loose tissue, and cover with a dry, sterile dressing, but do not apply any topical agents.

- If an acutely burned patient is a candidate for transfer to a burn center, consult with the receiving physician and facility for specific burn resuscitation procedures.

- The American College of Surgeons has refined the criteria previously developed by the American Burn Association for patients with burn injury to be transferred to a burn unit (**Table 12-8**).[42]

- Hyperbaric oxygen therapy may be considered for the treatment of specific inhalation injury (e.g., carbon monoxide inhalation). Hyperbaric oxygen therapy presumes that 100% oxygen delivered to the patient under high pressure further reduces the half-life of carboxyhemoglobin and thereby reduces cerebral edema and cerebral pressure.[18] Hyperbaric oxygen therapy may also be considered for patients who have been poisoned with cyanide, hydrogen sulfide, or carbon tetrachloride.[39]

- Administer medications, as prescribed, to treat hydrogen cyanide poisoning. The burning of polyurethane, wool, silk, and paper can be a source of hydrogen cyanide.[25] Cyanide has the ability to inactivate cytochrome oxidase, which is an important enzyme in cellular production of ATP. The administration of amyl nitrite by inhalation and sodium nitrite by intravenous injection converts the iron in hemoglobin to form methemoglobin, which cannot combine with oxygen but can attract the cyanide molecules. This process frees the cyanide from cytochrome oxidase, allowing it to participate in cellular activities; however, this process decreases oxygen transport. Sodium thiosulfate may be given to form thiocyanate. The use of sodium thiosulfate and hydroxocobalamin intravenously is recommended at the scene of the fire.[32]

Electrical Burn

- Monitor pH, PaO_2, $PaCO_2$, SaO_2, SpO_2, and serum bicarbonate levels.

- Ensure that ventilation and fluid replacement are adequate.

- Infuse intravenous fluid initially at a rate to maintain urinary output 75 to 100 ml/hour in adults. Fluid resuscitation estimates cannot be calculated accurately because although there may be obvious surface wounds to measure TBSA, there will also be "underlying deep muscle damage."[33,34]

- Observe the color of urine. Once it has been determined that pigment is not present in the urine, maintaining a urine output of 0.5 to 1.0 ml/kg is recommended.[34,38]

  - If urine is dark, pink, or red, myoglobin may be present. The administration of sodium

bicarbonate may be considered to facilitate excretion of these substances because they are excreted more readily in alkaline urine.[28,34] If urine color does not return to normal, anticipate administration of mannitol (hyperosmolar diuretic) to promote diuresis and excretion of myoglobin. Myoglobin, if not excreted, can precipitate in the renal tubules, which may result in renal failure.

- Monitor cardiac rate and rhythm for at least 24 hours.

- Monitor for signs and symptoms of compartment syndrome and prepare for fasciotomies, as indicated.

Chemical Burn

- Ensure protection of the trauma team from contamination by using gloves, gowns, masks, and goggles.

- Remove all dry/powder chemicals by brushing off with a dry towel before irrigating with water.

- Irrigate the burned area with water or normal saline; alkalies require longer irrigation times to neutralize and remove. Irrigation should continue until pain is resolved, possibly as long as 2 to 3 hours of hydrotherapy.

- Do not waste time identifying a neutralizing agent. However, surface burns caused by lime or lime-containing compounds, such as concrete,

Table 12-8: American Burn Association Burn Injury Referral Criteria

- Partial-thickness and full-thickness burns greater than 10% of the total BSA (body surface area) in patients younger than 10 years or older than 50 years of age
- Partial-thickness and full-thickness burns greater than 20% BSA in other age groups
- Partial-thickness and full-thickness burns involving the face, eyes, ears, hands, feet, genitalia, or perineum, or those that involve skin overlying major joints
- Full-thickness burns greater than 5% BSA in any age group
- Significant electrical burns, including lightning injury (significant volumes of tissue beneath the surface may be injured and result in acute renal failure and other complications)
- Significant chemical burns
- Inhalation injury
- Burn injury in patient with preexisting illness that could complicate management, prolong recovery, or affect mortality
- Any burn injury patient with concomitant trauma poses an increased risk of morbidity or mortality and may be treated initially in a trauma center until stable before transfer to a burn center
- Children with burn injuries who are seen in hospitals without qualified personnel or equipment to manage their care should be transferred to a burn center with these capabilities
- Burn injury in a patient who will require special social and emotional or long-term rehabilitative support, including cases involving suspected child abuse and neglect

Reprinted with permission from American College of Surgeons Committee on Trauma. (2004). Injuries due to burns and cold. In *Advanced trauma life support® for doctors* (Student provider manual) (7th ed., p. 238). Chicago: Author.

should **not** be initially irrigated with water because the combination of water and lime produces a corrosive substance that will cause further burning. After the lime powder is brushed off with a dry towel, the area can then be irrigated thoroughly.

- Surface burns with phenol contamination should be irrigated with copious amounts of water.[35] Irrigation with a lipid-soluble solvent (e.g., polyethylene glycol) is also recommended after water irrigation. Phenol absorption can produce serious systemic sequelae such as liver and kidney damage. Wear rubber gloves when caring for patients burned with phenol.[35]

- Hydrofluoric acid, which is used in glass etching, dental laboratories, industry, and electronic plants, may cause burns that are extremely serious and possibly life-threatening. Inhalation of this acid may lead to pulmonary edema. Local contact on the skin leads to deep penetration, causing tissue necrosis. The time from exposure to tissue damage can be seconds. This acid depletes serum calcium levels. Topical applications of 5% calcium gluconate-based gel are required.[35,38]

- For patients with moderate to large tar or asphalt burns, cool the area first and use petroleum products (e.g., neomycin sulfate, mineral oil) to dissolve the substance.

Evaluation and Ongoing Assessment

Refer to Chapter 3, Initial Assessment, for a description of the ongoing evaluation of the patient's airway, breathing, circulation, and disability. Additional evaluations include

- Monitoring urinary output.
- Assessing peripheral circulation around the area where the burn is located by palpating peripheral pulses and using a Doppler ultrasonic flow meter. Increase the frequency of checks with any noted diminution of pulse quality.
- Assessing progression of edema formation.
- Assessing wounds for bleeding, increasing drainage, and signs of infection.

Summary

Surface trauma can be defined as any disruption in the integumentary system; it can be a skin or a soft-tissue injury. Burns, lacerations, abrasions, avulsions, contusions, punctures, hematomas, and degloving injuries are forms of surface trauma often encountered in the acutely injured patient. Soft-tissue injuries can involve muscles, tendons, cartilage, ligaments, vessels, and nerves. Surface trauma can be the primary injury or a concurrent injury.

Burn injury and death from burn injury have declined dramatically over the past two decades, in part because of advances in medical technology, injury prevention programs, legislation, and other societal changes. The leading cause of death from being involved in a fire in a dwelling is inhalation of toxic substances. Regardless of the extent and depth of a thermal burn, adhere to the principles outlined in the initial assessment to correct any life-threatening compromises to airway, breathing, circulation, or all of these. Determine the severity of a burn by determining the depth, extent, and location of the burn and the age as well as the general preexisting health status of the patient.

After intervening to ensure airway clearance and adequate ventilation, initiate intravenous fluid replacement if the extent of the patient's burn is greater than 20% TBSA. Follow the guidelines for considering transfer of certain patients to a comprehensive burn unit or burn center.

Burn injury is traumatic not only to the patient, but also to the family and the caregivers. The burn patient may be facing a long, painful, and stressful recovery with devastating consequences to self-esteem, image, and equilibrium. The trauma nursing process, initiated in the emergency department, will affect the patient's response to the burn injury. The nursing process in collaboration with others is intended to prevent or correct those pathophysiologic changes, which could lead to serious sequelae, such as shock, pulmonary failure, infection, or all of these.

References

1. Porth, C. M. (2002). Alterations in fluid and electrolytes. In C. M. Porth (Ed.), *Pathophysiology: Concepts of altered health states* (6th ed., pp. 693–733). Philadelphia: Lippincott Williams & Wilkins.

2. Trott, A. T. (2005). Emergency wound care: An overview. In *Wounds and lacerations: Emergency care and closure* (3rd ed., p. 1). St. Louis, MO: Mosby.

3. McCaig, L. F., & Burt, C. W. (2005, May 26). Advance data from vital and health statistics. *National hospital ambulatory medical care survey: 2003 emergency department summary* (number 358). Retrieved June 20, 2006, from http://www.cdc.gov/nchs/data/ad/ad358.pdf

4. Trott, A. T. (2005). Surface injury and wound healing. In *Wounds and lacerations: Emergency care and closure* (3rd ed., pp. 19–27). St. Louis, MO: Mosby.

5. Singh, N., & McQuillan, K. A. (2002). In K. A. McQuillan, K. T. Von Rueden, R. L. Harstsock, M. B. Flynn, & E. Whalen (Eds.), *Trauma nursing: From resuscitation through rehabilitation* (3rd ed., pp. 690–716). Philadelphia: W. B. Saunders.

6. Trott, A. T. (2005). Complex wounds: Advanced repair technique. In *Wounds and lacerations: Emergency care and closure* (3rd ed., p. 145). St. Louis, MO: Mosby.

7. Trott, A. T. (2005). Wound cleansing and irrigation. *Wounds and lacerations: Emergency care and closure* (3rd ed., p. 88). St. Louis, MO: Mosby.

8. Flynn, M. B. (2002). Wound healing. In K. A. McQuillan, K. T. Von Rueden, R. L. Harstsock, M. B. Flynn, & E. Whalen (Eds.), *Trauma nursing: From resuscitation through rehabilitation* (3rd ed., pp. 260–281). Philadelphia: W. B. Saunders.

9. Li, J. (2006, April). *Antibiotics: A review of ED use.* Retrieved June 20, 2006, from http://www.emedicine.com/emerg/topic803.htm

10. Fry, D. E. (2004). Prevention, diagnosis, & management of infection. In E. E. Moore, D. V. Feliciano, & K. L. Mattox (Eds.), *Trauma* (5th ed., pp. 356–357). New York: McGraw-Hill.

11. U.S. Department of Health and Human Services, Centers for Disease Control and Prevention. (2005, September 9). *Tetanus prevention.* Retrieved September 22, 2005, from http://www.bt.cdc.gov/disasters/hurricanes/katrina/tetanus.asp

12. Anderson, R. N., & Smith, B. L. (2005). Deaths: Leading causes for 2002. *National Vital Statistics Reports, 53*(17), 1–92.

13. Pruitt, B. A., Goodwin, C. W., & Mason, A. D., Jr. (2002). Epidemiologic, demographic, and outcome characteristics of burn injury. In D. N. Herndon (Ed.), *Total burn care* (2nd ed., pp. 16–30). London: W. B. Saunders.

14. Rivera, F. P. (2000). Burns: The importance of prevention. *Injury Prevention, 6*(4), 243–244.

15. Schallom, L. (2002). Burns. In L. D. Urden, K. M. Stacy, & M. E. Lough (Eds.), *Thelan's critical care nursing: Diagnosis and management* (4th ed., pp. 965–992). St. Louis: Mosby.

16. Kochanek, K. D., Murphy, S. L., Anderson, R. N., & Scott, C. (2004). Deaths: Final data for 2002. *National Vital Statistics Report, 53*(5), 1–116.

17. American Burn Association. (2000). Burn *incidence and treatment in the US: 2000 fact sheet.* Retrieved February 25, 2006, from http://ameriburn.org/pub/BurnIncidenceFactSheet.htm

18. Price, D. P., Silverman, H., & Schwartz, G. R. (1999). Smoke inhalation. In G. R. Schwartz (Ed.), *Principles and practice of emergency medicine* (4th ed., pp. 1559–1565). Baltimore: Williams & Wilkins.

19. Dimick, A. R., & Wagner, R. G. Burns. (1999). In G. R. Schwartz (Ed.), *Principles and practice of emergency medicine* (4th ed., pp. 387–393). Baltimore: Williams & Wilkins.

20. Moritz, A. R., & Herriques, F. C., Jr. (1947). Studies of thermal injuries: The relative importance of time and surface temperature in the causation of cutaneous burns. *American Journal of Pathology, 23,* 695–720.

21. New York State Office of the Aging. (2004). *Fire safety checklist: Materials that burn.* Retrieved February 25, 2006, from http://www.agingwell.state.ny.us/safety/fire/fire3.htm

22. Rutherford, G. W., Marcy, N., & Mills, A. (2002). *U.S. Consumer Product Safety Commission special report: Emergency room injuries in adults 65 and older.* Retrieved December 18, 2005, from http://www.cpsc.gov/library/foia/foia05/os/older.pdf

23. Centers for Disease Control and Prevention. (2002). Lightning-associated injuries and deaths among military personnel—United States 1998–2001. *MMWR, 51*(38), 859–862.

24. Fish, R. M. (2004). Lightning injuries. In J. E. Tintinalli, G. D. Kelen, & J. S. Stapczynski (Eds.), *Emergency medicine: A comprehensive study guide* (6th ed., pp. 1235–1238). New York: McGraw-Hill.

25. Cancio, L. C., & Pruitt, B. A. (2002). Inhalation injury. In G. C. Tsokos & J. L. Atkins (Eds.), *Combat medicine: Basic and clinical research in military, trauma, and emergency medicine* (pp. 325–349). Totowa, NJ: Humana Press.

26. Mozingo, D. W., Cioffi, W. G., & Pruitt, B. A., Jr. (2003). Burns. In F. S. Bongard & D. Y. Sue (Eds.), *Current critical care diagnosis & treatment* (2nd ed., pp. 799–828). New York: McGraw-Hill.

27. Sheridan, R. L. (2002). Burns. *Critical Care Medicine, 30*(11 Suppl.), S500–S514.

28. Wolf, S. E., & Herndon, D. N. (2004). Burns and radiation injuries. In E. E. Moore, D. V. Feliciano, & K. L. Mattox (Eds.), *Trauma* (5th ed., pp. 1081–1097). New York: McGraw-Hill.

29. Kramer, G. C., Lund, T., & Herndon, D. N. (2002). Pathophysiology of burn shock and burn edema.

In D. N. Herndon (Ed.), *Total burn care* (2nd ed., pp. 78–87). London: W. B. Saunders.

30. Van Meter, K. W. (2004). Carbon monoxide poisoning. In J. E. Tintinalli, G. D. Kelen, & J. S. Stapczynski (Eds.), *Emergency medicine: A comprehensive study guide* (6th ed., pp. 1238–1242). New York: McGraw-Hill.

31. Schwartz, G. R. (1999). Pathophysiology of dying and reanimation. In G. R. Schwartz (Ed.), *Principles and practice of emergency medicine* (4th ed., pp. 1–32). Baltimore: Williams & Wilkins.

32. Traber, D. L., Herndon, D. N., & Soejima, K. (2002). The pathophysiology of inhalation injury. In D. N. Herndon (Ed.), *Total burn care* (2nd ed., pp. 221–231). London: W. B. Saunders.

33. Fish, R. M. (2004). Electrical injuries. In J. E. Tintinalli, G. D. Kelen, & J. S. Stapczynski (Eds.), *Emergency medicine: A comprehensive study guide* (6th ed., pp. 1231–1235). New York: McGraw-Hill.

34. Purdue, G. F., & Hunt, J. L. (2002). Electrical injuries. In D. N. Herndon (Ed.), *Total burn care* (2nd ed., pp. 455–460). London: W. B. Saunders.

35. Sanford, A. P., & Herndon, D. N. (2002). Chemical burns. In D. N. Herndon (Ed.), *Total burn care* (2nd ed., pp. 475–480). London: W. B. Saunders.

36. Fitzpatrick, J. C., & Cioffi, W. G. (2002). Diagnosis and treatment of inhalation injury. In D. N. Herndon (Ed.), *Total burn care* (2nd ed., pp. 232–244). London: W. B. Saunders.

37. Williams, W. G. (2002). Pathophysiology of the burn wound. In D. N. Herndon (Ed.), *Total burn care* (2nd ed., pp. 514–522). London: W. B. Saunders.

38. American Burn Association. (2005). *Advanced burn life support course manual.* (pp. 33–40). Chicago: Author.

39. Schwartz, G. R. (1999). The poisoned patient: Overview. In G. R. Schwartz (Ed.), *Principles and practice of emergency medicine* (4th ed., pp. 1607–1618). Baltimore: Williams & Wilkins.

40. American College of Surgeons Committee on Trauma. (2004). Injuries due to burns and cold. In *Advanced trauma life support® for doctors (instructor course manual)* (7th ed., pp. 143–151). Chicago: Author.

41. Warden, G. D. (2002). Fluid resuscitation and early management. In D. N. Herndon (Ed.), *Total burn care* (2nd ed., pp. 88–97). London: W. B. Saunders.

42. American College of Surgeons Committee on Trauma. (1998). Guidelines for the operation of a burn unit. In *Resources for the optimal care of the injured patient: 1999* (pp. 55–62). Chicago: Author.

In addition to the nursing diagnoses outlined in Chapter 3, Initial Assessment, the following nursing diagnoses are potential problems for the patient with surface and burn trauma. Once a patient has been assessed, diagnoses can be defined as either actual or risk. An actual nursing diagnosis is derived from a decision based on the patient's presenting signs and symptoms. A risk nursing diagnosis is a judgment the nurse makes based on a particular patient's risk and potential for developing certain problems.

Nursing Diagnoses	Interventions	Expected Outcomes
Airway clearance, ineffective, related to: • Edema of the airway, vocal cords, epiglottis, and upper airway • Irritation of the respiratory tract • Laryngeal spasm • Altered level of consciousness • Presence of an artificial airway • Direct trauma • Tracheobronchial secretions or obstruction • Aspiration of foreign matter • Inhalation of toxic fumes or substances	Ensure a patent airway: • Position patient to support maximum airway efficiency • Protect the cervical spine • Administer 100% oxygen • Use airway adjuncts to maintain airway • Prepare for early intubation • Suction to clear secretions • Reassess airway status frequently • Insert gastric tube • Obtain blood sample for arterial blood gases (ABGs), as indicated	**The patient will maintain a patent airway, as evidenced by:** • Regular rate, depth, and pattern of breathing • Bilateral chest expansion • Effective cough or gag reflex • Absence of signs and symptoms of airway obstruction: stridor, dyspnea, and hoarse voice • Clear sputum of normal amount without abnormal color or odor • Absence of signs and symptoms of retained secretions: fever, tachycardia, and tachypnea

Gas exchange, impaired, related to:
 	
• Alveolar damage
• Fluid shifts
• Decreased transport, release, and utilization of oxygen secondary to carbon monoxide inhalation
• Altered blood flow, oxygen-carrying capacity of the blood, oxygen supply
• Aspiration of foreign matter
• Hypo- or hyperventilation
• Inhalation of toxic fumes or substances
	• Administer 100% oxygen
	• Monitor level of consciousness
	• Assist with intubation as ordered
	• Monitor respiratory status frequently (rate, rhythm, depth, effort, chest wall movement)
	• Monitor color, temperature, and moisture of skin
	• Monitor pulse oximetry readings
	• Monitor cardiac rate and rhythm for at least 24 hours
	• Monitor results of blood gas studies
	• Monitor the sedated patient closely
	• Arrange hyperbaric oxygen (HBO) therapy, as ordered
		The patient will experience adequate gas exchange, as evidenced by:
		
		• ABG values within normal limits:
		  ▪ PaO_2 80 to 100 mm Hg (10.0 to 13.3 KPa)
		  ▪ SaO_2 > 95%
		  ▪ $PaCO_2$ 35 to 45 mm Hg (4.7 to 6.0 KPa)
		  ▪ pH between 7.35 and 7.45
		• Level of consciousness, awake and alert, age appropriate
		• Vital signs within normal limits for age
		• Decreasing carboxyhemoglobin level
		• Skin normal color, warm, and dry

Nursing Diagnoses	Interventions	Expected Outcomes

Breathing pattern, ineffective, related to:
 	
• Respiratory distress secondary to alveolar damage
• Pain
• Circumferential burns to thoracic cavity or neck
• Altered level of consciousness secondary to elevated carboxyhemoglobin level
	• Monitor rate, rhythm, depth, and effort of respirations
	• Elevate head of bed (if not contraindicated)
	• Insert gastric tube to decompress the stomach and evacuate contents
	• Administer 100% oxygen as indicated
	• Position the patient to support maximum airway efficiency
	• Prepare for escharotomy, as indicated
		The patient will have an effective breathing pattern, as evidenced by:
		
		• Normal rate, depth, and pattern of breathing
		• Symmetrical chest wall expansion
		• Absence of stridor, dyspnea, or cyanosis
		• Breath sounds present and equal bilateral
		• ABG values within normal limits:
		  ▪ PaO_2 80 to 100 mm Hg (10.0 to 13.3 KPa)
		  ▪ SaO_2 > 95%
		  ▪ $PaCO_2$ 35 to 45 mm Hg (4.7 to 6.0 KPa)
		  ▪ pH between 7.35 and 7.45

Fluid volume deficit, related to: • Hemorrhage • Increased capillary permeability • Protein shifts • Inflammatory processes • Evaporation losses	• Control external hemorrhage: Apply direct pressure over bleeding site; elevate affected extremity • Cannulate two veins with large-caliber intravenous catheters and initiate infusion of lactated Ringer's solution or normal saline; infuse fluid at a rate consistent with a replacement formula • Administer blood, as indicated • Monitor urine output, color, and specific gravity • Monitor patient's heart rate, peripheral pulses, color, temperature, moisture of skin, and capillary refill for perfusion status trends • Monitor vital signs, level of consciousness, and lung sounds frequently • Monitor results of laboratory studies; hemoglobin, hematocrit, electrolytes, and carbon monoxide	**The patient will have an effective circulating volume, as evidenced by:** • External hemorrhage controlled • Stable vital signs appropriate for age • Strong, palpable peripheral and central pulses • Level of consciousness, awake and alert, age appropriate • Skin color normal for individual, warm and dry • Urine output 30 to 50 ml/hr in adults > 30 kg; 1 ml/kg/hr in children < 30 kg • Capillary refill time of < 2 seconds • Serum electrolyte, hematocrit, and hemoglobin within normal limits
Hypothermia, risk, related to: • Impairment in skin integrity • Resuscitative procedures • Exposure • Ineffective thermoregulation • Consumption of alcohol • Decreased tissue perfusion	• Apply warm blankets • Avoid unnecessary exposure • Monitor temperature frequently • Use warming adjuncts (blankets, warming lights), as necessary • Increase room temperature • Use warmed intravenous fluids for infusion	**The patient will maintain a normal core body temperature, as evidenced by:** • Core temperature measurement of 98 to 99.5 °F (36 to 37.5 °C) • Vital signs within normal limits for age • Level of consciousness, awake and alert, age appropriate

Nursing Diagnoses	Interventions	Expected Outcomes
Tissue perfusion, altered renal, cardiopulmonary, cerebral, gastrointestinal, peripheral (specific type), related to: • Hypovolemia • Interruption of flow: arterial and/or venous • Vessel compression secondary to edema • Vessel compression secondary to compartment syndrome	• Assist with fasciotomies/escharotomies, as indicated • Monitor neurovascular status of areas with surface trauma • Use ultrasonic flow meter to measure tissue perfusion in burned distal digits • Monitor for signs and symptoms of compartment syndrome • Elevate injured extremities • Remove jewelry or constrictive clothing before • Control any uncontrolled bleeding • Cannulate two veins with large-caliber intravenous catheters and initiate infusion of lactated Ringer's solution or normal saline • Administer blood, as indicated	The patient will maintain adequate tissue perfusion, as evidenced by: • Vital signs within normal limits for age • Level of consciousness, awake and alert, age appropriate • Skin normal color, warm, and dry (central and distal to injury) • Strong and equal peripheral pulses • Absence of ischemic pain and motor paralysis • Normal sensation • Capillary refill time of < 2 seconds • Urine output of 30 to 50 ml in adults > 30 kg; 1 ml/kg/hr in children < 30 kg
Infection, risk, related to: • Impaired skin integrity • Presence of invasive lines • Interruption in perfusion • Grossly contaminated wounds • Presence of retained foreign debris • Immobility • Suppressed inflammatory response	• Maintain sterile technique during procedures • Maintain aseptic technique • Monitor vital signs, temperature • Assist with debridement of burned or devitalized tissue • Ensure maximum mobility for the patient • Apply topical ointments and dressings per hospital protocol • Properly clean wound • Irrigate wound thoroughly • Give antibiotics as soon as possible (if indicated) • Administer tetanus prophylaxis, as prescribed • Obtain wound/blood cultures	The patient will be free from infection, as evidenced by: • Core temperature measurement of 98 to 99.5 °F (36 to 37.5 °C) • Absence of systemic signs of infection: fever, tachypnea, tachycardia • White blood cell count within normal limits • Wound healing proceeds without signs/symptoms of infection: redness, swelling, purulent drainage, odor and tenderness

Nursing Diagnoses	Interventions	Expected Outcomes
Anxiety and fear (patient and family), related to: • Injury • Appearance (possible scarring, disfigurement) • Unpredictable nature of condition • Effects of actual or perceived loss of significant other • Threat to or change in health status, role functions, support systems, environment, self-concept, or interaction patterns • Threat of death, actual or perceived • Lack of knowledge • Loss of control • Disruptive family life • Pain • Threat to self-concept • Diagnostic/invasive procedures	• Explain procedures to patient and family in terms they can understand • Encourage verbalization of feelings and concerns • Listen attentively • Facilitate family presence during procedures per hospital protocol • Encourage patient and family to express concerns and ask questions • Provide information to patient and family as needed or requested • Provide appropriate referrals for social service or counseling • Administer analgesia/pain control, as prescribed	**The patient and family will experience decreasing anxiety and fear, as evidenced by:** • Orientation to surroundings • Ability to describe reasons for equipment and procedures used in treatment • Ability to verbalize concerns and ask questions of the health care team • Absence of fear-related behaviors: crying, agitation • Vital signs within normal limits for age • Use of effective coping skills • Reporting of relief or absence of pain
Pain, related to: • Burn trauma • Skin and soft-tissue trauma • Tissue stretching and edema • Neurovascular compromise • Experience during invasive procedures/diagnostic tests	• Administer intravenous analgesic medications as prescribed • Administer intravenous analgesic medications before procedures • Apply ice to soft-tissue trauma to reduce pain and swelling • Immobilize and elevate injured extremity • Use touch, positioning, or relaxation techniques to give comfort	**The patient will experience relief of pain, as evidenced by:** • Diminished or absent pain according to patient's self-report • Absence of physiologic indicators of pain: tachycardia, tachypnea, diaphoresis, pallor, elevation of blood pressure • Absence of nonverbal cues of pain: crying, grimacing, unable to assume a position of comfort • Verbalizing relief of pain during procedures and after administration of medications

Chapter 13

Special Populations: Pregnant, Pediatric, and Older Adult Trauma Patients

---

Objectives

On completion of this chapter/lecture, the learner should be able to:

1. Identify the common mechanisms of injury associated with special populations (pregnant, pediatric, and older adult trauma patients).

2. Describe the pathophysiologic changes as a basis for signs and symptoms.

3. Discuss nursing assessment with special considerations for pregnant, pediatric, and older adult trauma patients.

4. Plan appropriate interventions for special populations.

5. Evaluate the effectiveness of interventions for special populations with specific injuries.

Introduction to Special Populations

Pediatric patients should not be treated as little adults, nor should older adults receive the same nursing care as young adults. Pregnant patients are not one, but two patients to consider. Each special population reacts uniquely to traumatic injury. Their responses are not the same as the response of a young adult, which we characterize as a patient's typical response to trauma.

Consider a young man who has been involved in a motor vehicle crash. His response to hypovolemia is generally tachycardia, tachypnea, and hypotension. It is a classic picture that we recognize easily. However, the pediatric patient and the pregnant patient can only tolerate shock for a short time, so the typical picture is not seen. The older adult patient, who is often taking several prescribed medications for coexisting conditions such as hypertension or cardiac disease, may not respond to trauma with tachycardia. The older adult patient may also exhibit a normal blood pressure, which is actually hypotensive for that individual. Nurses caring for these patients need to understand the unique responses to traumatic injuries. Special consideration must be given to the assessment, planning, intervention, and evaluation of pregnant, pediatric, and older adult trauma patients.

Introduction

Epidemiology

Trauma affects 6% to 7% of pregnancies in the United States; 0.3 % of pregnant women require hospital admission because of trauma.[1] It is the leading cause of maternal death secondary to nonobstetric etiologies.[2] It is common for pregnant women to continue to travel, work, drive, and remain physically active throughout pregnancy. This exposure has increased the frequency of injury. Recent data indicate 3.7 traumatic fetal deaths per 100,000 live births.[3]

Young, African-American, and Hispanic pregnant women are at higher risk for trauma in pregnancy.[4] A recent study reported that 20% of injured pregnant patients tested positive for drugs and or alcohol, and approximately one third of those in motor vehicle crashes were not using seat belts.[4]

The resuscitation priorities for the injured pregnant patient are identical to those of the nonpregnant patient. The pregnant trauma patient, however, presents a challenge because resuscitation team members are faced with the simultaneous management of two patients. Because of the low incidence of injury to pregnant women, the trauma team may not be as familiar with the physiologic changes of pregnancy and fetal development, which may complicate the resuscitation process. Members of the trauma team should include both obstetricians and obstetrics nurses, who are present early in the resuscitation process.

Mechanisms of Injury and Biomechanics

Injury to the pregnant patient can result from forces causing blunt or penetrating trauma. The uterus has elastic fibers and, therefore, is not as susceptible to rupture as the placenta, which has no elastic fibers and is more susceptible to shearing forces. Energy applied to the abdomen of the pregnant patient is absorbed in part by the uterus, the amniotic fluid, and the fetus. Therefore, other abdominal organs are somewhat protected from energy loads. Blunt trauma is the most frequent cause of maternal and fetal injury. It may result from motor vehicle crashes, falls, or violence. Motor vehicle crashes are the leading cause of death for women in the childbearing years. In motor vehicle crashes, the most common cause of fetal death is maternal death.[2] Ejection from the vehicle and head injury are associated with a poorer fetal outcome.[2] Falls are the second most common cause of injury during pregnancy. Fatigue, laxity of ligaments in the pelvis, and the protruding abdomen contribute to an unstable gait. Physical violence occurs in as many as 10% to 11% of pregnant women.[2,4]

Penetrating trauma during pregnancy is most often caused by gunshot or knife wounds.[2,5] The incidence of uterine injury increases with each trimester. The enlarged uterus shields most of the abdominal organs from injury, making the uterus the most likely organ to be penetrated. Gunshot wounds cause transient shock waves and cavitations as the kinetic energy from the bullet is transferred to the high-density tissue of the body. Gunshot wounds cause more severe injury patterns than low-velocity knife wounds. The fetus is most at risk, with fetal injuries occurring in 66% of gunshot injuries to the uterus. Fetal mortality ranges from 40% to 70% and generally results from premature delivery or direct fetal injury. Stab wounds are less common than gunshot wounds and have a lower mortality for both the mother and the fetus.[5]

Anatomic and Physiologic Changes During Pregnancy as a Basis for Signs and Symptoms

Understanding the normal anatomic and physiologic changes during pregnancy is extremely important when caring for the pregnant trauma patient. The pregnant woman is normally in a hyperdynamic and hypervolemic state. During pregnancy, the heart rate increases 10 to 15 beats above the baseline.[5] Blood pressure decreases by approximately 15 to 20% during the earlier stages of pregnancy and returns to normal during the third trimester. Cardiac output increases 35% to 50% above baseline, reaching its maximum by 28 to 32 weeks' gestation.[2]

Maternal plasma volume increases 40% to 50% by the end of the first trimester. Production of red blood cells also increases, but to a lesser extent than plasma. This inequity results in a dilutional anemia with a small decrease in hematocrit. A mild to moderate blood loss (1500 to 2000 ml, or 30%) resulting from traumatic hemorrhage may be masked because of the normal physiology of pregnancy.[2] The fetus is compromised when maternal blood loss is 15% to 30%. Signs and symptoms of fetal distress include changes in fetal movement and either fetal tachycardia or bradycardia.

The uterus becomes an abdominal organ at approximately 12 weeks gestation. This location predisposes it to injury from blunt or penetrating forces. As the weight of the uterus continues to increase, it creates a hypotensive effect when the patient is placed in a supine position. The gravid uterus compresses both the inferior vena cava and the aorta, resulting in decreased preload and as much as a 25% decrease in cardiac output. Placing the severely injured pregnant patient in a supine position may result in hemodynamic instability. After 24 weeks gestation, supine positioning should be avoided.

Tidal volume (the amount of air moved in and out of the lungs with each breath) increases by 40%, and vital capacity (the maximum amount of air exhaled from the point of maximum inspiration) increases by 100 to 200 ml. The respiratory rate usually increases slightly. Oxygen consumption increases by 15% to 20%.[5] The elevated diaphragm decreases functional residual capacity (the volume of air in the lungs at the end of expiration). Arterial blood gases reflect hyperventilation and compensated respiratory alkalosis. Hypoxemia occurs more quickly in the pregnant trauma patient and is not tolerated well.[2]

During pregnancy, gastric motility decreases. Hormonal changes relax the gastroesophageal sphincter, increasing the risk of aspiration, especially in the second to third trimester of pregnancy.[2] The normal responses to peritoneal membrane irritation are changed because of stretching of the abdominal wall. Because of gradual compression of the viscera and stretching of the abdominal wall by the uterus, rebound tenderness and abdominal guarding may be decreased.[6] The usual methods of physical abdominal assessment may be less sensitive in detecting pain and injury.

Urinary frequency is common in pregnancy because of an increased glomerular filtration rate. In late pregnancy, the bladder is elevated anteriorly out of the pelvis into the abdomen. Hormonal changes cause a softening of most joints, with relaxation of the sacroiliac joint and widening of the symphysis pubis. Because of these changes, the pelvis is less susceptible to fractures.

The levels of fibrinogen and other clotting factors increase markedly during pregnancy. This change results in a hypercoagulable state of the blood. There is a modest decrease in the platelet count.[2] The injured patient is predisposed to disseminated intravascular coagulation if abruptio placentae or amniotic fluid embolus occurs. Fibrinogen in low normal levels may be indicative of abnormal consumption.

Selected Injuries

Premature Labor

Premature labor is the most frequent complication in the pregnant trauma patient. Premature labor usually can be detected in alert patients but may go unnoticed in an unconscious or intubated patient. Premature labor may indicate maternal injury that has not yet been diagnosed as well as fetal or uterine injury.[7] If premature labor is diagnosed, and the mother's condition is stable without rupture of the membranes, medications may be given to inhibit further uterine contractions.

Signs and Symptoms

- Uterine contractions > 6 per hour
  The patient may or may not sense the contractions.
- Back pain
- Clear or bloody vaginal discharge
- Cervical change (effacement or dilation)[7,8]

Abruptio Placentae

Abruptio placenta is the premature partial or total separation of the normally implanted placenta from the uterine wall. It is a common cause of fetal death after motor vehicle crashes. Suspect separation of the placenta if the patient presents with vaginal bleeding. The signs and symptoms can be vague, particularly with a partial separation. Changes in fetal heart rate may be the only indication. Abruptio placentae can develop as late as 48 hours after trauma. A formal ultrasound should be performed initially and repeated if signs and symptoms of maternal blood loss or fetal distress develop.

Signs and Symptoms

- Vaginal bleeding (may be present, or could be absent if the blood remains retroplacental)
- Uterine tenderness, tetany, or rigidity
- Premature labor
- Abdominal pain or cramps, back pain
- Maternal hemorrhage and evidence of hypovolemic shock; maternal coagulopathy[7]
- Fetal distress as evidenced by inadequate acceleration of the fetal heart rate after uterine contraction or late decelerations in fetal heart rate in response to uterine contraction. Fetal heart rate normally remains constant or accelerates during a contraction. Acceleration is considered a reassuring sign of fetal responsiveness. Inadequate acceleration can be a sign of hypoxia. Late decelerations, transient decreases after the peak of the contraction, may indicate hypoxia or compromised blood flow to the baby.
- Expanding or rising fundal height[7]

Uterine Rupture

Uterine rupture is rare, but it may occur in patients with extreme compression injury or with a history of cesarean sections. Uterine rupture may be associated with bladder rupture, indicated by blood or meconium in the urine. Uterine rupture often results in fetal demise. It is rarely repairable and generally requires a hysterectomy. Early detection and repair of minor lacerations or tears can prevent maternal hemorrhage and fetal compromise.

Signs and Symptoms

- Abdominal pain

The patient may have a history of acute pain followed by no pain.

- Uterine tenderness
- Difficulty identifying the fundal height
- Change or loss of the normal contour of the uterus

Fetal body parts may be more palpable.

- A palpable mass outside the uterus (may be the fetus)
- Vaginal bleeding
- Maternal hemorrhage and evidence of hypovolemic shock
- Fetal distress or absent fetal heart tones[7]

Maternal Cardiopulmonary Arrest/Fetal Delivery

The following conditions have been reported to contribute to the successful outcome of delivering a fetus by cesarean section from a pregnant trauma patient in cardiopulmonary arrest:[2]

- Estimation of gestational age and assessment of fetal heart activity should be done while cardiopulmonary resuscitation is being performed on the pregnant patient. This step should be done rapidly.
- Emergency cesarean section should be initiated within 4 to 5 minutes of maternal cardiopulmonary arrest.[1,2,9,10]
- Cardiopulmonary resuscitation should be continued throughout the cesarean section.
- A neonatal resuscitation team should be immediately available on delivery of the neonate.

Nursing Care of the Pregnant Trauma Patient

Assessment

History

- What was the mechanism of injury?
- Was the patient wearing a safety restraint device? How was it positioned?
- When was the last normal menstrual period (LNMP)?

Consider the possibility of pregnancy in any female of childbearing age. If the LNMP is more than 4 to 5 weeks ago, consider the patient as possibly pregnant.

- When is the expected date of confinement (EDC)?

To estimate the EDC, count back 3 months from the first day of the LNMP and add 7 days.

- What problems or complications have occurred during this or other pregnancies?
- Are uterine contractions or abdominal pain present?
- Is there fetal activity?
- Is there a possibility that injuries have been caused by domestic violence?

Physical Assessment

Inspection

- Observe the shape and contour of the abdomen.

A change in shape may indicate uterine rupture or concealed hemorrhage.

- Observe the abdomen for signs of fetal movement.
- Inspect the perineum.

Determine whether there is any vaginal bleeding or the presence of amniotic fluid. The patient may describe having had a sudden gush of fluid. This may be an indication of a spontaneous bladder void or premature rupture of amniotic membranes.

- Inspect the vaginal opening for crowning or any abnormal fetal presentation.

Prolapse of the umbilical cord is rare. If present, relieve cord compression immediately. If positioning the mother to relieve pressure on the cord is contraindicated, manual displacement of the presenting part of the cord may be needed.

Auscultation

- Auscultate fetal heart tones and rate.

Fetal heart rate is a precise indicator of the well-being of both the mother and the fetus. Fetal heart tones may be heard with a fetoscope at approximately 20 weeks gestation and by Doppler ultrasound at 10 to 14 weeks gestation. The normal range for fetal heart rate is between 120 and 160 beats per minute.[8]

Continuous fetal monitoring with cardiotocography is suggested for patients of more than 20 weeks gestation.[2]

Palpation

- Palpate and determine the height of the fundus.

Fundal height is an indicator of gestational age. The fundus is measured in centimeters from the symphysis pubis to the top of the fundus and approximates the number of weeks of gestation. The fundal height reaches the symphysis at 12 weeks, the umbilicus at 20 weeks, and costal margin at 36 weeks (**Figure 13-1**). Generally, a fundus that is palpable between the umbilicus and the xiphoid process is consistent with a viable fetus.[5]

- Palpate the uterus. Note any uterine tenderness or contractions.

Diagnostic Procedures

Radiographic Studies

Pregnant trauma patients may require several diagnostic imaging examinations to determine the definitive diagnosis of injury. Patients and members of the health care team are always concerned about possible adverse effects from radiation on the fetus. Exposure to less than 5 *rads* has not been associated with an increase of fetal anomalies or pregnancy loss.[11] A cervical spine x-ray is approximately 0.002 rads (**Table 13-1**). The fetus receives 30% of the radiation that the mother is exposed to during diagnostic imaging. It is important, then, to emphasize shielding of the fetus for all but pelvic and lumbar spine films/CT.[10] In addition, tests should be ordered only after careful consideration, and duplication of films should be avoided. The American College of Obstetricians and Gynecologists recommends that

consultation with a radiologist or radiation specialist should be considered to assist in calculation of estimated fetal dose when multiple diagnostic x-rays are performed or being considered.[10,11]

The Use of Ultrasound

For patients who do not know or cannot communicate that they are pregnant, results of a screening ultrasound test may be the first indication of pregnancy to the trauma team. Some trauma institutions have included uterine views with the Focused Assessment Sonography for Trauma (FAST) to screen for pregnancy. This test can be done more quickly and show results sooner than waiting for results from a urine pregnancy test. Very early pregnancies will still require laboratory testing for confirmation.[12]

Ultrasound involves the use of sound waves and is not a source of radiation. A formal ultrasound may be performed during the secondary assessment to determine:

- Gestational age
- Fetal weight
- Fetal heart rate and variability
- Placental location[1]

Laboratory Studies

- Prothrombin time (PT) and partial thromboplastin time (PTT) (serial coagulation studies)
- Beta human chorionic gonadotropin (βHCG)

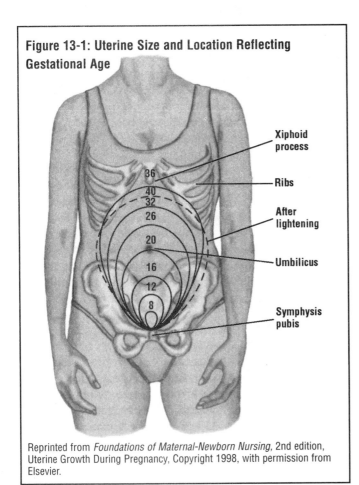

Figure 13-1: Uterine Size and Location Reflecting Gestational Age

- Xiphoid process
- Ribs
- After lightening
- Umbilicus
- Symphysis pubis

Reprinted from *Foundations of Maternal-Newborn Nursing*, 2nd edition, Uterine Growth During Pregnancy, Copyright 1998, with permission from Elsevier.

Table 13-1: Estimated Fetal Exposure for Various Radiographic Studies

Examination Type	Estimated Fetal Dose per Examination (rad)
Plain films	
Cervical spine	0.002
Chest (two views)	0.00007
Pelvis	0.040
Thoracic spine	0.009
Lumbosacral spine	0.359
CT scans	
Head	< 0.050
Chest	< 0.100
Abdominopelvic	2.60

Adapted with permission from Barraco, R. D., Chiu, W. C., Clancy, T. V., Como, J. J., Ebert, J. B., Hess, L. W., et al. (2005). Practice management guidelines for the diagnosis and management of injury in the pregnant patient: The EAST practice management guidelines work group. Retrieved June 26, 2006, from http://www.east.org/tpg/pregnancy.pdf

βHCG in blood confirms pregnancy as early as 1 to 2 weeks after conception and in urine, 2 to 4 weeks after conception.

- Kleihauer-Betke Test (KB)

The KB serum test detects fetal red cells in the maternal circulation, indicating hemorrhage of fetal blood through the placenta into the mother's circulation. This is particularly important when the woman is Rh negative and the fetus is Rh positive. Under these circumstances, hemorrhage can cause Rh sensitization that requires treatment with an appropriate amount of Rh immune globulin.[7,10] All pregnant Rh-negative trauma patients should be considered for Rh immune globulin therapy unless the injury is minimal (i.e., isolated distal extremity injury).[13]

Other Studies

- Diagnostic peritoneal lavage is safe in pregnant trauma patients. The open technique in which the peritoneum is visualized directly is used. Ensure that the stomach and bladder are emptied before the procedure.[7]

- Pelvic examination

Assess whether the cervix is open or closed and if membranes are intact. Any obvious vaginal fluid should be tested. The pH of amniotic fluid is 7.5; the pH of urine is 4.6 to 6. If amniotic fluid is observed, use a sterile speculum for the examination.

- Cardiotocography

Fetal monitoring should be initiated early in the resuscitation of the mother. Cardiotocography monitors both the fetal heart rate and uterine contractions by a sensor that is placed on the mother's abdomen. A nurse experienced in the interpretation of fetal monitoring should be present to assist in the care of the patient. Fetal monitoring is often continued for hours after the injury and may be the most sensitive indicator of initial fetal distress. An abnormal fetal heart rate or heart rate response to contraction may be the result of maternal hypovolemia, possible placental separation, or uterine rupture.

Trauma in Children

Introduction

Pediatric Epidemiology

Injuries are the leading cause of death among children in the United States between the ages of 1 and 14 years.[14] Each year there are 14 million episodes of injuries to children younger than 15 years, resulting in 9 million visits to the emergency department, 250,000 hospital admissions, and approximately 6,500 deaths.

Motor vehicle crashes are the leading cause of death. Despite seat belt laws in all 50 states, two thirds of children fatally injured in the United States were reported to be unrestrained or improperly restrained.[15] Falls remain the most common cause of severe injury in infants and toddlers. Bicycle-related incidents are a significant problem for children and adolescents. Additional causes of injury include burns, drowning, poisonings, firearms, and abuse.[16] Boys are injured twice as often as girls.[17]

Mechanisms of Injury and Biomechanics

Blunt trauma accounts for 80% of pediatric injuries;[16] the remaining injuries are penetrating in nature. In order of frequency, the most commonly injured body areas are the head, musculoskeletal system, abdomen, and thorax.

Penetrating mechanisms account for 20% of all injuries and 20% of deaths in those younger than 19 years of age. Penetrating injuries account for 10% of the admissions at most major pediatric trauma centers, with firearm injuries accounting for 7% of the patients.[18] The incidence of fatal stabbings in children has remained stable over the past two decades; however, nonfatal stabbings have increased.

Anatomic/Physiologic Differences in the Traumatically Injured Child

The trauma nursing process associated with the care of a pediatric trauma patient is based on knowledge of pediatric anatomy and physiology and the child's response to injury. Inherent in this process is the recognition of the distinct anatomic and physiologic differences between pediatric and adult patients.

Respiratory

- Infants, during the first several months of their lives, are obligatory nose breathers. Any nasal obstruction can cause respiratory distress.

- Small amounts of mucus, blood, or edema may occlude the airway because of its smaller diameter.

- The tongue and the pharyngeal tissue are softer and relatively larger when compared to the size of the oral cavity.[19] Edema of these structures is a cause of airway obstruction.

- Airway cartilage is soft, particularly the larynx in infants and small children. Flexion or hyperextension of the neck may cause airway compression.

- The larynx is higher and more anterior, increasing the risk of aspiration. The anterior position of the vocal cords makes direct visualization during intubation more difficult. The trachea is shorter, increasing the possibility of intubation of the mainstem bronchus.

- In children younger than 8 years of age, the cricoid cartilage is the narrowest portion of the trachea. Historically, uncuffed endotracheal tubes have been used in children younger than 8 years of age. Recent studies have demonstrated that in-hospital use of cuffed tubes is as safe as using uncuffed tubes for infants beyond the newborn period and in children.[19]

- Children younger than 8 years of age rely primarily on movement of the diaphragm for breathing because of their immature intercostal muscles. Excessive gastric air from crying or ventilatory assistance may affect the child's ability to ventilate adequately.[20]

- The chest wall in infants and young children is more pliable because the sternum and ribs are cartilaginous. A significant force may result in an injury to an underlying structure without concomitant rib fracture. The thin chest also allows for easy transmission of lung sounds from one side of the chest to the other. Intubation should be verified both clinically and radiographically.

- Normal respiratory rates vary according to the child's age. Generally, the younger the child, the faster the rate is (**Table 13-2**). A respiratory rate greater than 60 breaths per minute should be considered abnormal for any child.

- Children have lower glycogen stores but have increased metabolic demands, placing them at risk for hypoglycemia when under stress. In addition, they have less elastic tissue to keep the pulmonary alveoli expanded, lower tidal volumes,

and less residual capacity. Because of these factors and the underdevelopment of intercostal muscles, children may become fatigued during increased work of breathing. Respiratory failure may ensue.

Cardiovascular

- Normal blood pressure varies according to the child's age (**Table 13-2**).

- Children can compensate for a 25% blood loss by increasing the heart rate and peripheral vascular resistance, which maintains a normal systolic blood pressure; therefore, blood pressure is an unreliable indicator of shock.[21]

- Normal heart rates vary according to the child's age. Generally, the younger the child, the faster the heart rate is (**Table 13-2**). Tachycardia is one of the first signs of shock, but it can also be caused by many other factors, including anxiety and agitation. An increased heart rate caused by agitation and crying should return to normal when the child becomes calm. To maintain cardiac output during shock, the heart rate, rather than the stroke volume, increases.

- Blood volume is dependent on the size of the child. The circulating blood volume of an infant is approximately 90 ml/kg; in the child it is approximately 80 ml/kg.[21] Small blood losses can stimulate compensatory mechanisms.

Temperature Regulation

Children have a less-effective thermoregulatory mechanism, a greater ratio of body surface area to body mass, and less subcutaneous tissue for heat insulation. Hypothermia is not well tolerated. Infants and small children lose a significant amount of heat through their heads.

Table 13-2: Vital Signs by Age in Pediatric Patients

Age	Respiratory Rate/Minute	Heart Rate/Minute	Blood Pressure Systolic (mm Hg)
Preterm newborn	55–65	120–180	40–60
Term newborn	40–60	90–170	52–92
1 month	30–50	110–180	60–104
6 months	25–35	110–180	65–125
1 year	20–30	80–160	70–118
2 years	20–30	80–130	73–117
4 years	20–30	80–120	65–117
6 years	18–24	75–115	76–116
8 years	18–22	70–110	76–119
10 years	16–20	70–110	82–122
12 years	16–20	60–110	84–128
14 years	16–20	60–105	85–136

Reprinted from *Emergency Nursing Procedures*, 3rd edition, page 7, Procedure 2: Secondary Survey, Copyright 1999, with permission from Elsevier.

Other Anatomic and Physiologic Characteristics

- The metabolic demands of children are twice those of adults, and anxiety alone can increase the metabolic rate significantly.
- The neck is short in young children, which makes it difficult to evaluate neck veins and tracheal position.
- The head is heavier and larger in relation to the rest of the body, predisposing the child to head and neck trauma. The anterior and posterior fontanelles are open in infants. The cranium is thinner and more pliable in young children.
- The occiput is more prominent until approximately 10 years of age.
- The white matter is not well myelinated, making it more susceptible to shearing forces.
- The abdominal muscles are thinner, weaker, and less developed. The liver is more anterior and less protected by the ribs. The kidneys are mobile and not protected by fat.
- The bony spine is more flexible; spinal ligaments are lax.
- The bones of the extremities are more pliable and resilient to injury. Injuries to, or adjacent to, growth plates can potentially retard normal bone growth or alter bone development.

Nursing Care of the Pediatric Trauma Patient

Assessment

History

- Is the caregiver/parent present? If the child is a minor, obtain permission for treatment according to institutional protocols and state laws.
- What was the mechanism of injury? How has the child been acting since the injury? What does the caregiver think is wrong?
- If the pediatric patient was involved in a motor vehicle crash, was a safety restraint device used? Where was the lap belt positioned? Was the child in a booster seat? If in a bicycle incident, was the patient wearing a helmet?
- What was the child's most recent weight?
- Are immunizations up to date?

Physical Assessment

Inspection

- Assess for nasal flaring, intercostal retractions, or both.
- Assess the circulation for pallor or mottled skin or differences in central versus peripheral color.
- Inspect the abdomen for abrasions or ecchymosis from the seat belt.

Auscultation

- Auscultate breath sounds, especially at the anterior axillary lines. Breath sounds may be heard in all areas of the chest despite pneumothorax, because of the thinner chest in the child.
- Auscultate the apical heart rate and blood pressure. Remember that bradycardia is an ominous sign in a pediatric patient and can be a sign of impending cardiopulmonary arrest. Hypotension is a late sign of shock. Noninvasive blood pressure monitors (NIBP) should be used with caution. Ensure that parameters are specific for infants or children. Remember that the accuracy of NIBP is less in extremely high or low blood pressure measurements. Correlate the reading with the patient assessment.
- Auscultate bowel sounds.

Palpation

- Palpate the fontanelle in the infant for fullness or bulging. Dehydration will produce a sunken fontanelle. Full fontanelles in the infant positioned supine may not be clinically significant.
- Palpate central and peripheral pulses for comparison.
- Assess capillary refill. Determine the temperature of the extremities. Cool extremities with mottled skin and lethargy may be indications of shock.[22]
- Palpate the abdomen for distention. Children may swallow large amounts of air when crying. Distention may reflect gastric dilation from swallowed air.

The neurologic assessment must be tailored to the age and developmental stage of the child. The Pediatric Glasgow Coma Scale score (Table 13-3) is an adaptation of the Glasgow Coma Scale score and can be used to trend the neurologic assessment in an infant or child. A reliable caregiver or parent can be extremely helpful in determining changes in behavior or level of consciousness.

Diagnostic Procedures

Physical examination is often unreliable, especially in the infant or very young child or in those with head injury. Imaging of the patient can be helpful in identification of bony and organ injury. Children's x-rays cannot be interpreted the same way as those of the adult. Children may have significant spinal cord injury without radiographic abnormality (SCIWORA)[22] and other bony injuries when x-rays appear to be normal. Additional studies may need to be performed. Also, x-rays of extremities may need to include comparison views of the uninjured extremity.

The FAST ultrasound may be useful in the hypotensive child to assess for intra-abdominal fluid or pericardial tamponade.

Computerized tomography remains the imaging test of choice for accurate diagnostic evaluation of the injured child. Children should always be accompanied to the imaging department. Age-appropriate explanations may help decrease anxiety. Sedation may be needed to complete the exams.

Diagnostic peritoneal lavage is not commonly performed in children.[22] It may be used in instances where the FAST ultrasound is not available. Either the percutaneous or the open technique may be used with an infraumbilical approach. If gross blood is not obtained, 10 ml/kg of warmed lactated Ringer's solution is infused (up to 1,000 ml) through the peritoneal catheter.[23]

Introduction

Epidemiology

It is estimated that 12.5% of the population is aged 65 or older. These older adults are living longer and are more active because of various advances in health care. Trauma is the fifth leading cause of death in persons older than 65 years, and older adults account for 25% of the deaths from trauma.[24]

Motor vehicle crashes are the primary cause of injury for all patients up to age 75. After age 75, falls become the most common mechanism of injury. Every year, approximately 50% of people older than 80 years of age will fall and require medical treatment. One third to one half of older adults hospitalized after falls do not survive another year.[25] Those who have fallen become more careful and fearful of experiencing another fall. This fear greatly limits travel outside the home and enjoyment of life experiences.

Table 13-3: Pediatric Modification of Glasgow Coma Scale*

GCS Score		Pediatric Modification	
Eye Opening			
≥ 1 year	**0–1 year**		
4 Spontaneously	4 Spontaneously		
3 To verbal command	3 To shout		
2 To pain	2 To pain		
1 No response	1 No response		
Best Motor Response			
≥ 1 year	**0–1 year**		
6 Obeys			
5 Localizes pain	5 Localizes pain		
4 Flexion—withdrawal	4 Flexion—withdrawal		
3 Flexion—abnormal (decorticate rigidity)	3 Flexion—abnormal (decorticate rigidity)		
2 Extension (decerebrate rigidity)	2 Extension (decerebrate rigidity)		
1 No response	1 No response		
Best Verbal Response			
0–2 years	**2–5 years**	**> 5 years**	
5 Cries appropriately, smiles, coos	5 Appropriate words and phrases	5 Oriented and converses	
4 Cries	4 Inappropriate words	4 Disoriented and converses	
3 Inappropriate crying/screaming	3 Cries/screams	3 Inappropriate words	
2 Grunts	2 Grunts	2 Incomprehensible sounds	
1 No response	1 No response	1 No response	

*Score is the sum of the individual scores from eye opening, best verbal response, and best motor response, using age-specific criteria. GCS score of 13–15 indicates mild head injury, GCS score of 9–12 indicates moderate head injury, and GCS score of ≤ 8 indicates severe head injury.

Reprinted from *Emergency Pediatrics: A Guide to Ambulatory Care*, 6th edition, page 419, Head Trauma, Copyright 2003, with permission from Elsevier.

The injured older adult is much more likely to die than a younger patient. At lower injury severity scores, older adults do not die as a direct consequence of their injuries but as a result of secondary complications.[26] On the basis of this information, an aggressive treatment approach to the older adult trauma patient is justified to ensure the best long-term survival and functional outcomes. Seriously injured older adults are less likely to receive care in a trauma center than younger patients.[27] Age older than 55 years is suggested as a guideline by the American College of Surgeons as a factor to consider when triaging the trauma patient to a trauma center rather than a nontrauma center.[28]

Mechanisms of Injury and Biomechanics

Falls are the most common mechanism of injury in the older adult population. Falls are usually from a ground level and involve a slip, trip, or stumble. Changes in visual acuity, sensation and proprioception, and syncopal problems may be contributing factors to causing the fall.[29]

Motor vehicle crashes are the second most common mechanism of injury. Fourteen percent of all traffic fatalities involve older adult drivers.[30] Delayed reaction time as well as changes in visual acuity place the older driver at a higher risk.

Pedestrians struck by a motor vehicle represent the third most common mechanism of injury for the older adult population. Age-related changes including hearing impairment, visual changes, and alterations in mobility make it more difficult for older adults to hear and see traffic as well as cross the street quickly.

Comorbid disease is more commonly the precipitating factor for an injury in the older adult. These precipitating factors can include syncope, postural hypotension, cardiac dysrhythmia, and other factors. Falling may be the presenting mechanism of injury for patient problems such as dehydration, urinary tract infection, pneumonia, myocardial infarction, or adverse effects of medications.[25] As the nurse caring for the older adult, it is important to assess for these factors so that appropriate diagnostic testing and interventions can be initiated early.

Anatomic/Physiologic Differences in the Older Adult Trauma Patient

Normal aging is a gradual process that affects homeostasis and the integration of multiple body systems. Along with aging-related changes are the changes that result from comorbidities and medications used to treat those diseases. Because of these changes, older adults have a limited ability to respond to the stress of injury. There is a lack of physiologic reserve. Even a low-velocity impact may cause serious injury when an older adult has underlying disease.

Aging results in decreased cerebral blood flow. Brain mass shrinks with cerebral atrophy, and the dura adheres more tightly to the skull. The bridging veins are stretched between the brain and the dura, making them susceptible to injury. In addition, older adults have a higher incidence of coagulopathies as well as comorbid conditions treated with anticoagulant medications. For these reasons, a minor blow to the head may result in subdural hematoma. Cerebral atrophy allows intracerebral hemorrhage expansion, delaying early signs and symptoms associated with increased intracranial pressure. The ability of the brain to rapidly process, coordinate, and react to stimuli is diminished.

Aging-related loss of pulmonary reserve, coupled with the stress of trauma, predisposes the older adult patient to respiratory complications. This factor may be accentuated by a long history of smoking. There is a gradual decrease in the strength of the respiratory muscles, especially the diaphragm, along with a reduced cough reflex that is associated with aging. Any degree of hypoxia may be detrimental to the older adult. Supplemental oxygen must be administered to prevent hypoxia.[29] Blunt trauma frequently results in rib fractures. The slowness of healing combined with loss of pulmonary and immunologic reserve makes rib fractures a dangerous injury for the older adult. Each rib fracture is associated with a marked increase in mortality and the risk of pneumonia.[31]

Atherosclerosis may limit the ability of the vessels to respond in stress. Arterial elasticity decreases, increasing peripheral resistance and cardiac workload, resulting in the development of hypertension. Baroreceptors become less sensitive, and arterial and cardiac muscles are less responsive to beta-adrenergic stimulation. Changes in the myocardium cause the heart to pump less effectively. Cardiac output and stroke volume decrease with aging because of stiffness of the myocardium, a decreased conduction velocity, and a decrease in coronary artery blood flow. Beta-blockers, calcium channel blockers, and afterload-reducing medications impair myocardial responses to shock. The compensatory mechanism of an increased heart rate will not be seen. Shock may be present, with blood pressure readings remaining within standard normal limits.[29] Older adults may have a preexisting anemia. Trauma may cause a decrease in the oxygen transport to the tissues, precipitating angina or myocardial infarction. It is imperative that treatment be aggressive in preserving the oxygen-carrying capacity of the blood to maintain arterial oxygen saturation above 90%. Early placement of a pulmonary artery catheter and aggressive augmentation of hemodynamic parameters have been shown to improve outcomes for older adult trauma patients.[32]

Older adults often have preexisting malnutrition, which may alter the body's capacity to respond to a traumatic injury. Peristalsis and gastric motility slow with aging. Older adults have decreased fat stores and slowed basal metabolic rates.

The older adult has an impaired ability to concentrate urine, which makes urine output a poor indicator of intravascular volume. There is also a decrease in glomerular filtration rate, impaired water reabsorption, loss of the ability to buffer acids or bases, and delayed ability of the kidney to respond to stress. These changes in renal function must be considered when the nurse is thinking about drug dosages or the administration of ionic contrast in older adults.

With aging, the skin provides less cushioning against mechanical forces, making older adults more susceptible to shearing-type injuries, such as abrasions caused by lying on a backboard. A decrease in skin tensile strength associated with a decrease in skin thickness and subcutaneous fat all combine to impair the older adult's ability to tamponade underlying bleeding. The changes of aging result in a loss of thermoregulatory abilities, an impaired barrier to infection, and prolonged wound healing.

Older adults have a brittle skeleton, which is easily fractured. Pre-existing arthritis may limit mobility and joint flexibility. Dehydration of the intervertebral discs occurs, and joint cartilages atrophy. These degenerative joint changes as well as osteoporotic changes in the bony skeleton make radiographic diagnosis of vertebral fractures difficult.

Nursing Care of the Older Adult Trauma Patient

Assessment

History

- Does the patient have pre-existing medical conditions?
- What medications does the patient take? Do they include anticoagulants such as warfarin sodium (Coumadin), aspirin, or clopidogrel (Plavix)? Is the patient currently taking any over-the-counter agents?
- What were the events that led to the injury? Did the patient feel dizzy or have palpitations before the injury?
- What was the patient's neurologic status before the injury? What was the patient's functional mobility level before the injury?

- Was the patient living independently, or is someone else responsible for care?
- Does the patient have any advance directives?

Physical Assessment

Inspection

- Inspect the mouth for loose teeth, partial plates, or dentures that can obstruct the airway.
- Inspect the skin carefully for deformities, pressure areas, loss of skin integrity, and ecchymosis.

Auscultation

- Auscultate the apical heart rate and blood pressure. Assess for abnormal heart sounds, which may be indicative of fluid overload or incompetent valves. Certain medications such as beta-blockers or cardiac glycosides may decrease the heart rate. Tachycardia as a response to shock may not be seen in these patients.

  Hypertension is a disease seen frequently in older adults. A normal blood pressure reading may be indicative of shock in the patient with a history of hypertension.

Palpation

- Palpate the bony prominences of the spine, examining the patient for pain or tenderness as well as deformity. Deformity may be the result of injury or pre-existing arthritis. Fracture of the spine in the older adult may result from lesser mechanisms of injury because of osteoporosis. Collaborate with the physician to determine the need for imaging of the spine.

Diagnostic Procedures

An older patient's injury may be the result of a reaction to other symptoms that presented before the injury. Diagnostic procedures should include studies to rule out other factors such as myocardial infarction, dysrhythmia, stroke, or arterial insufficiency.

Laboratory Studies

- Serum electrolytes
- Serum magnesium
- Serum calcium
- Cardiac enzymes, troponin
- Therapeutic drug levels[30]
- PT, PTT

Other Studies

- Electrocardiogram
- Echocardiogram
- Carotid ultrasound

Assessment for Maltreatment in Special Populations

Trauma patients within these special populations are at a higher risk for maltreatment or physical/emotional abuse. Suspect maltreatment when there is an inconsistency between the stated mechanism of injury and the actual injury observed. Often there is a significant time lapse between the injury and the presentation to the emergency department. Other signs and symptoms of maltreatment may include unexplained bruises in various stages of healing, unexplained fractures, and unusual interactions between the patient and their caregiver, including fear, withdrawal, verbal abuse, and harassment.

Planning and Implementation

Refer to Chapter 3, Initial Assessment, for a description of the specific nursing interventions for patients with compromises to airway, breathing, circulation, and disability. Appendix 13-1 provides special considerations for pregnant, pediatric, and older adult patients.

Evaluation and Ongoing Assessment

Refer to Chapter 3, Initial Assessment, for a description of the ongoing evaluation of the patient's airway, breathing, and circulation. Additional evaluations include

- Assessing vital signs frequently to determine trends. This includes monitoring of fetal heart rate and uterine activity in the pregnant trauma patient.
- Monitoring cardiovascular and pulmonary response to intravenous therapy.
- Monitoring temperature frequently, especially in pediatric and older adult trauma patients.
- Assessing the level of anxiety of the patient and family and their ability to cope.

Summary

The care of special populations that have experienced trauma requires knowledge of their unique anatomic and physiologic differences. Trauma in pregnant, pediatric, and older adult patients must be treated differently. Assessment, intervention, and evaluation must be guided by the unique response to traumatic injury. It is recommended that nurses who care for pediatric patients attend the Emergency Nurses Association's Emergency Nursing Pediatric Course (ENPC). For those interested in more educa-

tion related to the care of older adults, it is recommended that nurses take the Geriatric Emergency Nursing Education (GENE) course.

References

1. Grossman, N. B. (2004). Blunt trauma in pregnancy. *American Family Physician, 70*(7), 1303–1310.

2. Van Hook, J. W. (2002). Trauma in pregnancy. *Clinical Obstetrics and Gynecology, 45*(2), 414–424.

3. Kolb, J. C., Carlton, F. B., Cox, R. D., & Summers, R. L. (2002). Blunt trauma in the obstetric patient: Monitoring practices in the ED. *American Journal of Emergency Medicine, 20*(6), 524–527.

4. Ikossi, D. G., Lazar, A. A., Morabito, D., Fildes, J., & Knudson, M. M. (2005). Profile of mothers at risk: An analysis of injury and pregnancy loss in 1,195 trauma patients. *Journal of the American College of Surgeons, 200*(1), 49–56.

5. Shah, A. J., & Kilcline, B. A. (2003). Trauma in pregnancy. *Emergency Medicine Clinics of North America, 21*(3), 615–629.

6. Chuidian, F. X., & Feeser, V. R. (2002). The pregnant trauma patient: A focused approach to assessment. *Journal of Critical Illness, 17*(12), 484–490.

7. Smith, L. G. (2002). The pregnant trauma patient. In K. A. McQuillan, K. T. Von Rueden, R. L. Hartsock, M. B. Flynn, & E. Whalen (Eds.), *Trauma nursing: From resuscitation through rehabilitation* (3rd ed., pp. 718–746). Philadelphia: W. B. Saunders.

8. Knudson, M. M., Rozycki, G. S., & Paquin, M. M. (2004). Reproductive system trauma. In E. E. Moore, D. V. Feliciano, & K. L. Mattox (Eds.), *Trauma* (5th ed., pp. 851–874). New York: McGraw-Hill.

9. Bridgeman, P. (2004). Management of pregnant trauma patients. *Emergency Nurse, 12*(5), 22–25.

10. Barraco, R. D., Chiu, W. C., Clancy, T. V., Como, J. J., Ebert, J. B., Hess, L.W., et al. (2005). *Practice management guidelines for the diagnosis and management of injury in the pregnant patient: The EAST Practice Management Guidelines Work Group.* Appendix 1. Charleston, SC: Eastern Association for the Surgery of Trauma (EAST). Retrieved June 26, 2006, from http://www.east.org/tpg/pregnancy.pdf

11. American College of Obstetricians and Gynecologists Committee Opinion # 299: Guidelines for diagnostic imaging during pregnancy. (2004). *Obstetrics and Gynecology, 104*(3), 647–651.

12. Brown, M. A., Sirlin, C. B., Farahmand, N., Hoyt, D. B., & Casola, G. (2005). Screening sonography in pregnant patients with blunt abdominal trauma. *Journal of Ultrasound Medicine, 24*(2), 175–181.

13. American College of Surgeons Committee on Trauma. (2004). Trauma in women. In *Advanced trauma life support® for doctors: Student course manual* (7th ed., pp. 275–282). Chicago: Author.

14. Segui-Gomez, M., Chang, D. C., Paidas, C. N., Jurkovich, G. J., MacKenzie, E. J., & Rivara, F. P. (2003). Pediatric trauma care: An overview of pediatric trauma systems and their practices in 18 US states. *Journal of Pediatric Surgery, 38*(8), 1162–1169.

15. Davies, K. L. (2004). Buckled-up children: Understanding the mechanism, injuries, management, and prevention of seat belt related injuries. *Journal of Trauma Nursing, 11*(1), 16–24.

16. Moloney-Harmon, P. A. (2002). Pediatric trauma. In K. A. McQuillan, K. T. Von Rueden, R. L. Hartsock, M. B. Flynn, & E. Whalen (Eds.), *Trauma nursing: From resuscitation through rehabilitation* (3rd ed., pp. 747–771). Philadelphia: W. B. Saunders.

17. Tepas, J. J., & Schinco, M. A. (2004). Pediatric trauma. In E. E. Moore, D. V. Feliciano, & K. L. Mattox (Eds.), *Trauma* (5th ed., pp. 1021–1039). New York: McGraw-Hill.

18. Cotton, B. A., & Nance, M. L. (2004). Penetrating trauma in children. *Seminars in Pediatric Surgery, 13*(2), 87–97.

19. American Heart Association. (2005). Part 12. Pediatric Advanced Life Support. *Circulation,* 112(24): IV-167–187.

20. Atkinson, C., & Bowman, A. (2003). Pediatric airway differences. *Journal of Trauma Nursing, 10*(4), 118–122.

21. Rzucidlo, S. E., & Shirk, B. J. (2004). Trauma nursing: Pediatric patients. *RN, 67*(6), 36–42.

22. DeRoss, A. L., & Vane, D. W. (2004). Early evaluation and resuscitation of the pediatric trauma patient. *Seminars in Pediatric Surgery, 13*(2), 74–79.

23. American College of Surgeons Committee on Trauma. (2004). Pediatric trauma. In *Advanced trauma life support® for doctors: Student course manual* (7th ed., pp. 243–262). Chicago: Author.

24. Kauder, D. R., Schwab, C. W., & Shapiro, M. B. (2004). Geriatric trauma: Patterns, care and outcomes. In E. E. Moore, D. V. Feliciano, & K. L. Mattox (Eds.), *Trauma* (5th ed., pp. 1041–1058). New York: McGraw-Hill.

25. Harrahill, M. (2001). Falls in the elderly: Making the difference. *Journal of Emergency Nursing, 27*(2), 209–210.

26. Newton, K. (2001). Geriatric trauma. *Topics in Emergency Medicine, 23*(3), 1–12.

27. Lane, P., Sorondo, B., & Kelly, J. J. (2003). Geriatric trauma patients—Are they receiving trauma center care? *Academic Emergency Medicine, 10*(3), 244–250.

28. American College of Surgeons Committee on Trauma (1998). Interhospital transfer and agreements. In *Resources for optimal care of the injured patient: 1999* (pp. 19–22). Chicago: Author.

29. Pudelek, B. (2002). Geriatric trauma: Special needs for a special population. *AACN Clinical Issues, 13*(1), 61–72.

30. Stevenson, J. (2004). When the trauma patient is elderly. *Journal of PeriAnesthesia Nursing, 19*(6), 392–400.

31. Bergeron, E., Lavoie, A., Clas, D., Moore, L., Ratte, S., Tetreault, S., et al. (2003). Elderly trauma patients with rib fractures are at greater risk of death and pneumonia. *Journal of Trauma—Injury, Infection and Critical Care, 54*(3), 478–485.

32. Jacobs, D. G., Plaisier, B. R., Barie, P. S., Hammond, J. S., Holevar, M. R., Sinclair, K. E., et al. (2003). Practice management guidelines for geriatric trauma: The EAST practice management guidelines work group. *The Journal of Trauma—Injury, Infection and Critical Care, 54*(2), 391–416.

Pregnant	Pediatric	Older Adult
Airway		
The pregnant trauma patient is at risk for aspiration because of the pressure of the enlarged uterus on diaphragm/chest contents and delayed gastric emptying. May need to intubate prophylactically to protect against aspiration.[2]	Because infants and young children have a large occiput, positioning them supine on a backboard causes their cervical vertebrae to flex and move anteriorly (**Figure 13-2**). This flexion may contribute to airway compromise and/or decreased effectiveness of the jaw thrust or chin lift maneuvers. Select an appropriately sized endotracheal tube. Tube size depends on the age and size of the child. The following formulas can be used to estimate the endotracheal tube size for children 1 to 10 years of age, based on the child's age: • Uncuffed endotracheal tube size (mm ID) = (age in years/4) + 4 • Cuffed endotracheal tube size (mm ID) = (age in years/4) + 3 Cuffed tubes are as safe for in-hospital use as uncuffed tubes for infants beyond the newborn period and in children. Cuffed tubes may be preferable in certain situations such as poor lung compliance, high airway resistance, or a large glottic air leak. Cuff inflation pressures should be kept < 20 cm H_2O.[19] Commercial pediatric resuscitation tapes used to measure the length of the child provide information regarding appropriately sized tubes also. LMAs may also be used by experienced providers.[19] When confirming placement, both clinical assessment and confirmatory devices must be used to ensure proper tube placement.	Remove partial plates or dentures to assist in opening and establishing a patent airway. Carefully consider the need to intubate the patient, because intubation increases the risk of pneumonia.
Spinal Immobilization		
If the patient is on a backboard, tilt the backboard 15 to 20 degrees to the left. If this is not possible, manually displace the uterus to the left side.	Place padding under the child's shoulders to bring the shoulders into horizontal alignment with the external auditory meatus. This position provides neutral alignment of the cervical spine (**Figure 13-3**).	• Pad bony prominences to protect the skin from pressure forces. • Remove splints, backboard, and cervical collar as soon as injuries are ruled out.

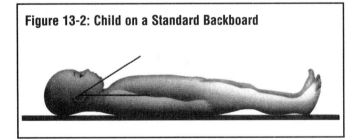

Figure 13-2: Child on a Standard Backboard

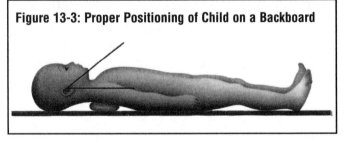

Figure 13-3: Proper Positioning of Child on a Backboard

Intervention	Pregnant	Pediatric	Older Adult
Breathing	Administer supplemental oxygen. Hypoxemia occurs more quickly in the pregnant patient and is not tolerated well.[2]	Administer oxygen via a pediatric non-rebreather mask at 12 to 15 L/min.	Supplemental oxygen must be administered to prevent hypoxia.[29]
Circulation	Initiate fetal monitoring early in the resuscitation.	Cardiopulmonary resuscitation is indicated if the child is pulseless or if the heart rate is less than 60 beats/minute AND systemic perfusion is poor. Cannulate two veins using the largest caliber catheter that the vessel can accommodate, and initiate infusion of crystalloid solution. Infuse a bolus of 20 ml/kg. Reassess circulation and initiate a second bolus, if indicated. Anticipate blood replacement. If the child remains hemodynamically unstable after two boluses, an infusion of red blood cells at 10 ml/kg may be indicated. If peripheral venous access cannot be readily established in a patient in shock, initiate intraosseous (IO) access with a 16- or 18-gauge bone marrow needle. The IO may be used to obtain an initial blood sample for type and crossmatch, as well as to provide a mechanism for the administration of fluids, blood products, and medications.	Assist with the insertion of hemodynamic monitoring devices, if indicated (i.e., central venous catheter, pulmonary artery catheter). These monitoring devices can assist in determining fluid requirements and assessing cardiovascular response. Care must be taken to monitor fluid infusions carefully to avoid overhydration. It has been recommended that older adult patients who have sustained blunt trauma be admitted to critical care as soon as possible for continued cardiovascular monitoring. For patients who are anticoagulated, laboratory studies should be initiated early in the resuscitation to evaluate coagulation. Reversal of anticoagulation may need to be initiated emergently before operative interventions.
Disability		Use the Pediatric Glasgow Coma Scale score for establishment of a baseline and for repeated assessment.	
Other: Temperature		Use warming lights and warm blankets, and apply a stockinette to the heads of infants and small children.	Keep the patient warm because older adults are prone to hypothermia and tolerate it poorly
Medication Administration	Determine the pregnancy safety category for all medications administered to the pregnant trauma patient.	Administer analgesics and other medications in doses recommended for the pediatric population.	Administer analgesics and other medications in doses recommended for older adults.
Urine Output		To evaluate the effectiveness of fluid resuscitation, monitor urinary output. Insertion of a Foley catheter may be helpful for precise measurements. Normal urinary output for infants is 2 ml/kg/hr. For small children, it is 1 ml/kg/hr.	

In addition to the nursing diagnoses outlined in Chapter 3, Initial Assessment, the following nursing diagnoses are potential problems for the pregnant patient with trauma. Once a patient has been assessed, diagnoses can be defined as either actual or risk. An actual nursing diagnosis is derived from a decision based on the patient's presenting signs and symptoms. A risk nursing diagnosis is a judgment the nurse makes based on a particular patient's risk and potential for developing certain problems.

Nursing Diagnoses	Interventions	Expected Outcomes

Aspiration, risk, related to:
 	
• Impaired cough and gag reflexes
• Increased risk of vomiting secondary to gastrointestinal changes of pregnancy
	• Position the patient to support maximum airway efficiency
	• Use airway adjuncts to maintain the airway
	• Administer 100% oxygen
	• Suction to clear secretions
	• Reassess airway status frequently
	• Insert a gastric tube, as indicated
	• Obtain blood sample for arterial blood gas (ABG), as indicated
		The patient will not experience aspiration, as evidenced by:
		
		• A patent airway
		• Clear and equal bilateral breath sounds
		• Regular rate, depth, and pattern of breathing
		• ABG values within normal limits:
		  ▪ PaO_2 101 to 104 mm Hg (13.5 to 13.9 KPa)
		  ▪ SaO_2 > 95%
		  ▪ $PaCO_2$ 25 to 30 mm Hg (3.3 to 4.0 KPa)
		  ▪ pH 7.35 to 7.45
		• Clear chest radiograph without evidence of infiltrates
		• Ability to handle secretions independently

Gas exchange, impaired, related to:
 	
• Increased oxygen consumption
• Altered blood flow, oxygen-carrying capacity of the blood, oxygen supply
• Aspiration of foreign matter
• Hypo- or hyperventilation
	• Administer 100% oxygen via nonrebreather mask
	• Monitor level of consciousness
	• Assist with intubation, as indicated
	• Reassess fetal heart tones frequently
	• Monitor respiratory status frequently: rate, depth, rhythm of respirations, ventilatory effort, chest wall movement
	• Monitor color, temperature, moisture of skin
	• Monitor pulse oximeter reading
	• Monitor results of blood gas studies
	• Monitor the patient closely if sedated
	• Maintain the patient in left lateral decubitus position
	• Administer blood, as indicated
		The patient will experience adequate gas exchange, as evidenced by:
		
		• ABG values within normal limits:
		  ▪ PaO_2 101 to 104 mm Hg (13.5 to 13.9 KPa)
		  ▪ SaO_2 > 95%
		  ▪ $PaCO_2$ 25 to 30 mm Hg (3.3 to 4.0 KPa)
		  ▪ pH 7.35 to 7.45
		  ▪ $SpO_2 \geq$ 95%
		• Skin normal color, warm, and dry
		• Improved level of consciousness
		• Regular rate, depth, and pattern of breathing
		• Fetal heart tones maintained between 120 and 160 beats/minute

Nursing Diagnoses	Interventions	Expected Outcomes

Tissue perfusion, altered, related to:
 	
• Increased oxygen consumption
• Hypovolemia
• Interruption of flow: arterial and/or venous
	• Administer 100% oxygen via nonrebreather mask
	• Monitor level of consciousness
	• Assist with intubation as indicated
	• Reassess fetal heart tones frequently
	• Monitor respiratory status frequently: rate, depth, rhythm of respirations, ventilatory effort, chest wall movement
	• Monitor color, temperature, moisture of skin
	• Monitor pulse oximeter reading
	• Monitor results of blood gas studies
	• Monitor the patient closely if sedated
	• Control any uncontrolled bleeding
	• Cannulate two veins with large-caliber catheters and initiate infusion of isotonic crystalloid solution
	• Administer blood, as indicated
	• Maintain the patient in left lateral decubitus position
	• Prepare for definitive care
		The patient will maintain adequate tissue perfusion, as evidenced by:
		
		• Vital signs with normal limits
		• Level of consciousness, awake and alert
		• Skin normal color, warm, and dry
		• Strong and equal peripheral pulses
		• Urine output of 1 ml/kg/hr
		• ABG values within normal limits:
		  ▪ PaO_2 101 to 104 mm Hg (13.5 to 13.9 KPa)
		  ▪ SaO_2 > 95%
		  ▪ $PaCO_2$ 25 to 30 mm Hg (3.3 to 4.0 KPa)
		  ▪ pH 7.35 to 7.45
		• Fetal heart tones maintained between 120 and 160 beats/minute
		• $SpO_2 \geq 95\%$

Fluid volume deficit, related to: • Hemorrhage secondary to maternal injury, uterine rupture, abruptio placentae • Fluid shifts • Alteration in capillary permeability • Vena cava compression by enlarged uterus	• Cannulate two veins with large-caliber catheters and initiate infusion of crystalloid solution • Monitor color, temperature, moisture of skin and capillary refill status • Administer blood, as indicated • Position the patient on her left side to relieve compression on the vena cava. (If on backboard, tilt backboard 15 to 20 degrees to the left. If this is not possible, manually displace the uterus to the left side.) • Monitor vital signs frequently • Monitor urinary output • Monitor level of consciousness • Control external hemorrhage with pressure dressings • Measure and record fundal height every 30 minutes	**The patient will have an effective circulating volume, as evidenced by:** • Stable vital signs appropriate for stage of pregnancy • Urine output of 1 ml/kg/hr • Level of consciousness, awake and alert • Skin normal color, warm, and dry • Maintenance of hematocrit of 30 ml/dl or hemoglobin of 12 to 14 g/dl or greater • Control of external hemorrhage

Nursing Diagnoses	Interventions	Expected Outcomes
Infection, risk, related to: • Premature rupture of membranes secondary to injury during pregnancy • Trauma • Amniotic fluid leak	• Maintain sterile technique during procedures (including vaginal examination) • Monitor temperature frequently • Assess the patient for signs of infection: fever, tachycardia, tachypnea, purulent drainage, odor	**The patient will be free from infection, as evidenced by:** • Core temperature measurement of 98 °F to 99.5 °F (36 °C to 37.5 °C) • Absence of systemic signs of infection: fever, tachypnea, tachycardia • Wounds free from redness, swelling, purulent drainage or odor • White blood cell count within normal limits • Level of consciousness, awake and alert, age appropriate • Uterus that is nontender to palpation
Anxiety and fear (patient and family), related to: • Threat of fetal injury or death	• Explain procedures to patient and family • Facilitate family presence according to hospital protocols • Encourage the patient and family to voice concerns and ask questions • Provide information to the patient and family as needed or requested	**The patient and family will experience decreasing anxiety and fear, as evidenced by:** • Decrease of fear-related behavior: crying, shouting, agitated behavior, noncommunicative behavior, blank stare; facial expressions, voice tone, and body posture normal for the patient and family • Appropriate use of coping mechanisms • Acknowledgment of fear and statement that there is decreasing fear • Absence of physiologic indicators of fear: palpitations, increased blood pressure, diaphoresis, tachycardia • The voicing of concerns and fears
Grieving, anticipatory, related to: • Actual or anticipated injury or death of fetus	• Encourage the patient and family to grieve • Promote hope when appropriate • Provide referrals to appropriate agencies: pastoral care, social service, rehabilitation • Encourage the patient and family to express feelings • Communicate acceptance of discussing loss	**The patient and family will begin the grieving process, as evidenced by:** • Expressing signs of the grieving process • Participating in decision making • Recognizing reasons for feelings • Sharing feelings of grief with family
Pain, related to: • Injury • Onset of labor • Experience during invasive procedures/diagnostic tests	• Administer pain medications as prescribed, preferably before procedures • Explain procedures in terms the patient and family can understand • Enlist the patient's cooperation • Use touch, positioning, or relaxation techniques to give comfort • Coach the patient in previously learned breathing techniques, as indicated, if in labor	**The patient will experience relief of pain, as evidenced by:** • Diminishing or absent level of pain through self-report • Absence of physiologic indicators of pain: tachycardia, tachypnea, pallor, diaphoretic skin, increased blood pressure • Absence of nonverbal cues of pain: crying, grimacing, unable to assume a position of comfort • Ability to cooperate with care or procedures

In addition to the nursing diagnoses outlined in Chapter 3, Initial Assessment, the following nursing diagnoses are potential problems for the pediatric patient with trauma. Once a patient has been assessed, diagnoses can be defined as either actual or risk. An actual nursing diagnosis is derived from a decision based on the patient's presenting signs and symptoms. A risk nursing diagnosis is a judgment the nurse makes based on a particular patient's risk and potential for developing certain problems.

Nursing Diagnoses	Interventions	Expected Outcomes
Fluid volume deficit, related to: • Hemorrhage • Fluid shifts • Alteration in capillary permeability • Alteration in vascular tone • Myocardial compromise	• Cannulate two veins using the largest caliber catheter that the vessel can accommodate, and initiate infusion of crystalloid solution • Initiate intraosseous access for fluid replacement, if necessary • Insert an indwelling urinary catheter • Administer blood, as indicated • Control external bleeding	**The patient will have an effective circulating volume, as evidenced by:** • Control of external hemorrhage • Stable vital signs appropriate for age • Urine output of 1 to 3 ml/kg/hr, age appropriate • Strong, palpable peripheral pulses • Level of consciousness, awake and alert, age appropriate: Pediatric Glasgow Coma Scale = ability to recognize caregivers, normal behavior for developmental age • Skin normal color, warm, and dry • Maintenance of normal hematocrit or hemoglobin for age • Capillary refill < 2 seconds
Tissue perfusion, altered renal, cardiopulmonary, cerebral, gastrointestinal, peripheral (specific type), related to: • Hypovolemia • Interruption of flow: arterial and/ or venous	• Initiate cardiopulmonary resuscitation, as indicated	**The patient will maintain adequate tissue perfusion, as evidenced by:** • Vital signs within normal limits for age • Level of consciousness, awake and alert, age appropriate • Skin normal color, warm, and dry • Strong and equal peripheral pulses • Urine output of 1 ml/kg/hr in children < 30 kg
Hypothermia, related to: • Rapid infusion of intravenous fluids • Decreased tissue perfusion • Exposure	• Cannulate two veins using the largest caliber catheter that the vessel can accommodate, and initiate infusion of crystalloid solution • Keep the child warm using blankets or overhead lamps • Monitor body temperature	**The patient will maintain a normal core body temperature, as evidenced by:** • Core temperature measurement of 98 °F to 99.5 °F (36 °C to 37.5 °C) • Skin normal color, warm, and dry

Nursing Diagnoses	Interventions	Expected Outcomes
Altered health maintenance, risk for altered (caregiver), related to: • Insufficient knowledge of care of wounds, casting material, immobilization devices, ambulatory aids • Restrictions to activity • Signs and symptoms of complications • Follow-up care	• Provide psychosocial support • Provide injury prevention teaching to caregivers	**The caregiver is knowledgeable about self-care and follow-up, as evidenced by:** • Recognizing and promptly reporting signs and symptoms that indicate serious complications • Stating necessity and planning for ongoing medical care • Describing and demonstrating proper use and care of ambulatory aids • Identifying how to reduce the risk of future trauma • Relaying an intent to comply with agreed-on restrictions
Anxiety and fear (patient and caregiver), related to: • Threat to or change in health status, role functions, environment, self-concept, or interaction patterns • Threat of death, actual or perceived • Lack of knowledge • Loss of control • Disruptive family life • Pain	• Threat to self-concept • Diagnostic/invasive procedures	• Provide psychosocial support • Prepare the child for operative intervention, hospital admission or transfer, as indicated • Administer analgesic medications, as prescribed • Facilitate family presence • Utilize comfort measures

In addition to the nursing diagnoses outlined in Chapter 3, Initial Assessment, the following nursing diagnoses are potential problems for the older adult trauma patient. Once a patient has been assessed, diagnoses can be defined as either actual or risk. An actual nursing diagnosis is derived from a decision based on the patient's presenting signs and symptoms. A risk nursing diagnosis is a judgment the nurse makes based on a particular patient's risk and potential for developing certain problems.

Nursing Diagnoses	Interventions	Expected Outcomes
Airway clearance, ineffective, related to: • Decreased level of consciousness • Secretions and debris in airway • Decreased strength of respiratory muscles • Presence of an artificial airway • Direct trauma • Tracheobronchial secretions or obstruction • Aspiration of foreign matter • Inhalation of toxic fumes or substances • Pain from decreased ability to cough	• Stabilize and/or immobilize the cervical spine • Assist with endotracheal intubation • Position the patient to support maximum airway efficiency • Use airway adjuncts to maintain open airway • Suction as needed to clear secretions • Insert gastric tube • Monitor oxygenation with continuous pulse oximetry	**The patient will have a patent airway, as evidenced by:** • Clear, bilateral breath sounds • Regular rate, depth, and pattern of breathing • Effective cough • Appropriate use of splinting techniques with coughing • Clear sputum of normal amount without color or odor • Absence of signs and symptoms of retained secretions: fever, tachycardia, tachypnea

Aspiration, risk, related to:
 	
• Reduced level of consciousness secondary to injury, drug interactions from multiple medications
• Impaired cough and gag reflex
• Trauma to head, face, and/or neck
• Secretions and debris in airway
• Increased intragastric pressure
• Impaired swallowing
	• Assist with endotracheal intubation
	• Obtain blood sample for arterial blood gases (ABGs), as indicated
	• Insert a gastric tube
	• Position the patient to support maximum airway efficiency
	• Monitor oxygenation with continuous pulse oximetry
		The patient will not experience aspiration, as evidenced by:
		
		• A patent airway
		• Clear and equal bilateral breath sounds
		• Regular rate, depth, and pattern of breathing
		• ABG values within normal limits:
		  ▪ PaO_2 80 to 100 mm Hg (10.0 to 13.3 KPa)
		  ▪ SaO_2 > 95%
		  ▪ $PaCO_2$ 35 to 45 mm Hg (4.7 to 6.0 KPa)
		  ▪ pH 7.35 to 7.45
		• $SpO_2 \geq$ 95%
		• Clear chest radiograph without evidence of infiltrates
		• Ability to handle secretions independently

Nursing Diagnoses	Interventions	Expected Outcomes

Gas exchange, impaired, related to:
 	
• Loss of integrity of thoracic cage and impaired chest wall movement secondary to injury, deterioration of ventilatory efforts
• Aspiration
• Altered blood flow, oxygen-carrying capacity of the blood, oxygen supply
• Aspiration of foreign matter
• Hypo- or hyperventilation
• Inhalation of toxic fumes or substances
• Weakened respiratory muscles
• Decreased compliance of chest wall
	• Assist with intubation, as indicated
	• Ventilate with bag-mask device or with a mechanical ventilator
	• Monitor oxygen saturation with continuous pulse oximetry
	• Administer blood, as indicated
	• Assist with insertion of hemodynamic monitoring devices
	• Administer 100% oxygen
	• Monitor level of consciousness
	• Monitor respiratory status: rate, rhythm, depth, effort, chest wall movement
		The patient will experience adequate gas exchange, as evidenced by:
		
		• ABG values within normal limits:
		  ▪ PaO_2 80 to 100 mm Hg (10.0 to 13.3 KPa)
		  ▪ SaO_2 > 95%
		  ▪ $PaCO_2$ 35 to 45 mm Hg (4.7 to 6.0 KPa)
		  ▪ pH 7.35 to 7.45
		• $SpO_2 \geq 95\%$
		• Skin normal color, warm, and dry
		• Level of consciousness, awake and alert
		• Regular rate, depth, and pattern of breathing

Fluid volume deficit, related to: • Hemorrhage • Fluid shifts • Alteration in capillary permeability • Alteration in vascular tone • Myocardial compromise • Decreased cardiopulmonary compensatory mechanisms secondary to the aging process	• Assist with insertion of hemodynamic monitoring devices • Control external hemorrhage • Cannulate two veins with large-caliber catheters and initiate infusion of crystalloid solution • Administer blood, as indicated • Monitor vital signs, level of consciousness • Monitor the patient's peripheral pulses, color, temperature, moisture of skin, capillary refill, and urine output • Monitor for possible fluid overload, especially with persisting heart or respiratory condition	The patient will have an effective circulating volume, as evidenced by: • Stable vital signs • Urine output of 1 ml/kg/hr • Strong, palpable peripheral and central pulses • Level of consciousness, awake and alert • Skin normal color, warm, and dry • Maintenance of hematocrit of 30 ml/dl or hemoglobin of 12 to 14 g/dl or greater, or at preinjury level • Hemodynamic values within normal limits • Control of external hemorrhage
Tissue perfusion, altered renal, cardiopulmonary, cerebral, gastrointestinal, peripheral (specific type), related to: • Hypovolemia • Interruption of flow: arterial and/or venous	• Control any uncontrolled bleeding • Cannulate two veins with large-caliber catheters and initiate infusion of crystalloid solution • Administer blood, as indicated • Prepare for definitive care • Monitor for possible fluid overload	The patient will maintain adequate tissue perfusion, as evidenced by: • Vital signs within normal limits for age • Level of consciousness, awake and alert • Skin normal color, warm, and dry • Strong and equal peripheral pulses • Urine output of 1 ml/kg/hr
Hypothermia, related to: • Rapid infusion of intravenous fluids • Decreased tissue perfusion • Exposure • Impaired thermoregulation and heat production secondary to aging • Decreased tissue perfusion	• Keep the patient warm • Apply warm blankets • Avoid any unnecessary exposure • Monitor temperature • Use warming adjuncts (blankets, warming lights) as necessary • Increase the room temperature • Use warmed intravenous solution for infusion	The patient will maintain a normal core body temperature, as evidenced by: • Core temperature measurement of 98 °F to 99.5 °F (36 °C to 37.5 °C) • Skin normal color, warm, and dry

Nursing Diagnoses	Interventions	Expected Outcomes
Pain, related to: • Effects of trauma/injury agents • Experience during invasive procedures/ diagnostic tests	• Pad bony prominences to protect the skin from pressure forces • Remove splints, backboards, and cervical collars as soon as injuries are ruled out • Administer analgesics and other medications, as prescribed • Provide psychosocial support • Use touch, positioning, or relaxation techniques to give comfort • Splint or immobilize suspected fractures • Facilitate family presence	**The patient will experience relief of pain, as evidenced by:** • Diminishing or absent level of pain through self-report • Absence of physiologic indicators of pain, which include tachycardia, tachypnea, pallor, diaphoretic skin, increasing blood pressure • Absence of nonverbal cues of pain: crying, grimacing, inability to assume position of comfort, and/or guarding • Ability to cooperate with care, as appropriate
Impaired skin integrity, risk, related to: • Pressure, shear, friction, maceration forces on skin and tissue • Mechanical irritants: fixation devices • Impaired mobility • Urinary and bowel incontinence • Sensory and motor deficits • Altered peripheral perfusion • Pre-existing nutritional deficiencies • Pre-existing chronic diseases • Lack of physiologic reserve secondary to the aging process	• Pad bony prominences to protect the skin from pressure forces • Remove splints, backboards, and cervical collars as soon as injuries are ruled out • Reposition frequently	**The patient will demonstrate absence or resolution of impaired skin integrity, as evidenced by:** • Absence of signs of irritation: redness, ulceration, blanching, itching • Signs of progressive healing of dermal layer • Understanding and willingness to participate in frequent movement to relieve pressure • Verbalization of an understanding of immobilization devices
Infection, risk, related to: • Contact with contagious agents (community-acquired and nosocomial) • Contamination of wounds from injury or instrumentation • Prolonged immobility • Lack of physiologic reserve secondary to aging process • Pre-existing nutritional deficiencies • Pre-existing chronic diseases	• Administer antibiotics, as prescribed • Provide meticulous wound care • Maintain aseptic technique • Administer tetanus prophylaxis, as prescribed	**The patient will be free from infection, as evidenced by:** • Core temperature measurement of 98 °F to 99.5 °F (36 °C to 37.5 °C) • Absence of systemic signs of infection: fever, tachypnea, tachycardia • Wounds free from redness, swelling, purulent drainage or odor • Level of consciousness, awake and alert, age appropriate • White blood cell count within normal limits
Anxiety and fear, related to: • Unfamiliar environment • Unpredictable nature of condition • Invasive procedures • Cognitive deficit	• Provide psychosocial support • Utilize institutional protocols to screen for, intervene, and report episodes of maltreatment • Minimize distracting stimuli • Provide frequent orientation to environment and plan of care • Facilitate family presence	**The patient and family will experience decreasing anxiety and fear, as evidenced by:** • Orientation to surroundings based on previous mental status • Ability to describe reasons for equipment and procedures used in treatment • Utilization of effective coping skills • Ability to verbalize concerns and ask questions of the health care team • Vital signs returning to normal limits

Chapter 14

Disaster Management

Objectives

On completion of this chapter/lecture, the learner should be able to:

1. Define and describe disasters, disaster management, and disaster planning.

2. Discuss the operational and medical management of disaster medicine and provide recommended resources for the health care team.

3. Review general principles of triage, including care and decontamination of patients involving potential chemical, biological, radiological, nuclear, and explosive (CBRNE) events.

4. Describe and discuss the types of illnesses or injuries that may occur as a result of disaster, as well as treatment options.

5. Describe the importance of the preplanning, training, and implementation of a centralized management system for dealing with mass casualties.

6. Describe and discuss various nursing roles and responsibilities relating to disaster management.

Preface

Disaster is defined as "an occurrence causing widespread destruction and distress."[1] This occurrence may be natural or man-made and results in temporary or permanent changes to the environment, ecosystem, or society. Disaster management, and the medical response to disasters, is a multifaceted and continuously evolving discipline. Disaster management is unique in that it requires a change in the paradigm of providing or utilizing the greatest number of resources for the greatest good of each individual patient to the allocation of limited resources for the greatest good of the greatest number of casualties.[2]

The number, severity, and variety of casualties that present to emergency departments after disasters occur often overwhelm local and regional health care systems. It is incumbent on all health care personnel to develop processes, train, and prepare for such events with a multidisciplinary approach.

Disasters affect the physical, psychological, emotional, and financial well-being of the community. They may result in numerous injuries, food and water shortages, infectious and vector-borne diseases, loss of homes, and devastation to the area affected. Multiple layers of the community and health care system are affected by a disaster (Table 14-1).

Epidemiology

The purpose of disaster epidemiology is to describe and measure the health effects of disasters. This data:

- Provides information about the needs of populations affected by disasters
- Helps providers plan for and prevent adverse health effects
- Helps providers plan for unforeseen events

According to the Centre for Research on the Epidemiology of Disasters (CRED), 255 million people worldwide were affected by disasters in 2003, representing a 180% increase from the 90 million who were affected in 1990.[3] Every year, natural disasters occur somewhere in the world. Natural disasters include earthquakes, wildfires, hurricanes, floods, heat waves, volcanic eruptions, and tsunamis. Natural disasters such as the eruption of Mount St. Helens, the devastating earthquake in Northridge, California, and Hurricanes Andrew and Katrina have contributed to the morbidity and mortality of thousands. The Indonesian government estimates that 100,000 people died and over 400,000 people were left homeless as a result of the tsunami of December 2004.[4]

Man-made disasters, such as the bombing of the Murrah Federal Building in Oklahoma City, the sarin attack in Japan, and the horrific attacks of September 11, 2001, on the Pentagon and New York City, demonstrate mankind's ability to wreak havoc and destruction on a wide scale. It is estimated that the September 11 attacks resulted in more fatalities than the worst tornado, earthquake, or hurricane of the previous century.[5] Natural and man-made disasters often overlap because of the disruptions to electrical power, structural collapse of buildings, and the release of hazardous chemicals into the environment secondary to explosions.

The aftereffects of disasters are far-reaching. Public health concerns include:

- Safety of drinking water
- Spread of infectious disease
- Availability of shelter
- Psychological impact on victims and community

The community infrastructure is also negatively affected. Hospitals, law enforcement agencies, and fire departments are often stressed beyond their normal operating capacities. There may be significant disruptions to communication, transportation, and other public works systems. Families and even entire communities may be displaced after a disaster.

Disaster Definitions

- **Institutional-based:** Any situation that results in a health care facility becoming partially or totally inoperable.[6]
- **Community-based:** Any situation, natural or man-made, that overwhelms a community's ability to respond with existing resources.[6]

In institutional disaster management, the words *internal* and *external* are used to determine whether or not a disaster has occurred within the hospital campus (internal) or in the community (external). This is an important distinction because it determines whether or not there is a need to prepare for casualty arrivals or manage resources within the hospital.

An internal disaster is an event that disrupts routine hospital functions. In an external disaster, if the health care needs exceed the immediate responders' or receiving hospital's ability to care for, or treat, the ill or injured victims, this is termed a disaster. It is incumbent on every hospital-based health care provider to know and understand their facility's roles within both the facility and community disaster plan. The primary focus of this chapter is external disaster management.

In community-based disasters, there are three classifications, regardless of whether the source is man-made or natural.[6]

- **Multiple-patient incident:** Fewer than 10 casualties (usually a single-hospital response)
  - Most common classification in disaster medicine
  - Significant, rapid increase in workload that can be absorbed by existing health care facilities

Table 14-1: Levels of Response to Disaster

Level	Responders
Level One	On-scene responders • Emergency medical services (EMS) • Law enforcement • General public
Level Two	Hospitals • Local receiving facilities • Regional trauma centers
Level Three	Government Agencies • Centers for Disease Control and Prevention (CDC) • Federal Emergency Management Agency (FEMA) • National Disaster Medical System (NDMS) • Military

- **Multiple-casualty incident:** Results in 100 or fewer casualties (may be single-hospital or multi-hospital response)
  - Existing health care facilities may be stressed but not overwhelmed.
  - Includes mass transportation such as bus or train crashes or natural events such as floods, tornadoes, snowstorms, or fires.
  - Radiation or biological contamination, hostage situations, or terrorist incidents are examples of man-made (external) environmental events.
- **Mass casualty incident:** Results in more than 100 casualties and involves responses from multiple hospitals
  - Existing health care facilities are significantly overwhelmed.
  - Major earthquakes, hurricanes, structural failures, hazardous materials, or radiation contamination are examples of mass casualty incidents.
  - Least common type of disaster.
  - Causes greatest amount of deaths, injuries, and property damage.

Types of Disasters

Natural

Natural disasters are prevalent, occur worldwide every year, and cause loss of life and limb, property damage, agriculture damage, loss of livestock, and disruption of the infrastructures of society. Over the past two decades, natural disasters resulted in the deaths of at least three million people and caused more than $50 billion in property damages.[7] Technologic advances are improving the ability to predict certain types of natural disasters based on season, measurement of geologic activity, ocean currents, or other instrumentation.

Earthquakes

Earthquakes are natural disasters during which large numbers of victims can perish in a short amount of time. Many earthquakes occur suddenly, violently, and without warning. Significant damage to roads, buildings, water, power, and gas lines (depending on the severity of the quake) may occur with accompanying floods or landslides. Injuries commonly associated with earthquakes include crush injuries from falling objects or structural failure. Aftershocks, seismic activity of lesser magnitude after the main earthquake, may cause further structural failures and additional injuries.

Hurricanes

A hurricane is defined as a tropical storm that has a constant wind speed of at least 74 miles per hour.[9] Hurricanes blow in a spiral pattern around an "eye," a calm center approximately 20 to 30 miles wide, but the storm itself may extend several hundred miles. As the hurricane approaches land, it is immediately preceded by torrential rainstorms, high winds, and storm surges.

Injuries and deaths during and after hurricanes result from drowning, electrocutions, and trauma related to structural failure and flying debris.[10]

Tornadoes

A tornado is a type of violent windstorm characterized by a funnel-shaped, twisting cloud (hence the nickname "twister") that contains winds up to 200 miles per hour and can occur with little or no warning. Tornados can destroy homes, power lines, and agriculture. More than 80% of tornados occur between noon and midnight and during the months from March through August.[11]

Deaths from tornadoes can result from either blunt or penetrating trauma from flying debris, falling objects, or structural collapse. Injuries and deaths are also common during the recovery and clean up phases.

Floods

With the exception of fire, floods are the most common of all natural disasters. Flooding can occur after heavy thunderstorms, hurricanes, or winter snow thaws. The National Flood Insurance Program defines flood as "a general and temporary condition of partial or complete inundation of two or more acres of normally dry land area or of two or more properties."[12] Despite this definition, flooding is known to cause long-term destruction due to the damage to roads and buildings. Infectious and vector-borne diseases are common public health concerns.

Fires/Wildfires

The United States continues to have fire death rates and property losses that are among the highest of industrialized nations. Burns and inhalation injuries are common multiple-patient incidents experienced throughout the United States.

Although wildfires are characterized as natural disasters, it is perhaps more accurate to classify them as man-made disasters. Careless smoking and arson are the two leading causes of wildfire that result in death. The majority of wildfires are small without significant mortality or financial losses. Wildfires result in increased numbers of patients reporting to emergency departments with inhalation injuries and exacerbations of pulmonary conditions such as asthma, bronchitis, shortness of breath, chest pain, and wheezing.[14]

Man-made

Traumatic and medical emergencies result from an extensive assortment of man-made causes. Examples include multivehicle crashes, the intentional or unintentional release of chemical or biological agents, and explosive or nuclear events. The increased concern and awareness of certain agents as weapons of mass destruction (WMDs) is now an important aspect of contemporary disaster management.

A chemical, biological, radiological, nuclear, or explosive (CBRNE) incident is a deliberate attack, whereas a hazardous materials (HAZMAT) incident is usually considered unintentional. Small amounts of CBRNE agents can produce large numbers of casualties. Biological agents are often contagious and not only infect those exposed, but can be transmitted to others. Identification may be difficult, relying on astute clinicians' awareness and recognition of signs and symptoms, unusual patterns of illness, and clustering of patients with similar symptoms. A CBRNE incident may require decontamination on a large scale. In addition, a significant psychological component to a CBRNE incident is common and requires both on-scene and follow-up monitoring. Widespread chaos and hysteria are frequently encountered, and first responders may have a difficult time with crowd control, scene safety, and scene security. Many community agencies need to be available to respond in the event of a CBRNE incident.

Chemical Agents

Depending on temperature and pressure, chemical agents can exist as solids, liquids, or gases. Chemical bioterrorism agents are hazardous chemicals designed to irritate, incapacitate, or kill an intended target. Most weaponized chemical agents are liquids, dispersed as aerosols.[15] Chemical agents are categorized by their physiological effects and chemical makeup, which can have both systemic and local effects on the body. **Table 14-2** lists several of the more common chemical agents. Special considerations for chemical-agent triage include recalling that many toxic chemicals do not have antidotes readily available and care of the casualties is primarily supportive.[15] Additionally, deceased casualties will still require decontamination.

Nerve Agents

Nerve agents, the most toxic of all weaponized chemical agents, are organophosphates, originally developed as pesticides. Sarin (GB) is the most well known agent, due in part to its use in the 1995 subway attack in Tokyo, Japan. There are two broad categories, the V-series and G-series agents. V-series agents evaporate more slowly, allowing them to last

for hours to days on objects, depending on the ambient temperature.

The most likely routes of exposure to nerve agents released during a terrorist attack are dermal or inhalation. Secondary contamination (exposure to others) is not a risk with inhalation exposure. Dermatological exposure may be a risk to rescuers through direct contact or by the release of vapors from clothing.

Nerve agents function by inhibiting the enzyme acetylcholinesterase (AChE), allowing excess accumulation of acetylcholine at neuromuscular junctions, causing overstimulation of the involved organs. The extent and severity of the symptoms depends on the agent, the method and duration of exposure, and the amount of agent. The observation of signs and symptoms is the primary means of diagnosing exposure to nerve agents. Common signs and symptoms are listed in **Table 14-3**. **Table 14-4** describes the "SLUDGEBBB" and "DUMBELS" mnemonics that are helpful to remember signs and symptoms of exposure to cholinesterase inhibitors.

Atropine and pralidoxime (2-PAM Cl) are the only antidotes for nerve agent exposure. The 2-PAM Cl must be administered within minutes to a few hours after exposure to be effective.[16]

Blister Agents (Vesicants)

The most common routes of vesicant exposure are inhalation or topical (liquid contact). Vesicants cause irritation and blistering of the skin and mucous membranes, particularly in the lungs. With high-dose exposure, systemic absorption of a vesicant may result in cardiovascular and central nervous system (CNS) effects.[17] Most vesicants will manifest symptoms within minutes of exposure, although some clinical findings may be delayed for several hours.[17] Although exposure is not usually fatal, it can cause incapacitation, leading to long-term hospitalization.[18] The two most common agents in this class are mustard (HD) and lewisite (L). **Table 14-5** lists common signs and symptoms of vesicants.

Treatment priorities include aggressive airway maintenance, administration of oxygen, removal of clothing, and thorough washing of skin. Although there are various protocols and guidelines for skin decontamination of chemical agents; the Centers for Disease Control and Prevention (CDC) recommends soap and water or a solution of 0.5% sodium hypochlorite.[19]

Pulmonary Agents

Chlorine and phosgene (CG) are commonly used in industry and were used as weaponized agents during World War I. Both cause pulmonary edema by injuring the small peripheral airways, which is clinically similar to inhalation burn injury. Signs and

Table 14-2: Chemical Agents

Category/Examples	Effects on Body	Treatment
Pulmonary Agents • Phosgene • Chlorine	• Irritation to the respiratory tract • Coughing • Sneezing • Watery eyes • Shortness of breath • Tachypnea • Dyspnea	• Decontamination • Aggressive airway and breathing management • No specific antidote
Blood Agents • Cyanide	• Cellular anoxia • Rapid breathing • Restlessness • Dizziness • Weakness • Headache • Nausea and vomiting • Rapid heart rate • Apnea • Cardiac arrest	• Decontamination • Aggressive airway and breathing management • Antidotes: Amyl nitrate, sodium thiosulfate, sodium nitrate, Hydroxocobolamin
Vesicants* • Mustard • Lewisite	• Rhinorrhea • Blepharospasm • Pruritus • Skin irritation • Damage to eyes and mucous membranes • Blisters to skin • Hoarseness • Cough • Dyspnea	• Decontamination • Aggressive airway and breathing management • Antidote for Lewisite: Dimercaprol (BAL)
Nerve Agents* • Tabun (GA) • Sarin (GB) • VX	• Miosis • Rhinorrhea • Lacrimation • Salivation • Nausea and vomiting • Fasciculations • Seizures • Death secondary to the inhibition of acetyl-cholinesterase	• Decontamination • Aggressive airway and ventilation management • Antidote: Atropine, 2-PAM Cl
Incapacitating Agents BZ	• Hallucinations • Illusions	Decontamination
Riot-control Agents CS (Mace)	• Irritation of upper respiratory tract • Lacrimation	Decontamination

*Other agents can also be systemically distributed through the bloodstream

symptoms are listed in **Table 14-6**. Pulmonary agents are heavy gases; therefore, immediate treatment includes moving to an area of fresh air and higher ground.[20] Patients may require mechanical ventilation and antibiotic therapy for pneumonia.

Blood Agents

Blood agents, such as carbon monoxide and cyanide, interfere with oxygenation at the cellular level. Inhalation is the usual route of entry; however, ingestion or absorption are possible.

Cyanide is a rapidly acting, deadly chemical that can be found in a variety of sources:

- Certain foods or plants (e.g., almonds, millet, lima beans, soy, spinach, fruit seeds/pits)
- Cigarette smoke
- Pesticides
- Multiple industrial settings (e.g., plastics, photography, textiles, paper)

After absorption through the skin, eyes, or respiratory tract, cyanide is rapidly distributed to the tissues. The hallmark of cyanide toxicity is metabolic acidosis.

Cells are forced into anaerobic metabolism with resultant accumulation of hydrogen ions and lactate.

Clinicians should be alert for key historic features of cyanide contact, which include

- Specific odors (nearly 50% of patients exposed report the odor of bitter almonds after exposure to hydrogen cyanide). [21]
- Effects on surroundings (e.g., dead animals, multiple casualties).
- Time, route, and nature of the exposure. Refer to **Table 14-7** for more information on cyanide exposure, signs and symptoms, and treatment.

Biological Agents

Biological agents are characterized as bacterial, viral, or toxins. The CDC has organized biological agents into three categories—A, B, and C—based on their virulence, ability to be spread from person to person, and availability (**Table 14-8**).[22] Because they are easily reproduced and difficult to detect, biological agents are increasingly described as possible weapons of mass destruction. These agents can be spread via:

- Aerosol
- Explosives
- Food or water supplies

Table 14-3: Signs and Symptoms of Organophosphate/Nerve Agent Exposure

Body Area Affected	Symptom
Cardiovascular	• Bradydysrhythmias • Tachydysrhythmias • Ventricular dysrhythmias • Heart block(s) • Hypertension
Central nervous system	• Seizures • Loss of consciousness • Coma • Irritability • Restlessness
Respiratory	• Copious secretions • Rhinorrhea • Wheezing • Dyspnea
Gastrointestinal/ genitourinary	• Increased saliva production • Nausea • Vomiting • Diarrhea • Abdominal pain • Urinary incontinence
Musculoskeletal	• Weakness • Fasciculations
Integumentary	• Sweating
Other	• Lacrimation

Table 14-4: Mnemonics for Symptoms of Organophosphate/Nerve Agent Exposure

SLUDGE/BBB	
S =	Salivation
L =	Lacrimation
U =	Urination
D =	Diarrhea
G =	Gastrointestinal distress
E =	Emesis
B =	Bronchorrhea
B =	Bronchospasm
B =	Bradycardia

DUMBELS	
D =	Diaphoresis & diarrhea
U =	Urinary incontinence
M =	Myosis (Miosis)
B =	Bradycardia, Bronchorrhea, Bronchospasm
E =	Emesis
L =	Lacrimation
S =	Salivation and Secretion

Because of the delay from exposure to onset of symptoms, outbreaks can resemble a naturally occurring phenomenon, rather than an attack. Diagnosis of a biological attack requires a high index of suspicion and will challenge even the most perceptive clinician. Health care providers should be observant for patterns of illness and diagnostic clues that may indicate an outbreak of infectious disease associated with the intentional release of a biological agent. Signs that indicate exposure to biological agents include

- A number of patients presenting with the same signs and symptoms
- Unusual age distribution for a common disease[23]

Table 14-9 provides an overview of signs and symptoms that might be encountered after the release of an infectious agent.

Anthrax

Anthrax (also known as woolsorter's disease, black bane, or fifth plague) is a disease caused by an aerobic gram-positive rod, *Bacillus anthracis*, which forms a spore that is resistant to light, heat, desiccation, and many disinfectants. The spores become virulent once they are introduced to a human or animal. Humans usually contract this disease accidentally through contact with infected animals, meat, or the hides of animals that contain the spores. Anthrax infection can be cutaneous, inhalational, or gastrointestinal.

Table 14-5: Vesicant Agents

Body Area Affected	Signs and Symptoms
Respiratory	• Clear rhinorrhea • Nasal irritation/pain • Sore throat • Cough • Dyspnea (shortness of breath) • Chest tightness • Tachypnea • Hemoptysis
Dermatological	• Itching • Immediate blanching (phosgene oxime) • Erythema (immediate with lewisite and phosgene oxime, may be delayed for 2 to 24 hours with mustards) • Blisters (within 1 hour with phosgene oxime, delayed for 2 to 12 hours with lewisite, delayed for 2 to 24 hours with mustards) • Necrosis and eschar (over a period of 7 to 10 days)
Ocular	• Conjunctivitis • Lacrimation • Eye pain/burning • Photophobia • Blurred vision • Eyelid edema • Corneal ulceration • Blindness
Cardiovascular	• Hypotension (with high-dose exposure to lewisite) • Atrioventricular block and cardiac arrest (with high-dose exposure)
Central nervous system (with exposures to high doses)	• Tremors • Convulsions • Ataxia • Coma

Adapted from Centers for Disease Control and Prevention (CDC). (2005). Vesicant/blister agent poisoning. Retrieved August 10, 2006, from http://www.bt.cdc.gov/ agent/vesicants/tsd.asp

Table 14-6: Pulmonary Agents

Chlorine	Phosgene (CG)
Signs & Symptoms	
• Coughing	• Coughing
• Chest tightness	• Burning sensation in the throat and eyes
• Burning sensation in the nose, throat, and eyes	• Watery eyes
• Watery eyes	• Blurred vision
• Blurred vision	• Difficulty breathing or shortness of breath
• Nausea and vomiting	• Nausea and vomiting
• Burning pain, redness, and blisters on the skin if exposed to gas, skin injury similar to frostbite if exposed to liquid chlorine	• Skin contact can result in lesions similar to those from frostbite or burns
• Difficulty breathing or shortness of breath (may appear immediately if high concentrations of chlorine gas are inhaled, or may be delayed if low concentrations of chlorine gas are inhaled)	• Following exposure to high concentrations of phosgene, a person may develop fluid in the lungs (pulmonary edema) within 2 to 6 hours.
• Fluid in the lungs (pulmonary edema) within 2 to 4 hours	**Delayed effects** that can appear for up to 48 hours include the following:
	• Difficulty breathing
	• Coughing up white to pink-tinged fluid (a sign of pulmonary edema)
	• Low blood pressure
	• Heart failure

Treatment

• Leave area of exposure and get to fresh air; seek out higher ground; chlorine and phosgene gases are heavier than air and will sink to lower ground area

• Remove clothing and double bag in plastic bags

• Copious irrigation and skin cleansing with soap & water

Adapted from Centers for Disease Control and Prevention (CDC). (2005). Choking/lung/pulmonary agents. Retrieved August 10, 2006, from http://www.bt.cdc.gov/agent/agentlistchem-category.asp#choking

Table 14-7 Cyanide Exposure

Signs and Symptoms	Decontamination	Emergency Treatment
• Rapid breathing	• Removal of clothing	• Speed is critical. For symptomatic victims, provide treatment with 100% oxygen and specific antidotes as needed
• Restlessness	• Double bag clothing	
• Dizziness	• Copious irrigation and skin cleansing with soap and water	
• Weakness		• Cyanide antidotes include amyl nitrite and intravenous infusions of sodium nitrite and sodium thiosulfate—are packaged in the cyanide antidote kit.
• Headache		
• Nausea and vomiting		
• Rapid heart rate		• New antidote approved in 2007 is intravenous infusion of hydroxocobalamin (Cyanokit®)
Exposure to a large amount of cyanide by any route may cause these other health effects		
• Convulsions		
• Low blood pressure		
• Slow heart rate		
• Loss of consciousness		
• Lung injury		
• Respiratory failure leading to death		

Adapted from Centers for Disease Control and Prevention (CDC). (n.d.). Cyanide. Retrieved August 10, 2006, from http://www.bt.cdc.gov/agent/cyanide

Plague

Plague is an infectious disease caused by a gram-negative bacillus, *Yersinia pestis*. Plague bacillus is one of the most potent biological warfare agents in the world. The incubation period and clinical symptoms vary by mode of transmission. The bubonic form is the most common presentation (85%) of naturally occurring plague in the United States, followed by septicemic (10–15%) and pneumonic (1%).[24] Because patient-to-patient transmission is common and highly fatal, contact and droplet precautions are appropriate.

Table 14-8: Categories of Biological Agents

Category A	Category B	Category C
High-priority agents include organisms that pose a risk to national security because they: • Can be easily disseminated or transmitted from person to person • Result in high mortality rates and have the potential for major public health impact • Might cause public panic and social disruption, and require special action for public health preparedness. • Examples: anthrax, plague, botulism	Second-highest-priority agents include those that: • Are moderately easy to disseminate • Result in moderate morbidity rates and low mortality rates • Require specific enhancements of CDC's diagnostic capacity and enhanced disease surveillance. • Examples: brucellosis, Q fever, ricin	Third-highest-priority agents include emerging pathogens that could be engineered for mass dissemination in the future because of: • Availability • Ease of production and dissemination • Potential for high morbidity and mortality rates and major health impact. • Examples: infectious diseases such as hantavirus

Adapted from Centers for Disease Control and Prevention (CDC). (n.d.). Bioterrorism Agents/Diseases. Retrieved August 10, 2006, from http://www.bt.cdc.gov/agent/agentlist-category.asp#catdef

Table 14-9: Symptom Clusters Suggestive of the Release of an Infectious Agent

Disease (Agent)	Symptoms
Anthrax	• Inhalational—Nonspecific prodrome (fever, dyspnea, cough) after inhalation of infectious spores followed by respiratory failure and hemodynamic collapse; may note thoracic edema and widened mediastinum on chest radiographs • Growth of gram-positive bacilli in blood cultures • Cutaneous—Area of local edema developing into a pruritic macule or papule that will enlarge and ulcerate within 1–2 days; evolves into painless, depressed, black eschar
Plague	• Fever, cough with mucopurulent sputum, hemoptysis, and chest pain • Bronchopneumonia noted on chest radiograph • Gram-negative rods noted in sputum
Botulism	• Symmetric cranial neuropathies (drooping eyelids, weakened jaw clench, difficulty swallowing or speaking), blurred vision, symmetric descending weakness following a proximal to distal pattern • Respiratory dysfunction from respiratory muscle paralysis
Smallpox (Variola)	• Initially nonspecific prodrome of fever, myalgias precedes rash • Vesicular-pustular rash most prominent on face and extremities at the same stage of development
Tularemia	• Acute onset of nonspecific febrile illness reported 3–5 days after inhalation of agent; pleuropneumonitis develops within days
Hemorrhagic fever (Ebola or Marburg viruses)	• Incubation period of 5–10 days; acute onset of fever, myalgias and headaches often accompanied by nausea, vomiting, abdominal pain, diarrhea, chest pain, cough • Maculopapular rash prominent on the torso • Petechiae, ecchymoses, and hemorrhages

Adapted from Centers for Disease Control and Prevention (CDC). (2001, October 19). Morbidity and Mortality Weekly Report. Retrieved August 10, 2006, from http://www.cdc.gov/mmwr/preview/mmwrhtml/mm5041a2.htm

Large numbers of previously healthy patients presenting with acute fulminant pneumonia should prompt suspicions of plague infection. Mortality for untreated plague is high, but antibiotic therapy can be effective if it is begun within 24 hours of symptom onset.[25]

Smallpox

Variola virus is the causative agent of smallpox, one of the most dreaded and feared diseases worldwide. Clinical presentation postexposure includes

- Viral prodrome (e.g., malaise, fever, cephalgia, and gastrointestinal upset).

- Erythematous rash that develops 2 to 3 days postexposure. The rash progresses into maculopapular lesions that evolve into vesicles and eventually pustules (**Table 14-10**). The rash begins on the face, progresses to the extremities, and then to the torso.

Patients should be placed on airborne and contact precautions. There is no cure for smallpox; the care is supportive in nature. However, if the vaccine is administered up to 4 days after exposure to the virus and before appearance of the rash, there is some protection and prevention of infection or limitation of disease severity.[26] Immune globulin, available through the CDC, may be administered concurrently with the vaccine.

Table 14-10: Smallpox Rash Features

Duration/Contagion	Rash Feature
Incubation period (Duration: 7 to 17 days) **Not** contagious	• Asymptomatic after exposure
Initial symptoms (Prodrome) (Duration: 2 to 4 days) Sometimes contagious*	• Initial symptoms include fever, malaise, head and body aches, and sometimes vomiting. • High fevers, ranging from 101 °F to 104 °F (38 °C to 40 °C). Generally lasts 2 to 4 days.
Early rash (Duration: about 4 days) Most contagious	• The rash begins with small red spots on the tongue and in the mouth that will develop into sores that open and spread the virus throughout the mouth and oropharynx. • After the sores break down, the erythematous rash begins on the face and spreads to the extremities. The rash usually spreads to all parts of the body within 24 hours. During this time, the fever may resolve and the person may feel slightly better. • The rash becomes maculopapular (raised) the third day and fills with a thick, opaque fluid with a "pit" or depression in the center. This is a significant distinguishing characteristic of smallpox. • The patient will experience a return of high fevers until scabs form over the bumps.
Pustular rash (Duration: about 5 days) Contagious	• The maculopapular rash evolves into pustules.
Pustules and scabs (Duration: about 5 days) Contagious	• The pustules begin to form a crust and then scab. After 2 weeks most of the sores have scabbed over.
Resolving scabs (Duration: about 6 days) Contagious	• As the scabs begin to fall off, they leave marks that eventually become pitted scars. • Three weeks after the rash appears, most scabs will have fallen off, but the person remains contagious until all the scabs have fallen off.
Scabs resolved. Not contagious. Scabs have fallen off. Person is no longer contagious.	• Smallpox may be contagious during the prodrome phase, but is most infectious during the first 7 to 10 days following rash onset.*

Adapted from Centers for Disease Control and Prevention (CDC). (2004). Smallpox disease overview. Retrieved August 10, 2006, from http://www.bt.cdc.gov/agent/smallpox/overview/disease-facts.asp

Ricin

Ricin is an extremely toxic poison made from the byproducts of castor bean processing. It can be distributed as pellets, as powder, or in mist form. Effective orally or by injection, ricin cannot be absorbed by exposure through intact skin. Toxic effects are dose-dependent and cause symptoms by inhibiting intracellular protein synthesis, resulting in cell death. Oral ingestion results in nausea, vomiting, diarrhea, dehydration, and gastrointestinal hemorrhage, although fatalities are rare because of poor absorption. Pulmonary and systemic effects are secondary to inhalational exposure, with widespread and nonspecific symptoms including fever, tachypnea, tachycardia, hypotension, hepatitis, pancreatitis, myocardial damage, vomiting, diarrhea, and bone marrow suppression. Manifestations of symptoms occur within 8 to 24 hours, with death after several days or a protracted hospitalization.[27]

Botulinum

The botulinum toxin, produced by the bacterium *Clostridium botulinum* is considered the most lethal substance known.[28] The toxin's effect is dependent on whether the agent is ingested, inoculated, or inhaled. The onset of symptoms varies between hours and days, depending on the initial dose and route of exposure. The toxin prevents the release of acetylcholine, prohibiting muscular contraction, and resulting in flaccid paralysis.

The hallmark symptom of descending flaccid paralysis begins with the facial nerves and expands to include the muscles of chewing, swallowing, and eventually respiration.

Improperly canned or preserved food is the usual source of food-borne botulism. Inhalational botulism can only occur through the intentional release of aerosolized *C. botulinum*. Because the toxin cannot cross the blood–brain barrier, symptoms are confined to the peripheral nervous system and result in mild anticholinergic symptoms such as dry mouth, dilated pupils, and decreased bowel and bladder motility.

Radiological/Nuclear

The potential use of radiological weapons remains an ongoing concern. Terrorist use of a radiological device may occur in several ways.[29]

- Simple radiological device—the intentional spread of radioactive materials without an explosive device, such as placing radioactive material in a populated area
- Radiological dispersal device—an explosive device used to scatter radioactive materials, such as a dirty bomb
- Reactor—although unlikely because of high security, a terrorist attack at a nuclear plant would result in significant release of radioactive materials if the terrorists were able to disable the cooling system
- Improvised nuclear device—nuclear detonation from a device other than a military weapon

Injuries that may occur as a result of detonation of a nuclear device include

- Thermal burns
- Injuries secondary to radiation exposure

Nuclear/radiological exposure can produce complex injuries, which may present immediately or have a delayed onset. Ionizing radiation is a form of electromagnetic energy that can occur naturally or be machine-generated. The most common types of ionizing radiation are alpha and beta particles, gamma rays, x-rays, and neutrons (**Table 14-11**). Radiation

Table 14-11: Types of Ionizing Radiation

Types of Ionizing Radiation	Definition
Alpha particles	Composed of two neutrons and two protons with a relatively large mass and charge; do not penetrate skin and can be repelled by a thin layer of clothing. Alpha particles would present a risk if ingested or inhaled but are not considered an external hazard.
Beta particles	Considered moderately penetrating and can penetrate human skin to the germinal layer where new skin is produced. May result in severe burns if left on the skin.
Gamma rays	High-energy rays with a short wavelength. Able to penetrate through many centimeters of human tissue and most materials; require dense materials to shield body from this penetrating radiation.
Neutron particles	Neutral particle within the atom. Very penetrating and cause damage by imparting energy to other particles ("billiard ball" effect) or by being captured by elements within the body, such as sodium.
X-rays	Similar to gamma rays but have a longer wavelength. They are produced by high-energy electrons passing through a positive nucleus. Very penetrating and considered an external hazard.

Reprinted from *Disease-a-Month*, 49(8), A Primer for Nuclear Terrorism, pages 485–516, Copyright 2003, with permission from Elsevier.

exposure is commonly measured in rads (radiation absorbed dose) or rems (radiation equivalent-man) in the United States and in gray (Gy) or sievert (Sv) internationally.[29]

Irradiation and contamination are important terms to understand in radiation exposure management. An individual becomes irradiated when the body is exposed to penetrating radiation from an external source. This radiation is either absorbed or passes through the body. Similar to a patient receiving a diagnostic x-ray; the individual is not radioactive. Contamination occurs internally or externally, when radioactive materials (gases, liquids, or solids) are inhaled, ingested, or deposited on the body. Radioactive materials are distributed throughout the body based on the type of radiation. Effects of radiation exposure are also time- and dose-dependent.

Acute Radiation Syndrome

Acute radiation syndrome (ARS) is an acute illness that follows a generally predictable course, over a time period ranging from hours to weeks, after exposure to ionizing radiation. Acute radiation syndrome is most significant in tissues with rapidly proliferating cells. The symptoms develop because of damage to the stem cell line, which results in altered cell replication processes and loss of normal cells. Symptoms may subside as is often the case during the course of medical radiotherapy.[30]

Symptoms are determined by the total dose of radiation exposure.[29,30] Because of the insult to the hematopoietic system, the absolute lymphocyte count is an important indicator of severity of illness and prognosis. If the total lymphocyte count is greater than 1,200 at 48 hours, it is unlikely that the patient has received a lethal dose of radiation. If at 48 hours the absolute lymphocyte count is between 300 and 1,200, a significant exposure has occurred. The development of gastrointestinal symptoms within 2 hours is an indicator of significant exposure with a probable fatal outcome.[29] Treatment and supportive care should be promptly initiated for patients exhibiting signs and symptoms of ARS.

Management of Nuclear Explosion Casualties

Management priorities secondary to a nuclear explosion focus on the recognition of signs and symptoms of radiation exposure and decontamination of casualties. A contaminated patient, with radioactive material on their clothes or body, poses some risk for spread of the material to others and the environment. An irradiated victim poses little risk to health care providers.[29] Because it is rare for an irradiated patient to infect health care workers, lifesaving treatments take precedence over decontamination.[31] Patients can be organized into three categories based on signs and symptoms:

- Survival probable—dose less than 100 rads (< 1Gy)
- Survival possible—dose 200–800 rads (2–8 Gy)
- Survival improbable—dose greater than 800 rads (> 8 Gy)

The medical management of radiation casualties includes triage and emergency lifesaving care. Victims are identified as having either internal or external contamination during the initial assessment and triage. A radiation-contaminated victim is treated in the same manner as any hazardous material incident victim. Treatment includes

- Stabilization, assessment, and maintenance of the ABCs
- Decontamination
  - The emergency department is divided into dirty and clean areas. The floor of the dirty area is covered by an inexpensive, easily removable product. All unnecessary equipment is removed from the dirty area or draped. Contaminated patient clothing is removed from the department after double-bagging and labeling. Removal of patient clothing can eliminate up to 90% of the external contamination.[31,32] Personal protective equipment (PPE) required for hospital staff includes
    - Surgical gown, cap, mask, and overshoes
    - Surgical face shield
    - Two pairs of surgical gloves with the inner set taped to the gown
    - Shoes taped to surgical trousers
    - Plastic apron

A Geiger-Muller survey meter is used to assess external contamination. Intact skin is decontaminated with soap and water, working from the periphery to the center. Several washings may be required. Wounds should be masked with waterproof surgical drapes to prevent further contamination.

Explosives

Explosions are the most common cause of casualties associated with terrorist attacks.[33] Victims from explosions sustain more severe injuries and have a higher mortality rate when compared with any other form of trauma.[34]

Blast Injury

The injury pattern that results from explosive devices is a unique entity within trauma care. In the United States, most blast injuries are unintentional, the result of fireworks mishaps, occupational accidents, or industrial disasters. Around the world, undetonated land mines, hand grenades, and military explosive devices are responsible for many civilian and military casualties.[35,36] Four categories describe blast injuries: primary, secondary, tertiary, and quaternary[36,37] (**Table 14-12**).

The combination of mechanisms acting concurrently causes the unique clinical picture of bombing/explosive victims (**Table 14-13**). Victims in a confined space have an increased mortality rate, a higher significance of primary blast injuries, and more extensive burn injuries.[34,36,37] The most common fatal condition from primary blast injury is pulmonary barotrauma.[36,38] One particularly common (and potentially fatal) consequence of the overpressurization wave is blast lung, which is characterized by the clinical triad of apnea, bradycardia, and hypotension.[38]

Psychological Casualties and Psychosocial Issues

Whether the source of a disaster is natural or manmade, there is often widespread social, behavioral, and psychological morbidity following the event. Psychosocial casualties may arrive at the emergency department in large numbers immediately following a disaster and may continue to present for months afterwards.[39] Primary prevention begins with:

- An awareness of the need for realistic information regarding the threat
- A planned response

Secondary prevention begins during the initial triage and treatment stage. All first responders, including mental health providers, should be prepared to provide supportive treatment for patients who present with acute emotional distress.

Triage of psychiatric patients presents a number of dilemmas to the triage officer. Many patients will attribute symptoms such as tachycardia, shortness of breath, shivering, and myalgias to toxic agent expo-

Table 14-12: Mechanisms of Blast Injury

Category and Characteristics	Body part injured	Types of injuries

Primary
• Injury caused by the blast itself
• Results from the impact of the overpressurization wave with body surfaces
	• Gas-filled structures are most susceptible:
	  ▪ Lungs
	  ▪ GI tract
	  ▪ Middle ear
		• Blast lung (pulmonary barotrauma)
		• Tympanic membrane rupture and middle ear damage
		• Abdominal hemorrhage and perforation
		• Globe (eye) rupture
		• Concussion (traumatic brain injury without physical signs of head injury)

Secondary • Injury caused by projectiles from the blast • Results from flying debris and bomb fragments	Any body part	• Penetrating ballistic (fragmentation) or blunt injuries • Eye penetration (can be occult)
Tertiary • Injury caused from the force of throwing the victim against stationary objects • Results from individuals being thrown by the blast wind	Any body part	• Fracture and traumatic amputation • Closed and open brain injury
Quaternary • All explosion-related injuries, illnesses, or diseases not due to primary, secondary, or tertiary mechanisms. • Includes exacerbation or complications of existing conditions	Any body part	• Burns (flash, partial, and full thickness) • Crush injuries • Closed and open brain injury • Asthma, COPD, or other breathing problems from dust, smoke, or toxic fumes • Angina • Hyperglycemia, hypertension

Centers for Disease Control and Prevention (CDC). (2003). *Explosions and blast injuries: A primer for clinicians.* Retrieved August 10, 2006, from http://www.bt.cdc.gov/masscasualties/explosions.asp

sure and demand postexposure treatment. Because psychogenic symptoms can imitate symptoms of an actual exposure, it is important to elicit a careful history and perform a thorough exam to determine if an exposure has actually occurred.

Psychiatric interventions initiated immediately after the disaster tend to focus on the symptoms and psychological reactions that have not yet become actual disorders. Many symptoms are normally expected behaviors and include sleep disorders, appetite disturbances, and generalized anxiety. Other symptoms include

- Increased fear related to potential use of weapons of mass destruction
- Fear of contact with others
- Paranoia

The judicious use of antipsychotic and anxiolytic medications may help to mediate the acute manifestations of psychoses and delirium after a disaster.

Table 14-13: Overview of Explosive-Related Injuries

System	Injury or Condition
Auditory	Tympanic membrane rupture, ossicular disruption, cochlear damage, foreign body
Eye, orbit, face	Perforated globe, foreign body, air embolism, fractures
Respiratory	Blast lung, hemothorax, pneumothorax, pulmonary contusion and hemorrhage, AV fistulas (source of air embolism), airway epithelial damage, aspiration pneumonitis, sepsis
Digestive	Bowel perforation, hemorrhage, ruptured liver or spleen, sepsis, mesenteric ischemia from air embolism
Circulatory	Cardiac contusion, myocardial infarction from air embolism, shock, vasovagal hypotension, peripheral vascular injury, air embolism-induced injury
CNS injury	Concussion, closed and open brain injury, stroke, spinal cord injury, air embolism-induced injury
Renal injury	Renal contusion, laceration, acute renal failure due to rhabdomyolysis, hypotension, and hypovolemia
Extremity injury	Traumatic amputation, fractures, crush injuries, compartment syndrome, burns, cuts, lacerations, acute arterial occlusion, air embolism-induced injury

Centers for Disease Control and Prevention (CDC). (2003). *Explosions and blast injuries: A primer for clinicians.* Retrieved August 10, 2006, from http://www.bt.cdc.gov/masscasualties/explosions.asp

Treatment should be kept as simple as possible. Establishing a secure location, somewhat removed from the chaos of the triage spaces and from other patients, can be very helpful. Nurses, social workers, chaplains, mental health workers, and other ancillary personnel can be utilized more effectively in a controlled setting. **Table 14-14** provides a review of the goals for disaster psychiatry.

Medical personnel and first responders are particularly at risk with repeated exposure to trauma, multiple deaths, and infectious or contaminated agents. They must be provided an adequate rest–work rotation, support groups, and regular debriefing through the use of critical incident stress management (CISM) teams.

Planning and Implementation

The DISASTER Paradigm

A mnemonic to guide the approach to an actual or potential disaster is described in the *Basic Disaster Life Support Provider Manual.*[40] The DISASTER paradigm mnemonic (**Table 14-15**) provides a framework to organize and guide health care providers' preparation and response to a disaster.

Detection

The key to detection is awareness. This is the ability to recognize a situation that has the potential to overwhelm available resources. An example is an infectious disease outbreak. Once identified, it must be determined whether or not this was a natural occurrence or the deliberate release of a biological agent. The cause of the event will most likely be

Table 14-14: Goals of Disaster Psychiatry

- Psychological first aid: minimize the immediate emotional and psychological impact of disasters by providing education, support, and treatment.
- Help casualties return to the level of functioning prior to the disaster.
- Observe and understand that all casualties of a disaster may benefit from the expertise of mental health professionals.
- Identify casualties at risk for long-term mental health disorders secondary to the disaster.
- Be available to treat the long-term mental health problems secondary to the disaster until community resources are established to meet this need.
- Provide consultations to other responders and facilities.

Reprinted from *Psychiatric Clinics of North America,* 27(3), General Disaster Psychiatry, pages 391–406, Copyright 2004, with permission from Elsevier.

unknown to initial emergency responders. Questions that focus on detection include the following.

- Is there suspicion of a threat and what is it?
- Can anything unusual be seen, heard, or smelled?

Incident Command

The purpose of the incident command system is to develop a standardized command and control system to direct the emergency response. Five functional elements within the organizational structure include incident command, operations, planning, logistics, and finance.[40,41]

Use of the Hospital Emergency Incident Command System (HEICS) (**Figure 14-1**) serves to improve coordination between the various agencies and hospitals responding to the event. HEICS is a set of procedures that fits within a hospital's emergency preparedness plan. A hospital disaster plan is required, but HEICS provides the hospital with a chain of command, a flexible organizational chart, prioritized checklists, and a common language to better facilitate communication with other community facilities and agencies. Within HEICS, a single incident commander is responsible for the overall leadership and guidance. A chain of command delegates authority through several integrated divisions such as operations, finance, logistics, and planning. Within the emergency depart-

Table 14-15: DISASTER Paradigm

D = **D**etect	Can we **detect** the reason for the disaster?
I = **I**ncident Command	Do we need **incident command**, and if so, where?
S = **S**cene Security and **S**afety	Is a **safety** or **security** issue present?
A = **A**ssess hazards	Have we **assessed** the possible **hazards** present?
S = **S**upport Required	What **support** in terms of people and supplies are needed?
T = **T**riage and Treatment	Do we need to **triage** and how much **treatment** is needed?
E = **E**vacuation	Can we **evacuate**/transport the victims to another location?
R = **R**ecovery	What are the **recovery** issues?
	Is there a disaster or mass casualty present?
	• Is the need greater than our resources?

Courtesy of Dallas, C. E., Coule, P. L., James, J. J., Lillibridge, S., Pepe, P. E., Schwartz, R. B., et al. (Eds.). (2004). Basic disaster life support provider manual, v 2.5. Chicago: American Medical Association..

ment, triage, decontamination, and initial treatment are assigned to teams with an overall supervisor to coordinate the process.

Safety and Security

Safety and security begin with proper training and preparation. The health care worker must ask questions such as, "What situations might be encountered?" Maintaining the safety of all personnel is important because injuries to health care workers reduce the available resources and increase patient load.

There are considerable safety risks to prehospital personnel after a natural disaster. There are often fallen trees, downed power lines, flooding, structural fires, and the risk of explosions. The loss of electrical power is a safety risk for hospital workers and patients who require life-support and resuscitative equipment. Water management must also be considered because the water supply may be compromised.

Assess Hazards

The key to hazard detection is awareness. Personal protective equipment (PPE) should be readily available and utilized by all members of the team. Exposure to chemical, biological, or radiological hazards is a concern for all health care workers.

Support

Disaster management and preparedness includes maintaining an adequate amount of supplies, facilities, vehicles, and essential personnel to respond to the event. Preplanning is crucial to all aspects of support. Support includes additional hospital personnel, EMS units, law enforcement, public health personnel, private contractors, and possibly military or other government agencies.

Ensuring adequate supplies and other consumables is a crucial aspect of disaster support planning. There should be prearranged orders for supplies and goods, such as health care supplies, water, and food, which are necessary after a disaster.

Triage and Treatment

Triage

Triage during a mass casualty event is significantly different than standard prehospital or emergency department triage procedures. Mass casualty triage is often decentralized and performed at multiple sites with more frequent reassessments. There is a utilitarian approach to triage in disaster management in which the greatest good is provided to the greatest number, based on available resources.

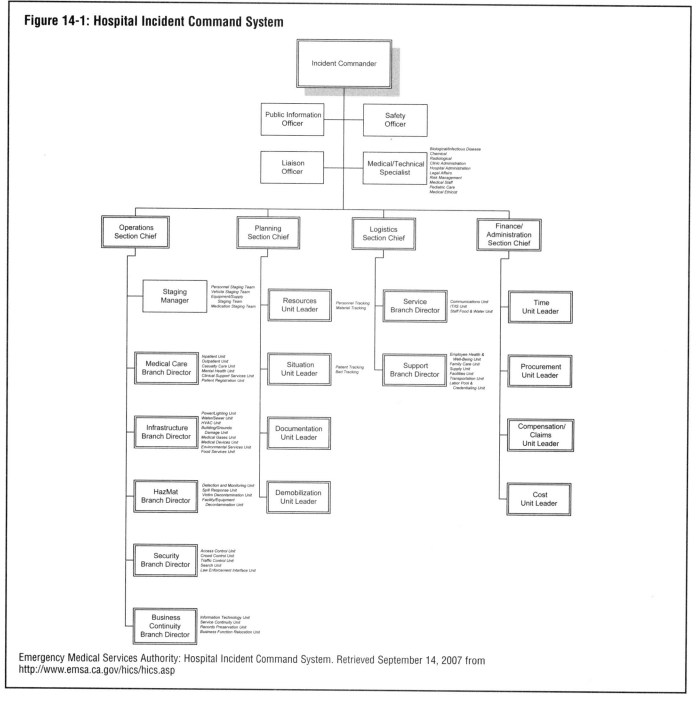

Figure 14-1: Hospital Incident Command System

Emergency Medical Services Authority: Hospital Incident Command System. Retrieved September 14, 2007 from http://www.emsa.ca.gov/hics/hics.asp

Treatment

Traumatic injuries following a disaster are common, ranging from uncomplicated lacerations and fractures, to significant blunt and penetrating wounds, and multisystem injuries. Anticipate extensive orthopedic services, including surgical and postoperative supplies and personnel. Adequate supplies for wound care, irrigation, debridement, and dressings must be stocked and available. Tetanus and antibiotic prophylaxis are also important wound management issues after a disaster.

Preexisting medical conditions such as asthma and chronic obstructive pulmonary disease may be exacerbated by dust and debris. Acute cardiac events have been noted to increase after disasters.[42,43] Disaster management plans should include measures to ensure adequately staffed and supplied intensive care units.

The lack of adequate potable water supplies, loss of power to provide refrigeration, lack of waste removal, and the inability of the chronically ill to access their medications or treatments are known to contribute to increased cases of respiratory and gastrointestinal illnesses.[44,45] Disaster management plans should also address a strategy for dealing with disease vectors such as mosquitoes, rats, and fleas.

Decontamination

Whether a disaster is natural or man-made, victims may have been exposed to chemical, biological, or radiological contaminants. Health care workers can be exposed to hazardous materials or chemicals in many different ways. Understanding basic decontamination procedures is important to reduce the risk to the health care worker. The goal of decontamination is to eradicate all harmful substances from the skin, hair, mucosa, lungs, and gastrointestinal tract to prevent further harm to the patient and rescuer(s). The practice of decontamination is a physical skill that requires considerable and continual hands-on training.[46]

The first step in decontamination is recognition of an unusual substance. Once identified, containment measures must be implemented to minimize the spread of the potential threat. It is crucial that health care providers understand, practice, and can perform their tasks while utilizing the appropriate level of PPE (Table 14-16). Most prehospital decontamination procedures have been patterned after the military concepts of hot, warm, and cold zones[46] (Table 14-17).

Decontamination at the hospital site is quite different. Many patients will have transported themselves rather than using EMS. These patients have traveled away from the exposure and hot zone. The hospital disaster plan should clearly identify the hospital's decontamination hot zone, such as an ambulance or parking area. Only the most basic of emergency medical treatments (e.g., opening and maintaining the airway, applying dressings) are provided in this area. Decontamination should take place in the warm zone. Patients should not be sent into the emergency department until they are considered clean and decontaminated. Environmental issues need to be considered; therefore, warming measures (e.g., lights, warmed fluids, blankets) should be readily available.

Initial decontamination procedures include

- Removal of contaminated clothing
- Double bagging and labeling contaminated clothing
- Washing the skin thoroughly with soap and warm water or flushing the skin with copious amounts of water

Hospital disaster planners must ensure that the decontamination team has access to water and application equipment (e.g., shower setups, hoses) along with a means for controlling water runoff.

Evacuation

Disaster preparedness must also consider evacuation scenarios. There are multiple ways to evacuate and transport victims from a disaster. EMS will be the primary mode of evacuation for more seriously ill/injured victims. Public transportation may be used to transport large numbers of minimally injured patients to appropriate treatment facilities.

Multiple difficulties encountered in the evacuation process including the structural instability of buildings, collapsed debris, flooding, and the inability to utilize regular traffic routes may impede evacuation.

Recovery

Planning for disasters includes addressing the means and process of recovery. The recovery phase is the process to return the community to its normal, predisaster state. This includes cleanup, removal of debris, and construction and restoration of the infrastructure. The reestablishment of local and routine health care, communication structures, food and water supplies, sanitation systems, and shelter for displaced victims of disaster is paramount.

Table 14-16: Personal Protective Equipment (PPE)

Level	Protects against	Respiratory Equipment	Skin protection
A	Gases, vapors, aerosols, oxygen-deficient areas, liquids, and solids	Self-contained breathing apparatus (SCBA) (protection from gas, vapor, or oxygen-deficient environment)	Fully encapsulated, chemical resistant suit (protection from vapor)
B	Vapors, aerosols, oxygen-deficient areas, solids, and liquids	SCBA or positive pressure supplied-air respirator (SAR) (protection from gas, vapor or oxygen-deficient environments)	Splash-proof, chemical resistant suit (protection from splashes)
C	Most vapors and aerosols, solids, and liquids	(Powered) Air-purifying respirator (APR or PAPR) or face cartridge mask	Splash-proof chemical resistant suit (protection from splashes)
D	None	HEPA filter protects against particulate matter	Minimal

Adapted from U.S. Environmental Protection Agency (EPA). (2006). *Personal protective equipment*. Retrieved August 11, 2006, from http://www.epa.gov/superfund/programs/er/hazsubs/equip.htm

Table 14-17: Zones of Decontamination

Hot zone	Area of highest contamination; may be the area immediately surrounding the point of contact with the contaminant(s). Minimal medical care provided here; basic airway, hemorrhage control or the administration of specific antidotes. Patients taken from the hot zone to the warm zone.
Warm zone	Preferably positioned uphill and upwind of the hot zone; there is some contamination, but less so than the hot zone. There is limited medical care provided, enough to stabilize the patient long enough to be decontaminated and moved into the cold zone.
Cold zone	Safe and free from contamination; all patients are assumed to be properly decontaminated and available for full medical treatment.

Reprinted from *Critical Care Clinics*, 21, Decontamination, pages 653–672, Copyright 2005, with permission from Elsevier.

Nursing Roles in Disaster Management

Nurses have varied and crucial roles in multiple aspects of disaster management. Emergency nurses participate in a wide variety of activities that are intimately connected to disaster management such as triage and provision of care to critically ill or injured patients. In addition, nurses can influence policymakers, undertake research efforts, and participate in systems training involved in disaster management.[47] Fundamental aspects of nursing such as caring, education, patient advocacy, and prevention can all be applied to the disaster model.

Planning

Nurses must be part of the emergency and disaster plans within the community and workplace. They should be an integral component of the planning, training, and execution of disaster plans. Nurses are generally adept at defining and describing surge capacity and what resources are available during such

Figure 14-2: Modified Simple Triage and Rapid Treatment (START) Method

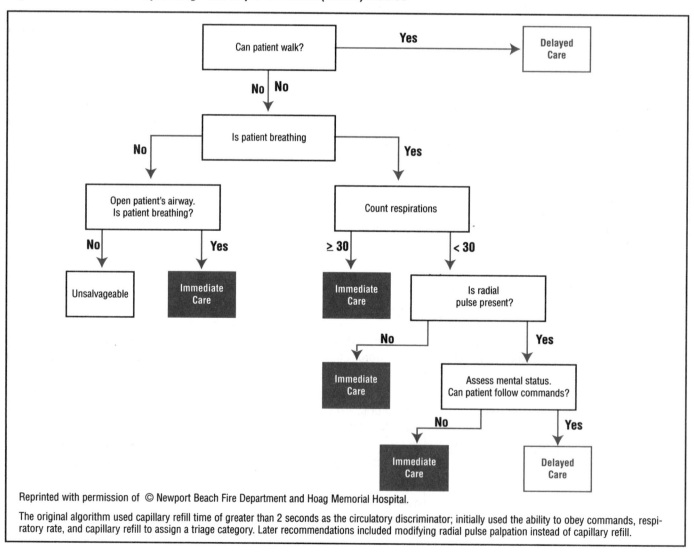

Reprinted with permission of © Newport Beach Fire Department and Hoag Memorial Hospital.

The original algorithm used capillary refill time of greater than 2 seconds as the circulatory discriminator; initially used the ability to obey commands, respiratory rate, and capillary refill to assign a triage category. Later recommendations included modifying radial pulse palpation instead of capillary refill.

an event. It is crucial that emergency nurses become aware of the disaster plan of the facility and the community in which they practice.

Clinical Skills/Tasks

After a disaster, emergency and critical care nurses may be assigned to out-of-hospital locations to serve as triage officers, first responders, or care providers under extreme conditions. Within the hospital, the loss of power, equipment, and/or personnel may cause a significant strain on resources, both human and system. Daily nursing care of inpatients may require reprioritization. Nurses must be able to perform all the ordinary aspects of their nursing jobs, including proper first aid, basic airway management, and use of ventilators.

Triage Principles

The word *triage* comes from the French word *trier*, which means "to sort." The primary goals of triage are

- Rapid assessment of patients who present for emergency care
- Determination of the severity of illness or injury and the corresponding need for emergency care

The four components that compose the framework for any triage system are

- Across-the-room assessment
- Subjective assessment
- Objective assessment
- Triage decision

The across-the-room assessment precedes the other components. It involves a quick, visual overview of the patient's general appearance, airway, breathing, circulation, and disability (brief neurologic assessment). Subjective and objective assessments follow.

The triage decision is based on analyzing the data collected and determining the most appropriate plan of care for the patient. The patient is classified into an acuity level based on the triage system being utilized.

It is important to recognize that the principles of triage remain the same whether there are one or many patients; however, the method of triage may change. Currently, triage is divided into two categories: nondisaster and multicasualty/disaster.

The purpose of nondisaster triage is to provide the best care for each patient. There are a number of hospital-based, nondisaster triage classification methods, including three-level, four-level, and five-level systems.

The purpose of multicasualty/disaster triage differs from nondisaster triage as available resources are

allocated to benefit the greatest number of patients. A number of different methods have evolved to direct triage during a mass casualty incident. Both colors and familiar terms have been used to categorize patients (Tables 14-18 and 14-19). The Simple Triage and Rapid Treatment (START) method has been used in several disaster settings (Figure 14-2). Nurses must be familiar with the disaster triage methods used in their communities or region. Some states are attempting to standardize the method of disaster triage used for the entire state. This is particularly beneficial for communication and access to available resources during a disaster.

Once a patient is triaged, determination of definitive care is made. During routine emergency department operations, this may be in an "acute" treatment area, "nonacute" treatment area, or minor

Table 14-18: Color-coded Disaster Triage Categories

Category	Definitions
Emergent (Red)	• Life-threatening injuries • Often an airway or surgical issue that can be corrected in the emergency department
Urgent (Yellow)	• Major illness or injury that requires treatment within 30 to 60 minutes such as open fractures
Non-urgent (Green)	• Walking wounded • Can self-treat
Expectant (Black)	• Dead or expected to die; full arrest, massive full-thickness burns.

Table 14-19: M.A.S.S. Triage and ID-ME! System

M.A.S.S. Triage

M = **M**ove

A = **A**ssess

S = **S**ort

S = **S**end

ID-ME!

I = **I**mmediate

D = **D**elayed

M = **M**inimal

E = **E**xpectant

Courtesy of Dallas, C. E., Coule, P. L., James, J. J., Lillibridge, S., Pepe, P. E., Schwartz, R. B., et al. (Eds.). (2004). Basic disaster life support provider manual, v 2.5. Chicago: American Medical Association.

care area. In multicasualty/disasters, definitive treatment may occur in a variety of locations including trauma centers, community hospitals, urgent care centers, and public health clinics.

Summary

Disaster management is a complex and multifaceted process that requires a great deal of advance preparation, training, and a systems-level view of the community, hospital, and staff. It is a dynamic process that involves input and participation from local, state, and federal components. A wide variety of nursing functions and roles are performed during a disaster. Nurses are an integral part of the planning, implementation, and response to disasters, whether natural or man-made, and must be aware of the various roles and responsibilities that are common to disaster planning. For further reading refer to the references for this chapter.

References

1. *The American Heritage Dictionary of the English Language: Fourth Edition.* (2000). Disaster definition. Retrieved November 6, 2006, from http://www.bartleby.com/61/19/D0251900

2. American College of Surgeons Committee on Trauma. (2003, November 1). Position statement on disaster and mass casualty management. *Journal of the American College of Surgeons, 197*(5), 855–856.

3. Guha-Sapir, D., Hargitt, D., & Hoyois, D. (2004). *Thirty years of natural disasters 1974–2003: The numbers.* Retrieved August 7, 2006, from http://www.em-dat.net/documents/Publication/publication_2004_emdat.pdf

4. Zipperer, M. (2005). Post-tsunami Banda Aceh-on the road to recovery. *The Lancet Infectious Diseases, 5*(3), 134.

5. Lovejoy, J. C. (2002). Initial approach to patient management after large-scale disasters. *Clinical Pediatric Emergency Medicine, 3,* 217–223.

6. Emergency Nurses Association. (2000). *Emergency nursing core curriculum* (5th ed., pp. 695–719). Philadelphia: W. B. Saunders.

7. Kaji, A. H., & Waeckerle, J. F. (2003). Disaster medicine and the emergency medicine resident. *Annals of Emergency Medicine, 41*(6), 865–870.

8. Federal Emergency Management Agency (FEMA). (2006). *Earthquake.* Retrieved November 6, 2006, from http://www.fema.gov/hazard/earthquake/usquakes.shtm

9. Federal Emergency Management Agency (FEMA). (2006). *Hurricane.* Retrieved August 8, 2006, from http://www.fema.gov/hazard/hurricane/

10. Centers for Disease Control and Prevention (CDC). (2004, September 17). Preliminary medical examiner reports of mortality associated with Hurricane Charley—Florida, 2004. *Morbidity and Morality Weekly Report, 53*(36), 835–837. Retrieved August 8, 2006, from http://www.cdc.gov/mmwr/preview/mmwrhtml/mm5336a1.htm

11. Federal Emergency Management Agency (FEMA). (2006). *Tornado.* Retrieved August 8, 2006, from http://www.fema.gov/hazard/tornado/index.shtm

12. The National Flood Insurance Program. (2006). *What is a flood?* Retrieved August 8, 2006, from http://www.floodsmart.gov/floodsmart/pages/whatflood.jsp

13. U.S. Fire Administration. (2004). *Fire in the United States 1992–2001* (13th ed.). Emmitsburg, MD: Author.

14. Centers for Disease Control and Prevention (CDC). (1999, February 5). Surveillance of morbidity during wildfires—Central Florida. *Morbidity and Morality Weekly Report, 48*(04), 78–79. Retrieved August 8, 2006, from http://www.cdc.gov/mmwr/preview/mmwrhtml/00056377.htm

15. Gum, R. M., & Hoyle, J. D. (2006). *CBRNE—Chemical warfare mass casualty management.* Retrieved August 8, 2006, from http://www.emedicine.com/emerg/topic895.htm

16. Agency for Toxic Substances and Disease Registry. (2006). *Medical management guidelines (MMGs) for nerve agents: Tabun (GA); sarin (GB); soman (GD); and VX.* Retrieved August 8, 2006, from http://www.atsdr.cdc.gov/MHMI/mmg166.html

17. Centers for Disease Control and Prevention (CDC). (2005). *Case definition: Vesicant (mustards, dimethyl sulfate, and lewisite).* Retrieved August 8, 2006, from http://www.bt.cdc.gov/agent/vesicants/casedef.asp

18. Takafuji, E. T., & Kok, A. B. (1997). The chemical warfare threat and the military healthcare provider. In F. R. Sidell, E. T. Takafuji, & D. R. Franz (Eds.). *Textbook of military medicine: Medical aspects of chemical and biological warfare.* Washington, DC: Office of the Surgeon General.

19. Centers for Disease Control and Prevention (CDC). (2002). *Emergency response card: Information for first responders—Blister agent: Lewisite.* Retrieved August 8, 2006, from http://www.bt.cdc.gov/agent/lewisite/ctc0020.asp

20. Centers for Disease Control and Prevention (CDC). (2005). *Choking/lung/pulmonary agents.* Retrieved August 10, 2006, from http://bt.cdc.gov/agent/agentlistchem-category.asp

21. Schraga, E. D., & Pennardt, A. (2006). *CBRNE—Cyanides, hydrogen.* Retrieved August 8, 2006, from http://www.emedicine.com /EMERG/topic909.htm

22. Centers for Disease Control and Prevention (CDC). (n.d.). *Bioterrorism Agents/Diseases.* Retrieved August 10, 2006, from http://www.bt.cdc.gov/agent/agentlist-category.asp

23. Centers for Disease Control and Prevention (CDC). (2001). Recognition of illness associated with the intentional release of a biologic agent. *Morbidity and Morality Weekly Report, 50*(41), 893–897. Retrieved August 8, 2006, from http://www.cdc.gov/mmwr/preview/mmwrhtml/mm5041a2.htm

24. Lazarus, A. A., & Decker, C. F. (2004). Plague. *Respiratory Care Clinics of North America, 10*(1), 83–98.

25. Bozeman, W. P., Dibero, D., & Schauben, J. L. (2002). Biologic and chemical weapons of mass destruction. *Emergency Medicine Clinics of North America, 20*(4), 975–993, xii.

26. World Health Organization. (n.d.). Smallpox. Retrieved August 8, 2006, from http://www.who.int/mediacentre/factsheets/smallpox/en/

27. Spivak, L., & Hendrickson, R. G. (2005). Ricin. *Critical Care Clinics, 21,* 815–824.

28. Horowitz, B. Z. (2005). Botulinum toxin. *Critical Care Clinics, 21*(4), 825–839, viii.

29. Leikin, J. B., McFee, R. B., Walter, F. G., & Edsall, K. (2003). A primer for nuclear terrorism. *Disease-a-Month, 49*(8), 485-516.

30. Stone, H. B., Coleman, C. N., Anscher, M. S., & McBride, W. H. (2003). Effects of radiation on normal tissue: Consequences and mechanisms. *The Lancet Oncology, 4*(9), 529–536.

31. American Medical Association (AMA). (2004). *Core disaster life support provider manual, v. 2.0.* Chicago: Author.

32. Koenig, K. L., Goans, R. E., Hatchett, R. J., Mettler, F. A., Jr., Schumacher, T. A., Noji, E. K., et al. (2005). Medical treatment of radiologic casualties: Current concepts. *Annals of Emergency Medicine, 45*(6), 643–652.

33. Arnold, J. L., Halpern, P., Tsai, M. C., & Smithline, H. (2004). Mass casualty terrorist bombings: A comparison of outcomes by bombing type. *Annals of Emergency Medicine, 43*(2), 263–273.

34. Singer, P. (2005). Conventional terrorism and critical care. *Critical Care Medicine, 33*(1 Suppl.), S61–S65.

35. Nelson, T. J., Wall, D. B., Stedje-Larsen, E. T., Clark, R. T., Chambers, L. W., & Bohman, H. R. (2006). Predictors of mortality in close proximity blast injuries during operation Iraqi freedom. *Journal of the American College of Surgeons, 202*(3), 418–422.

36. Lavonas, E., & Pennardt, A. (2006). Blast injuries. Retrieved August 8, 2006, from http://www.emedicine.com/emerg/topic63.htm

37. Kluger, Y., Peleg, K., Daniel-Aharonson, L., Mayo, A., & The Israeli Trauma Group. (2004). The special injury pattern in terrorist bombings. *Journal of the American College of Surgeons, 199*(6), 875–879.

38. Centers for Disease Control and Prevention (CDC). (2006). *Explosions and blast injuries: A primer for clinicians.* Retrieved August 8, 2006, from http://www.bt.cdc.gov/masscasualties/explosions.asp

39. Benedek, D. M., Holloway, H. C., & Becker, S. M. (2002). Emergency mental health management in bioterrorism events. *Emergency Medical Clinics of North America, 20,* 393–407.

40. Dallas, C. E., Coule, P. L., James, J. J., Lillibridge, S., Pepe, P. E., Schwartz, R. B., et al. (Eds.). (2004). *Basic disaster life support provider manual, v 2.5.* Chicago: American Medical Association.

41. Schultz, C. H., Koenig, K. L., & Noji, E. K. (2002). Disaster preparedness. In J. A. Marx, R. S. Hockberger, & R. M. Walls (Eds.). *Rosen's emergency medicine: Concepts and clinical practice* (5th ed., pp. 2631–2640). St. Louis, MO: Mosby.

42. Stalnikowicz, R. & Tsafrir, A. (2002). Acute psychosocial stress and cardiovascular events. *American Journal of Emergency Medicine, 20*(5), 488–491.

43. Chi, J. S., Speakman, M. T., Poole, W. K., Kandefer, S. C., & Kloner, R. A. (2003). Hospital admissions for cardiac events in New York City after September 11, 2001. *The American Journal of Cardiology, 1,* 61–63.

44. Noji, E. K. (2005). Public health issues in disasters. *Critical Care Medicine, 33*(1 Suppl), S29–S33.

45. Orellana, C. (2005). Tackling infectious disease in the tsunami's wake. *The Lancet Infectious Diseases, 5*(2), 73.

46. Houston, M., & Hendrickson, R. G. (2005). Decontamination. *Critical Care Clinics, 21,* 653–672.

47. Garfield, R., Dresden, E., & Rafferty, A. M. (2003). Commentary: The evolving role of nurses in terrorism and war. *American Journal of Infection Control, 31*(3), 163–167.

I. Preparation

A. Allow students to become comfortable; explain that this will be an interactive discussion session without practical (hands-on) skills to practice.

II. Introduction

A. Purpose

The instructor and learners will discuss two different mass casualty scenarios and describe the appropriate management of these scenarios.

B. Format

1. Small-group format

a. Principles of triage

b. Difference between mass casualty triage and "bricks-and-mortar" (single casualty/patient) triage

c. Role-playing

III. Principles of Triage

A. General principles

1. Airway, breathing and circulation precedence

2. Humanitarian triage

3. Utilitarian triage

B. Mass casualty triage algorithms/methods

1. Color-coded triage tags

2. START

3. JumpSTART

4. MASS and ID-ME

IV. Case Scenarios

A. Triage Scenario 1

A multivehicle collision has occurred on the local interstate. Various prehospital responders are on scene. Several victims have already been flown to the local Level 1 trauma center. Five victims (from the same family) have arrived simultaneously at the ambulance bay. Prehospital report stated that the adults were unrestrained, while the pediatric patients were restrained in the back seat of a minivan that rear-ended another vehicle at highway speeds and was then rear-ended by another vehicle. There is one resuscitation bed available.

Once the participant has identified the problem(s) there should be discussion and a decision over the order in which patients should be treated.

Patient A: An obese 38-year-old female complaining of shortness of breath; obvious upper thigh deformity. She is asking repeatedly about her children and her mother-in-law.

Patient B: A minimally responsive, pale 40-year-old male with shallow respirations, bleeding from mouth; nasal airway in place.

Patient C: An unresponsive elderly patient that is properly immobilized on a backboard with bag-mask ventilation occurring. Large open scalp wound with a lot of blood on backboard.

Patient D: A 14-year-old female properly immobilized on a backboard; screaming hysterically "My back, my back, please help me."

Patient E: An 8-year-old male in a cervical collar and properly immobilized on a long backboard who is quietly crying; bloody gauze to left forehead.

1. Place patients in the order of priority for additional treatment and/or interventions:

Patient A _____

Patient B _____

Patient C _____

Patient D _____

Patient E _____

2. Provide a justification/rationale for the decision made in #1.

Patient A _____

Patient B _____

Patient C _____

Patient D _____

Patient E _____

3. Describe potential interventions for the patients.

B. Triage Scenario 2

An explosion has occurred at a local factory. The on-scene commander reports approximately 25 patients with several fatalities. You are the triage nurse at the nearest hospital that is accepting the first five casualties. Decontamination has been completed on scene. Several of the patients had to be extricated from the rubble after the explosion.

Once the participant has identified the problem(s) there should be discussion and a decision over the order that patients should be treated in.

Patient A: 44-year-old unresponsive male. CPR is in progress and there is an endotracheal tube in place.

Patient B: 38-year-old male, moaning; his left hand is splinted against his chest with a bloody dressing. He arrives on a gurney in high-Fowler's position with a large-caliber IV infusing a crystalloid solution. There is also bleeding from the ears.

Patient C: 40-year-old male who is screaming; he is immobilized on a long back board with a cervical collar and nonrebreather face mask; obvious partial and full-thickness burns to torso, upper extremities. There is a large-caliber IV infusing a crystalloid solution.

Patient D: 26-year-old female, high-Fowler's position on a gurney; crying silently, holding her lower extremity with a penetrating foreign body noted to her lower leg, distal pulses intact.

Patient E: 28-year-old male restrained on a long backboard with a rigid cervical collar; multiple abrasions noted to his face, upper extremities. He has bleeding from his ears.

1. Place patients in the order of priority for additional treatment and/or interventions:

   Patient A _____

   Patient B _____

   Patient C _____

   Patient D _____

   Patient E _____

2. Provide a justification/rationale for the decision made in #1.

   Patient A _____

   Patient B _____

   Patient C _____

   Patient D _____

   Patient E _____

3. Describe potential interventions for the patients.

References

1. Dara, S. I. (2005). Worldwide disaster medical response: An historical perspective. *Critical Care Medicine 33*(1 Suppl), S2–S6.

2. Army Medical Department Center and School, Borden Institute. (2004). *Emergency war surgery* (3rd ed., Chapter 3, Triage). Winnetka, IL: Brookside Associates.

3. Agency for Healthcare Research and Quality (AHRQ) and the Office of the Assistant Secretary for Public Health Emergency Preparedness, U.S. Department of Health and Human Services (HHS). (2006). *Bioterrorism and other public health emergencies: Altered standards of care in mass casualty events*. Retrieved from http://www.ahrq.gov/research/altstand/

Chapter 15

Psychosocial Aspects of Trauma Care

Objectives

On completion of this chapter/lecture, the learner should be able to:

1. Define stress, crisis, and grief.

2. Define three specific psychosocial needs of a trauma patient and the patient's family.

3. Identify two ethical issues that affect the care of the trauma patient.

4. Discuss the psychosocial assessment of a trauma patient and/or family experiencing crisis and/or grief.

5. Plan appropriate interventions for a trauma patient and/ or family experiencing crisis and grief.

6. Define a critical incident.

7. Discuss the assessment of trauma team members experiencing a reaction to a critical incident.

8. Plan appropriate interventions for trauma team members experiencing a reaction to a critical incident.

Introduction

Injury often occurs without warning and results in changes to the lives of patients, their families, and their friends. "Family" defines an individual's support system and may include, but is not limited to, relatives, friends, and significant others. Frequently, the coping methods people use on a daily basis do not enable them to handle the intense emotional, physical, social, and spiritual needs produced by a trauma event. Understanding the concepts of stress, crisis, and grief will assist the emergency nurse in caring for the trauma patient and family.

Ethical issues also may need to be considered when caring for the injured patient. These include the futile resuscitation of a critically injured patient and end-of-life care. Studies have shown that 10% to 15% of injured patients will die of their injuries. In addition, persons older than 65 years of age are the fastest-growing age group that has injuries. Because of these issues, palliative care must now become an important concept in trauma management.[1]

Stress

Stress is "the body's arousal response to any demand, change, or perceived threat. A stressor is the circumstance or event that elicits this response."[2] The definition of stress suggests "a relationship between an individual and their environment that is perceived by the person as taxing or exceeding their resources and therefore endangering his or her well-being."[3] However, "stress is an essential component of life, and need not always have negative connotations. The negative aspect of stress could, perhaps, be more accurately described as distress."[4]

Stress may contribute to health by providing an individual with a challenge for personal growth. Conversely, stress may be harmful when the response leads to functional problems. Whether a particular event or circumstance leads to harmful stress depends on the individual's perception of the stressor.[5] The response to stress has been described biologically as a general adaptation syndrome with three stages: the alarm reaction, the stage of resistance, and the stage of exhaustion.[5] Adaptation, or the healthy response to stress, prevents advancing to stage III, which is only initiated by a serious threat.[6]

Crisis

Crisis is not synonymous with stress. A crisis is a sudden unexpected threat to, or loss of, basic resources or life goals. These situations are often new to individuals, and they find that their usual coping methods are ineffective and that immediate interventions are required. It is not the event(s) that constitute the crisis, but how the person perceives the event(s). The person in crisis perceives a loss of control and feelings of helplessness and is usually more vulnerable and open to assistance than he or she was previously.

People who have experienced previous crises may be able to cope with less intervention because of behaviors learned and used in the past. In addition to being stressful, a crisis is an opportunity to strengthen positive coping mechanisms and even to develop new strategies.[7] However, these strategies cannot be sustained for long periods of time because of the intense feelings of distress and disorder.[5]

Crisis may occur at any time, depending on a person's perception of the event. Trauma patients and their families may experience crisis when usual methods of coping and problem solving are either unavailable or inadequate to resolve the situation. Other potential factors contributing to a crisis situation are the overwhelming stimuli of the event and the personal experiences and perceptions brought by each individual person. Crisis can lead to intense periods of psychological, behavioral, and physical disarray.[5]

Crisis may occur
- Immediately after the injury

  The patient may be concerned for his or her life or the potential death of others involved in the incident. A lack of information or inappropriate perception of information may produce crisis.

- When usual methods of coping and problem solving are unavailable or inadequate to resolve the situation

  This is of particular significance if the patient or family is from out of town, is alone, or has no previous experience with such events.

- As time passes

  Pain and discomfort increase, and physical and mental energy are depleted.

Additionally, crisis states tend to have the following characteristics:
- Sudden onset (no warning for most trauma events)
- A nonspecific response that varies from individual to individual
- Short-lived and self-limiting status (a period of vulnerability is amenable to interventions, and acute escalation of crisis can be prevented)
- An opportunity to increase emotional strength when the crisis has been successfully resolved[7]
- The potential to produce dangerous, self-destructive, or socially unacceptable behaviors if not resolved

Concepts of Psychosocial Needs

The psychosocial needs of trauma patients and their families are centered on three concepts:
- Need for information
- Need for compassionate care
- Maintenance of hope

Providing accurate and understandable information to the patient and family in a timely and frequent manner is essential. When information is not provided, the patient and family may have inaccurate perceptions. The family will benefit from seeing the patient in the treatment environment as soon as possible.

Patients and families need to feel that care is being rendered in a compassionate manner. Touch, tone of voice, personal reference to the patient by name, words, and behaviors of the nurse contribute to this perception. In addition, some people attribute the nurse's presence, the amount of information provided, and the amount of time spent with the patient as indicators of caring.[8,9]

Pain control is another indicator of caring; suffering in others is distressing not only to the family but also to caregivers. Families often believe that a nurse who is gentle and caring with them will also show similar behaviors to the patient.[8,9]

No matter how critical the situation, the patient and family need to maintain a sense of hope. Hope may be for recovery, for the individual as a spiritual and physical whole, or for an afterlife. The nurse should allow the patient or the family (or both) to realistically hold on to hope. Hope may be the only positive emotion they feel while listening to discouraging and frightening facts.[8,10]

Ethical Issues in Trauma Care

The evolution of trauma care has caused those who provide care to focus on the quality of life that many patients may experience after resuscitation. Early access to the emergency medical services system, trauma centers, and advanced critical care units have allowed resuscitation of critically injured patients who may not have survived in the past. As pointed out earlier, a certain percentage of patients will not survive despite aggressive care, and a growing number of persons older than 65 with preexisting health problems are increasingly being injured.

Because traumatic injury is usually sudden, advanced care planning related to whether a patient would like to be resuscitated is generally not considered unless do-not-resuscitate documents are available at the scene or in the emergency department (ED).

This is usually not the case. Most states and hospitals do not have guidelines related to futile resuscitation. However, it is important to evaluate the end points of resuscitation in fairness to the patient, family, and staff caring for the patient.[11] These types of decisions should be determined long before the trauma team is faced with making a decision during a patient resuscitation.

The concept of palliative care is now being considered in trauma care. The philosophy of palliative care includes[12]

- Providing relief from pain and suffering
- Identifying death as a normal and natural part of life
- Recognizing that the dying process is individualized and should occur within the dynamics of the family
- Enhancing the quality of life and integrating the physical, psychological, social, and spiritual aspects of care

- Providing interventions that affirm life and neither hasten nor postpone death

Palliative care is a different and difficult philosophy for those involved in trauma care in both the field and the emergency department However, trauma patients should be allowed the same compassionate care as others who have approached the end of life through a chronic or incurable illness.

Nursing Care of an Individual Experiencing a Crisis

Assessment

History

Refer to Chapter 3, Initial Assessment, for a description of general information that should be collected regarding every trauma patient. Only pertinent questions specific to psychosocial alterations are described following.

After physiologic stability is ensured, the following additional information should be obtained from the patient or family, if possible:

- What is the patient's perception of the precipitating event or present situation?

  Ask the patient to recount the event and the present situation. Has anything else happened in the recent past to trigger this crisis? The injury may have been triggered by another event (e.g., a recent job loss, a change in marital status, a quarrel, or financial stress). Determine stressors or critical incidents that may have preceded the present situation.

- Is there a concurrent maturational crisis (e.g., birth, marriage, separation, death, retirement)?[6]

- What was the patient's previous level of functioning and ability to solve problems?

  Has anything like this ever happened before, and if so, what happened? How did the patient respond in handling the situation? Determine problem-solving or coping strategies used previously.

- Is there any recent, actual or perceived, loss or change in body appearance?

- Are there any persistent stressors (e.g., frequent injuries, chronic illness, or change in job or family status)?

Physical Assessment

Conduct a cursory mental status examination to initially rule out psychiatric disturbances, if indicated. If the patient shows a need for definitive psychiatric care, especially after crisis intervention steps have been taken, obtain a psychiatric consultation. Always rule out organic causes of psychological disequilibrium.

The physical signs often seen as an emotional response to trauma can range from anxiety to withdrawal (Box 15-1). Patients with ongoing ineffective coping will exhibit additional findings (Box 15-2).

Planning and Implementation

Refer to Chapter 3, Initial Assessment, for a description of the specific nursing interventions for patients with compromises to airway, breathing, circulation, and disability.

Crisis intervention requires immediate help for people to reestablish some balance to their life or equilibrium. It is short term and focuses on solving immediate problems to restore the previous level of functioning. The long-term goal is functional equilib-

---

Box 15-1: Physical Signs of Emotional Response

- Talks fast, loudly, profanely
- Paces; is demanding or restless
- Avoids eye contact
- Is withdrawn, isolates self
- Denies obvious injury or emotions
- Is overly compliant or noncompliant with instructions
- Has tachycardia, sweaty palms, dry mouth, and/or hyperventilation because of sympathetic nervous system activation
- Shows helplessness
- Cannot identify resources and solutions. Cannot state how to notify spouse, family, or friends about the incident. May not be able to make necessary arrangements for transportation, child, or elder care, if needed.
- Has a diminished ability to solve problems (e.g., states, "I don't know what to do about the baby-sitter at home or the children, or informing my workplace.").
- Shows increased frustration, decreased coping and decision-making ability. Says, "I can't make these decisions, stop asking me."
- Expresses negative feelings about self
- Feels responsibility for negative things happening. Says, "I can't do anything right."
- Shows self-destructive behavior. This is a higher risk if the patient has a history of suicidal behavior or recent suicidal thoughts.

Box 15-2: Additional Findings of Ineffective Coping

- Lack of concern about appearance
- Lack of concern about dried blood, dirt on uninjured parts of body, or the need for privacy or modesty
- Behavior changes
- Altered mood or affect, flat affect, denies obvious pain, tense and rigid, compulsive, agitated, or restless after pain medications
- Garbled or irrational thought pattern
- Diminished impulse control (e.g., pulls out intravenous catheters, shows aggressive or assaultive behavior)

Box 15-3: Crisis Intervention Strategies for Trauma Patients

- Encourage coping skills used successfully in the past but not being used now (e.g., allow individual to cry, use the phone to call for help, use healthy denial, and provide the opportunity to talk or remain quiet).[7]
- Identify friends or relatives who can provide support.[7]
- Encourage the patient to express feelings that may decrease tension, explore new coping mechanisms, and re-establish social interactions.[7]
- Clarify any misconceptions the patient or family may perceive.[7]
- Do not discourage expressions of anger.[7]
- Actively listen and provide opportunities for verbalization and privacy.
- Establish a trusting relationship.
- Promote the patient's sense of self-esteem.
- Give the patient as many choices as possible (e.g., what name to be called, choice of positioning, when to see family).
- Structure the environment.
  - Set approximate time frames. Give patient instructions on how to comply with recommendations and what to report to nurse (e.g., an increased level of pain).
- Explain procedures and the diagnosis in clear and understandable language.
- Give realistic information without taking away hope.
- Identify the most pressing psychosocial needs in collaboration with the patient.
- Assist in establishing realistic short-term goals.
  - It may be necessary to frequently repeat information, explanations, and encouragement because the patient's attention span may be short and recollection of information may be limited.
- Assist the patient in establishing an actual plan for coping or resolving the crisis.[7]
- Facilitate implementation of the plan.
  - Give positive feedback for compliance with the plan.

TNCC Sixth Edition

rium higher than the pre-crisis level.[13] **Box 15-3** lists several crisis intervention strategies for patients, and **Boxes 15-4** and **15-5** identify several strategies for families of trauma patients.

Family Presence During Resuscitation

The issue of family presence during active resuscitation has long been contentious. A British study concluded that families excluded from the resuscitation room had more psychological problems during bereavement than those allowed to witness an unsuccessful resuscitation.[14]

Research has found that family members of critically ill or injured patients feel that the most important needs of the patient are for the family to[15-17]

- Be with the patient.
- Be helpful to the patient.
- Be informed of the patient's condition, including if the patient is going to die.
- Be comforted and supported by their family members.

Box 15-4: Crisis Intervention Strategies for Families of Trauma Patients Before Hospital Arrival

Notify the family.

- If the family was present at the scene, the police may have already given them some information and transported them to the hospital. Generally, it is not appropriate to notify the family over the phone that the patient has died unless the family has to travel a long distance. In this case, tell the family the exact time of death to decrease potential guilt they may feel for not being present.[10,15]

If the family is notified by telephone:

- Verify the identity and relationship of the person being notified.
- Provide clear, concise information, including a general description of the patient's condition, injuries, and hopeful findings (e.g., "He is able to move both arms and legs; the patient is alert").
- Provide the hospital name, address, phone number, and directions.
- Obtain unknown patient information (e.g., allergies, immunization status, current medications, and medical history). Providing this information might make the family feel more useful and alleviate some of the feelings of helplessness.
- Before ending the conversation, ask if there are any questions and determine the relative's understanding of the patient's condition. Provide directions to the hospital, and confirm transportation plans to the hospital.[18]

- Be accepted, comforted, and supported by health care personnel.
- Feel that the patient is receiving the best possible care.

The notion of allowing family members to make an informed decision to witness resuscitation still leaves many health care professionals with feelings of trepidation. Pre-established institutional protocols or guidelines will ensure a consistent practice that facilitates the decision to allow family presence and precludes individual preference by various members of the trauma team.

The Emergency Nurses Association supports the option of family presence during resuscitation efforts.[18] Ultimately, the patient and family members are the individuals who have the most vested interests in the outcomes of invasive procedures and resuscitation. Therefore, these individuals in collaboration with health care providers should make the decision regarding family presence.[18]

A mounting body of evidence not only identifies the benefits for families to witness resuscitation but also suggests they have every right to do so. Families who witness resuscitation are reported to have fewer symptoms of grief and distress during the first 6 months after their bereavement.[14]

If family-based holistic care for patients and families is the goal, it is time to be open and honest about the activities of the resuscitation room.[18] A summary of how to implement family presence during resuscitation is presented in **Box 15-6**.[19,20]

Nursing Care of Families Experiencing Grief

Grief

Grief is the physical, emotional, spiritual, cognitive, social, and behavioral response to loss. It is often precipitated by the death of someone close, but it can also be caused by loss of function or change in body image. Various theoretical models have proposed that responses to loss include the following stages: grieving (shock, disbelief, anger, protest); mourning (depression, isolation, sadness, frustration); and bereavement (awareness and acceptance).[21] The final adaptation to loss is restitution, whereby the individual renews and invests in new relationships.[21] Although the stages appear to be sequential, few people pass through them in an orderly fashion. Grief reactions related to injury and loss are experienced not only by patients and families but also by the trauma team members.

Physical Assessment

People who are grieving may have a variety of reactions. Patient and family reactions should be supported and not thwarted. Usually these reactions help to begin the grieving process. The family's reactions may include[22]

- Shock or disbelief
- Denial
- Anger
- Hostility
- Physical complaints
- Guilt
- Panic

Box 15-5: Crisis Interventions Strategies for Families of Trauma Patients After Arrival at the Hospital

- Have a health care team member meet the family.
- Determine whether any family member wishes to be present in the resuscitation area, based on institutional protocols.[18]
- Take other family members to a private place.[14]
- Identify each family member and his or her relationship to the patient, and then refer to patient and family by name.
- Sit comfortably next to the closest relative and make eye contact. Touching may or may not be appropriate.
- Speak in quiet soothing tones.
- Introduce yourself and describe the role of other trauma team members.
- Determine what information is already known. Verify and provide an update on the patient's condition, including diagnostic and therapeutic interventions.
- Describe what the patient will look like when the family enters the room.
- Allow periods of silence to give the family time to grasp information.
- Encourage the family to express their feelings; do not discourage crying.
- Assure the family that someone is currently with the patient and is providing care.
- Give the family a realistic time as to when they can expect more information and from whom.
- Ask if there are any more questions and provide short, clear, and factual answers.
- Encourage the family to visit the patient when feasible.
- Allow the family to touch and talk to the patient.
- Identify potential coping skills. If the family reports few coping skills, identify potential support systems (e.g., friends, clergy).
- Provide periodic updates regarding the patient's condition.
- Encourage the family to seek periodic fresh air and rest breaks, nutrition, and hydration to help them focus and concentrate.
- Continually assess maladaptive behaviors shown by the family.
- Seek assistance from security personnel, if necessary, to provide a safe environment.

Box 15-6: Implementing Family Presence During Resuscitation

- A support person who is a member of the trauma team discusses with the family how they would like to be involved, and whether they would like to be in the trauma room. If the family chooses not to be present during resuscitation, there is no judgment made about the decision.
- Explain that family members will be accompanied by someone specifically to care for them. Once in the resuscitation room, they will be directed to a place that is not a barrier to patient care.
- Give clear and honest explanations of what has happened in terms of the injury and warn them of what they can expect to see and hear when they enter the room, particularly the procedures they may witness. For example, the patient may be intubated and on a ventilator, which will not allow the patient to speak. Sedation and neuromuscular blocking agents may have been administered to improve oxygenation, and because of this the patient will not be able to move.
- The support person is responsible for establishing boundaries, such as limiting the number of family members that may be in the resuscitation room. All communication should go through the support person, and family members may ask questions through the support person during the resuscitation.
- Ensure that family members understand that they will be able to leave and return at any time and will always be accompanied.
- Ask the family not to interfere, for the good of the patient and their own safety. They will be allowed the opportunity to touch the patient when it is safe to do so.
- Explain procedures as they occur in terms the family can understand. Ultimately, this may mean explaining that the patient has failed to respond, that resuscitation has been discontinued, and that the patient has died. This discussion should include the attending physician(s).
- Advise that once the patient has died, there will be a brief interval while the equipment is removed, after which they can return to be with the deceased in private.
- Offer the family time to think about what has happened, and give them the opportunity to ask further questions.

Interventions

In addition to the interventions listed in Boxes 15-3 to 15-5, the following are aimed at supporting the grieving process.

- Place the family in a private but safe environment that provides an escape route for the trauma team members or a method to summon assistance if help is needed.
- Never deliver news about the patient alone.
- If there is concern about physical violence, have a security or police officer accompany the trauma team members who will be talking with the family.
- Reinforce reality (e.g., use words such as dead, death, or has died). Avoid words such as expired, passed on, or left us.[18]
- Be supportive and use silence immediately after the notification of death to allow the family to react.
- Avoid statements negating or minimizing the family's feelings and thoughts. Do not use statements such as "It was really for the best." Instead of offering solutions, simply say you are sorry.
- Do not reinforce denial.
- If a family member displays aggressive behavior, have the security or police officer remove that person from the room. Additional counseling for this person may be needed.
- Prepare the family for the condition of the room and the patient. It may not be necessary to totally clean the room before the family sees the patient.
- Allow the family to see the patient, and suggest touching and holding the patient.
- Show acceptance of the body, even if severely injured.
- Assist any family member who feels sick or is likely to faint.
- Acknowledge and respect cultural variations in the expression of grief. Outward displays of emotion and traditional beliefs surrounding death should not be discouraged.
- Provide the family with the opportunity to leave the ED when they are ready.

Organ and Tissue Donation

In 1968, the Uniform Anatomical Gift Act was passed to ensure that a national method was used to obtain organs for transplant. This law allowed individuals 18 years and older to be organ donors. Minors could be donors with parental permission. In 1986, the Omnibus Reconciliation Act encompassed legislation that required hospitals that received Medicare or Medicaid funding to (1) have written protocols for identifying potential donors and (2) make families of potential donors aware of the option of organ and tissue donation. However, individuals and families can always decline.

Despite these regulations, organ donation still remained limited. Additionally, nurses, physicians, and other health care professionals expressed discomfort about discussing organ donation with families when they were responsible for providing patient care to a family member. In 1998, the Routine Referral Law stated that all hospitals that received Medicare and Medicaid funding needed to notify their local organ procurement organizations (OPO) of every death or imminent death. Only donor network staff or specially trained individuals can now approach families of potential donors. One further act that passed in 2004, the Organ Donation and Recovery Improvement Act, provided grant monies to further increase the awareness and need for organ donation.

By statute, consent to allow organ donation if the patient's wishes are not known may be obtained from these individuals in the following order of priority:

1. Spouse
2. Adult child
3. Parent
4. Adult sibling
5. Legal guardian

Many critically injured trauma patients may be potential organ donors. It is important for the nurse and other trauma team members to keep this in mind and ensure that the appropriate persons are notified early in the provision of care.[23]

Care of Trauma Team Members

A critical incident is any situation experienced by trauma team members that causes them to feel unusually strong emotional reactions that have the potential to interfere with their ability to function. Some common examples of critical incidents that may trigger these reactions are[24]

- Any event with significant emotional power to overwhelm usual coping mechanisms
- Death of a child or a child injured by malicious or careless adults
- Patients who are relatives or friends of the trauma team member
- Events that threaten the safety or life of trauma team members
- Events that attract excessive media attention

- Incidents with unusual circumstances and/or distressing sights, sounds, or smells
- Mass casualty situations

The trauma team members may also need help in identifying potential coping skills during or after caring for trauma patients. The following may aid effective coping skills.

- Ongoing peer support and understanding.[20]
- The opportunity to discuss difficult situations.
- The choice not to participate in debriefing sessions. It can be equally as detrimental to force an individual to openly discuss a situation as it is to not provide the opportunity to express anxieties. A team member should acknowledge that it is acceptable to say, "I am able to cope with this in my own way, and I will ask for help if and when I need it."

Critical Incident Stress Management

If the situation has been a critical incident for the team or an individual team member, intervention from a critical incident stress management (CISM) team may be helpful. The CISM team usually consists of mental health professionals and peer support personnel. The primary purposes of the CISM team are to

- Prepare the staff to manage their job-related stress.
- Provide assistance for staff members who are experiencing the negative effects of stress.
- Provide education and prevention programs.

Physical Assessment

Critical incidents may produce a characteristic set of physical, cognitive, emotional, and behavioral symptoms.[24] Reactions to a critical incident may appear immediately, within a few hours or days, or several weeks or months later. Reactions may last an indefinite period of time. These reactions (**Table 15-1**) reflect a normal response to an abnormal event.

Interventions

CISM may include utilization of defusing or debriefing techniques. Defusings are gatherings after a stressful situation and are primarily informational.[25] They provide an opportunity to discuss the impact of a difficult event. Defusings are shorter, less formal, and less structured than debriefings. They allow for ventilation of feelings regarding the incident.[25]

Debriefings provide an early opportunity (within 24 to 72 hours of the incident) for the nurse to be a part of an organized debriefing group that will deal with these stress responses. The goal is to provide an opportunity for trauma team members to effectively deal with their intense emotions in a supportive environment, thus enabling them to return to a productive level of functioning. Debriefings provide staff with time to express anger, frustrations, and grief, thereby facilitating closure of the incident.[25] The following are debriefing interventions:

- Promote the ventilation of feelings.
- Provide support and reassurance.
- Mobilize resources. Additional support may be required after a debriefing.[19]
- Do not criticize anyone's performance.
- Conduct the debriefing (**Table 15-2**) with specially trained facilitators.

Table 15-1: Signs and Symptoms of Stress Caused by Critical Incidents

Physical	Cognitive	Emotional	Behavioral
• Fatigue	• Confusion	• Anxiety	• Withdrawal
• Nausea	• Intrusive images	• Guilt	• Emotional outbursts
• Muscle tremors	• Nightmares	• Grief	• Suspiciousness
• Chest pain	• Cognitive deficits in:	• Denial	• Alcohol consumption
• Dyspnea	▪ Decision making	• Fear	• Inability to rest
• Elevated blood pressure	▪ Concentration	• Uncertainty	• Pacing
• Tachycardia	▪ Memory	• Loss of emotional control	• Nonspecific somatic complaints
• Thirst	▪ Problem solving	• Depression	• Change in sexual function
• Headaches	▪ Abstract thinking	• Apprehension	• Changes in activity and speech
• Visual disturbances		• Intense anger	
• Dizziness		• Irritability	
		• Agitation	

Table 15-2: Steps in the Debriefing Process

Initial phase

People in attendance are introduced, and the rules of debriefing are discussed. Only those involved in the event are allowed to attend. Issues discussed are considered confidential.

Fact phase

Individuals involved discuss their role in the event and describe what they experienced through the senses.

Thought phase

Persons willing to speak are asked to share what they felt during the incident and how they personalized their experience.

Reaction phase

Participants describe the worst part of the incident and how they reacted. This allows a safe environment to discuss the psychologic and physiologic effects of the incident.

Symptom phase

Participants discuss any reactions to stress they have experienced since the incident. Mental health professionals determine the need for additional help for any of the group members.

Teaching phase

Team members talk about stress management strategies and methods to support one another during a crisis.

Reentry phase

Group is given an opportunity to ask any additional questions. The events of the crisis are summarized, and referrals are made for additional help, if needed.

Source: Emergency Nurses Association. (1998). Crisis intervention. In *Emergency nursing pediatric course provider manual* (pp. 341–354). Park Ridge, IL: Author.

Summary

The psychosocial aspects of trauma include, but are not limited to, stress, crisis, and grief. Sustaining an injury is a stressor not only to the patient but also to family and significant persons related to the patient. Whether a particular event or circumstance leads to stress depends on the individual's perception of the stressor. Only in rare circumstances would a patient not perceive any degree of trauma as a stressor. Adaptation is the healthy response to stress.

Ethical issues such as futility of resuscitation and integration of palliative care also provide unique challenges in the care of the trauma patient.

Relating to families of trauma patients poses additional responsibilities for the trauma nurse. There needs to be provision of personal or telephone communication in a manner that recognizes the patient's and family's needs for accurate and understandable information, compassion, care, and hope.

Interventions to reduce the effects of a crisis are aimed at restoring one's previous level of function and, in the long term, may also enhance functional equilibrium to a level higher than the pre-crisis level.

Trauma team members may perceive certain environmental events or circumstances as stressors.

Critical incident stress management is a method to assist trauma team members in coping with the effects of stress or crisis. Despite criticisms, CISM has been found to be one of the most efficacious methods available to assist all members of the trauma team with the management of the stress that can occur with the care of trauma.[25]

References

1. Mosenthal, A. C., & Murphy, P. A. (2003). Trauma care and palliative care: Time to integrate the two? *Journal of the American College of Surgeons, 197,* 509–516.

2. Landrum, P. A., Beck, K., Rawlins, R. P., & Williams, S. R. (1993). The person as a client. In R. P. Rawlins, S. R. Williams, & K. Beck (Eds.), *Mental health & psychiatric nursing: A holistic life-cycle approach* (3rd ed., p. 31). St. Louis, MO: Mosby–Year Book.

3. Townsend, M. C. (1993). *Psychiatric/mental health nursing: Concepts of care* (p. 10). Philadelphia: F. A. Davis.

4. Selye, H. (1978). *The stress of life* (2nd ed.). New York: McGraw-Hill.

5. Wright, B. (1996). *Sudden death* (2nd ed.). New York: Churchill Livingstone.

6. Townsend, M. C. (1993). *Psychiatric/mental health nursing: Concepts of care* (p. 4). Philadelphia: F. A. Davis.

7. Aguilera, D. C. (1990). *Crisis intervention theory and methodology.* St. Louis, MO: Mosby–Year Book.

8. Belinger, J. E. (1983). Coping tasks in critical care. *Dimensions of Critical Care Nursing, 2,* 80–88.

9. Brown, L. (1986). The experience of care: Patient perspectives. *Topics in Clinical Nursing, 8,* 56–62.

10. Hickey, M. (1985). What are the needs of families of critically ill patients? *Focus on Critical Care, 12,* 41–43.

11. Kinlaw, K. (2005). Ethical issues in palliative care. *Seminars in Oncology Nursing, 21,* 63–68.

12. Kuebler, K. K., Lynn, J., & Von Rohen, J. (2005). Perspectives in palliative care. *Seminars in Oncology Nursing, 21,* 2–10.

13. Williams, S. R. (1993). Crisis intervention. In R. P. Rawlins, S. R. Williams, & K. Beck (Eds.), *Mental health & psychiatric nursing: A holistic life-cycle approach* (3rd ed., pp. 542–560). St. Louis, MO: Mosby–Year Book.

14. Robinson, S. M., Mackenzie-Ross, S., Campbell Hewson, G. L., Egleston, C. V., & Prevost, A. T. (1998). Psychological effect of witnessed resuscitation on bereaved relatives. *Lancet, 352,* 614–617.

15. McLaughlan, C. (1990). Handling distressed relatives and breaking bad news. *British Medical Journal, 301,* 1145–1150.

16. McQuay, J. E. (1995). Support of families who had a loved one suffer a sudden injury, illness, or death. *Critical Care Nursing Clinics of North America, 7,* 541–547.

17. Moreland, P. (2005). Family presence during invasive procedures and resuscitation in the emergency department: A review of the literature. *Journal of Emergency Nursing, 31,* 58–72.

18. Emergency Nurses Association. (2005). *Position statement: Family presence at the bedside during invasive procedures and/or resuscitation.* Park Ridge, IL: Author.

19. Resuscitation Council UK. (1996). *Should relatives witness resuscitation?* London: Author.

20. Nibert, L. N., & Ondrejka, D. (2005). Family presence during pediatric resuscitation: An integrative review of evidence-based practice. *Journal of Pediatric Nursing 20,* 145–147.

21. Newman, A. M. (1993). Loss. In R. P. Rawlins, S. R. Williams, & K. Beck, (Eds.), *Mental health & psychiatric nursing: A holistic life-cycle approach* (3rd ed., pp. 239–256). St. Louis, MO: Mosby–Year Book.

22. Pritchett, K. T., & Lucas, P. M. (1997). Grief and loss. In B. S. Johnson (Ed.), *Adaptation and growth: Psychiatric-mental health nursing* (4th ed., pp. 199–218). Philadelphia: W. B. Saunders.

23. New York Organ Donor Network. (2005). Organ and tissue donation—legislation passed into law. Retrieved August 9, 2005, from www.nyodn.org/organ/l/legispass.html

24. Mitchell, J. T., & Bray, G. P. (1990). *Emergency services stress.* Englewood Cliffs, NJ: R. J. Brady/Prentice Hall.

25. Mitchell, A., Sakraida, T., & Kameg, K. (2003). Critical incident stress debriefing: Implications for best practice. *Disaster Management and Response, 1,* 46–51.

In addition to the nursing diagnoses outlined in Chapter 3, Initial Assessment, the following nursing diagnoses are potential problems for the patient or family with a psychosocial alteration. Once a patient has been assessed, diagnoses can be defined as either actual or risk. An actual nursing diagnosis is derived from a decision based on the patient's presenting signs and symptoms. A risk nursing diagnosis is a judgment the nurse makes based on a particular patient's risk and potential for developing certain problems.

Nursing Diagnoses	Interventions	Expected Outcomes
Anxiety (patient and family), related to • Situational crisis • Knowledge deficit • Actual or perceived threat of death • Threat to change in health status, socioeconomic status, relationships, role functioning, support systems, environment, self-concept, or interaction patterns • Loss of control • Feelings of failure • Disruptive family life • Threat to self-concept	• Encourage coping skills used successfully in the past • Identify friends or relatives who can provide support • Actively listen and provide opportunities for verbalization and privacy • Establish a trusting relationship • Promote the patient's sense of self-esteem • Give the patient as many choices as possible • Explain procedures and diagnosis in clear and understandable language • Give realistic information without taking away hope • Assist the patient in establishing an actual plan for coping • Assure the family that someone is currently with the patient providing care • Facilitate family presence • Give the family a realistic time as to when they can expect more information • Identify potential coping skills • Provide periodic updates • Encourage the family to seek periodic fresh air and rest breaks, nutrition, and hydration to help them focus and concentrate • Provide referrals to appropriate agencies: pastoral care, social services	**The patient and family will experience decreasing anxiety, as evidenced by:** • Questioning expected routines and treatments • Participating in decision making and self-care whenever possible • Relating a decrease in anxiety • Having the absence of physiologic indicators of anxiety: increased heart rate, increased respiratory rate, increased arousal

Nursing Diagnoses	Interventions	Expected Outcomes
Fear (patient and family), related to: • Actual or perceived threat of death • Separation from support systems • Unfamiliar environment • Invasive procedures and therapeutic treatments • Pain • Effects of loss of body part or function • Language barrier • Knowledge deficit	• Clarify any misconceptions • Provide referrals to appropriate agencies: pastoral care, social services • Administer analgesic medications, as prescribed • Provide comfort measures	**The patient and family will experience decreasing fear, as evidenced by:** • Showing a decrease in fear-related behavior: crying, shouting, agitated behavior, noncommunicative behavior, blank stares • Demonstrating effective use of coping mechanisms • Having facial expressions, voice tone, and body posture within normal range for patient and family • Acknowledging fear and stating they have decreasing fear • Having an absence of physiologic indicators of fear: palpitations, increased blood pressure, diaphoresis, tachycardia
Grieving, related to: • Actual or anticipated losses associated with recent injury (patient and family) • Actual or potential loss of family member	• Do not discourage expressions of anger • Assist in establishing realistic short-term goals • Encourage the family to express their feelings • Allow patient and family to grieve • Promote hope when appropriate • Provide referrals to appropriate agencies: pastoral care, social service, rehabilitation	**The patient and family will begin to manifest grieving behavior, as evidenced by:** • Expressing signs of the grieving process • Participating in decision making • Recognizing reasons for feelings • Sharing feelings of grief with significant others • Expressing feelings about loss • Seeking social support • Progressing through stages of grief • Verbalizing reality of loss • Accepting referrals, as appropriate
Violence, risk, related to: • Fear and anxiety secondary to crisis event • Concomitant substance abuse	• Structure the environment • Continually assess maladaptive behaviors • Seek assistance from security personnel, if necessary, to provide a safe environment	**The patient and family will not be violent toward persons or objects, as evidenced by:** • Displaying behavior that demonstrates increased trust of health care providers • Verbally expressing feelings of frustration • Demonstrating control of behavior with assistance from others • Having the absence of indicators of aggressive behavior: clenched fists, pacing, shouting
Knowledge deficit, related to: • Injury, procedures, equipment	• Explain procedures and equipment used in terms the patient and family can understand	**The patient and family will experience reduced knowledge deficit, as evidenced by:** • Verbalizing an understanding of procedures and equipment use • Cooperating during procedures

Chapter 16

Transition of Care for the Trauma Patient

Objectives

On completion of this chapter/lecture, the learner should be able to:

1. Describe the trauma system components related to the stabilization and transfer of critical trauma patients.

2. Identify indications for transfer of trauma patients to a designated or verified trauma center.

3. Discuss the specific interventions to stabilize the condition of trauma patients before transfer.

4. Explain the precautions to be observed during intrahospital transport of trauma patients.

5. Discuss the care required for critically injured patients who must remain in the emergency department before admission.

Introduction

Research done in the late 1970s and early 1980s reported that survival is improved if severely injured patients are cared for in trauma facilities with dedicated resources and staff to meet their special needs.[1-3] More recent studies in the United States,[4] Australia,[5] and Canada[6] continue to support this claim. In Canada, researchers demonstrated a statistically significant reduction in mortality for trauma patients transported directly from the scene to three Level 1 trauma centers compared to mortality in patients transferred from lower-level initial receiving facilities to the Level 1 trauma centers.[7] The American College of Surgeons Committee on Trauma (ACS-COT) recommends that "no longer should the trauma patient be transferred to the closest hospital, but rather to the closest appropriate hospital, preferably a designated trauma center."[8]

Trauma systems also include planning for appropriate and adequate emergency medical services (EMS) response, prehospital triage, transfer criteria, and transfer agreements between hospitals.[9] Trauma is a worldwide problem and needs to be addressed globally. The Essential Trauma Care Project, which is a combined effort of the World Health Organization and the International Association of the Surgery of Trauma and Surgical Intensive Care (IATSIC), has developed *Guidelines for Essential Trauma Care*. These guidelines are summarized in **Table 16-1**.[10]

Table 16-1: Essential Trauma Care Services

- Obstructed airways are opened and maintained before hypoxia leads to death or permanent disability.
- Impaired breathing is supported until the injured person is able to breathe adequately without assistance.
- Pneumothorax and hemothorax are promptly recognized and relieved.
- Bleeding (external or internal) is promptly stopped.
- Shock is recognized and treated with intravenous fluid replacement before irreversible consequences occur.
- The consequences of traumatic brain injury are lessened by timely decompression of space-occupying lesions and prevention of secondary brain injury.
- Intestinal and abdominal injuries are promptly recognized and repaired.
- Potentially disabling extremity injuries are corrected.
- Potentially unstable spinal cord injuries are recognized and managed appropriately, including early immobilization.
- The consequences to the individual of injuries that result in physical impairment are minimized by appropriate rehabilitation services.
- Medications for the above services and for the minimization of pain are available when needed.

Reprinted with permission from Mock, C., Lomand, J. D., Goosen, J., Joshipura, M., & Peden, M. (2004). *Guidelines for essential trauma care.* Geneva, Switzerland: World Health Organization.

To evaluate whether a facility has the necessary resources to care for a trauma patient, consider not only those resources for initial care but also those needed for subsequent hospitalization. If the initial receiving hospital does not have the necessary resources or if it takes a significant amount of time to mobilize them, resuscitation should be provided to stabilize the patient's condition and at the same time consideration given to transferring the patient to a more comprehensive facility.

The mode of transportation also has an influence on patient outcome. Research has shown that rapid, organized transport can make a difference in mortality and morbidity in the injured patient.[11-13] Air or ground transport may decrease the amount of time needed to get the patient to definitive care, depending on the location of the injured patient and the availability of resources and trained personnel. Helicopter transport is especially valuable in rural areas. Determining the best method of transport is an important component of patient management.

As the number of patients seen and cared for in the emergency department (ED) has increased and the number of nursing staff and critical care beds has decreased, many injured patients must remain in the emergency department until a bed becomes available and staff are able to provide care.[14-16] This means that emergency nurses must be able to care for patients who may require complicated ventilatory support and monitoring. It will require additional ED staff as well as increased training and a reorganization of the hospital system to move these patients as soon as possible to critical care units.

Finally, transport within the hospital from the emergency department to locations for diagnostic or other procedures and transfer to definitive-care units requires skilled team members and appropriate equipment to provide the care that patients may need when they are out of the emergency department.

Emergency Medical Treatment and Active Labor Act (EMTALA)

The Emergency Medical Treatment and Active Labor Act (EMTALA) was enacted in 1986 as part of the Consolidated Omnibus Budget Reconciliation Act (COBRA) of 1985. This act was passed in response to concerns that patients were being refused treatment or being transferred to other hospitals based on their ability to pay.[17] Any person who works in the emergency department or is involved in patient transfer and transport must be aware of the implications of EMTALA. Under the EMTALA laws and regulations, hospitals that participate in the federal Medicare programs and offer emergency services must provide all patients seeking medical care with a medical screening examination (triage is not considered a medical screening) followed by the necessary care needed to stabilize the patient's emergency condition. If the hospital does not have the capabilities to stabilize the patient's condition, or if the patient requests, an appropriate transfer should be made to a facility that can provide stabilizing treatment.[17]

Although EMTALA requirements pertain only to facilities receiving Medicare funding, they are considered the standard of care, are incorporated into interfacility transfer guidelines and principles that have been developed, and have been incorporated in both medical and nursing organizations involved in patient transport. Noncompliance with EMTALA requirements may result in civil penalties for Medicare-participating hospitals and physicians. The administrative, legal, and clinical aspects of interfacility transfer should be addressed in hospital policies and procedures as well as in written transfer agreements between facilities. The main components of an appropriate interfacility transfer should include the following:[16-19]

- A medical screening examination should be performed by an independent practitioner for patients seeking medical treatment in the emergency department.

- Necessary stabilization and resuscitation of patients with an emergency medical condition should be provided within the capacity of the transferring hospital.

- Informed consent should be obtained from the patient before the transfer. The patient (or guardian in the case of an incompetent patient) should be informed of the potential risks and benefits of transfer.

- The physician at the transferring hospital should contact the physician at the receiving facility to obtain approval to accept the transfer. The receiving hospital must have the capability to provide the level of care the patient needs.

- A report of the patient's condition, transfer arrangements, and other significant information should be provided to the appropriate nursing staff at the receiving hospital before transfer.

  - All patient care, diagnostics, laboratory results, medical records, and patient consent should be documented and accompany the patient to the receiving hospital when possible.

  - Actual and anticipated patient needs during interfacility transfer should be assessed, and transport team configuration as well as mode of transportation should be chosen by the transferring physician. These decisions should be based on factors such as patient acuity, level of care needed during transfer, weather conditions, time constraints concerning patient care, and availability of personnel and resources.

Trauma Systems

A systematic and organized approach to trauma care has proved effective in decreasing death and disability because of injury.[6,11] Established plans and protocols that ensure rapid access to care by personnel with expertise in trauma care at facilities with dedicated resources help to protect the public from premature death and disability. A trauma system addresses the continuum of care from injury prevention to acute care through rehabilitation and reintegration into society. Different states and countries may utilize trauma system guidelines developed by the ACS-COT or by other national and statewide agencies.

The ACS-COT has endorsed a trauma system as consisting of four administrative components: leadership, system development, finances, and legislation.[12] The operational components of a comprehensive trauma system are

- Medical direction
- Prevention
- Communication
- Training
- Triage
- Prehospital care
- Transportation
- Hospital care
- Public education
- Rehabilitation
- Medical evaluation

The development and legislation of a comprehensive trauma system is a major challenge for the community. To legislate trauma systems, public support and clinical expertise from health professionals are required.[12] A model plan is available to aid states in planning and implementing trauma systems.[12] This is usually the responsibility of state EMS or health agencies.

Levels of Trauma Centers

Trauma centers are distinguished from other hospitals by a strong commitment to provide 24-hour availability of dedicated resources for trauma care. Nurses, physicians, and ancillary personnel with specialized knowledge in trauma care must be immediately available. Hospital resources such as surgical services, critical care units, and diagnostic services must also be readily available.

In the United States, the ACS has designated levels of trauma care and identified characteristics that should be present for each level. For example,

- A dedicated trauma service
- A trauma director
- In-house 24-hour surgeon availability
- Emergency resuscitation equipment for patients of all ages
- Performance improvement program
- Coordination and/or participation in community prevention programs

The current challenges faced in the delivery of health care have affected and will continue to affect trauma care. Nurses who care for trauma patients need to be aware of the level of care that is available in their institution and be actively involved in evaluating it and improving it.

Interfacility Transfer

Interfacility transfer presents the challenge of maintaining quality of care with the least amount of risk to the patient. Transport is not without risk. Potential risks include

1. Changes in patient stability and acuity
2. Difficulties due to vehicle movement
3. Problems related to limited space and resources
4. Complications due to extended out-of-hospital time
5. The potential for ground or air ambulance incidents

The potential risks versus benefits must be weighed when deciding whether or how the patient should be transferred.[20,21]

Indications for Transfer

The ACS-COT has established guidelines to identify patients to be considered for early transfer[12] (**Table 16-2**). These criteria are based on specific injuries that should prompt the trauma team to consider transfer to a facility with comprehensive resources.

Protocols and Procedures

Interfacility transfer of trauma patients involves both administrative and clinical aspects. Policies, procedures, protocols, and interfacility transfer agreements must be in place and operational before

Table 16-2: Interhospital Transfer Criteria When the Patient's Needs Exceed Available Resources

Clinical Considerations

Central Nervous System
- Head injury
  - Penetrating injury or depressed skull fracture
  - Open injury with or without a cerebrospinal fluid leak
  - GCS score < 15 or neurologically abnormal
  - Lateralizing signs
- Spinal cord injury or major vertebral injury

Chest
- Widened mediastinum or signs suggesting great vessel injury
- Major chest wall injury or pulmonary contusion
- Cardiac injury
- Patient who may require prolonged ventilation

Pelvis/Abdomen
- Unstable pelvic-ring disruption
- Pelvic-ring disruption with shock and evidence of continuing hemorrhage
- Open pelvic injury
- Solid organ injury

Extremity
- Severe open fractures
- Traumatic amputation with potential for replantation
- Complex articular fractures
- Major crush injury
- Ischemia

Multisystem Injury
- Head injury with face, chest, abdominal, or pelvic injury
- Injury to more than two body regions
- Major burns or burns with associated injuries
- Multiple, proximal long-bone fractures

Comorbid factors
- Age > 55 years
- Children ≤ 5 years of age
- Cardiac or respiratory disease
- Insulin-dependent diabetes, morbid obesity
- Pregnancy
- Immunosuppression

Secondary Deterioration (Late Sequelae)
- Mechanical ventilation required
- Sepsis
- Single or multiple organ system failure (deterioration in central nervous, cardiac, pulmonary, hepatic, renal, or coagulation systems)
- Major tissue necrosis

Adapted with permission. *American College of Surgeons Committee on Trauma: Resources for Optimal Care of the Injured Patient*, in publication.

the need for transfer arises. The decision to transfer and preparation for transfer occur simultaneously during patient stabilization.

Protocols and procedures include

- The criteria to identify patients who should be transferred
- Identification of the medical authority responsible for the transfer
- Identification of facilities with specific clinical resources (e.g., burn centers, pediatric trauma centers)
- Type of available transport services
- Necessary personnel and equipment to accompany the patient
- Clinical protocols and/or standing orders for transport
- Steps to arrange transfer
- Guidelines to include the family and significant others in the transfer process
- Transfer forms and required documentation
- Identification of medical reports and clinical records that should accompany the patient
- Recommendations for handling special situations during the transport (e.g., vehicle breakdown, long detours, patient deterioration or death)

Transfer Agreements

Written transfer agreements facilitate effective communication, establish treatment protocols, and define a patient follow-up process. Transfer agreements are established between transferring and receiving facilities. Transfer agreements that outline specific treatment and transfer protocols are suggested for the following clinical categories:

- Burns
- Head injuries
- Spinal cord and vertebral column injuries
- Multiple system traumas
- Limb and digit amputations
- Children, pregnant females, elderly patients, or patients with pre-existing disease (cardiac, pulmonary, or other chronic disease)

Transferring Hospital

The transferring hospital is responsible for performing treatments and diagnostic studies requested by the receiving facility. The physician in the transferring facility is responsible for activating the transfer process by first obtaining approval from a physician willing to accept the patient at the receiving facility.[22] The transferring facility is responsible for ensuring that the appropriate personnel and equipment are available to maintain care en route.

It is important to note that if it is part of an EMS guideline that an air ambulance may be activated by an EMS agency to transport a trauma patient to an appropriate trauma center, the EMS agency may meet the helicopter and the transport team on the hospital's helipad. The hospital has no EMTALA obligation to the patient unless the hospital personnel are asked to evaluate the patient.[17-19,23]

Modes of Transportation

The transferring and receiving facilities must make a collaborative decision regarding the most appropriate transport service. When choosing between ground and air transport, consider the following factors:

- Equipment availability
- Work space
- Qualifications of transport personnel
- Weather and road conditions or obstacles
- Patient's response to mode of transport

Ground ambulances, because of their increased availability, are the most commonly used interhospital transport service. Basic life support (BLS) ambulances are typically not equipped for the complex care necessary for the severely injured trauma patient. Advanced life support (ALS) ambulances are staffed by personnel trained to perform more definitive care, such as endotracheal intubation, intravenous therapy, and drug administration. The transferring facility must send appropriate personnel with equipment to provide the patient with ALS. Most injured patients require at a minimum a registered nurse and another qualified transport team member.[20,21]

Two types of aircraft are used for air transport: helicopters and fixed-wing planes. Transport teams are composed of some combination of a pilot(s), nurse, physician, respiratory therapist, or paramedic. Helicopters can be used in most communities without a significant delay in overall transfer time. Fixed-wing aircraft may be utilized for transfer of the trauma patient when the transport distances exceed the fuel and distance range of a helicopter.

Nursing Interventions Before Interfacility Transfer

Refer to Chapter 3, Initial Assessment, for a description of the assessment and interventions for airway, breathing, circulation, and disability.

Adequate preparation of patients being transferred from one hospital to another requires that patients be in a stable condition and interventions be done to address anticipated problems en route.[14]

Interventions may include the following:

- Secure a patent airway.
- Immobilize the vertebral column.

  It is safer to transport the trauma patient with full spinal immobilization.

- Ensure adequate breathing.

  - Have a bag-mask device and a portable ventilator available. Ensure there is an adequate supply of supplemental oxygen available in the transport vehicle. It is a good idea to connect the patient to the ventilator before transport and monitor the patient's ability to tolerate the device.

  - Assist with chest tube insertion before transport, as indicated.

    Connect the chest tube to a chest drainage system or Heimlich valve. Avoid chest drainage systems that use glass bottles. Ensure that an additional suction device is available in the transport vehicle.

  - Attach a pulse oximeter.

- Ensure adequate circulation.

  - Use plastic intravenous fluid bags.

  - Ensure that additional intravenous fluids are available in the transport vehicle.

  - Connect extension sets to intravenous tubing to allow more flexibility during patient movement.

  - Consider positioning an uninflated pneumatic antishock garment under the patient. Inflate, if indicated.

- Insert an indwelling urinary catheter and attach it to a closed urinary drainage system.
- Insert a gastric tube.
- Administer methylprednisolone to a patient with a suspected spinal cord injury, as prescribed.
- Splint suspected fractures.

  Do not use air splints.

- Cover wounds with sterile dressings.

  - Do not suture superficial lacerations.

  - Cover large burns with a dry sterile sheet.

    Follow wound care as described in Chapter 12, Surface and Burn Trauma.

- Administer tetanus and antibiotic prophylaxis, as prescribed.
- Administer analgesic and antianxiety medications, as prescribed.

- Obtain the radiographic and laboratory studies outlined in Chapter 3, Initial Assessment, as time permits.
- Prepare copies of medical records, results of diagnostic studies, and radiographs.
- Obtain consent for transfer if required.

  After discussing the need for transfer with the patient and family, obtain consent for the transfer. Use clear and simple explanations to describe the need to transfer, as well as the risks.

- Complete a transfer checklist, according to institutional protocol.
- Explain to the patient special circumstances surrounding the transfer (e.g., use of a helicopter).
- Call the receiving facility and give a brief report.
- Allow the family to see the patient.

  If the patient's prognosis is poor, it may be the last time the family will see the patient alive.

- Suggest that the family stay at the referring hospital until the patient has left with the transport team for the receiving hospital.
- Provide written directions or maps to the receiving facility.

  Reinforce the need for the family and others to observe all traffic laws. Caution the family not to attempt to follow the transport vehicle.

- Provide psychosocial support to the patient and family.

Intrafacility Transport

Transport of the trauma patient out of the emergency department is inevitable. Intrafacility transport of trauma patients may occur between the following treatment areas:

- Radiology/special procedures department
- Operating suite
- Critical care unit
- Step-down unit
- Medical/surgical unit

Several factors place the patient at risk for instability during intrahospital transport:[14]

- Inadequate airway maintenance
- Dysrhythmias
- Physiologic instability
- Rapid, rough, or disorganized transport
- Inadequate monitoring or reassessment
- Long distances between treatment areas

- Discontinuance of the effects of sedation or anesthesia
- Position of the patient

Written policies and procedures usually outline the qualifications of personnel accompanying the patient during intrahospital transport, the minimal equipment needed for transport, communication protocols, and monitoring guidelines.[16]

Table 16-3 lists the minimal equipment that should accompany a patient during intrafacility transport. This equipment should be routinely checked and individualized to the types of patients who require interfacility transport.

Select the type of personnel to conduct the transport based on the patient's clinical status, distance, and destination. A registered professional nurse, with trauma care knowledge and skills, is an appropriate person to accompany all actual and potentially unstable patients during the transport. It is important to remember that documentation about patient condition and interventions should be continued until the patient arrives at the definitive unit and a report is given to the receiving nurse.

Nursing Interventions During Intrafacility Transport

Recommended nursing interventions to increase safety before intrahospital transport include the following:

- Ensure definitive airway control.
- Suction airway and endotracheal tube, as indicated.

Table 16-3: Intrafacility Transport Equipment

- Airway equipment
- Suction
- Oral airways
- Endotracheal tubes
- Laryngoscope blades and handles
- Supplies to secure the endotracheal tube
- Failed airway equipment
- Bag-mask device
- Medications for airway management
- Pain medication
- Sedation agents
- Intravenous access supplies
- Intravenous fluids
- Monitor/defibrillator
- Restraints
- Resuscitation medications

- Maintain breathing; provide assisted ventilation, as indicated.
- Ensure patency and flow rate of intravenous infusions.
- Assess neurologic status before transfer.
- Secure all monitoring devices and equipment.
- Explain the logistics of the transport to the patient and family.
- Give a report to the receiving nurse. Include the following:
  - Mechanism of injury
  - Prehospital history
  - Patient assessment and interventions
  - Results of diagnostic procedures
  - Vital signs
  - Planned interventions or procedures

Care of the Critically Injured Patient in the Emergency Department

There may be times when a critical care bed is not immediately available for an injured patient. If a patient must be cared for in the emergency department, policies and procedures should be developed that address how this might be accomplished. Additional skills may be required to manage ventilators and invasive monitors that are not routinely used in the emergency department. Recommended interventions may include the following:

- Development of specific protocols for the management of:
  - Ventilated patients
  - Invasive monitoring
- Medication administration protocols, for example:
  - Sedation and pain management of the injured patient
  - Sedation for the mechanically ventilated patient
- Procedures that should be performed in the emergency department
- Staffing needs for "boarded" patients

Summary

Stabilization, Transfer, and Transport

Most trauma patients (80%) are not critically injured; however, approximately 15% of all trauma patients are seriously injured, with another 5% being critically injured. Trauma systems that coordinate prehospital and hospital services into an integrated regional program for the optimal care of the more critically and seriously injured patients have proved to be effective in reducing mortality and morbidity.

Staff in any hospital that receives a trauma patient must decide whether to stabilize and admit the patient or stabilize and transfer the patient to a facility with more comprehensive resources. Once a decision is made to transfer a patient, the administrative policies, procedures, and protocols to facilitate the transfer must be activated. Resuscitation and stabilization of the patient are carried on simultaneously with implementing the transfer.

Predetermined protocols, written transfer agreements with tertiary facilities, and advance identification of qualified personnel for interfacility transfers will enhance the transfer process once it is initiated by the transferring physician. Intrafacility transfers require adherence to standards of care previously identified by institutional protocols and procedures.

References

1. Cales, R. H. (1984). Trauma mortality in Orange County: The effect of implementation of a regional trauma system. *Annals of Emergency Medicine, 13,* 1–10.

2. West, J. G., Trunkey, D., & Lim, R. C. (1979). Systems of trauma care: A study of two counties. *Archives of Surgery, 114,* 455–459.

3. West, J. G., Cales, R. H., & Gazzaniga, A. B. (1983). Impact of regionalization: The Orange County experience. *Archives of Surgery, 118,* 740–744.

4. Cayten, C. G., Quervalu, I., & Agarwal, N. (1999). Fatality analysis reporting system demonstrates association between trauma system initiatives and decreasing death rates. *Journal of Trauma, 46,* 751–756.

5. Cooper, D. J., McDermott, F. T., Cordner, S. M., Tremayne, A. B., & the Consultative Committee on Road Traffic Fatalities in Victoria. (1998). Quality assessment of the management of road traffic fatalities at a level 1 trauma center compared with other hospitals in Victoria, Australia. *Journal of Trauma, 45,* 772–779.

6. Sampalis, J. S., Denis, R., Lavoie, A., Frechette, P., Boukas, S., Nikolis, A., et al. (1999). Trauma care regionalization: A process-outcome evaluation. *Journal of Trauma, 46,* 565–581.

7. Sampalis, J. S., Denis, R., Frechette, P., Brown, R., Feliszer, D., & Mulder, D. (1997). Direct transport to tertiary trauma centers versus transfer from lower level facilities: Impact on mortality and morbidity among patients with major trauma. *Journal of Trauma, 46,* 288–296.

8. American College of Surgeons Committee on Trauma. (1997). Transfer to definitive care. In *Advanced trauma life support® for doctors: Instructor course manual* (6th ed., pp. 389–399). Chicago: Author.

9. Mock, C., Kobusingye, O., Joshipura, M., Nguyen, S., & Arreola-Risa, C. (2005). Strengthening trauma and critical care globally. *Current Opinion in Critical Care, 11,* 568–575.

10. Mock, C., Lomand, J. D., Goosen, J., Joshipura, M., & Peden, M. (2004). *Guidelines for essential trauma care.* Geneva, Switzerland: World Health Organization.

11. Demetriafes, D., Kimbrell, B., Salim, A., Velmahos, G., Rhee, P., Preston, C., et al. (2005). Trauma deaths in a mature urban trauma system: Is tri-modal distribution a valid concept? *Journal of American College of Surgeons, 201,* 343–348.

12. American College of Surgeons Committee on Trauma. (1998). Interhospital transfer and agreements. In *Resources for optimal care of the injured patient: 1999* (p. 21). Chicago: Author.

13. Davis, D., Peay, J., Serrano, J., Buono, C., Vilke, G., Sise, M., et al. (2005). The impact of aeromedical response to patients with moderate to severe traumatic brain injury. *Annals of Emergency Medicine, 46,* 115–122.

14. Lazear, S. E. (2003). Air and ground transport. In L. Newberry (Ed.), *Sheehy's emergency nursing principles and practice* (5th ed., pp. 98–114). St. Louis, MO: Mosby–Year Book.

15. Gavin-Fought, S., & Nemeth, L. (1992). Intrahospital transport: A framework for assessment. *Critical Care Nursing Quarterly, 15,* 87–90.

16. Warren, J., Fromm, R., Orr, R., Rotello, L., Horst, H., & American College of Critical Care Medicine. (2004). Guidelines for the inter- and intrahospital transport of critically ill patients. *Critical Care Medicine, 32,* 256–262.

17. Centers for Medicare & Medicaid Service (CMS). (2005). Emergency Medical Treatment & Active Labor Act (EMTALA) Resource. Retrieved December 17, 2005, from http://www.cms.hhs.gov/providers/emtala/default.asp

18. Department of Health and Human Services (DHHS), Centers for Medicare and Medicaid Services (CMS), 42 CRF Parts 413, 482, and 489. (2003, September 9). Medicare program: Clarifying policies related to the responsibilities of Medicare-participating hospitals in treating

individuals with emergency medical conditions. Final rule. *Federal Register.*

19. American College of Surgeons Committee on Trauma. (2002). Interfacility transfer of injured patients: Guidelines for rural communities. Retrieved December 17, 2005, from www.facs.org/trauma/publications/ruralguidelines.pdf

20. Bledsoe, B. E., & Smith, M. G. (2004). Medical helicopter accidents in the United States: A 10-year review. *Journal of Trauma, 56,* 1325–1329.

21. Commission on Accreditation of Medical Transport Systems (CAMTS). (2004). *Sixth edition accreditation standards.* Anderson, SC: Author.

22. American College of Surgeons Committee on Trauma. (1998). Interhospital transfer and agreements. In *Resources for optimal care of the injured patient: 1999* (pp. 19–22). Chicago: Author.

23. American College of Emergency Physicians (ACEP). (2004). Appropriate interhospital patient transfer. *Annals of Emergency Medicine, 43,* 685–686.

Chapter 17

Demonstration of the Trauma Nursing Process Station

Objectives

On completion of this demonstration, the learner should be able to:

1. Demonstrate a primary assessment.

2. Identify life-threatening conditions recognized during the primary assessment.

3. Identify the interventions to manage life-threatening conditions recognized during the initial assessment.

4. Demonstrate a secondary assessment.

5. Based on data from the secondary assessment, identify appropriate diagnostic studies and interventions.

Introduction

The phases of the Trauma Nursing Process are integrated into a scenario-driven psychomotor skill station in the *Trauma Nursing Core Course*.

Assessment, diagnosis, outcome identification, planning, and implementation are the first five steps in the nursing process. Evaluation, the last step, is an ongoing process once the patient arrives in the emergency department.

During actual patient care, all personnel who anticipate direct patient contact or contact with the patient's bodily fluids must wear personal protective equipment. (**Note:** Since TNCC skill stations are simulated situations, the use of personal protective equipment is optional.)

Assessment

Primary Assessment

All elements assessed during the primary assessment are of such a critical nature that major deviations from normal require immediate intervention. Do not proceed until all major life-threatening conditions have been treated. The primary assessment addresses airway (A), breathing (B), circulation (C), disability or neurologic status (D), and exposure and environmental control (E).

Secondary Assessment

The secondary assessment is completed after the primary assessment. It includes F–I as described in **Table 17-1**. The focus of the secondary assessment is to identify ALL injuries in order to determine the priorities for the planning and implementation phases of the nursing process.

During the Trauma Nursing Process skill station, learners should state they would obtain additional information from prehospital providers, patient-generated information, and past medical history, if available. The learner must demonstrate and describe the head-to-toe assessment by describing appropriate inspection techniques, (e.g., noting lacerations, abrasions, contusions, ecchymosis, etc.), demonstrating appropriate palpation techniques, and demonstrating appropriate auscultation techniques.

Analysis, Nursing Diagnoses, Expected Outcomes, Planning, and Implementation

The severity of the patient's condition may require simultaneous assessment, diagnosis, and intervention. Appropriate nursing diagnoses are based on assessment findings. Specific patient outcomes are then identified, and a plan is developed to achieve them. For the purposes of this station, the learner will NOT be asked to identify nursing diagnoses or outcomes. The priorities for intervention will depend on the complexity of the patient's injuries, and the availability and qualifications of the emergency department staff and/or trauma nurse. Priority is given to injuries that have the greatest potential to compromise airway, breathing, circulation, and/or disability.

Ongoing Evaluation

Evaluate the patient's responses to any interventions to determine the need for further interventions. Evaluate the effectiveness of any intervention expected to have an immediate effect on the patient. Any abnormalities identified in the primary assessment and the vital signs must be re-evaluated at the completion of the secondary assessment.

Evaluation

Instructors will use a form to evaluate each learner's performance during the Trauma Nursing Process Station. There are specific forms for each case scenario. The * and ** steps indicated on this form are consistent for all case scenarios. Each step counts for one point.

The single-starred (*) steps are essential skill steps. The single-starred steps must be performed during the skill station demonstration, but their sequence is not critical.

Table 17-1: Trauma Assessment Mnemonic

A =	Airway with simultaneous cervical spine stabilization and/or immobilization
B =	Breathing
C =	Circulation
D =	Disability (neurologic status)
E =	Expose patient/environmental control
F =	Full set of vital signs/focused adjuncts/facilitate family presence
G =	Give comfort measures
H =	History/Head-to-toe assessment
I =	Inspect posterior surfaces

The double-starred (**) steps must be demonstrated in order during the primary assessment. No points are granted for double-starred steps performed after the primary assessment. Failure to perform any of the double-starred steps results in unsuccessful completion of the psychomotor skill station. Learners cannot return to the primary assessment during the secondary assessment and identify double-starred steps.

The following performance information is important for successful completion of the Trauma Nursing Process skill stations:

1. Learners must demonstrate both criteria if two criteria are listed (e.g., auscultates breath sounds **AND** heart tones; inspects **AND** palpates).

2. Learners must demonstrate appropriate assessment techniques (i.e., auscultation and palpation). It is not acceptable for the learner to state, "I would palpate the abdomen," without actually touching the model. The correct method to auscultate breath sounds is dependent on whether the patient is intubated or not.

3. Learners must be specific regarding inspection and palpation (i.e., "I am inspecting and palpating for injuries.").

4. Learners must use the appropriate equipment in each station.

5. To assess airway patency in the unconscious patient, the learner should simultaneously manually open the airway using a jaw thrust or chin lift maneuver while assessing for airway patency.

6. For scenarios that include the patient arriving immobilized on a backboard with a rigid cervical collar, the learner is awarded credit for maintaining spinal protection as long as none of the immobilization devices is completely removed.

7. Learners must evaluate the effectiveness of interventions which are expected to have an immediate effect on the patient (e.g., auscultation of breath sounds after intubation).

8. In the primary assessment, observation of skin color is appropriate for assessment of breathing effectiveness and circulation. The learner only has to state the need to observe skin color once to receive credit in both steps.

9. When needle thoracentesis is indicated, the learner will describe the technique (landmarks and equipment).

10. Learners must assess the level of consciousness according to the AVPU mnemonic.

11. Learners must state the need to assess pupils (PERRL), but do not need to demonstrate the PERRL examination.

12. When learners ask for vital signs, instructors will respond with specific blood pressure, pulse, respirations, and temperature measurements.

13. To obtain the patient history, learners should obtain any one of the following: any additional information from prehospital providers, patient-generated information, or past medical history, if available.

14. Learners need not restate all of the simulated injuries identified during the assessment. Restating the injuries at the end of the assessment is the option of the instructor.

15. If a learner states any additional appropriate diagnostic studies or interventions during the primary or secondary assessments, these will count toward the total of five required for performance of the skill step.

Demonstration

Two instructors will demonstrate how to perform a trauma nursing assessment through role-play or use of the training video, and will identify examples of interventions for each step of the assessment. During the skill station rotation, learners will have the opportunity to practice these skills based on specific case scenarios. For further explanation of specific assessments and interventions, refer to each clinical chapter in the manual. The following tables serve as guidelines to conduct the assessment and identify appropriate interventions (see **Tables 17-2** to **17-4**).

During the learner's evaluation in the Trauma Nursing Process station, the learner will be asked to identify five additional diagnostic studies and/or interventions based on the case scenario. Be specific with regard to the radiographic studies.

Evaluate the effectiveness of the interventions that are expected to have an immediate effect on the patient (e.g., auscultation of breath sounds after intubation). Re-evaluate all primary assessment interventions, vital signs, and pain at the completion of the secondary assessment.

Summary

The Trauma Nursing Process is a standard of care endorsed by the American Nurses Association and the Emergency Nurses Association. The Trauma Nursing Process involves six phases: assessment, nursing diagnosis, expected outcomes, planning, implementation, and evaluation. The Trauma Nursing Process skill station is an opportunity for learners to demonstrate their knowledge and understanding of trauma nursing.

Table 17-2: Primary Assessment

Assessments	Interventions
A = Airway with simultaneous cervical spine protection (stabilization and/or immobilization) While maintaining cervical spine protection: • Vocalization • Tongue obstructing airway • Loose teeth or foreign objects • Blood, vomitus, or other secretions • Edema	• Position the patient • Jaw thrust or chin lift • Remove any foreign objects • Suction blood, vomitus, or secretions • Insert oropharyngeal or nasopharyngeal airway • Endotrachael intubation • Needle or surgical cricothyrotomy
B = Breathing • Spontaneous breathing • Rise and fall of chest • Rate and pattern of breathing • Use of accessory muscles and/or diaphragmatic breathing • Skin color • Integrity of the soft tissue and bony structures of the chest wall • Bilateral breath sounds	• Supplemental oxygen • Bag-mask ventilation • Needle thoracentesis/decompression • Chest tube • Nonporous dressing taped on three sides
C = Circulation • Palpates central pulse for rate and quality • Skin color, temperature, and moisture • External bleeding	• Direct pressure over uncontrolled bleeding sites • Insert two large-caliber intravenous catheters with warmed isotonic crystalloid solution • Infuses fluid rapidly with blood tubing • Blood sample for typing • Blood administration • Pericardiocentesis • Emergency thoracotomy • Surgery • Cardiopulmonary resuscitation and advanced life support measures
D = Disability • Level of consciousness (AVPU) • Pupils (PERRL)	• Perform further investigation • Hyperventilation, if indicated
E = Expose Patient and Environmental Control (remove clothing and keep patient warm) • Obvious wounds/deformities • Temperature control	• Remove clothing • Preserve clothing for evidence if indicated (don't cut though bullet wounds, use paper bags) • Cover with blankets • Warming lights • Increase ambient temperature

Table 17-3: Secondary Assessment

F = Full Set of Vital Signs/Focused Adjuncts/Facilitate Family Presence

- Obtain a complete set of vital signs
- Consider the focused adjuncts
  - Cardiac monitor
  - Pulse oximeter (SpO_2)
  - Urinary catheter if not contraindicated
  - Gastric tube
  - Laboratory studies
- Facilitate family presence

G = Give Comfort Measures

- Assesses pain using an appropriate pain scale
- Verbal reassurance
- Initiates a nonpharmacologic pain intervention
- Considers obtaining order for pain medication

H = History

- MIVT
- Patient-generated information
- Past medical history

H = Head-To-Toe Assessment

Head and face
- Inspect for wounds, ecchymosis, deformities, drainage from nose and ears, and checks pupils
- Palpate for tenderness, note bony crepitus, deformity

Neck
- Remove anterior portion of the rigid cervical collar to inspect and palpate the neck
- Another team member must hold the patient's head while the collar is being removed and replaced
- Inspect for wounds, ecchymosis, deformities, and distended neck veins
- Palpate for tenderness, note bony crepitus, deformity, subcutaneous emphysema, and tracheal position

Chest
- Inspect for breathing rate and depth, wounds, deformities, ecchymosis, use of accessory muscles, paradoxical movement
- Auscultate breath sounds and heart sounds
- Palpate for tenderness, note bony crepitus, subcutaneous emphysema, and deformity

Abdomen and flanks
- Inspect for wounds, distention, ecchymosis, and scars
- Auscultate for bowel sounds
- Palpate all four quadrants for tenderness, rigidity, guarding, masses, and femoral pulses

Pelvis and perineum
- Inspect for wounds, deformities, ecchymosis, priapism, blood at the urinary meatus or in the perineal area
- Palpate the pelvis and anal sphincter tone

Extremities
- Inspect for ecchymosis, movement, wounds, and deformities
- Palpate for pulses, skin temperature, sensation, tenderness, deformities, and note bony crepitus

I = Inspect Posterior Surfaces

- Maintain cervical spine protection and support injured extremities while the patient is logrolled
- Inspect the posterior surfaces for wounds, deformities, and ecchymosis
- Palpate the posterior surfaces for tenderness and deformities
- Palpate anal sphincter tone (if not performed previously)

Table 17-4: Planning and Implementation

Area	Diagnostic Studies	Interventions

General	• Laboratory studies
	  ▪ Type and screen or crossmatch
	  ▪ Hemoglobin and hematocrit
	  ▪ Blood alcohol
	  ▪ Serum lactate level
	  ▪ Serum pregnancy test as indicated
	  ▪ Kleihauer-Betke test as indicted
	• Arterial blood gases
		• Operative intervention
		• Admission or transfer
		• Glasgow Coma Scale score and Revised Trauma Score
		• Psychosocial support of patient and family
		• Pain control
		• Nonpharmacological pain intervention
		• Medications as indicated
		  ▪ Tetanus prophylaxis
		  ▪ Antibiotics
		  ▪ Pain medications
		  ▪ Neuromuscular blockers
		  ▪ Sedation

Head and face	• Plain radiographic studies • Computed tomography (CT) scan • Magnetic resonance imaging (MRI) • Angiography	• Position patient • Medications, as prescribed • Intracranial pressure monitoring • Suctioning
Neck	• Plain radiographic studies • CT scan • MRI • Angiography	• Spinal protection with vertebral column immobilization • Steroids, per institutional protocols
Chest	• Plain radiographic studies • CT scan • MRI • Arteriography or aortography • Focused assessment sonography for trauma (FAST) • Bronchoscopy • Esophagoscopy • Electrocardiogram • Hemodynamic monitoring	• Chest tube • Autotransfusion • Needle thoracentesis/decompression • Pericardiocentesis • Prepare for possible thoracotomy
Abdomen and flanks	• Plain radiographic studies • CT scan • MRI • FAST • Intravenous pyelogram (IVP) • Diagnostic peritoneal lavage (DPL) • Cystogram or urethrogram • Angiography	• Urinary catheter • Gastric tube • Consider pelvic antishock garment for intraabdominal or pelvic bleeding
Pelvis and perineum	• Plain radiographic studies • CT scan • MRI • Focused assessment sonography for trauma (FAST)	• Urinary catheter • Pneumatic antishock garment for splinting • External pelvic stabilization device

Table 17-4: Planning and Implementation (continued)

Area	Diagnostic Studies	Interventions
Extremities	• Plain radiographic studies • CT scan • MRI • Measurement of compartment pressures	• Immobilization/traction devices • Elevation • Ice
Posterior surfaces	• Plain radiographic studies • CT scan • MRI	• Spinal protection with vertebral column immobilization
Surface trauma		• Irrigation • Wound care • Ice • Care for amputated parts • Tetanus prophylaxis • Antibiotics

The skill steps to complete the Trauma Nursing Process are listed below. In the actual Trauma Nursing Process skill stations, specific case scenarios will be used. In the skill stations, an intervention may not necessarily be required for each step in the primary assessment, but will be based on the actual case scenario.

Two instructors will demonstrate, or the video will be used to demonstrate, the skill steps in the Trauma Nursing Process. The skill steps will include a demonstration of the primary and secondary assessment. Actual case scenarios are presented in each of the Trauma Nursing Process teaching and evaluation scenarios.

Prehospital MIVT Report

An ambulance is en route with a 22-year-old unhelmeted motorcyclist who struck an automobile at 45 mph (60 kph) and was thrown 20 feet (6 m) onto the road. Prehospital personnel report the patient is unresponsive with a blood pressure of 100/60 mm Hg, strong pulse of 128 beats/minute, and spontaneous respirations of 24 breaths/minute. Cervical spine protection was initiated and the patient is in complete spinal immobilization. The patient has one large-caliber intravenous catheter with isotonic crystalloid solution infusing, oxygen via nonrebreather mask is being administered, and both wrists are splinted. The patient has just arrived in the emergency department. Please proceed with your primary and secondary assessments and interventions.

Focus of this teaching station: Need for intubation, assessment of possible head and neck injury.

In the interest of model comfort and safety, assume the model is in complete spinal immobilization and that the team is adhering to Standard Precautions.

Skill Steps	Instructor Responses	Demonstrated Yes	No
1. Assesses airway patency; **AND** if unresponsive, manually opens the airway using a jaw thrust or chin lift (states at least 3 of the following): • Vocalization • Tongue obstructing airway • Loose teeth or foreign objects • Blood, vomitus, or other secretions • Edema	 • Does not vocalize • No obstruction by the tongue • No loose teeth or foreign objects present • No bleeding • No edema noted	**____	____
2. Maintains spinal immobilization.		____	____
3. Assesses breathing effectiveness (states at least 3 of the following): • Spontaneous breathing • Rise and fall of chest • Rate and pattern of breathing • Use of accessory muscles and/or diaphragmatic breathing • Skin color • Integrity of the soft tissue and bony structures of the chest wall • Bilateral breath sounds	 • Present • Bilateral and shallow • Very slow and shallow • None • Pale • No open wounds, chest wall intact • Severely diminished	**____	____
4. States need for assisted ventilation with bag-mask device.		____	____

Instructor response: *"The physician decides to intubate the patient. Intubation has just been accomplished. What is your next step?"*

Skill Steps	Instructor Responses	Demonstrated Yes	No
5. Assesses endotracheal tube placement (states at least 2 of the following):		____	____
• Observes for rise and fall of the chest with bag-valve ventilations	• Chest rises and falls		
• Auscultates over the epigastric area, **AND** then auscultates bilateral breath sounds	• No gurgling over the epigastrium; breath sounds equal bilaterally		
• Uses an exhaled CO_2 detector or esophageal detector device (EDD)	• Exhaled CO_2 detector color change confirms placement; or no resistance is felt when pulling back on syringe of EDD		
6. Palpates central pulse.	• Pulse present and rapid	** ____	____
7. Inspects **AND** palpates skin (states at least 2 of the following):			
• Color	• Pale		
• Temperature	• Cool		
• Moisture	• Dry		
8. Inspects for external bleeding.	• No uncontrolled external bleeding	** ____	____
9. Assesses patency of prehospital intravenous line.	• Intravenous line is patent	____	____
10. States need to cannulate additional vein with a large-caliber intravenous catheter	• If learner elects to obtain blood samples for typing and other lab studies, credit should be given in Facilitates lab studies.	** ____	____
11. Administers warmed, isotonic crystalloid solution with blood tubing **AND** at a rapid rate.		____	____
12. Assesses level of consciousness (AVPU).	• Now responsive to pain	** ____	____
13. Assesses pupils (PERRL).	• PERRL but sluggish • Neurological evaluation has been requested	____	____
14. Removes all clothing.		** ____	____
15. States one measure to prevent heat loss (blankets, warming lights, increase room temperature).		** ____	____

If learner did not intervene to correct life-threatening findings in the primary assessment, stop and review the purpose of the primary assessment.

Secondary Assessment			
16. States need to get a full set of vital signs.	• BP = 110/60 mm Hg • P = 100 beats/minute • R = assisted at 20 breaths/minute • T = 98 °F (36.8 °C)	____	____
17. Attaches patient to cardiac monitor.	• ECG = sinus rhythm	____	____
18. Places pulse oximeter on patient.	• SpO_2 = 98%	____	____
19. States need to consider insertion of a urinary catheter.	• No contraindications *If learner elects to insert urinary catheter here, give credit in #35 for inspecting the perineum.*	____	____
20. States need to consider insertion of a gastric tube.	• No contraindications	____	____
21. Facilitates laboratory studies, if not already done.		____	____

Skill Steps	Instructor Responses	Demonstrated Yes	No
22. Facilitates family presence per institutional protocols		____	____
23. Assesses pain using an appropriate pain scale.	• Patient responds to painful stimuli	* ____	____
24. Gives comfort measures (states at least one measure). • Verbal reassurance, touching • Initiates a nonpharmacologic pain intervention such as applying ice to swollen areas, repositioning, or padding uncomfortable areas, if not contraindicated.	• Deferred • Checked wrist splints; patient repositioned	____	____
25. Considers obtaining order for an analgesic medication.	• An appropriate dose of a narcotic analgesic has been ordered by the physician.	____	____
26. History: States the pertinent history to be obtained (states at least one of the following): • MIVT • Patient-generated information • Past medical history	• Landed on head • Not available • Not available	____	____

Demonstrates and describes the head-to-toe assessment by: describing appropriate inspection techniques (e.g., lacerations, abrasions, contusions, ecchymosis), demonstrating appropriate palpation techniques, and demonstrating appropriate auscultation techniques

Skill Steps	Instructor Responses	Demonstrated Yes	No
27. Inspects **AND** palpates head **AND** face for injuries.	• Multiple abrasions and contusions	____	____
28. Inspects **AND** palpates neck for injuries.	"I'll maintain stabilization while you assess the neck." • Step-off deformity and crepitus palpated at C4 to C6 *"I'll replace the collar."*	____	____
29. Inspects **AND** palpates chest for injuries.	• No abnormalities	____	____
30. Auscultates breath sounds **AND** heart sounds.	• Breath sounds clear and equal bilaterally • Normal heart sounds	____	____
31. Inspects the abdomen for injuries.	• No abnormalities	____	____
32. Auscultates bowel sounds.	• Bowel sounds present	____	____
33. Palpates all four quadrants of the abdomen for injuries.	• No abnormalities	____	____
34. Inspects **AND** palpates the pelvis for injuries.	• No abnormalities	____	____
35. Inspects the perineum for injuries.	• No abnormalities *If learner elects to insert urinary catheter here, give credit in #19.*	____	____
36. Inspects **AND** palpates all four extremities for neurovascular status and injuries. • Right upper extremity • Left upper extremity • Right lower extremity • Left lower extremity	• Both wrists swollen and deformed • Normal neurovascular status in all extremities	____	____
37. Describes method to maintain spinal stabilization when patient is log-rolled.		* ____	____
38. Inspects **AND** palpates posterior surfaces for injuries.	• Sphincter tone, checked by physician, is normal • No other abnormalities	____	

Skill Steps	Instructor Responses	Demonstrated Yes	No
39. Identifies all simulated injuries. • Possible head injury • Possible cervical spine injury • Possible fractured wrists	*If the learner has not mentioned all of the simulated injuries, ask him or her to identify all simulated injuries.*	* ___	___

Instructor response: *"You identified certain injuries during the assessment. Now that you have completed the secondary assessment, list 5 additional diagnostic studies or interventions for this patient."*

Note to Instructors: If the learner has previously identified any of the appropriate diagnostic studies or interventions listed, include the diagnostic study or intervention into the total of 5.

Skill Steps	Instructor Responses	Demonstrated Yes	No
40. Identifies appropriate diagnostic studies or interventions (states at least (five) 5 of the following): • Head CT scan • Cervical spine radiograph or CT scan • Chest radiograph or CT scan • Abdominal CT scan • Focused assessment sonography for trauma (FAST) exam • Pelvis radiograph • Wrist radiographs • Other • Arterial blood gases • Serum lactate level • Type and screen or crossmatch for blood • Glasgow Coma Scale score • Revised Trauma Score • Pain control • Psychosocial support • Tetanus prophylaxis • Prepare for admission, surgery, or transfer	Suggested interventions specific to this station are listed at the top in head-to-toe order. Interventions common to all TNP stations are listed at the bottom.	* ___	___

Instructor response: *"What findings need to be re-evaluated?"*

Skill Steps	Instructor Responses	Demonstrated Yes	No
41. States need to re-evaluate primary assessment.		___	___
42. States need to re-evaluate vital signs.		___	___
43. States need to re-evaluate pain.		___	___
44. States need to re-evaluate all identified injuries.		___	___

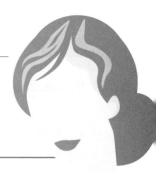

Psychomotor

Objectives

In a simulated situation with patients requiring the nursing skills associated with the trauma nursing process, airway and ventilation interventions, or spinal immobilization, the learner will be able to:

1. Identify the priorities of care for the simulated patient.

2. Correctly demonstrate the required nursing skills for the simulated patient.

3. Evaluate the patient's response to the demonstrated nursing skills.

4. The instructor will explain psychomotor skill station evaluation:

   • Double-starred (**) steps must be performed **during the primary assessment** to successfully complete the station.

   • Single-starred (*) steps are critical and must be performed **during the station.**

   • Criteria for completion: 70% of total points and completion of all * and ** steps.

   • Sample evaluation sheets: lists all * and ** steps and station requirements.

   • Principles: learners must "talk through" the cases and demonstrate skills.

   • Case progression: the instructor will provide patient information in response to the learner's demonstration.

Skill Stations

The order of the skill stations is as follows:

I. Introduction

A. Instructor and learner introductions

B. Purpose

1. Each learner will demonstrate a primary and secondary assessment and initiate appropriate interventions on a simulated patient.

C. Teaching format

1. The Demonstration of the Trauma Nursing Process Station, Chapter 17, previously provided the learner with a general discussion and demonstration of the trauma nursing assessment and interventions.

2. During the Trauma Nursing Process Skill Stations, the learners in each group will be presented specific case scenarios. Each learner will demonstrate and/or describe a trauma assessment and identify appropriate interventions following the designated case.

3. The instructor will guide learners through the scenarios, clarify questions, assist learners to perfect their skills, and will provide additional information as requested by the learner.

D. Evaluation

1. Each learner will be evaluated separately at one Trauma Nursing Process Evaluation Station. Do not attempt to memorize the specific teaching scenarios as a new scenario will be used for evaluation.

2. Certain critical steps must be identified during the primary assessment. They are marked with a double star (**) on the evaluation form.

3. Additional critical steps are marked with a single star (*) on the evaluation form. All of these steps must be demonstrated.

4. During testing, instructors cannot use prompts, but will answer specific questions and provide assessment data.

5. At least 70% of the total points must be demonstrated.

6. At the completion of the demonstration, the learner will be asked if there is anything he or she wants to add or revise. Learners may not add or revise any of the ** steps.

II. Principles of the Trauma Nursing Process

A. General principles

1. Assessment, nursing diagnosis, outcome identification, planning, and implementation are the first five steps of the nursing process. Evaluation, the last step, is an ongoing process once the patient arrives in the emergency department.

2. In actual patient care, all personnel who anticipate direct patient contact or contact with the patient's body fluids must wear personal protective equipment. (Note: Since TNCC skill stations are simulated situations, the use of personal protective equipment is optional.)

B. Primary assessment

1. All elements assessed during the primary assessment are of such a critical nature that any major deviations from normal require immediate intervention. Do not proceed until all major life-threatening conditions have been treated. The primary assessment addresses airway (A), breathing (B), circulation (C), disability, neurologic status (D), and expose patient/environmental control (E).

C. Secondary assessment

1. The secondary assessment is completed after the primary assessment. It includes F through I as described below. The focus of the secondary assessment is to identify all injuries in order to determine the priorities for the planning and intervention phases of the nursing process.

Trauma Assessment Mnemonic

A =	Airway with simultaneous cervical spine stabilization and/or immobilization
B =	Breathing
C =	Circulation
D =	Disability (neurologic status)
E =	Expose patient/environmental control
F =	Full set of vital signs/focused adjuncts/facilitate family presence
G =	Give comfort measures
H =	History\Head-to-toe assessment
I =	Inspect posterior surfaces

D. Nursing diagnoses, outcome identification, planning, and implementation
   1. The severity of the patient's condition may require simultaneous assessment, diagnosis, and implementation. Appropriate nursing diagnoses are based on assessment findings. Specific patient outcomes are then identified and a plan is developed. The priorities for intervention will depend upon the complexity of the patient's injuries and the availability and qualifications of the emergency department staff and/or trauma nurse. Give priority to those injuries with the greatest potential to compromise airway, breathing, circulation, and/or disability. For the purposes of these stations, the learner is NOT expected to identify nursing diagnoses or outcomes.
E. Ongoing evaluation
   1. Evaluate the patient's response to any interventions to determine further interventions. The learner should evaluate the effectiveness of any intervention expected to have an immediate effect on the patient. Any abnormalities identified in the primary assessment and the vital signs must be re-evaluated at the completion of the secondary assessment.

III. Summary

A. Trauma Nursing Process Stations
   1. The Trauma Nursing Process Skill Stations present the learners with six patient scenarios. The purpose of these stations is to allow the participants time to observe and practice the Trauma Nursing Process assessments and interventions.
   2. During evaluation, the learner must demonstrate all critical steps designated with one and two stars (* and **), and 70% of the total number of points. The learner will be evaluated using a new and different scenario. Therefore, concentrate on understanding the principles of the Trauma Nursing Process during the Skill Stations and not memorizing the specific teaching case scenarios.
B. Critical step review
   1. Critical steps are indicated by a double star (**)

   Certain critical steps must be demonstrated/described during the primary assessment.

The total number of possible critical steps may vary based on the scenario.
   a. Assesses airway patency
   b. Identifies one appropriate airway intervention
   c. Assesses breathing effectiveness
   d. Identifies one appropriate intervention for ineffective breathing
   e. Palpates a pulse
   f. Inspects for external bleeding
   g. Identifies one appropriate intervention for ineffective circulation
   h. Assesses level of consciousness (AVPU)
   i. Identifies one appropriate intervention for altered level of consciousness
   j. Removes all clothing
   k. States one measure to prevent heat loss
   2. Critical steps as indicated by *

   Additional critical steps demonstrated and/or described during the remainder of the station are designated with a * on the evaluation form. All of these steps must be performed to successfully complete the Trauma Nursing Process station.
   a. Assess for pain using an appropriate pain scale
   b. Describes method to maintain spinal stabilization when patient is logrolled
   c. Identify all simulated injuries
   d. Identify at least five appropriate diagnostic studies and/or interventions
C. Principles and points to remember
   1. Correlate the mechanism of injury with potential injuries
   2. Address all life-threatening conditions before the secondary assessment
   3. Maintain cervical spine protection during all steps of the nursing process
   4. Caring for a multiple trauma patient requires a team approach and is more efficient when the leader is well identified
   5. Delineate trauma team roles prior to receiving the patient
   6. Assign one team member the responsibility for recording all assessment findings and interventions

Trauma Nursing Process Scenario: Teaching Case A (Fall)

Prehospital MIVT Report

An ambulance is en route with a 24-year-old who fell 20 feet (6 m) from a roof, landing on concrete. The patient is moaning, complaining of difficulty breathing, and pain to his left chest, head, abdomen, left knee, and back. There is a large, actively bleeding scalp laceration. Blood pressure is 120/70 mm Hg, pulse 120 beats/minute, and respirations 32 breaths/minute and shallow. Cervical spine protection was initiated, and the patient is in complete spinal immobilization. The patient has two large-caliber intravenous catheters with isotonic crystalloid solution infusing, and oxygen via nonrebreather mask is being administered. A pressure dressing has been applied to the scalp laceration. The patient has just arrived in the emergency department. Please proceed with your primary and secondary assessments and interventions.

Focus of this teaching station: Control of external hemorrhage and pain management

In the interest of model comfort and safety, assume the model is in complete spinal immobilization and that the team is adhering to Standard Precautions.

Skill Steps	Instructor Responses	Demonstrated Yes	Demonstrated No
1. Assesses airway patency (states at least 3 of the following):		** ___	___
• Vocalization	• Patient is moaning; gurgling sounds present		
• Tongue obstructing airway	• No obstruction by the tongue		
• Loose teeth or foreign objects	• Loose teeth present		
• Blood, vomitus, or other secretions	• Blood and secretions are present		
• Edema	• No edema noted		
2. Maintains spinal immobilization.		___	___
3. Suctions the airway.		** ___	___
4. Reassesses airway patency.	• After suctioning, the airway is patent	___	___
5. Assesses breathing effectiveness (states at least 3 of the following):		** ___	___
• Spontaneous breathing	• Present		
• Rise and fall of chest	• Bilateral and shallow		
• Rate and pattern of breathing	• Rapid and shallow, approximately 32 breaths/minute		
• Use of accessory muscles and/or diaphragmatic breathing	• Accessory muscle use noted		
• Skin color	• Pale		
• Integrity of the soft tissue and bony structures of the chest wall	• No open wounds, chest wall intact, ecchymotic area on left lower anterior chest. *Patient holding hand over left chest, complaining of pain.*		
• Bilateral breath sounds	• Diminished on left		
6. Maintains oxygen via nonrebreather mask.		___	___
7. Palpates central pulse.	• Pulse present and rapid	** ___	___

Skill Steps	Instructor Responses	Demonstrated Yes	No
8. Inspects **AND** palpates skin (states at least 2 of the following):		____	____
• Color	• Pale		
• Temperature	• Cool		
• Moisture	• Moist		
9. Inspects for external bleeding.	• Scalp laceration dressing saturated; continues to actively bleed	** ____	____
10. Applies direct pressure to laceration.	• Bleeding controlled with pressure; dressing reapplied. **OR** • If learner does not address bleeding from scalp, pulse rate increases to 140 beats/minute.		
11. Assesses patency of prehospital intravenous lines.	• Both IVs are patent	____	____
12. Administers warmed, isotonic crystalloid solution **AND** at a rapid rate.		** ____	____
13. Reassesses circulation.		____	____
• Color	• If learner orders fluid at a rapid rate, pulse decreases to 110 beats/minute. Skin pale, warm and dry. **OR**		
• Temperature			
• Moisture	• If learner does not order fluid at a rapid rate, pulse rate increases to 140 beats/minutes. Skin pale, cool and clammy.		
• Pulse			
If learner gives fluid at a rapid rate after reassessing circulation (step 13), give credit for step 12.			
14. Assesses level of consciousness (AVPU).	• Alert; patient complains of pain with inspiration	** ____	____
15. Assesses pupils (PERRL).	• PERRL	____	____
16. Removes all clothing.	• Abrasions and bruising on left lower chest, left upper quadrant of abdomen, and left knee	** ____	____
17. States one measure to prevent heat loss (blankets, warming lights, increase room temperature).		** ____	____
If learner did not intervene to correct life-threatening findings in the primary assessment, stop and review the purpose of the primary assessment.			
Secondary Assessment			
18. States need to get a full set of vital signs.	• BP = 112/60 mm Hg • P = 110 beats/minute • R = 32 breaths/minute • T = 98 °F (36.8 °C)	____	____
19. Attaches patient to cardiac monitor.	• ECG = sinus tachycardia without ectopy	____	____
20. Places pulse oximeter on patient.	• SpO_2 = 96%	____	____
21. States need to consider insertion of a urinary catheter.	• No contraindications *If learner elects to insert urinary catheter here, give credit in #37 for inspecting the perineum.*	____	____
22. States need to consider insertion of gastric tube.	• No contraindications	____	____
23. Facilitates laboratory studies, if not already done.		____	____
24. Facilitates family presence per institutional protocols	• Wife is in the waiting room.	____	____
25. Assesses pain using an an appropriate pain scale.	• Pain is 10 out of 10.	* ____	____

Skill Steps	Instructor Responses	Demonstrated Yes	Demonstrated No
26. Gives comfort measures (states at least one measure). • Verbal reassurance, touching • Initiates a nonpharmacologic pain intervention such as applying ice to swollen areas, repositioning, or padding uncomfortable areas, if not contraindicated.	• Verbal reassurance is ineffective—patient continues to complain of pain	___	___
27. Considers obtaining order for an analgesic medication.	An appropriate dose of a narcotic analgesic has been ordered by the physician.	___	___
28. History: States the pertinent history to be obtained (states at least one of the following): • MIVT; what position did he land in? • Patient-generated information • Past medical history	 • Landed on concrete striking head, then landed on left side of body • Complains of difficulty breathing and pain to left forehead, left chest, left knee, abdomen, and back • No significant past medical history	___	___
Demonstrates and describes the head-to-toe assessment by: describing appropriate inspection techniques (e.g., lacerations, abrasions, contusions, ecchymosis), demonstrating appropriate palpation techniques, and demonstrating appropriate auscultation techniques			
29. Inspects AND palpates head AND face for injuries.	• Small contusions and ecchymosis • 5-cm laceration over left frontal-temporal scalp • Pressure dressing has controlled bleeding.	___	___
30. Inspects AND palpates neck for injuries.	*"I'll maintain stabilization while you assess the neck."* • No abnormalities *"I'll replace the collar."*	___	___
31. Inspects AND palpates chest for injuries.	• Ecchymosis and pain noted to left lower anterior chest.	___	___
32. Auscultates breath sounds AND heart sounds.	• Breath sounds diminished bilaterally • Breathing improves following administration of pain medication • Normal heart sounds	___	___
33. Inspects the abdomen for injuries.	• Ecchymosis left upper quadrant	___	___
34. Auscultates bowel sounds.	• Bowel sounds absent	___	___
35. Palpates all four quadrants of the abdomen for injuries.	• Left upper and lower quadrants tender to palpation	___	___
36. Inspects AND palpates the pelvis for injuries.	• No abnormalities	___	___
37. Inspects the perineum for injuries.	• No abnormalities *If learner elects to insert urinary catheter here, give credit in #21.*	___	___
38. Inspects AND palpates all four extremities for neurovascular status and injuries. • Right upper extremity • Left upper extremity • Right lower extremity • Left lower extremity	 • Left knee swollen and tender • Normal neurovascular status in all extremities	___	___

Skill Steps	Instructor Responses	Demonstrated Yes	No
39. Describes method to maintain spinal stabilization when patient is logrolled.		*_____	_____
40. Inspects **AND** palpates posterior surfaces for injuries.	• Lumbar spine tender to palpation • Sphincter tone, checked by the physician, is normal • No other abnormalities	_____	_____
41. Identifies all simulated injuries. • Facial contusions and scalp laceration • Left chest ecchymosis • Possible rib fracture • Possible abdominal injury • Possible injury to lumbar spine • Possible left knee injury	*If the learner has not mentioned all of the simulated injuries, ask him or her to identify all simulated injuries.*	*_____	_____

Instructor response: *"You identified certain injuries during the assessment. Now that you have completed the secondary assessment, list 5 additional diagnostic studies or interventions for this patient."*

Note to Instructors: If the learner has previously identified any of the appropriate diagnostic studies or interventions listed, include the diagnostic study or intervention into the total of 5.

Skill Steps	Instructor Responses	Demonstrated Yes	No
42. **Identifies appropriate diagnostic studies or interventions (states at least 5 of the following):** • Head CT scan • Ice to face • Laceration repair • Cervical spine radiograph or CT scan • Chest radiograph or CT scan • Abdominal CT scan • Focused assessment sonography for trauma (FAST) exam • Lumbar spine radiograph • Pelvis radiograph • Left knee radiograph • Splint left knee • Other • Arterial blood gases • Serum lactate level • Type and screen or crossmatch for blood • Glasgow Coma Scale score • Revised Trauma Score • Pain control • Psychosocial support • Tetanus prophylaxis • Prepare for admission, surgery, or transfer	Suggested interventions specific to this station are listed at the top in head-to-toe order. Interventions common to all TNP stations are listed at the bottom.	*_____	_____

Instructor response: *"What findings need to be re-evaluated?"*

Skill Steps	Instructor Responses	Demonstrated Yes	No
43. States need to re-evaluate primary assessment.		_____	_____
44. States need to re-evaluate vital signs.		_____	_____
45. States need to re-evaluate pain.		_____	_____
46. States need to re-evaluate all identified injuries.		_____	_____

Trauma Nursing Process Scenario: Teaching Case B (Gunshot)

Prehospital MIVT Report

An ambulance is en route to a small community hospital with a 32-year-old victim of a shooting. The patient is alert and has a gunshot wound to the right anterior chest. A nonporous dressing taped on three sides has been placed over the wound. EMS personnel report that the patient's skin is pale, blood pressure is 110/82 mm Hg, pulse 122 beats/minute, and respirations are 28 breaths/minute. Oxygen via nonrebreather mask is being administered, and two large-caliber intravenous catheters are infusing isotonic crystalloid solution at a fast rate. The patient has just arrived in the emergency department sitting in high-Fowler's position and yelling. Please proceed with your primary and secondary assessments and appropriate interventions.

Focus of this teaching station: Assessment of penetrating trauma to chest and preservation of forensic evidence

In the interest of model comfort and safety, assume that the team is adhering to Standard Precautions.

Skill Steps	Instructor Responses	Demonstrated Yes	Demonstrated No
1. Assesses airway patency (states at least 3 of the following):		******_____	_____
• Vocalization	• Patient is yelling loudly		
• Tongue obstructing airway	• No obstruction by the tongue		
• Loose teeth or foreign objects	• No loose teeth or foreign objects		
• Blood, vomitus, or other secretions	• No secretions present		
• Edema	• No edema noted		
If learner attempts to initiate cervical spine protection, it is not indicated at this time.			
2. Assesses breathing effectiveness (states at least 3 of the following):		******_____	_____
• Spontaneous breathing	• Present but labored		
• Rise and fall of chest	• Symmetrical		
• Rate and pattern of breathing	• Tachypneic at 40 breaths/minute; rapid and shallow		
• Use of accessory muscles and/or diaphragmatic breathing	• Accessory muscle use present		
• Skin color	• Pale		
• Integrity of the soft tissue and bony structures of the chest wall	• Open wound to right chest, 5th intercostal space (ICS), anterior axillary line		
• Bilateral breath sounds	• Diminished on right side		
3. Maintains oxygen via nonrebreather mask.		_____	_____
4. States suspects right pneumothorax or hemothorax and describes location and equipment needed for chest tube insertion.	• Assists with chest tube insertion **OR** • If learner elects to needle decompress or remove the occlusive dressing, the instructor should ask for the definitive intervention (chest tube).	******_____	_____
Instructor response: "The physician places a chest tube on the right side. What is your next step?"			

Skill Steps	Instructor Responses	Demonstrated Yes	No
5. Reassess breathing effectiveness.	• Breathing improved. • 200 ml bloody drainage from chest tube	_____	_____
6. Palpates central pulse.	• Pulse strong and rapid	** _____	_____
7. Inspects **AND** palpates skin (states at least 2 of the following):		_____	_____
• Color	• Pale		
• Temperature	• Warm		
• Moisture	• Dry		
8. Inspects for external bleeding.	• No uncontrolled bleeding	** _____	_____
9. Assesses patency of prehospital intravenous lines.	• Intravenous lines patent	_____	_____
10. Administers warmed isotonic crystalloid solution **AND** at a rapid rate.		_____	_____
11. Assesses level of consciousness (AVPU).	• Alert	** _____	_____
12. Assesses pupils (PERRL).	• PERRL	_____	_____
13. Removes all clothing.		** _____	_____
14. Places clothing in separate paper bags and labels appropriately for evidence collection.	• "The clothing is preserved as evidence."	_____	_____

If learner fails to appropriately collect and preserve clothing for evidence, instructor should stop scenario and discuss evidence preservation.

Skill Steps	Instructor Responses	Demonstrated Yes	No
15. States one measure to prevent heat loss (blankets, warming lights, increase room temperature).		** _____	_____

If learner did not intervene to correct life-threatening findings in the primary assessment, stop and review the purpose of the primary assessment.

Secondary Assessment			
16. States need to get a full set of vital signs.	• BP = 110/68 mm Hg • P = 112 beats/minute • R = 20 breaths/minute • T = 97 °F (36.2 °C)	_____	_____
17. Attaches patient to cardiac monitor.	• ECG = sinus tachycardia without ectopy	_____	_____
18. Places patient on pulse oximeter.	• SpO_2 = 94%	_____	_____
19. States need to consider insertion of urinary catheter.	• No contraindications *If the learner elects to insert urinary catheter here, give credit in #35 for inspecting the perineum*	_____	_____
20. States need to consider insertion of gastric tube.	• No contraindications	_____	_____
21. Facilitates laboratory studies, if not already done.		_____	_____
22. Facilitates family presence per institutional protocols. • Need to consider maintaining staff and patient safety measures. • Limit patient visitors.	• Family notified	_____	_____

Skill Steps	Instructor Responses	Demonstrated Yes	Demonstrated No
23. Assesses pain using an appropriate pain scale.	• Pain in 6 out of 10.	* _____	_____
24. Gives comfort measures (states at least one measure). • Verbal reassurance, touching • Initiates a nonpharmacologic pain intervention such as applying ice to swollen areas, repositioning, or padding uncomfortable areas, if not contraindicated.	• Less anxious since chest tube insertion and relief of hemothorax.	_____	_____
25. Considers obtaining order for an analgesic medication.	• An appropriate dose of a narcotic analgesic has been ordered by the physician.	_____	_____
26. History: States the pertinent history to be obtained (states at least one of the following): • MIVT • Patient-generated information • Past medical history	• No new information • Complains of mild difficulty breathing • No significant past medical history	_____	_____
Demonstrates and describes the head-to-toe assessment by describing appropriate inspection techniques (e.g., lacerations, abrasions, contusions, ecchymosis), demonstrating appropriate palpation techniques, and demonstrating appropriate auscultation techniques.			
27. Inspects AND palpates head AND face for injuries.	• No abnormalities	_____	_____
28. Inspects AND palpates neck for injuries.	• No abnormalities. There is no cervical collar in place in this scenario and would not recommend placing a collar.	_____	_____
29. Inspects and palpates chest for injuries.	• Chest tube present in right chest wall (total of 300 ml of drainage from chest tube) • Gunshot wound noted to right chest, 5th intercostal space, midaxillary line; dressing intact • Subcutaneous emphysema palpated on right anterolateral chest wall	_____	_____
30. Auscultates breath sounds AND heart sounds.	• Breath sounds slightly diminished on the right • Normal heart sounds	_____	_____
31. Inspects the abdomen for injuries.	• No abnormalities	_____	_____
32. Auscultates bowel sounds.	• Bowel sounds present	_____	_____
33. Palpates all four quadrants of the abdomen for injuries.	• No abnormalities	_____	_____
34. Inspects AND palpates the pelvis for injuries.	• No abnormalities	_____	_____
35. Inspects the perineum for injuries.	• No abnormalities *If learner elects to insert urinary catheter here, give credit in #19.*	_____	_____
36. Inspects and palpates all four extremities. for neurovascular status and injuries • Right upper extremity • Left upper extremity • Right lower extremity • Left lower extremity	• Dried blood to both hands, otherwise, no abnormalities • Normal neurovascular status to all extremities	_____	_____

Skill Steps	Instructor Responses	Demonstrated Yes	No
37. Turns patient and inspects and palpates posterior surfaces for injuries.	• Open wound right scapular area • Sphincter tone, checked by physician, is normal	___	___
38. Identifies all simulated injuries. • Right chest wound (hemo-pneumothorax) • Open scapular wound to right back	*If the learner has not mentioned all the simulated injuries, ask him or her to identify all simulated injuries.*	* ___	___

Instructor response: *"You identified certain injuries during the assessment. Now that you have completed the secondary assessment, list 5 additional diagnostic studies or interventions for this patient."*

Note to Instructors: If the learner has previously identified any of the appropriate diagnostic studies or interventions listed, include the diagnostic study or intervention into the total of 5.

Skill Steps	Instructor Responses	Demonstrated Yes	No
39. Identifies appropriate diagnostic studies or interventions (states at least 5 of the following): • Chest radiograph (first) • CT scan of chest (second) • Echocardiogram • Focused assessment sonography for trauma (FAST) exam (controversial in penetrating trauma) • Bag hands for forensic evidence–<u>do not wash hands</u> • Clean and dress open wounds • Antibiotics • Notify law enforcement • Other • Arterial blood gases • Serum lactate level • Type and screen or crossmatch for blood • Glasgow Coma Scale score • Revised Trauma Score • Pain control • Psychosocial support • Tetanus prophylaxis • Prepare for admission, surgery, or transfer	Suggested interventions specific to this station are listed at the top in head-to-toe order. Interventions common to all TNP stations are listed at the bottom.	* ___	___

Instructor response: *"What findings need to be re-evaluated?"*

Skill Steps	Instructor Responses	Demonstrated Yes	No
40. States need to re-evaluate primary assessment.		___	___
41. States need to re-evaluate vital signs.		___	___
42. States need to re-evaluate pain.		___	___
43. States need to re-evaluate all identified injuries.		___	___

Trauma Nursing Process Scenario: Teaching Case C (Geriatric)

Prehospital MIVT Report

An ambulance is en route with an 83-year-old female patient who was struck by an automobile and thrown approximately 20 feet (6 m) landing on grass. The patient is alert, but exhibits repetitive questioning. The patient complains of pelvic and bilateral leg pain. Blood pressure is 102/76 mm Hg, pulse 72 beats/ minute, and respirations 26 breaths/minute. Cervical spine protection was initiated, and the patient is now in complete spinal immobilization. Oxygen via nonrebreather mask is being administered, and one large-caliber intravenous catheter is infusing isotonic crystalloid solution at a controlled rate. Medication list indicates she is on Coumadin and a beta-blocker. The patient has just arrived in the emergency department. Please proceed with your primary and secondary assessments and appropriate interventions.

Focus of this teaching station: Assessment of geriatric patient, medication effects, shock, and end-of-life issues

In the interest of model comfort and safety, assume the model is in complete spinal immobilization and that the team is adhering to Standard Precautions.

Skill Steps	Instructor Responses	Demonstrated? Yes	No
1. Assesses airway patency (states at least 3 of the following): • Vocalization • Tongue obstructing airway • Loose teeth or foreign objects • Blood, vomitus, or other secretions • Edema	• Patient has garbled speech with repetitive questioning • No obstruction by the tongue • Dentures loose • Blood in mouth; no vomitus or other secretions • No edema noted	** ___	___
2. Maintains spinal immobilization.		___	___
3. States need to suction patient and remove dentures.		** ___	___
4. Reassesses airway patency after suctioning and removal of dentures.	• Airway is patent	___	___
5. Assesses breathing effectiveness (states at least 3 of the following): • Spontaneous breathing • Rise and fall of chest • Rate and pattern of breathing • Use of accessory muscles and/or diaphragmatic breathing • Skin color • Integrity of soft tissue and bony structures of the chest wall • Bilateral breath sounds	• Present • Symmetrical • 26 breaths/minute and shallow • No use of accessory muscles • Pale • No open wounds, chest wall intact • Equal and clear bilaterally	** ___	___
6. Maintains oxygen via nonrebreather mask		___	___

Skill Steps	Instructor Responses	Demonstrated? Yes	No
7. Palpates central pulse.	• Pulse present, 72, and irregular	** ____	____
8. Inspects **AND** palpates skin (states at least 2 of the following):		____	____
• Color	• Very pale		
• Temperature	• Cool		
• Moisture	• Moist		
9. Inspects for external bleeding.	• No uncontrolled bleeding		
10. Assesses patency of prehospital intravenous line.	• Intravenous line patent	____	____
11. States need to cannulate additional vein with a large-caliber intravenous catheter using blood tubing.	*If the learner elects to obtain blood samples for typing and other lab studies, credit should be given in Facilitates lab studies.*	** ____	____
12. Infuses warmed, isotonic crystalloid solution **AND** at a rapid rate		** ____	____
13. Assesses level of consciousness (AVPU).	• Alert, but confused with repetitive questioning	** ____	____
14. Assesses pupils (PERRL).	• PERRL	____	____
15. Removes all clothing.	• Open left tibia/fibula fracture	** ____	____
	• Deformity of right thigh and pain with movement of leg		
	• Multiple abrasions, skin tears		
16. States one measure to prevent heat loss (blankets, warming lights, increase room temperature).		** ____	____

If learner did not intervene to correct life-threatening findings in the primary assessment, stop and review the purpose of the primary assessment.

Secondary Assessment			
17. States need to get a full set of vital signs.	• BP = 128/82 mm Hg	____	____
	• P = 76 beats/minute; irregular		
	• R = 24 breaths/minute		
	• T = 97 °F (36.2 °C)		
18. Attaches patient to cardiac monitor.	• ECG = atrial fibrillation	____	____
19. Places pulse oximeter on patient.	• SpO$_2$ = 95%	____	____
20. States need to consider insertion of urinary catheter.	• Contraindicated—blood at the meatus. Will report findings to physician.	____	____
	If learner considers insertion of a urinary catheter here, give credit in #36 for inspecting the perineum.		
21. States need to consider insertion of gastric tube.	• No contraindications	____	____
22. Facilitates laboratory studies, if not already done.		____	____
23. Facilitates family presence per institutional protocols.	• Son and daughter have just arrived.	____	____

Skill Steps	Instructor Responses	Demonstrated? Yes	No
24. Assesses pain using an appropriate pain scale.	• Severe pain to pelvis and legs with movement	*____	____
25. Gives comfort measures (states at least one measure) • Verbal reassurances, touching • Initiates a nonpharmacologic pain intervention such as applying ice to swollen areas, repositioning, or padding uncomfortable areas, if not contraindicated.	 • Verbal reassurances given. • Ice to right thigh deformity • Immobilize left lower leg fracture	____	____
26. Considers obtaining order for an analgesic medication.	• An appropriate dose of a narcotic analgesic has been ordered by the physician.	____	____
27. History: States the pertinent history to be obtained (states at least one of the following): • MIVT • Patient-generated information • Past medical history	 • No new information • Patient complains of pain in pelvis and bilateral lower extremities. • CAD, HTN, MI, chronic atrial fib; Current medications include a beta-blocker and Coumadin; family brought advanced directives paperwork	____	____
Demonstrates and describes the head-to-toe assessment by describing appropriate inspection techniques (e.g., lacerations, abrasions, contusions, ecchymosis), demonstrating appropriate palpation techniques, and demonstrating appropriate auscultation techniques.			
28. Inspects **AND** palpates head **AND** face for injuries.	• Multiple abrasions on head and face • No uncontrolled bleeding	____	____
29. Inspects **AND** palpates neck for injuries.	*"I'll maintain stabilization while you assess the neck."* • Tenderness to palpation at C6 to C7 *"I'll replace the collar."*	____	____
30. Inspects **AND** palpates chest for injuries.	• No abnormalities	____	____
31. Auscultates breath sounds **AND** heart sounds.	• Breath sounds equal and clear bilaterally • Normal heart sounds; irregular	____	____
32. Inspects abdomen for injuries.	• No abnormalities	____	____
33. Auscultates bowel sounds.	• Bowel sounds present	____	____
34. Palpates all four quadrants of abdomen for injuries.	• Tenderness on palpation of lower quadrants	____	____
35. Inspects **AND** palpates pelvis for injuries.	• Pelvic instability noted	____	____
36. Inspects perineum for injuries.	• Blood at meatus	____	____
37. Inspects **AND** palpates all four extremities for neurovascular status and injuries. • Right upper extremity • Left upper extremity • Right lower extremity • Left lower extremity	 • Open left tib/fib deformity with no active bleeding • Obvious deformity right thigh • Normal neurovascular status in all extremities	____	____
38. Describes method to maintain spinal stabilization when patient is logrolled.		*____	____
39. Inspects **AND** palpates posterior surfaces for injuries.	• Pain with palpation in lower lumbar spine and sacral area • Sphincter tone, checked by physician, is normal	____	____

Skill Steps	Instructor Responses	Demonstrated? Yes	No
40. Identifies all simulated injuries. • Possible head injury • Possible cervical spine injury • Possible right femur fracture/leg injury • Possible left lower leg open fractures • Possible pelvic fracture	*If the learner has not mentioned all the simulated injuries, ask him or her to identify all simulated injuries.*	*_____	_____

Instructor response: *"You identified certain injuries during the assessment. Now that you have completed the secondary assessment, list 5 additional diagnostic studies or interventions for this patient."*

Note to Instructors: If the learner has previously identified any of the appropriate diagnostic studies or interventions listed, include the diagnostic study or intervention into the total of 5.

Skill Steps	Instructor Responses	Demonstrated? Yes	No
41. Identifies appropriate diagnostic studies or interventions (states at least 5 of the following): • Head CT scan • Cervical spine radiographs or CT scan • Chest radiograph • 12-lead ECG • Abdominal CT scan • Lumbar spine radiograph • Pelvis radiograph or CT scan • Pelvic stabilization device • Left lower leg radiographs • Right upper leg radiographs • Splint right femur • Splint and wound care to left leg • Coagulation profile • Antibiotics • Other • Arterial blood gases • Serum lactate level • Type and screen or crossmatch for blood • Glasgow Coma Scale score • Revised Trauma Score • Pain control • Psychosocial support • Tetanus prophylaxis • Prepare for admission, surgery, or transfer	Suggested interventions specific to this station are listed at the top in head-to-toe order. Interventions common to all TNP stations are listed at the bottom.	*_____	_____

Instructor response: *"What findings need to be re-evaluated?"*

Skill Steps		Yes	No
42. States need to re-evaluate primary assessment.		_____	_____
43. States need to re-evaluate vital signs		_____	_____
44. States need to re-evaluate pain.		_____	_____
45. States need to re-evaluate all identified injuries.		_____	_____

Discuss the use of advanced directives, especially if the patient deteriorates.

Trauma Nursing Process Scenario: Teaching Case D (Peds)

Caregiver-generated Information

A 24-month-old toddler is brought in by parents stating the child was struck by a vehicle that was backing out from a driveway and fell back hitting his head on the cement. There was a witnessed brief loss of consciousness. There was a large amount of blood at the scene. Scalp laceration identified and dressing was applied by parents. The patient has just arrived in the emergency department. Please proceed with your primary and secondary assessments and appropriate interventions.

Focus of this teaching station: Management of head injury; pediatric assessment, fluid resuscitation, and environmental control; pediatric immobilization

In the interest of model comfort and safety, assume that the team is adhering to Standard Precautions.

Skill Steps	Instructor Responses	Demonstrated? Yes	No
1. Assesses airway patency (states at least 3 of the following):		** ___	___
• Vocalization	• Patient is crying		
• Tongue obstructing airway	• No obstruction by the tongue		
• Loose teeth or foreign objects	• No teeth or foreign objects		
• Blood, vomitus, or other secretions	• No bleeding, vomitus, or secretions		
• Edema	• No edema noted		
2. Initiates age-appropriate spinal immobilization.	Complete spinal immobilization is performed	___	___
3. Assesses breathing effectiveness (states at least 3 of the following):		** ___	___
• Spontaneous breathing	• Present		
• Rise and fall of chest	• Normal, symmetrical		
• Rate and pattern of breathing	• 36 breaths/minute with normal depth		
• Use of accessory muscles and/or diaphragmatic breathing	• No use of accessory muscles		
• Skin color	• Pale		
• Integrity of the soft tissues and bony structures of the chest wall	• Scattered abrasions, chest wall intact		
• Bilateral breath sounds	• Equal and clear bilaterally		
4. States need to administer 100% oxygen via non-rebreather mask or age-appropriate equipment as tolerated.		___	___
5. Palpates pulse (central AND peripheral).	• Pulses present and rapid, centrally and peripherally	** ___	___
6. Inspects AND palpates skin (states at least 2 of the following):		___	___
• Color	• Pale		
• Temperature	• Cool		
• Capillary refill	• Capillary refill 4 seconds		
	Instructor note: Capillary refill is only used in the pediatric population to assess circulation.		

Skill Steps	Instructor Responses	Demonstrated? Yes	No
7. Inspects for external bleeding.	• Blood oozing from scalp laceration. Dressing intact. • No uncontrolled external bleeding	_____	_____
8. States need to cannulate at least one vein using the largest caliber catheter that the vessel can accommodate.	• IV established • If learner elects to obtain blood samples for typing and other lab studies, credit should be given in Facilitates lab studies.	** _____	_____
9. Administers warmed, isotonic crystalloid solution at 20 ml per kilogram.		** _____	_____
10. Reassesses circulatory status.	• Capillary refill is now less than 3 seconds and skin in warm **OR** • If learner does not administer fluid bolus, capillary refill 4–5 seconds and skin remains cool	_____	_____
11. Assesses level of consciousness (AVPU).	• Alert, crying, irritable, cannot be consoled by his parents	** _____	_____
12. Assesses pupils (PERRL).	• PERRL	_____	_____
13. Removes all clothing.	• Abrasions on arms, chest, and lower extremities	** _____	_____
14. States one measure to prevent heat loss (blankets, warming lights, increase room temperature).		** _____	_____

If learner did not intervene to correct life-threatening findings in the primary assessment, stop and review the purpose of the primary assessment.

Secondary Assessment			
15. States need to get a full set of vital signs.	• BP = 96/70 mm Hg • P = 120 beats/minute • R = 28 breaths/minute, crying • T = 97 °F (36.2 °C) • Weight = 12 kg	_____	_____
16. Attaches patient to cardiac monitor.	• ECG = sinus tachycardia without ectopy	_____	_____
17. Places pulse oximeter on patient.	• SpO_2 = 99%	_____	_____
18. States need to consider insertion of a urinary catheter.	• No contraindications. *If learner elects to insert urinary catheter here, give credit in #34 for inspecting the perineum.*	_____	_____
19. States need to consider insertion of gastric tube.	• No contraindications.	_____	_____
20. Facilitates laboratory studies, if not already done.		_____	_____
21. Facilitates family presence per institutional protocols.	• Mom at bedside	_____	_____
22. Assesses pain using an appropriate pain scale.	• Pain is 9 out of 10 on a pediatric pain scale.	* _____	_____

Skill Steps	Instructor Responses	Demonstrated Yes	Demonstrated No
23. Gives comfort measures (states at least one measure). • Verbal reassurances, touching • Initiates a nonpharmacologic pain intervention such as applying ice to swollen areas, repositioning, or padding uncomfortable areas, if not contraindicated.	• Allow parents to remain with child. • Explain all procedures and plan of care with parents.	___	___
24. Considers obtaining order for analgesic medication.	• An appropriate dose of a narcotic analgesic has been ordered by the physician.	___	___
25. History: States the pertinent history to be obtained (states at least one of the following): • MIVT • Caregiver-generated information • Past medical history	• No new information • No new information • Immunizations up to date	___	___
Demonstrates and describes the head-to-toe assessment by: describing appropriate inspection techniques (e.g., lacerations, abrasions, contusions, ecchymosis), demonstrating appropriate palpation techniques, and demonstrating appropriate auscultation techniques.			
26. Inspects **AND** palpates head **AND** face for injuries.	• Ecchymosis and hematoma to right occipital area; flap laceration oozing, dressing intact. • No drainage from ears or nose.	___	___
27. Inspects **AND** palpates neck for injuries.	*"I'll maintain stabilization while you assess the neck."* • No abnormalities *"I'll replace the immobilization devices."*	___	___
28. Inspects **AND** palpates chest for injuries.	• Multiple scattered abrasions on chest wall with no crepitus, deformity, or instability palpated.	___	___
29. Auscultates breath sounds **AND** heart sounds.	• Breath sounds equal and clear bilaterally • Normal heart sounds	___	___
30. Inspects the abdomen for injuries.	• No abnormalities	___	___
31. Auscultates bowel sounds.	• Bowel sounds present	___	___
32. Palpates all four quadrants of the abdomen for injuries.	• No abnormalities	___	___
33. Inspects **AND** palpates pelvis for injuries.	• No abnormalities	___	___
34. Inspects perineum for injuries.	• No abnormalities *If learner elects to insert urinary catheter here, give credit in #18*	___	___
35. Inspects and palpates all four extremities for neurovascular status and injuries. • Right upper extremity • Left upper extremity • Right lower extremity • Left lower extremity	• Abrasion to right shoulder • Abrasions on bilateral lower extremities • Normal neurovascular status in all extremities.	___	___
36. Describes method to maintain spinal stabilization when patient is logrolled.		*___	___

Skill Steps	Instructor Responses	Demonstrated Yes	No
37. Inspects **AND** palpates posterior surfaces for injuries.	• Multiple abrasions on back • Sphincter tone, checked by physician, is normal	_____	_____
38. Identifies all simulated injuries • Right occipital scalp laceration • Head injury • Multiple abrasions on chest, extremities and back.	*If the learner has not mentioned all simulated injuries, ask him or her to identify all simulated injuries.*	*_____	_____

Instructor response: *"You identified certain injuries during the assessment. Now that you have completed the secondary assessment, list 5 additional diagnostic studies or interventions for this patient."*

Note to Instructors: If the learner has previously identified any of the appropriate diagnostic studies or interventions listed, include the diagnostic study or intervention into the total of 5.

Skill Steps	Instructor Responses	Demonstrated Yes	No
39. Identifies appropriate diagnostic studies or interventions (at least 5 of the following): • Head CT scan • Skull radiographs (controversial; not indicated if head CT scan is obtained) • Dressing for scalp laceration • Cervical spine radiographs or CT scan • Chest radiograph or CT scan • Abdominal CT scan • Pelvic radiograph • Ice • Wound care • Consider sedation for diagnostic studies • Other • Arterial blood gases • Serum lactate level • Type and screen or crossmatch for blood • Pediatric Glasgow Coma Scale score • Pediatric Trauma Score • Pain control • Psychosocial support • Tetanus prophylaxis • Prepare for admission, surgery, or transfer	Suggested interventions specific to this station are listed at the top in head-to-toe order. Interventions common to all TNP stations are listed at the bottom.	*_____	_____

Instructor Response: *"What findings need to be re-evaluated?"*

Skill Steps	Instructor Responses	Demonstrated Yes	No
40. States need to re-evaluate primary assessment		_____	_____
41. States need to re-evaluate vital signs		_____	_____
42. States need to re-evaluate pain		_____	_____
43. States need to re-evaluate all identified injuries.		_____	_____

If time permits, discuss age-appropriate pediatric immobilization techniques.

Trauma Nursing Process Scenario:
Teaching Case E (OB and Intimate Partner Violence)

Prehospital MIVT Report

An ambulance is en route with a 19-year-old woman who is 34 weeks pregnant. She told EMS that she fell backward down 10 concrete steps while carrying groceries into her home. There was a brief loss of consciousness. The patient is tearful and complains of head, face, neck, left ankle, and abdominal pain. Blood pressure is 100/60 mm Hg, pulse 138 beats/minute, and respirations 26 breaths/minute. Cervical spine protection was initiated, and the patient is now in complete spinal immobilization. Oxygen via nonrebreather mask is being administered, and one large-caliber intravenous catheter is infusing isotonic crystalloid solution at a controlled rate. The patient has just arrived in the emergency department. Please proceed with your primary and secondary assessments and appropriate interventions.

Focus of this teaching station: Assessment and spinal immobilization of pregnant patient, intimate partner violence assessment

In the interest of model comfort and safety, assume the model is in complete spinal immobilization and that the team is adhering to Standard Precautions.

Skill Steps	Instructor Responses	Demonstrated Yes	No
1. Assesses airway patency (states at least 3 of the following):		**	
• Vocalization	• Patient is talking		
• Tongue obstructing airway	• No obstruction by the tongue		
• Loose teeth or foreign objects	• No loose teeth or foreign objects		
• Blood, vomitus, or other secretions	• No bleeding, vomitus, or secretions		
• Edema	• No edema noted		
2. Maintains spinal immobilization.			
3. Assesses breathing effectiveness (states at least 3 of the following):		**	
• Spontaneous breathing	• Present		
• Rise and fall of chest	• Symmetrical		
• Rate and pattern of breathing	• Rapid and shallow; pain on inspiration		
• Use of accessory muscles and/or diaphragmatic breathing.	• No use of accessory or abdominal muscles		
• Skin color	• Pale		
• Integrity of soft tissue and bony structures of the chest wall	• Chest wall intact with contusions noted		
• Bilateral breath sounds	• Equal and clear; diminished bilaterally *(may be normal finding in a 34-week pregnant patient)*		
4. Maintains oxygen via nonrebreather mask.			
5. Palpates central pulse.	• Pulse present and rapid	**	

Skill Steps	Instructor Responses	Demonstrated Yes	Demonstrated No
6. Inspects **AND** palpates skin (states at least 2 of the following):		____	____
• Color	• Very pale		
• Temperature	• Cool		
• Moisture	• Moist		
Patient states she feels anxious and uncomfortable and complains of nausea.			
7. **Tilts the backboard 15 to 20 degrees to the left to displace the uterus. If unable to tilt board, manually displaces the uterus to the left side.**		** ____	____
8. **Reassess central pulse and skin.**	• Pulse present		
	• Skin pale and warm		
	• States feels better		
9. **Inspects for external bleeding.**	• No uncontrolled bleeding	____	____
10. **Assesses patency of prehospital intravenous line.**	• Intravenous line patent	____	____
11. **States need to cannulate additional vein with large-caliber intravenous catheter and blood tubing.**	• If learner elects to obtain blood samples for typing and other lab studies, credit should be given in Facilitates lab studies.	** ____	____
12. **Infuses warmed, isotonic crystalloid solution AND at a rapid rate.**		** ____	____
13. **Assesses level of consciousness (AVPU).**	• Alert, but anxious and withdrawn. Gives short answers to questions. Worried about baby.	** ____	____
14. **Assesses pupils (PERRL).**	• PERRL	____	____
15. **Removes all clothing.**	• Multiple bruises/contusions in different stages of healing across chest and abdomen	** ____	____
	• Contusions/abrasions to right side of face		
	• Deformity left ankle		
16. **States one measure to prevent heat loss (blankets, warming lights, increase room temperature)**		** ____	____

If learner did not intervene to correct life-threatening findings in the primary assessment, stop and review the purpose of the primary assessment.

Skill Steps	Instructor Responses	Demonstrated Yes	No
Secondary Assessment			
17. States need to get a full set of vital signs and fetal heart tones.	• BP = 110/76 mm Hg • P = 116 beats/minute • R = 24 breaths/minute • T = 99 °F (37.2 °C) • Fetal heart tones = 150 beats/minute *(normal is 120 to 160)*	____	____
18. Attaches patient to cardiac monitor.	• ECG = sinus tachycardia without ectopy	____	____
19. Places pulse oximeter on patient.	• SpO_2 = 97%	____	____
20. States need to consider insertion of urinary catheter.	• No contraindications *If learner elects to insert urinary catheter here, give credit in #37 got inspecting the perineum.*	____	____
21. States need to consider insertion of gastric tube.	• No contraindications	____	____
22. Facilitates laboratory studies, if not already done.		____	____
23. Facilitates family presence per institutional protocols.	• Husband in the waiting room. He is pacing and demanding to be with patient for the exam. • Patient does not want visitors at present. Security is notified of situation.	____	____
24. Assesses pain using an appropriate pain scale.	Pain is 4 out of 10.	*____	____
25. Gives comfort measures (states at least one measure). • Verbal reassurances, touching • Initiates a nonpharmacologic pain intervention such as applying ice to swollen areas, repositioning, or padding uncomfortable areas, if not contraindicated.	• Patient responds to verbal reassurances • Ice pack for right facial contusion	____	____
26. Considers obtaining order for analgesic medication	• An appropriate dose of a narcotic analgesic has been ordered by the physician	____	____
27. History: States the pertinent history to be obtained (states at least one of the following): • MIVT • Patient-generated information • Past medical history	• No new information • Patient changes story to having tripped while walking up the steps and fell. Patient says she falls all the time. • This is her first pregnancy (Gravida 1). • Unsure of last menstrual period • Patient states she is 34 weeks pregnant; she has received prenatal care; records not available.	____	____
Demonstrates and describes head-to-toe assessment by describing appropriate inspection techniques (e.g., lacerations, abrasions, contusions, ecchymosis), demonstrating appropriate palpation techniques, and demonstrating appropriate auscultation techniques.			
28. Inspects and palpates head and face for injuries.	• Contusion and hematoma to right forehead • Small abrasions to right side of face • Right periorbital ecchymosis is present	____	____

Skill Steps	Instructor Responses	Demonstrated Yes	No
29. Inspects **AND** palpates neck for injuries.	*"I'll maintain stabilization while you assess the neck."* • Tenderness to right lateral neck • No point tenderness of cervical spine *"I'll replace the collar."*	_____	_____
30. Inspects **AND** palpates chest for injuries.	• Contusions to the chest wall in various colors • Pain with palpation to right chest	_____	_____
31. Auscultates breath sounds **AND** heart sounds.	• Clear and diminished bilaterally (may be a normal finding for 34 weeks pregnant) • Normal heart sounds	_____	_____
32. Inspects the abdomen for injuries.	• Multiple contusions to abdomen in different stages of healing	_____	_____
33. Auscultates bowel sounds.	• Bowel sounds decreased	_____	_____
34. Palpates all four quadrants of the abdomen for injuries.	• Tender across upper abdomen, pain with palpation to right upper quadrant	_____	_____
35. Assesses fundal height and correlates with reported gestational age.	• Fundal height appropriate for reported gestational stage	_____	_____
36. Inspects **AND** palpates the pelvis for injuries.	• No abnormalities	_____	_____
37. Inspects the perineum for injuries.	• No bulging, bleeding, or other fluids noted *If learner elects to insert catheter here, give credit in #20*	_____ _____	_____ _____
38. Inspects **AND** palpates all four extremities for neurovascular status and injuries. • Right upper extremity • Right lower extremity • Left lower extremity • Left upper extremity	 • Multiple bruises in different stages of healing. • Normal neurovascular status in all extremities • Left ankle deformed and tender	_____	_____
39. Describes method to maintain spinal stabilization when patient is logrolled.		*_____	_____
40. Inspects **AND** palpates posterior surfaces for injuries.	• Multiple bruises to lower back and buttocks in different stages of healing	_____	_____
41. Identifies all simulated injuries. • Right forehead contusion/hematoma • Chest wall contusions • Left ankle injury • Periorbital ecchymosis • Right lateral neck injury • Abdominal contusions and injury • Contusions to back and buttocks • Possible intimate partner violence injury pattern	If the learner has not mentioned all simulated injuries, ask him or her to identify all simulated injuries.	*_____	_____

Instructor response: *"You identified certain injuries during the assessment. Now that you have completed the secondary assessment, list 5 additional diagnostic studies or interventions for this patient."*

Note to Instructors: If the learner has previously identified any of the appropriate diagnostic studies or interventions listed, include the diagnostic study or intervention into the total of 5.

Skill Steps	Instructor Responses	Demonstrated	
		Yes	No
42. Identifies appropriate diagnostic studies or interventions (states at least 5 of the following): • Radiographs with shielding • Head CT scan • Facial bones radiographs • Cervical spine radiographs or CT scan • Chest radiograph • Thoracic or lumbar spine films • Focused assessment sonography for trauma (FAST) exam • Abdominal CT scan • Fetal monitoring • Splint left ankle • Clean and dress abrasions • Screen for intimate partner violence and make appropriate referrals; provide information so the patient can stay safe • Obtain advocate for the patient • Consultation with obstetrician/OB nurses to assist with management and monitoring • Other • Arterial blood gases • Serum lactate level • Type and screen or crossmatch for blood • Glasgow Coma Scale score • Revised Trauma Score • Pain control • Psychosocial support • Tetanus prophylaxis • Prepare for admission, surgery, or transfer	Suggested interventions specific to this station are listed at the top in head-to-toe order. Interventions common to all TNP stations are listed at the bottom.	*___	___
Instructor response: *"What findings need to be re-evaluated?"*			
43. States need to re-evaluate primary assessment.		___	___
44. States need to re-evaluate fetal assessment.		___	___
45. States need to re-evaluate vital signs.		___	___
46. States need to re-evaluate pain.		___	___
47. States need to re-evaluate all identified injuries.		___	___

Trauma Nursing Process Scenario: Teaching Case F (MVC)

Prehospital MIVT Report

An ambulance is en route with a 28-year-old male unrestrained driver involved in a motor vehicle crash. Another vehicle impacted the driver's side door at a high rate of speed. He is responding to painful stimuli only. His skin is pale, and he has deformities of the left upper arm and left upper leg. Blood pressure is 90/60 mm Hg, pulse 130 beats/minute, and respirations 10 breaths/minute spontaneously. He is now being assisted with bag-mask device. Cervical spine protection was initiated, and the patient is now in complete spinal immobilization. He has one large-caliber intravenous catheter with isotonic crystalloid solution infusing at a controlled rate. The patient has just arrived in the emergency department. Please proceed with your primary and secondary assessments and appropriate interventions.

Focus of this teaching station: Airway management, management of shock, pain management, and immediacy of operative intervention.

In the interest of model comfort and safety, assume the model is in complete spinal immobilization and that the team is adhering to Standard Precautions.

Skill Steps	Instructor Responses	Demonstrated Yes	No
1. **Assesses airway patency; AND** due to unresponsiveness, manually opens the airway using a jaw thrust or chin lift (states at least 3 of the following):		** ___	___
• Vocalization	• Patient does not vocalize.		
• Tongue obstructing airway	• Tongue obstruction present		
• Loose teeth or foreign objects	• Loose teeth present		
• Blood, vomitus, or other secretions	• Bleeding noted; no vomitus		
• Edema	• No edema noted		
2. **Maintains spinal immobilization.**		___	___
3. **States need to suction patient.**		** ___	___
4. **Reassesses airway patency after suctioning,**	• Airway remains compromised due to decreased level of consciousness and tongue obstruction.	___	___
5. **States need to measure and insert an oral airway and continue assisted ventilations.**	• An oral airway has been inserted and the airway is now patent. • Continue with your primary assessment.	** ___	___
6. **Assesses breathing effectiveness (states at least 3 of the following):**		** ___	___
• Spontaneous breathing	• Present		
• Rise and fall of chest	• Symmetrical		
• Rate and pattern of breathing	• Slow (10 breaths/minute) and shallow		
• Use of accessory muscles and/or diaphragmatic breathing	• No use of accessory muscles		
• Skin color	• Pale		
• Integrity of soft tissue and bony structures of the chest wall	• No open wounds, chest wall intact		
• Bilateral breath sounds	• Equal and clear but diminished bilaterally		
The emergency department physician or trauma surgeon has elected to intubate the patient using rapid sequence intubation (RSI) due to his decreased level of consciousness and to provide for airway protection. Now that the patient has been intubated what is your next step?			

Skill Steps	Instructor Responses	Demonstrated Yes	Demonstrated No
7. Assesses endotracheal tube placement (states at least 2 of the following):		** ____	____
• Observes for rise and fall of the chest with bag-valve ventilations.	• Equal rise and fall of chest with bag-valve ventilation		
• Auscultates over the epigastric area, **AND** then auscultates bilateral breath sounds.	• No gurgling heard over epigastric area; equal breath sounds auscultated bilaterally		
• Uses an exhaled CO_2 detector or esophageal detector device (EDD).	• Exhaled CO_2 detector color change confirms placement; or no resistance felt when pulling back on syringe of EDD		
8. States need to secure endotracheal tube and continues ventilating patient with bag-valve device until ventilator arrives.	• Cuff is inflated and tube is secured.	____	____
9. Palpates central pulse.	• Pulse present and rapid	** ____	____
10. Inspects **AND** palpates skin (states at least 2 of the following):		____	____
• Color	• Pale		
• Temperature	• Cool		
• Moisture	• Moist		
11. Inspects for external bleeding.	• No uncontrolled external bleeding	____	____
12. Assesses patency of prehospital intravenous line.	• IV is patent	____	____
13. States need to cannulate additional vein with large-caliber intravenous catheter.	If learner elects to obtain blood for typing and other lab studies, credit should be given in Facilitates lab studies.	** ____	____
14. Infuses warmed crystalloid solution with blood tubing **AND** at a rapid rate.	• 1000 ml of warmed crystalloid solution has been infused.	** ____	____
15. Reassesses circulation.	• Skin is pale, cool, and dry.	____	____
16. Assesses level of consciousness (AVPU).	• Patient remains unresponsive to painful stimuli due to effects of medications used for RSI.	** ____	____
17. Assesses pupils (PERRL).	• PERRL, but sluggish	____	____
18. Removes all clothing.	• Deformity left upper arm and left upper leg • Discoloration to left upper quadrant of abdomen	** ____	____
19. States one measure to prevent heat loss (blankets, warming lights, increase room temperature).		** ____	____

If learner did not intervene to correct life-threatening findings in the primary assessment, stop and review the purpose of the primary assessment.

Secondary Assessment			
20. States need to get a full set of vital signs.	• BP = 92/58 mm Hg • P = 126 beats/minute • R = 16 breaths/minute-assisted • T = 96 °F (35.5 °C)	____	____

If learner chooses to intervene based on vital signs, state fluid resuscitation is ongoing and the physician has been notified. Please proceed with your assessment.

21. Attaches patient to cardiac monitor.	• ECG = sinus tachycardia without ectopy	____	____
22. Places pulse oximeter on patient.	• SpO_2 = 97%	____	____

Skill Steps	Instructor Responses	Demonstrated Yes	Demonstrated No
23. States need to consider insertion of urinary catheter.	• No contraindications *If learner elects to insert urinary catheter here, give credit in #39 for inspecting the perineum.*	____	____
24. States need to consider insertion of a gastric tube.	• No contraindications	____	____
25. Facilitates laboratory studies, if not already done.		____	____
26. Facilitates family presence per institutional protocols.	• Family is in transit to the hospital	____	____
27. Assesses pain using an appropriate pain scale.	• Physical signs indicate that the patient is experiencing moderate pain.	*____	____
28. Gives comfort measures (states at least one measure). • Verbal reassurances, touching • Initiates a nonpharmacologic intervention such as applying ice to swollen areas, repositioning, or padding uncomfortable areas, if not contraindicated.	•Immobilizes left upper arm and left upper leg	____	____
29. Considers obtaining order for an analgesic medication.	• An appropriate dose of a narcotic analgesic has been ordered by the physician.	____	____
30. History: States the pertinent history to be obtained (states at least one of the following): • MIVT • Patient-generated information • Past medical history	 • No additional information • None • Unknown	____	____

Demonstrates and describes the head-to-toe assessment by describing appropriate inspection techniques (e.g., lacerations, abrasions, contusions, ecchymosis), demonstrating appropriate palpation techniques, and demonstrating appropriate auscultation techniques.

Skill Steps	Instructor Responses	Demonstrated Yes	Demonstrated No
31. Inspects **AND** palpates head **AND** face for injuries.	• Hematoma on forehead • Multiple facial abrasions	____	____
32. Inspects **AND** palpates neck for injuries.	*"I'll maintain stabilization while you assess the neck."* • No abnormalities *"I'll replace the collar."*	____	____
33. Inspects **AND** palpates the chest for injuries.	• No abnormalities	____	____
34. Auscultates breath sounds **AND** heart sounds bilaterally.	• Breath sounds equal and clear • Normal heart sounds	____	____
35. Inspects the abdomen for injuries.	• Ecchymosis to left upper quadrant • Abdomen distended	____	____
36. Auscultates bowel sounds.	• Bowel sounds absent	____	____
37. Palpates all four quadrants of the abdomen for injuries.	• Abdomen is rigid	____	____
38. Inspects **AND** palpates the pelvis for injuries.	• No abnormalities	____	____
39. Inspects the perineum for injuries.	• No abnormalities *If learner elects to insert urinary catheter here, give credit in #23.*	____	____

Skill Steps	Instructor Responses	Demonstrated Yes	No
40. Inspects AND palpates all four extremities for neurovascular status and injuries. • Right upper extremity • Left upper extremity • Right lower extremity • Left lower extremity	• Left upper arm deformed with ecchymosis • Left upper leg swollen with obvious deformity • Pulses and brisk capillary refill present in all four extremities.	____	____
41. Describes method to maintain spinal stabilization when patient is logrolled.		*____	____
42. Inspects AND palpates posterior surfaces for injuries.	• No abnormalities • Sphincter tone, checked by physician, is normal	____	____
43. Identifies all simulated injuries. • Possible head injury • Deformity left upper arm • Deformity left upper leg • Possible abdominal injury	If the learner has not mentioned all simulated injuries, ask him or her to identify all simulated injuries.	*____	____

Instructor response: *"You identified certain injuries during the assessment. Now that you have completed the secondary assessment, list 5 additional diagnostic studies or interventions for this patient."*

Note to Instructors: If the learner has previously identified any of the appropriate diagnostic studies or interventions listed, include the diagnostic study or intervention into the total of 5.

Skill Steps	Instructor Responses	Demonstrated Yes	No
44. Identifies appropriate diagnostic studies or interventions (states at least 5 of the following): • Head CT scan • Cervical spine radiographs or CT scan • Chest radiograph • Abdominal CT scan • Focused assessment sonography for trauma (FAST) exam • Diagnostic peritoneal lavage (DPL) • Left upper arm radiographs • Immobilize left arm • Left femur radiographs • Splint left femur • Clean and dress abrasions • Consider orthopedic consult • Other • Arterial blood gases • Serum lactate level • Type and screen or crossmatch for blood • Glasgow Coma Scale score • Revised Trauma Score • Pain control • Psychological support • Tetanus prophylaxis • Prepare for admission, surgery, or transfer	Suggested interventions specific to this station are listed at the top in head-to-toe order. Interventions common to all TNP stations are listed at the bottom.	*____	____

Instructor response: "What findings need to be re-evaluated?"

Skill Steps	Instructor Responses	Demonstrated	
		Yes	No
45. States need to re-evaluate primary assessment.		___	___
46. States need to re-evaluate vital signs.		___	___
47. States need to re-evaluate pain.		___	___
48. States need to re-evaluate all identified injuries.		___	___

Airway & Ventilation Interventions

I. Introduction to the Skill Station

A. Instructor and learner introductions

B. Purpose

Each learner will demonstrate an assessment of airway patency, identify the appropriate interventions to obtain and maintain a patent airway, and demonstrate and describe interventions to ensure effective ventilation.

C. Teaching Format

1. The instructor will discuss and/or demonstrate:

   a. Principles of airway and ventilation assessment and management

   b. Jaw thrust and chin lift maneuvers

   c. Oropharyngeal suctioning

   d. Insertion of oropharyngeal or nasopharyngeal airway

   e. Oxygen delivery methods

   f. Bag-mask ventilation

   g. Assessment of endotracheal tube placement

   h. End-tidal CO_2 monitoring

   i. Alternative airways

   j. Needle thoracentesis

   k. Nurse's role in chest tube insertion

   l. Management of chest drainage systems

   m. Preparation for rapid sequence intubation

   n. Pulse oximetry, esophageal detector devices, and surgical airways are optional components.

2. The learners will practice:

   a. Jaw thrust and chin lift maneuvers

   b. Insertion of an oropharyngeal airway

   c. Bag-mask ventilation

   d. Assessment of endotracheal tube placement

D. Evaluation

1. This is not a testing station. Learners will receive verbal feedback and participate in a question and answer session related to specific techniques and topics.

2. Material presented in this skill station may be included on the written exam and in the Trauma Nursing Process Evaluation.

II. Principles of Airway and Ventilation

A. General principles

1. The first priority in nursing care of the trauma patient is the establishment of a patent airway.

2. Airway management for the trauma patient must be achieved without hyperextension or flexion of the neck. This may cause additional damage in the presence of cervical spine trauma.

3. Refer to Chapter 4, Airway and Ventilation, for more information related to assessment of airway and ventilation.

4. In actual patient care, all personnel who anticipate direct patient contact or contact with the patient's bodily fluids must wear personal protective equipment. (***Note:*** *Since TNCC skill stations are simulated situations, the use of personal protective equipment is optional.*)

B. Maneuvers to open and clear the airway

1. Assess airway patency in the conscious patient. In the unresponsive patient, manually open the airway using a jaw thrust or chin lift maneuver. Then assess for airway patency by checking the following:

   a. Vocalization

   b. Tongue obstructing airway

   c. Loose teeth or foreign objects

   d. Blood, vomitus, or other secretions

   e. Edema

2. Lifting the patient's mandible lifts the tongue and opens the airway. To position the mandible without hyperextending or flexing the cervical spine, use a jaw thrust or chin lift maneuver.

   a. Jaw thrust maneuver—Stand at the patient's head and lift the mandible forward (see **Figure 4-6**).

b. Reassess airway patency

or

c. Chin lift maneuver—Stand at the side of the patient and place one hand on the victim's forehead to stabilize the head and neck. Grasp the mandible between the thumb and index finger with the other hand and lift the mandible (see **Figure 4-7**).

d. Reassess airway patency

3. Suction to clear the airway of blood, mucus, foreign objects, vomitus, or other materials. Avoid stimulation of the gag reflex.

C. Airway adjuncts

1. Once a patent airway has been established, an airway adjunct may be required to maintain the airway in an open position.

2. A nasopharyngeal airway can be used in responsive or unresponsive patients, but not in patients with facial trauma or a basilar skull fracture.

   a. Use the largest size that will fit in the patient's nostril. Measure the correct length of nasopharyngeal airway by holding the proximal end of the airway at the nares and the distal end should reach the tip of the earlobe.[1]

   b. Lubricate the airway with a water-soluble lubricant prior to insertion

   c. Insert the nasopharyngeal airway with the bevel facing the nasal septum. Direct the airway posteriorly and slightly rotate it toward the ear until the flange rests against the nostril. Avoid inserting the airway into a nostril obstructed by septal deviation, polyps, etc. The majority of available nasal airways are made to insert in the right nostril.[2] If the left nares must be used, the airway must be turned upside down to be sure the bevel faces the septum.[2]

   d. Reassess airway patency

3. An oropharyngeal airway can only be used in unresponsive patients.

   a. Measure the airway by holding the proximal end of the airway at the corner of the mouth and the distal end should reach the tip of the earlobe.

   b. Insert the airway with the distal tip of the oropharyngeal airway turned toward the roof of the mouth. As the airway device passes across the back of the tongue, gently rotate the airway 180 degrees. Do not use this technique on children.

or

   c. Use a tongue depressor to hold the tongue against the floor of the mouth and insert the airway following the curvature of the mouth. The flange should rest against the patient's lips. This technique is recommended for pediatric patients; however, the other method is recommended if a tongue depressor is unavailable.[3]

   d. Reassess airway patency

D. Assess breathing effectiveness

1. Spontaneous breathing
2. Rise and fall of chest
3. Rate and pattern of breathing
4. Use of accessory muscles and/or diaphragmatic breathing
5. Skin color
6. Integrity of the soft tissue and bony structures of the chest wall
7. Bilateral breath sounds

E. Oxygen delivery methods

1. A tight-fitting nonrebreather mask delivers the highest concentration of oxygen to a spontaneously breathing nonintubated patient.

2. A patient with inadequate or absent respirations will require manual ventilation before definitive airway control. See **Table AV-1** Oxygen Delivery Devices[4] for additional information regarding oxygen delivery devices.

F. Bag-mask ventilation

1. A bag-mask device must have an oxygen reservoir system and be connected to an oxygen source.

2. Effective bag-mask ventilation requires a tight seal of the face mask, in conjunction with adequate compression of the bag. Achieving this seal may require two people.

   a. Bag-mask ventilation by one person: Stand at the patient's head and place the narrow end of the mask over the bridge of the patient's nose. Hold the mask firmly with the thumb over the patient's nose; grasp and lift the mandible with the fingers. Compress the bag with the other hand. Individuals with small hands may be able to generate a larger tidal volume by compressing the bag against their bodies.

b. Bag-mask ventilation by two persons: One person stands at the patient's head and places the thumbs on each side of the mask; he or she then grasps and lifts the mandible with the fingers of both hands. The second person stands to the patient's side and compresses the bag.

3. Maintain an oxygen flow rate sufficient to keep the reservoir bag inflated; usually requires 12 to 15 L/minute.

4. Assess for effective ventilation by inspecting for chest rise and fall and skin color.

G. Endotracheal tube placement

1. Once the endotracheal tube cuff has been inflated, proper placement can be confirmed by the following:

a. Observing for the rise and fall of the chest with ventilations.

b. Auscultation over the epigastric area. Endotracheal tube placement is assessed immediately by auscultating over the epigastrium while observing for rise and fall of the chest wall.

c. If stomach gurgling occurs and chest wall expansion is not evident, inadvertent esophageal intubation should be assumed and no further breaths delivered.[5]

d. If the chest rises and falls symmetrically and gastric insufflation is not heard, auscultate the lungs at the sec- ond intercostal space, midclavicular line and at the fifth intercostal space anterior axillary line bilaterally.

e. Equal breath sounds indicate proper endotracheal tube placement. Secure the tube, and continue ventilations.

f. Absent or decreased breath sounds on one side may indicate improper tube placement or a pneumothorax.

g. To rule out improper tube placement, slightly withdraw the tube and reassess breath sounds.

h. Absence of bilateral breath sounds probably indicates esophageal placement; immediately remove the tube and hyperventilate the patient.

2. Additional indicators of correct tube placement include:

a. Direct visualization of the endotracheal tube passing through the cords

b. Normal oxygen saturation (SpO_2 is slow to respond to incorrect tube placement)

c. Many detectors change to n ormal exhaled CO_2 measurement.

Exhaled CO_2 devices are adjuncts, but not substitutes, for determining correct placement of an endotracheal tube. In emergency settings, monitoring carbon dioxide levels to assure proper endotracheal tube placement usually refers to monitoring exhaled carbon dioxide ($PetCO_2$) in a patient who has been endotracheally intubated. After the endotracheal tube has been inserted, a disposable exhaled CO_2 detector can be placed on the end of the tube. The color of the detector changes based on the concentration of carbon dioxide exhaled. Many detectors change to:

• Purple—during inspiration when CO_2 is very low

Table AV-1: Oxygen Delivery Devices

Device	Oxygen Concentration Delivered	Liter Flow (L/min)	Comments
Nasal cannula	24 to 44%	1 to 6	Difficult to tolerate flow > 6 L
Simple face mask	40 to 60%	8 to 10	Minimum flow rate is 5 L per minute
Nonrebreather mask	60 to 90%	12 to 15	Prevents accumulation of CO_2
Bag-mask with oxygen reservoir	60 to 100%	15	Delivers highest concentration of O_2

- Yellow—during expiration when CO_2 is high
- Beige—intermediate concentrations of CO_2

If the device is purple during expiration, the tube is most likely misplaced in the esophagus. Patients who have consumed carbonated beverages may have false (yellow) readings because there is enough carbon dioxide in gastric air. Other exhaled CO_2 sensing devices are available. These devices use a disposable (or reusable if properly cleaned) sensor attached to a portable recording machine. More sophisticated capnometers and capnographs that continuously monitor carbon dioxide concentrations during each breath are used in operating rooms and intensive care units to monitor the patient's respiratory, metabolic, and ventilation to perfusion ratios.[6]

Capnometry measures both inspired and exhaled CO_2 (PetCO$_2$) and is a measured calculation. Capnography equipment displays a wave form of CO_2 as a function of time during ventilation.[7] Some facilities may choose to use capnometers instead of disposable exhaled detectors.

    d.   Chest radiograph confirmation

  3. Inflate the cuff, if not already inflated, and secure endotracheal tube

H. Pulse oximetry

1. Pulse oximetry is an available method to monitor a patient's oxygen saturation or the percentage of hemoglobin saturated with oxygen (SpO$_2$). Pulse oximeters do not measure oxygen tension (PO$_2$) or alveolar ventilation. However, the oxyhemoglobin dissociation curve demonstrates that when the PO$_2$ is 60 mm Hg (8 KPa), the oxygen saturation is approximately 90%, and when the PO$_2$ is 40 mm Hg (5.3 KPa), the oxygen saturation is approximately 75%. Normally, 98% of hemoglobin is saturated with oxygen. At the higher range of oxygen saturation (i.e., 94 to 98%) the oxyhemoglobin dissociation curve is relatively flat; therefore, a small change in oxygen saturation could correlate with significant changes in oxygen tension. The usefulness of pulse oximetry is related to detection of unsuspected hypoxemia.[8]

2. The pulse oximeter probe attached to the patient (usually to a finger) contains light-emitting diodes (LEDs), a photo diode, and a microprocessor that interprets the amount of light in the sensor during a pulse beat. The oxygen saturation is calculated by the oximeter based on the differential absorption of light by the patient's oxyhemoglobin. The probe attached to the patient is connected by a cord to a machine that digitally displays the SpO$_2$ and the pulse (which is also audible).

3. Pulse oximetry has certain limitations related to conditions that may not generate an adequate signal (e.g., vasoconstriction, hypothermia, malplacement of the probe, low tissue perfusion, or dark nail polish). Additionally, certain circumstances may be interpreted by the oximeter as pulsations (e.g., flickering fluorescent lights, hand tremors, or positive pressure ventilation).[8,9] Methemoglobin (oxidation of the iron molecule in the blood from the ferrous to the ferric state caused by injury or toxic substances) and carboxyhemoglobin (hemoglobin combined with carbon monoxide) cannot be distinguished from oxyhemoglobin. If any alteration of hemoglobin is suspected, monitor blood gasses, pH, and oxygen saturation from arterial blood samples.

4. Advantages of pulse oximetry:
   a. Noninvasive and painless
   b. Portable, lightweight, and compact
   c. Less costly as compared to arterial blood gas testing
   d. Adjunct for monitoring the need for intubation, deterioration or improvement of a patient's respiratory status
   e. Can be attached to a finger, earlobe, toe, corner of the mouth, or other available body part

I. Alternative Airways

1. The Combitube™ is a dual-lumen, dual-cuff airway that can be placed blindly into the esophagus (see **Figure 4-9**). Ventilation can occur through either lumen depending on whether it is positioned in the trachea or esophagus. It is

not considered a definitive airway. Its use is contraindicated in patients with an intact gag reflex.[10] Steps for insertion of a Combitube™ include the following:

a. Both cuffs should be completely deflated—check integrity of cuffs prior to insertion

b. Lubricate the tube with a water-soluble lubricant.

c. Hold the tube with the curve in the same direction as the curve of the pharynx. Insert the tip into the patient's mouth until the two black rings on the tube are between the teeth. If the tube does not advance easily, remove it.

d. Inflate the proximal blue cuff (pharyngeal) with 100 ml of air. Inflate the distal white/clear cuff (tracheal) with 15 ml air.

e. Ventilate through the distal blue tube. If there is a rise and fall of the chest, the tube is in the esophagus. Continue to ventilate through the distal tube. Decompress the stomach by placing a gastric tube through the proximal tube.

f. If the chest does not rise and fall, attempt ventilation through the proximal white/clear tube. If the chest rises and falls, the tube is in the trachea (rare). Continue to ventilate through the proximal tube.[10]

g. Complications may include perforation of the esophagus, inadequate ventilation, or aspiration.[10]

2. The laryngeal mask airway (LMA) looks like an endotracheal tube but is equipped with an inflatable, elliptical, silicone rubber collar at the distal end. It is designed to cover the supraglottic area and allow for ventilation. It is not considered a definitive airway.[11] Steps for insertion of an LMA include the following:

a. Check the integrity of the cuff.

b. Coat the posterior surface with a water-soluble lubricant.

c. Position your index finger in the crease between the airway tube and the mask

d. Insert the LMA with the cuff tip gliding against the posterior pharyngeal wall.

e. Use your index finger to push the LMA along the anatomical curve of the pharynx.

f. Advance until you feel resistance.

g. Remove the index finger, but apply slight pressure to the tube so it does not dislodge.

h. Inflate the cuff with air. Release the tube during inflation to ensure proper placement. There should be a slight outward movement of the tube with inflation. You should also note a slight swelling at the cricoid area, equal breath sounds bilaterally, and no visible cuff in the mouth.

i. Some LMAs allow intubation with an endotracheal tube through the LMA.[11]

3. In the rare event that endotracheal intubation cannot be performed, surgical cricothyrotomy may be considered. This procedure is indicated when intubation is necessary but not possible or is contraindicated (i.e., massive facial trauma, fractured larynx, or severe oropharyngeal hemorrhage which obstructs the glottic opening). This procedure is not recommended in children under age 12.[12]

Surgical cricothyrotomy is accomplished by making an incision into the cricothyroid membrane (see **Figure 4-13**) and inserting an endotracheal or tracheostomy tube into the trachea (usually a size 5 or 6 mm tube).[12]

4. When intubation or surgical cricothyrotomy are contraindicated or not possible, needle cricothyrotomy is performed to establish a temporary airway. A large-caliber (12- or 14-gauge) over-the-needle intravenous catheter is inserted through the cricothyroid membrane (see **Figures 4-11 and 4-12**).[12]

5. Several ventilation methods may be used. Transtracheal jet insufflation provides a temporary means of providing oxygen and ventilation to the patient with an airway obstruction until a definitive airway is established. Transtracheal jet insufflation consists of inserting a large-caliber plastic over-the-needle catheter (12- or 14-gauge), through the cricothyroid membrane. The needle is inserted at a 45-degree angle into the trachea, below the oropharyngeal obstruction. Using a plastic "Y" connecting

device inserted into the over-the-needle catheter, oxygen is delivered at a high pressure (30 to 60 psi) in an intermittent fashion (1 insufflation every 5 seconds).[1,12] Since inadequate exhalation results in the patient gradually retaining carbon dioxide, transtracheal jet insufflation should be used for a limited time (not to exceed 45 minutes), especially in the patient with alterations in consciousness. Observe the patient for any signs of complications associated with high pressure ventilation (e.g., tension pneumothorax), especially if the patient is suspected of having an obstruction of the glottis.[12]

J. Learners may practice skills as time permits.

III. Principles of Chest Trauma Interventions

A. General principles

1. A needle thoracentesis may be required to rapidly correct a tension pneumothorax.

2. A chest tube thoracostomy is required to evacuate air or blood from the pleural cavity.

3. Autotransfusion is a procedure to transfuse patients with their own shed blood.

4. Preparation and maintenance of chest drainage systems is a nursing responsibility. Trauma nurses must be familiar with the specific chest drainage units and autotransfusion systems used at their facilities.

B. . Needle thoracentesis

1. Indications: A tension pneumothorax. Signs and symptoms include respiratory distress, hypotension, hypoxia, unilaterally decreased or absent breath sounds, jugular venous distention, and tracheal shift. Cardiac arrest may result if a tension pneumothorax is not promptly decompressed.

2. Precautions:

a. In the absence of a tension pneumothorax, a needle thoracentesis may create a pneumothorax or injure the lung.[13,14]

b. Diaphragmatic rupture with herniation of abdominal contents into the thoracic cavity may mimic a pneumothorax. Needle thoracentesis is not indicated and, if performed, may result in intestinal content contamination of the pleural cavity.[14]

3. Steps for needle thoracentesis

a. The insertion-site is the second intercostal space, midclavicular line. Insert the needle on the same side as the decreased/absent breath sounds, and on the opposite side of the tracheal shift.

b. Insert a 10- to 16-gauge over-the-needle catheter, 3 to 6 cm in length, over the top of the third rib into the pleural space until air escapes.[13,14] Air should exit under pressure. Remove the needle and leave the catheter in place until replaced by a chest tube.

c. Prepare for chest tube insertion since needle thoracentesis is a temporary measure.

C. Chest tube insertion and chest drainage systems

1. Indications: Open or closed pneumothorax or hemothorax. Signs and symptoms of pneumothorax include respiratory distress, decreased or absent breath sounds, and hyperresonance on the injured side. Hemothorax has similar signs and symptoms, except percussion produces dullness. Chest tubes may also be inserted in patients with "substantial chest injury" who require positive pressure ventilation or those who require transfer to another facility.[13]

2. Contraindications: The only contraindication is the need for an immediate open thoracotomy.

3. Chest drainage systems: If air or blood accumulates in the pleural cavity, negative pressure is lost and the lung collapses. The therapeutic goal of drainage devices is restoration of negative pressure. There are two types of chest drainage systems

a. In underwater systems, the water in the water seal chamber has a one-way valve allowing blood or air to escape while preventing backflow.

b. The waterless drainage systems have a mechanical valve in place of water to allow blood and/or air drainage. The one-way valve prevents backflow.

4. Steps for insertion of a chest tube

a. Assemble the chest drainage unit, per manufacturer's directions, by placing sterile water in the water seal chamber (if necessary) and in the suction chamber (if necessary).

b. Ensure the patient has at least one large-caliber intravenous catheter infusing a crystalloid solution.

c. Assist with chest tube insertion by positioning the patient supine, with the head of the bed elevated 45 degrees (if possible) and the arm over the head. Clean the insertion-site, fourth or fifth intercostal space, anterior or midaxillary line.

d After the chest tube is inserted, connect the chest tube to the drainage tubing.

e. Attach suction chamber tubing to wall suction. In water systems, regulate the wall suction to maintain a gentle continuous bubbling action.

f. Tape all tubing connections between the patient and underwater seal or chest drainage unit to prevent inadvertent disconnection.

g. Apply a petroleum-impregnated, occlusive dressing (dressing may vary by institutional protocol) around the chest tube insertion-site and cover with 4 × 4 (10 cm × 10 cm) gauze dressings. Secure the tube with heavy tape.

h. Document correct tube placement by obtaining a chest radiograph to confirm correct tube placement.

i. Managing a chest drainage system

1) Maintain the chest drainage unit below the level of the chest to facilitate the flow of drainage and prevent reflux into the chest cavity. With water seal chest drainage units, keep the unit upright to prevent the loss of the water seal.

2) The tubing should be gently coiled without dependent loops or kinks.

3) Assess and document fluctuation, output, color of drainage, and air leak (FOCA)

4) Consider notifying the physician if initial chest drainage output is > 1,000 ml or there is continued blood loss > 200 ml/hour for 3-4 hours

j. Assessing for an air leak

1) The water level in the water seal chamber should gently rise and fall with each breath. Assess for an air leak by looking for bubbling in the water seal chamber. Constant bubbling in the water seal chamber indicates an air leak either in the lung or in the chest drainage unit or tubing.

2) An air leak is an expected finding with an unexpanded lung.

3) Leaks may originate from[15]
   • The chest tube drainage system
   • A continued air leak in the lung
   • Injury to the esophagus or bronchus
   • A malpositioned chest tube

4) If an air leak is suspected, assess that all connections are tight. Turn off suction and reassess after one minute.

5) To assess the location of the leak, intermittently occlude the chest tube or drainage tubing beginning at the dressing site, progressing to the chest drainage unit, if needed. If the bubbling in the water seal chamber immediately stops when the chest tube is occluded at the dressing site, the air leak is inside the patient's chest or under the dressing. Reinforce the occlusive dressing and notify the physician.[16]

6) If the bubbling does not stop when the chest tube is occluded at the dressing site, continue to intermittently occlude down the tubing at various positions until the bubbling stops. When the bubbling stops, the air leak is between the occlusion and the patient's chest.

7) If the bubbling does not stop with occlusion, replace the chest drainage unit.

k. Assessing tube patency

If a clot is suspected, as when fresh bleeding suddenly stops or slows, gently manipulate the tube by squeezing the drainage tubing in a proximal to distal direction. Do not squeeze or "milk" the tube enough to collapse it as it may increase the negative pressure. The need to dislodge a suspected clot is the only indication for squeezing the drainage tubing.[16]

l. Clamping the chest tube

During patient transport, clamping of chest tubes is not necessary. Clamping a chest tube if there is an ongoing air leak from the original injury may lead to the development of a tension pneumothorax.

m. Using a one-way valve

A one-way valve is used primarily during transport to ensure one-way drainage in the event the chest drainage unit is damaged or placed above the level of the chest. The one-way valve may also be used temporarily until a chest drainage unit is obtained. In addition, it is sometimes used instead of a chest drainage unit for a small, spontaneous pneumothorax (see **Figure 4-15**).

D. Autotransfusion

1. Indications: To transfuse patients with their own shed blood. In the emergency department, autotransfusion is usually limited to blood drained from a hemothorax. In significant chest trauma, autotransfusion should be anticipated and the collection device prepared before chest tube insertion, if possible.

2. Precautions/contraindications:

a. Blood contaminated with bowel contents or infection at the site of blood retrieval. Blood salvaged from a bacteria-contaminated cavity is considered in dire emergencies or when no alternative source of blood is available.[17]

b. Blood potentially contaminated with malignant cells[17]

c. Carefully consider autotransfusion in patients with hepatic or renal dysfunction

IV. Summary

A. The Airway and Ventilation Interventions Skill Station presents learners with information regarding the assessment of and interventions for airway and ventilation.

B. Principles and points to remember

1. The first priority in trauma care is the establishment of a patent airway.

2. Avoid stimulation of the gag reflex during suctioning

3. Avoid nasal airways in patients with severe head and/or facial trauma

4. Do not use oropharyngeal airways in a patient with a gag reflex

5. To confirm endotracheal placement observe for rise and fall of the chest and auscultate over the epigastrium. If the chest rises and falls symmetrically and gastric insufflation is not heard, auscultate the lungs at the second intercostal space, midclavicular line, and at the fifth intercostal space anterior axillary line bilaterally.

6. Breath sounds that are consistently louder on one side despite efforts at repositioning the endotracheal tube may signal a pneumothorax or hemothorax.

7. Ventilate the patient between all intubation attempts

8. Prolonged clamping of a chest tube is contraindicated because it may precipitate the development of a tension pneumothorax if there is an ongoing air leak.

9. Obtain chest radiographs following chest tube insertion to document tube placement and verify lung re-expansion

10. Avoid squeezing the chest tube to the point of collapse as it may cause lung injury

References

1. Gupton, C., & Dalton, A. (1999). Airway. In B. D. Browner, L. M. Jacobs, & A. N. Pollack (Eds.), *American academy of orthopedic surgeons* (7th ed., pp. 166–197). Boston: Jones and Bartlett.

2. Clark, D. Y. (2004). Nasal airway insertion. In J. A. Proehl (Ed.), *Emergency nursing procedures* (3rd ed., pp.21–23). St. Louis, MO: W. B. Saunders.

3. Emergency Cardiac Care Committee and Subcommittees, American Heart Association. (2005). Pediatric advanced life support. *Circulation*, 112, 167–187.

4. Branson, R. D. (1995). Gas delivery system: Regulators, flow meters and therapy devices. In R. D. Branson, D. R. Heff, & R. L. Chatburn (Eds.), *Respiratory care equipment* (pp. 48–72). Philadelphia: Lippincott.

5. Emergency Cardiac Care Committee and Subcommittees, American Heart Association. (2005). Adjuncts for airway control and ventilation. *Circulation*, 112, 51–57.

6. Bongard, F. S., & Sue, D. Y. (1994). Critical care monitoring. In F. S. Bongard & D. Y. Sue (Eds.), *Current critical care diagnosis and treatment* (pp. 170–190). Norwalk, CT: Appleton & Lange.

7. Heff, D. R., & Branson, R. D. (1995). Noninvasive respiratory monitoring equipment. In R. D. Branson, D. R. Heff, & R. L. Chatburn (Eds.), *Respiratory care equipment* (pp. 184–215). Philadelphia: Lippincott.

8. Hedges, J. R., Baker, W. E., Lanoix, R., & Field, D. L. (2004). Use of monitoring devices for assessing ventilation and oxygenation. In J. R. Roberts & J. R. Hedges (Eds.), *Clinical procedures in emergency medicine* (4th ed., pp. 29–50). Philadelphia: W. B. Saunders.

9. Padolina, R. M., & Siler, J. N. (1993). Monitoring for trauma anesthesia. In C. M. Grande (Ed.), *Textbook of trauma anesthesia and critical care* (pp. 432–444). St. Louis, MO: Mosby-Year Book.

10. Clark, D. Y. (2004). Combitube airway. In J. A. Proehl (Ed.), *Emergency nursing procedures* (3rd ed., pp.65–68). St. Louis, MO: W. B. Saunders.

11. Clark, D. Y. (2004). Laryngeal mask airway. In J. A. Proehl (Ed.), *Emergency nursing procedures* (3rd ed., pp.24–32). St. Louis, MO: W. B. Saunders.

12. American College of Surgeons Committee on Trauma. (2004). Airway and ventilatory management. In *Advanced trauma life support for doctors®: Student course manual* (7th ed., pp.41–68). Chicago: Author.

13. American College of Surgeons Committee on Trauma. (2004). Thoracic trauma. In *Advanced trauma life support program for doctors®*: Student course manual (7th ed., pp.103–129). Chicago, IL: Author.

14. Upton, D. A. (2004). Emergency needle thoracentesis. In J. A. Proehl (Ed.), *Emergency nursing procedures* (3rd ed., pp.178–181). St. Louis, MO: W. B. Saunders.

15. Livingston, D. H., & Hauser, C. J. (2004). Trauma to the chest wall and lung. In E. E. Moore, D. V. Feliciano, & K. L. Mattox (Eds.), *Trauma* (5th ed., pp. 507–538). New York: McGraw-Hill.

16. Upton, D. A. (2004). Management of chest drainage systems. In J. A. Proehl (Ed.), *Emergency nursing procedures* (3rd ed., pp. 187–188). St. Louis, MO: W. B. Saunders.

17. Upton, D. A. & Proehl, J. A. (2004). General principles of autotransfusion. In J. A. Proehl (Ed.), *Emergency nursing procedures* (3rd ed., pp. 354–356). St. Louis, MO: W. B. Saunders.

Airway and Ventilation Station: Teaching Scenario 1

Prehospital MIVT Report

A 22-year-old male hit a tree while riding his motorcycle. He was thrown 20 feet (6 m), was not wearing a helmet, and had multiple facial fractures. EMS reports that the patient was unconscious at the scene. The basic responders are assisting respirations using a bag-mask device. Cervical spine protection was initiated, and the patient is in complete spinal immobilization. The patient has just arrived in the emergency department and remains unresponsive. Please proceed with your assessment and appropriate interventions.

Focus of this teaching station: Review of rapid sequence intubation and airway rescue after failed RSI

Skill Steps	Instructor Responses	Demonstrated Yes	No
1. Assesses airway patency; AND if unresponsive, manually opens the airway using a jaw thrust or chin lift (states at least 3 of the following):		* ___	___
• Vocalization	• Patient does not vocalize		
• Tongue obstructing airway	• No obstruction by the tongue		
• Loose teeth or foreign objects	• No loose teeth or foreign objects		
• Blood, vomitus, or other secretions	• Blood and vomitus are present in the oropharynx		
• Edema	• No edema noted		
2. Maintains spinal immobilization.		___	___
3. Suctions the airway.	• When the learner performs the skill correctly, say: *"The airway has been suctioned."*	* ___	___
4. States need for an airway adjunct.		* ___	___
5. Demonstrates AND inserts an oral airway		* ___	___
• Measures to determine appropriate size	• Airway is patent (Use of a nasopharyngeal airway is not appropriate in a patient with facial fractures)		
• Inserts oral airway using tongue blade			
6. Assesses breathing effectiveness (states at least 3 of the following):		* ___	___
• Spontaneous breathing	• Poor respiratory effort		
• Rise and fall of chest	• Symmetrical		
• Rate and pattern of breathing	• Respiratory rate is slow, 6 breaths/minute		
• Use of accessory muscles and/or diaphragmatic breathing	• Minimal respiratory effort—no accessory muscle use or diaphragmatic breathing present		
• Skin color	• Pale with circumoral cyanosis		
• Integrity of the soft tissue and bony structures of the chest wall	• Multiple ecchymotic areas noted across anterior chest; chest wall intact		
• Bilateral breath sounds	• Decreased breath sounds bilaterally		

Skill Steps	Instructor Responses	Demonstrated Yes	No
7. States need for intubation. Continues assisted ventilation while preparing for intubation.	*"There is good rise and fall of the chest with assisted ventilations. Skin is pale."*	*___	___
"The physician elects to intubate the patient using rapid sequence intubation. What is your preparation for rapid sequence intubation?"			
8. Verbalizes preparation criteria for rapid sequence intubation: • Preparation • Preoxygenation • Pretreatment • Paralysis with induction • Protection and positioning • Placement with proof (of successful intubation) • Postintubation management ▪ Ordering a chest radiograph ▪ Acquiring a ventilator		*___	___
"Rapid sequence intubation medications have been administered. After several attempts the emergency care practitioner is unable to intubate. What are your next steps?"			
9. Resumes assisted ventilation. • Replaces oral airway, **AND** • Ventilates patient with bag-mask device, **AND** • Assesses effectiveness of ventilation	*"Ventilation is adequately maintained."*	___	___
"What are alternative methods for airway control?"			
10. States alternative methods to facilitate airway capture/control (states at least 2 of the following): • Contact alternate provider experienced in intubation (e.g., anesthesiologist) • Use different type of airway device (laryngeal mask airway [LMA™], Combitube™) • Consider duration of action of neuromuscular blocking agent and continue assisting the patient's ventilations until spontaneous respirations return • Consider the need for a surgical airway	Instructor and learners will discuss alternative airway management methods	___	___

Airway and Ventilation Station: Teaching Scenario 2

Prehospital MIVT Report

A 62-year-old female fell down four steps at the post office, hit her head, and lost consciousness. She was found apneic and was intubated by emergency medical services. History given by her family revealed that she is receiving anticoagulant therapy (warfarin sodium) for atrial fibrillation. Cervical spine protection was initiated, and the patient is in complete spinal immobilization. The patient has just arrived in the emergency department. Please proceed with your assessment and appropriate interventions.

Focus of this teaching station: Endotracheal tube patency and position

Skill Steps	Instructor Responses	Demonstrated Yes	No
1. Assesses airway patency (states at least 3 of the following):		*____	____
• Vocalization	• Patient does not vocalize		
• Tongue obstructing airway	• No obstruction by the tongue		
• Loose teeth or foreign objects	• No loose teeth or foreign objects		
• Blood, vomitus, or other secretions	• None noted in the oropharynx		
• Edema	• None noted		
The patient had a 7.5 endotracheal tube placed by EMS. What additional parameters need to be assessed to determine airway patency?			
2. Blood, vomitus, or other secretions in the endotracheal tube	• Visible secretions are present in the tube	____	____
3. States need to suction the endotracheal tube and oropharynx.	"The endotracheal tube has been suctioned."	*____	____
4. Reassesses endotracheal tube patency after suctioning	• No blood in the endotracheal tube or oropharynx	*____	____
5. Assesses endotracheal tube placement (states at least 2 of the following):		*____	____
• Observes for rise and fall of the chest with bag-valve ventilations	• No rise and fall of the chest with bag-valve ventilations		
• Auscultates over the epigastric area, **AND** then auscultates bilateral breath sounds	• No breath sounds are heard on auscultation of chest. Gurgling sounds are heard over the epigastrium with assisted ventilation		
• Uses an exhaled CO_2 detector	• Exhaled CO_2 detector shows no color change, numerical value of 8, dampened wave form.		
	• Abdomen is grossly distended		
If learner elects to use esophageal detector device (EDD), state that it is only used to verify tube placement immediately after intubation.			

Skill Steps	Instructor Responses	Demonstrated	
		Yes	No
6. Recognizes improper endotracheal tube placement, makes sure suction is available and removes endotracheal tube.		* ___	___
7. Places oropharyngeal airway.		___	___
8. Ventilates patient via bag-mask device.		___	___
9. Assesses effectiveness of ventilations (states at least 3 of the following): • Spontaneous breathing • Rise and fall of chest • Rate and pattern of breathing • Use of accessory muscles and/or diaphragmatic breathing • Skin color • Integrity of the soft tissue and bony structures of the chest wall • Breath sounds	 • No spontaneous respirations • Equal rise and fall with assisted ventilations •Assisted ventilations with bag-valve device • No use of accessory muscles or diaphragmatic breathing note • Pale • Chest wall intact without any ecchymosis • Bilateral breath sounds present	* ___	___
Instructor response: *"The physician has reintubated the patient. What is your next step?"*			
10. Assesses endotracheal tube placement (states at least 2 of the following): • Observes for rise and fall of the chest with bag-valve ventilations. • Auscultates over the epigastric area, **AND** then auscultates bilateral breath sounds. • Uses an exhaled CO_2 detector or esophageal detector device (EDD).	 • Bilateral rise and fall of the chest are observed with assisted ventilation • Breath sounds are equal and clear bilaterally. No gurgling sounds heard over the epigastrium. • Exhaled CO_2 detector changes color; or no resistance is felt when pulling back on syringe of EDD	* ___	___
11. States need to secure endotracheal tube and continue ventilations.		___	___
12. Considers insertion of gastric tube to decompress the patient's abdomen		___	___

Airway and Ventilation Station: Teaching Scenario 3

Prehospital MIVT Report

A 35-year-old male was involved in an explosion in which he was thrown 15 feet (4.5 m) and hit a wall. He sustained blunt chest trauma and facial burns and was noted to have soot around his mouth. Prehospital providers report that at the scene the patient had a decreased level of consciousness and respiratory distress, which required intubation. Cervical spine protection was initiated, and the patient is in complete spinal immobilization. Blood pressure is 70/40 mm Hg, pulse 120 beats/minute, and the patient is being ventilated with a bag-valve device. Prehospital providers report he is becoming more difficult to ventilate. The patient has just arrived in the emergency department. Please proceed with your assessment and appropriate interventions.

Focus of this teaching station: Management of tension pneumothorax in an intubated patient

Skill Steps	Instructor Responses	Demonstrated Yes	No
1. Assesses airway patency (states at least 3 of the following): • Vocalization • Tongue obstructing airway • Loose teeth or foreign objects • Blood, vomitus, or other secretions • Edema	• Patient does not vocalize • No obstruction by the tongue • None seen • No secretions noted • No edema • A 7.5 endotracheal tube is in place	* ____	____
2. Maintains spinal immobilization.		____	____
Airway is patent. Proceed with assessment of endotracheal tube placement.			
3. Assesses endotracheal tube placement (states at least 2 of the following): • Observes for rise and fall of the chest with bag-valve ventilations • Auscultates over the epigastric area **AND** then auscultates bilateral breath sounds • Uses an exhaled CO_2 detector	• No chest rise noted on the right and difficulty ventilating. • No gurgling over epigastrium. No breath sounds heard on right. • Exhaled CO_2 detector color change confirms placement. • The physician has visualized that the tube is through the cords. • Tube remains secured.	* ____	____

Skill Steps	Instructor Responses	Demonstrated	
		Yes	No
4. Assesses effectiveness of ventilations (states at least 3 of the following):		* ___	___
• Spontaneous breathing	• No spontaneous respirations		
• Rise and fall of chest	• No chest rise on the right		
• Rate and pattern of breathing	• Assisted ventilations with bag-valve device; increased difficulty ventilating the patient		
• Use of accessory muscles and/or diaphragmatic breathing	• No use of accessory muscles or diaphragmatic breathing noted		
• Skin color	• Pale		
• Integrity of the soft tissue and bony structures of the chest wall	• Ecchymosis and abrasions to right chest		
• Bilateral breath sounds	• No breath sounds on the right side		
If the student continues to assess endotracheal tube placement, emphasize that the tube is patent but that ventilating the patient is becoming increasingly difficult.			
5. Identifies tension pneumothorax and states need for needle decompression.	• Please proceed with demonstration of needle decompression.	* ___	___
6. Describes procedure for needle decompression.	• Needle decompression has been completed	* ___	___
• Identifies equipment needed - large (14- or 16-gauge) needle or pneumothorax decompression kit			
• Identifies landmarks for insertion—second intercostal space midclavicular line on the side of the pneumothorax			
• Identifies angle of insertion—90° angle			
7. Reassesses effectiveness of ventilations.	• Patient is easier to ventilate	___	___
	• Color improves		
	• Breath sounds improved on right side		
"What is your next step?"			
8. Prepare for chest tube insertion.		___	___

Airway and Ventilation Station: Teaching Scenario 4

Patient Information

A 28-year-old female arrived in the emergency department after falling off her horse. She was wearing a helmet. There was no loss of consciousness. The patient complained of shortness of breath upon arrival and was diagnosed with a left pneumothorax. A chest tube was inserted, with improvement noted. The cervical spine has been cleared. Oxygen via nonrebreather mask is being administered. The patient is waiting for admission to the floor. When the emergency nurse assesses the patient after change of shift report, the patient is found to be anxious and complaining of shortness of breath. Her heart rate increased from 80 beats/minute to 110 beats/minute, her respiratory rate increased from 16 to 28 breaths/minute, and her SpO_2 decreased from 98% to 90%. Her skin is moist and she is anxious. Please proceed with your assessment and appropriate interventions.

Focus of this teaching station: Management of chest tube malfunction

Skill Steps	Instructor Responses	Demonstrated Yes	No
1. **Assesses airway patency (states at least 3 of the following):**		*_____	_____
• Vocalization	• Patient speaking		
• Tongue obstructing airway	• No obstruction by the tongue		
• Loose teeth or foreign objects	• No loose teeth or foreign objects		
• Blood, vomitus, or other secretions	• No secretions noted		
• Edema	• No edema		
Instructor states that the patient's airway is patent.			
2. **Assesses breathing effectiveness (states at least 3 of the following):**		*_____	_____
• Spontaneous breathing	• Spontaneous breathing, patient is anxious		
• Rise and fall of chest	• Symmetrical rise and fall of the chest		
• Rate and pattern of breathing	• Rapid at 28 breaths/minute		
• Use of accessory muscles and/or diaphragmatic breathing	• Use of accessory muscles noted		
• Skin color	• Color is pale; SpO_2 90%		
• Integrity of the soft tissue and bony structures of the chest wall	• Chest tube on the left		
• Bilateral breath sounds	• Breath sounds are decreased on the left side		
3. **Identifies need to assess the patency of the chest tube**		*_____	_____
4. **Evaluates chest tube set-up.**		*_____	_____
• Looks for bubbling in the collection device.	• No bubbling		
• Evaluates patency of the chest tube.	• No drainage		
• Looks for fluctuation of fluid in the chest tube	• No fluctuation noted		
• Evaluates position of the chest tube.	• Tubing is kinked		

Skill Steps	Instructor Responses	Demonstrated	
		Yes	No
5. Straightens tubing and reassesses	• Patient improves—less anxious and respiratory rate improved • Bubbling present • Drainage now present • Fluctuation noted in tubing	_____	_____

6. Discusses other causes of chest tube malfunction
D: Displacement
O: Obstruction
P: Pneumothorax
E: Equipment failure
	• Discuss trouble shooting techniques for chest tubes.
	• Discuss other problem that may occur with chest tubes:
	  ▪ Chest tube inadvertently pulled out during transfer
	  ▪ Closed chest tube system kicked over and broken
	  ▪ Large amount of bleeding from chest tube
	  ▪ Thick drainage in tube—how to assist with drainage and avoid milking the tube
		_____	_____

Spinal Protection, Helmet Removal, and Splinting

I. Introduction to the Skill Station

A. Instructor and learner introductions

B. Purpose

1. The instructor will discuss and demonstrate:

   a. Principles of spinal protection

   b. Importance of the leader in direction of the procedure and instructing assistants

   c. Helmet removal method

   d. Application of a rigid cervical collar

   e. Logrolling the patient

   f. Removing the patient from the backboard

   g. Application of traction splint device

2. Each learner will:

   a. Act as the team leader

   b. Demonstrate helmet removal

   c. Demonstrate the application of a rigid cervical collar

   d. Demonstrate logrolling the patient off of the backboard

3. It is highly recommended that the participants also rotate as the patient on teaching day unless contraindicated.

C. Evaluation

1. This is not a testing station. Learners will receive verbal feedback and participate in a question and answer session related to the specific techniques and topics.

2. Material presented in this skill station may be included on the written exam.

II. Principles of Spinal Protection

A. General principles

1. The leader is responsible for verbally directing the procedure and instructing assistants.

2. The leader is responsible for stabilizing the patient's head and cervical spine during the removal of the helmet, application of the rigid cervical collar, and logrolling the patient off the backboard.

3. Additional assistants are required to perform this skill utilizing a team approach.

4. All unresponsive trauma patients must have their cervical spines protected. An unresponsive trauma patient is assumed to have a spinal injury until definitive evaluation is completed. Although cervical spine injury is a fairly infrequent occurrence (1 to 3% of blunt trauma cases), the results can be devastating.[1] Absence of fracture on a lateral cervical spine radiograph does not necessarily rule out cervical spine injury. All responsive patients that are assessed and treated on scene or who arrive in the emergency department with a significant mechanism of injury and complaint of neck pain should be immobilized. For the patient with a suspected spinal injury, it is important for the emergency nurse to be knowledgeable regarding care and movement of the patient while immobilized.

5. Patients should receive a thorough physical exam by a qualified provider and the appropriate imaging studies completed prior to the removal of any spinal immobilization devices.

6. Cervical collars alone do not immobilize the cervical spine. The head and torso must also be immobilized to prevent flexion, extension, rotation, and lateral movements. The backboard acts as a splint for the entire vertebral column. Straps secure the patient to the backboard.

7. There are no contraindications to helmet removal.[2] With a helmet in place, the airway cannot be monitored and it is difficult to correctly position the patient. Any patient who has been injured while wearing protective head gear should have the gear removed.

8. In actual patient care, all personnel who anticipate direct patient contact or contact with the patient's bodily fluids must wear gown, gloves, masks, and eye protection per institutional protocols.

B. Indications

1. Any patient whose mechanism of injury, symptoms, or physical findings suggest a spinal injury.

2. The following are associated with potential spinal injury:

   a. Mechanisms of injury

      1) Motor vehicle crash

      2) Falls

      3) Diving injury

      4) Near-drowning

      5) Direct force applied to spine or head

      6) Missile and other penetrating trauma to spine

      7) Ejection from vehicle

      8) Spontaneous structural failure from preexisting bone disease (e.g., compression fracture due to osteoporosis or cancer)

   b. Symptoms

      1) Neck pain and tenderness: posterior or anterior

      2) Occipital headache

      3) Back pain

      4) Paresthesia

      5) Paralysis/weakness

   c. Physical findings

      1) Head injury: laceration, contusion, hematoma, fracture

      2) Alteration in level of consciousness

      3) Edema and tenderness over spine

      4) Muscle spasm of neck/back/shoulders

      5) Penetrating wounds of neck or vertebral column

      6) Impaled object in neck or vertebral column

      7) Respiratory compromise

      8) Loss of urinary and/or sphincter tone

      9) Bradycardia and hypotension

C. Contraindications

1. Patients with a compromised airway (e.g., facial trauma) who sit up and lean forward, or stand and lean over, must not be forced to immediately lie down. Prepare for immediate and definitive control of their airway.

2. Insufficient number of assistants

3. Massive neck swelling as a result of tracheal injury or hemorrhage may preclude cervical collar use. The compression effect of the collar may compromise the airway or affect cerebral perfusion and intracranial pressure. Stabilization with a bilateral head support device is indicated.

III. Steps in Skill Performance

A. Leader approaches the patient and initiates cervical spine protection by placing one hand on the mandible (chin) and the other under the occiput.

Tell the learner: "I am going to demonstrate, and then I will have you return the demonstration."

1. Leader approaches the patient and applies manual in-line stabilization by placing his/her hands on the side of the patient's helmet with the fingers on the mandible. Leader will introduce self and instruct patient not to move his/her head throughout the procedure. Assistant #1 will cut or remove the helmet straps.

2. Assistant #1 will place one hand along the mandible, with thumb on one side and the remaining fingers on the other side while simultaneously using the other hand to support and place pressure on the occipital ridge. With this maneuver, Assistant #1 assumes control of in-line stabilization of the patient's head and neck.

   Warning: *"the head drops as the helmet is removed unless adequate support is provided posteriorly to the occipital ridges."*[3]

3. The leader will now be responsible for removing the helmet. The Leader positions his/her hands on each side of the helmet, applying firm, gentle lateral (outwards) pressure to the helmet.

4. The Leader removes helmet in a longitudinal direction (straight back). A full-face helmet will require tipping the helmet up and backward in order to clear the nose of the patient.[3]

5. It is recommended that a pad or folded towel be placed beneath the Leader's hand supporting the occiput.

6. Assistant #1 is responsible for ensuring that in-line stabilization is maintained throughout the removal procedure.

7. Once the helmet is removed, the Leader will then place his/her hands on the side of the patient's head with palms over ears and fingers under the edge of the mandible.[4]

B. Application of a rigid cervical collar

1. The Leader maintains in-line stabilization from above while Assistant #1 sizes and applies the rigid cervical collar.

2. A properly fitted collar will fit between the point of the chin and the suprasternal notch, resting on the clavicles and supporting the lower jaw.
   The Stifneck Select© collar is one type of rigid collar. To properly size and apply a Stifneck Select© collar:

   a. Determine the appropriate size by measuring from the patient's chin to the top of the shoulder. Place your fingers on the top of the shoulder where the collar will rest, and measure the distance to the point of the chin (not the angle of the jaw). Compare this distance on the collar by placing the same number of fingers on the hard plastic edge by the size windows. The correct size collar is equal to the measurement between the hard plastic edge (not the foam portion) and the size window at the top of the fingers.

   b. Adjust the chin support to the appropriate size and lock both sides by pressing the two lock tabs.

   c. Pre-form the collar.

   d. Slide the rear panel of the collar under the patient's neck until the Velcro® can be seen on the patient's other side.

   e. Slide the collar up the sternum until the chin piece fits snugly under the chin.

   f. Secure and fasten the Velcro®.
      Note: *Always follow the manufacturer's directions for correct application of the cervical collar.*

C. Logrolling of patient off backboard

1. The Leader directs Assistant #1 and Assistant #2 to position themselves on the same side with one at the patient's shoulders and one at the hips.

   a. On the Leader's count, the patient is then logrolled toward the assistants.

2. It is imperative that the spine remains straight, without a twisting motion. The Leader should ensure that the patient's nose remains in line with the umbilicus.

3. On the Leader's count, the patient will be rolled back to the supine position.

4. The Leader continually maintains manual stabilization of the head and neck until the rigid cervical collar has been applied and the patient has been logrolled from the board.

5. The Leader will release the manual in-line stabilization.

IV. Traction Splint Application

A. Discussion

1. Life-threatening conditions are always assessed and treated first.

2. Femur fractures may result in:

   a. Spasms of large thigh muscles

   b. Deformity of the extremity with shortening of affected limb

   c. Vascular injury

   d. Significant blood loss
      Blood loss of 750 to 1500 ml in an adult can result in hypovolemic shock.

   e. Pain

3. Complications of femur fractures include:

   a. Nerve injury

   b. Fat embolism

   c. Chronic pain

   d. Infection

4. Consider pain medication prior to application of the splint, based upon patient's hemodynamic status.

5. Traction provides immobilization by producing enough opposing force (counter traction) to stabilize the leg and prevent further injury. It does not realign ends of the fractured bones. Traction decreases the diameter of the thigh by increasing the length of the thigh compartment; this provides a tamponade effect. The upper body is used as the counter traction to the device.

6. Do not attempt to reposition protruding

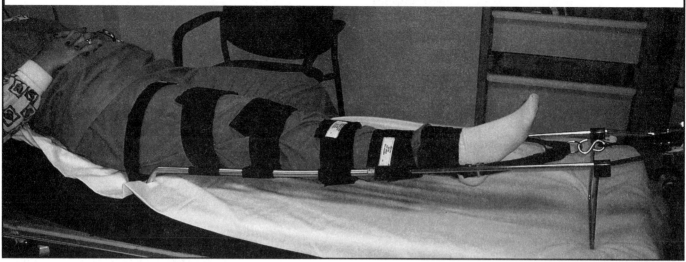

Hare traction splint in place to stabilize a femoral shaft fracture and aid in transport.

bone ends. If the bone end retracts under the skin while traction is being applied, do not apply any further traction.

7. Cover any wound with a dry, sterile dressing. Tetanus immunization status and antibiotic administration should be considered.

8. Radiographs can be taken with the splint in place.

9. Contraindications to traction splinting

   a. Injury to hip

   b. Injury to pelvis

   c. Any additional fracture to the injured extremity

   d. Injury close to or involving the knee

   e. Any leg injury involving a partial amputation

B. Key steps in the Demonstration of Traction Splinting

1. Display traction splint (as guided by local practice)

2. An assistant is required to perform this skill.

3. Assess neurovascular status before applying traction splint.

4. Measure patient and adjust traction splint along the uninjured leg.

5. Remove the patient's shoe and clothing from the injured leg. Ensure contents of pockets are empty and valuables secured.

6. Apply manual traction to injured leg and

maintain until traction splint is applied.

7. Apply splint per manufacturer's instructions.

8. Assess distal neurovascular status after splinting. If neurovascular function is present before, but not after splinting, remove the splint, re-evaluate, and re-splint.

9. Once traction has been applied to extremity, do not release until definitive care has begun.

   Note: Always follow the manufacturer's directions for correct application of the traction splint device that is used at a specific facility.

V. Summary

A. This skill station allows learners to practice the techniques of helmet removal, manual stabilization of a patient's neck, application of a rigid cervical collar, protection of patient's spinal column, and the application of a traction splint (optional).

B. Principle points to remember

1. An unresponsive trauma patient is assumed to have a spinal injury until definitive evaluation is completed.

2. Absence of fracture on a lateral cervical spine radiograph does not necessarily rule out cervical spine injury.

3. A patient with suspected spinal injury or in a high-risk category for spinal injury that is not on a backboard needs to be

evaluated first for life-threatening injuries.

4. If patient is pregnant, she will need to be secured to the backboard in a side-tilted position-approximately 15° to 20° to the left.

5. Maintaining the patient on a backboard for longer than two hours may increase the risk for skin breakdown. Apply padding to bony prominences (occiput, scapulae, sacrum, and heels) as soon as possible, and the patient should be removed from the backboard as soon as his or her condition warrants.[5]

6. Traction splints should be kept in place during transport and traction should not be released until more definitive care is available.

References

1. Cydulka, R. K. (2004). Severity of cervical spine ligamentous injury correlates with mechanism of injury, not with severity of blunt head trauma. *Annals of Emergency Medicine*, 43(1), 144–145.

2. Remz, R. (2001). Training medical personnel in techniques for proper motorcycle helmet removal. Washington, DC: The Motorcycle Riders Foundation.

3. Madigan, K. & Proehl, J. (2004). Helmet removal. In J. Proehl (Ed.), *Emergency nursing procedures* (3rd ed., pp. 533–535). St. Louis, MO: Elsevier.

4. American College of Surgeons. (1997). Helmet removal from injured patients. Retrieved October 21, 2006, from http://www.facs.org/trauma/publications/helmet.pdf

5. American College of Surgeons. (2004). Spine & spinal cord trauma. In *Advanced trauma life support® for doctors:* Student course manual (7th ed., pp. 197–203). Chicago: American College of Surgeons.

Websites:

http://www.haretractionsplint.com/hare_splint_users_guide.pdf

http://www.sagersplints.com/pages/instruct-pack.html

Spinal Protection and Helmet Removal Teaching Scenario

Prehospital MIVT Report

A 24-year-old male arrives in the emergency department after being thrown over the handlebars while riding his motorcycle. He is on a backboard and is still wearing his motorcycle helmet. There was no loss of consciousness but there is obvious scraping along the side of the helmet. He is alert, oriented, in no acute respiratory distress, and he is complaining of neck pain.

Skill Steps-Leader	Demonstrated	
	Yes	No
1. Approaches patient, applies manual in-line stabilization, and informs patient not to turn neck or head.	❑	❑
2. Explains the procedure to the patient to alleviate anxiety.	❑	❑
3. Assesses baseline motor and sensory function.	❑	❑
4. Calls for assistant(s) and appropriate supplies.	❑	❑
5. Directs Assistant #1 to place one hand along the mandible, with thumb on one side and the remaining fingers on the other side while simultaneously using the other hand to support and place pressure on the occipital ridge.	❑	❑
6. Positions his or her hands on each side of the helmet, applying firm, gentle lateral (outwards) pressure.	❑	❑
7. Removes helmet in longitudinal direction; if full-face helmet, will have to be tipped upwards and backwards	❑	❑
8. Assumes control of the patient's head by applying manual in-line stabilization by placing hands on the side of patient's head and fingers underneath mandible.	❑	❑
9. Directs Assistant #1 to measure and apply a rigid cervical collar on the patient.	❑	❑
10. Directs Assistant #1 and #2 to the one side of patient's body at shoulders and pelvis. Directs Assistant #3 to the opposite side.	❑	❑
11. On Leader's count, Leader directs logrolling of patient off of backboard while maintaining in-line manual stabilization. Directs assistant #3 to inspect and palpate along length of patient's spinal processes and then remove backboard.	❑	❑
12. On Leader's count, slowly returns the patient to the supine position, maintaining in-line manual stabilization.	❑	❑
13. Reassesses the sensory and motor functions.	❑	❑

Physical Assessment Station

Optional for courses in the United States

I. Introduction To The Skill Station

A. Purpose

1. Each learner will have an opportunity to practice the skills of inspection, palpation, percussion, and auscultation while performing a physical assessment.

2. The instructor will assist the learner to describe and demonstrate assessment of

   a. Head, neck, ears, and eyes

   b. Chest

   c. Abdomen

   d. Pelvis and external genitalia

   e. Extremities

   f. Posterior surfaces

3. This is a teaching station only

II. Principles of Physical Assessment

A. General principles

1. The assessment of injured patients is sequential, cumulative, and collaborative.

2. The physical assessment of a trauma patient consists of two components, the primary assessment and the secondary assessment.

3. The primary assessment is directed toward identifying the life-threatening injuries and implementing immediate interventions.

4. The secondary assessment that follows is cumulative, adding more detailed and extensive assessments directed toward identifying the less obvious injuries that may have been sustained.

5. Four basic skills are used during physical assessment: inspection, palpation, percussion, and auscultation.

B. Inspection

1. Inspection is the first assessment skill used. A quick general inspection of the patient is done followed by a more detailed inspection. Inspection is the use of vision and smell to detect characteristics or significant physical signs of injury.

Generally, inspection is the simplest technique to perform, but is under-appreciated in physical assessment. It is important to recognize variations among people that are considered normal variants.

2. Inspect every body part thoroughly and systematically. To do this effectively, good lighting and exposure are required. Each area of the body is inspected for size, shape, color, position, and symmetry with the opposite side of the body. The presence of any abnormalities is noted.

3. Inspection is generally considered a visual skill, but also can include smell because the sense of smell can sometimes detect abnormalities that may not be recognized by other means. For example, certain smells, such as alcohol, petroleum products, or other chemicals may have clinical significance in the patient's ongoing management. While smells, in many cases, are difficult to describe, experience is generally the best guide in making judgments about odors detected during assessment.

4. Inspection includes observing a patient's behavior, nonverbal cues, and indicators of anxiety, stress and/or fears.

C. Palpation

1. Palpation is the use of hands to touch body parts, resulting in sensitive assessments and measurements. Palpation is used to examine all body parts to detect characteristics of texture, shape, temperature, response, and movement.

2. To effectively palpate any area of the body, the patient must be relaxed and comfortably positioned to avoid muscle tension that may distort palpation findings. Areas that are known to be tender or painful should be palpated last.

3. The fingertips are the most sensitive parts of the examiner's hand. Alterations in the characteristics of texture, shape, size, and consistency can be detected because of

this sensitivity.

4. Other parts of the hand also serve important assessment functions. The back of the hand is used to assess temperature. The palm of the hand is most sensitive to the vibration produced when sound travels through fluids or solid structures.

5. Palpation and tactile pressure should be performed in a slow, gentle, and deliberate manner. It is extremely important to follow an organized approach and move from region to region. Any tender areas identified should be examined further.

6. The three basic methods of palpation are:

   a. Light palpation in which fingers are gently applied over the skin surface, the skin is depressed to 1 cm, and the outline or sensitivity of a region determined.

   b. Deep palpation is a technique used to examine the condition of organs, the size of masses, and the presence of rebound tenderness. Using one hand, the skin is depressed 2 to 3 cm. When using this method of assessment, always remain mindful that the patient may experience significant pain when an internal injury or organ abnormality is detected. For this reason, caution is needed to prevent unnecessary discomfort. Deep palpation may be contraindicated in the trauma patient. Avoid continuous deep palpation; intermediate deep palpation is less painful and less likely to interfere with the examiner's sense of touch.[1]

   c. Bimanual palpation is also a deep palpation technique. Both hands are used to palpate deeply by placing one hand (the sensing hand) in a relaxed and lightly placed position on the patient's skin. The other hand applies pressure to the sensing hand. This hand placement allows the lower sensing hand to remain sensitive and detect organ characteristics. Although two hands (bimanual) are used for this technique, the phrase bimanual palpation usually refers to the examination of pelvic adnexa while fingers from one hand are inserted into the vagina and the other hand deeply palpates the abdomen to locate the ovaries.[1,2] This is an advanced assessment technique not performed by nurses during a trauma assessment unless qualified to do so.

7. The specific palpation technique used depends on the body area examined and the patient's condition. For example, a patient with a fractured rib will only require light palpation, and should be examined with care to avoid producing pain or further injury.

D. Percussion

1. Percussion involves striking the body's surface with a finger to produce sound and vibration in order to determine the location, size, and density of underlying structures to verify normality or abnormalities assessed by palpation and auscultation. Percussion also allows the examiner to determine if the underlying tissue is solid, air-filled, or fluid-filled.

2. There are five percussion sounds that can be produced: resonant, hyperresonant, dull, flat, and tympany. The sites at which they are normally heard and the sound characteristics are summarized in (Table PA-1).

3. Knowledge of normal organ densities allows the examiner to locate an organ or mass and determine its size by percussing its boundaries.

Table PA-1 Characteristics and Location of Percussion Sounds

Tissue Type	Amplitude	Pitch	Quality	Duration
Normal lung	Medium to loud	Low	Resonant	Moderate
Lung with more air (e.g., COPD)	Louder	Lower	Hyperresonant	Longer
Hepatic/splenic	Soft	High	Dull	Short
Muscle, bone	Softer	High	Flat	Shorter
Air-filled organ (i.e., intestine)	Loud	High	Tympanic	Longest

Reprinted from *Physical Examination and Health Assessment,* 4th edition, page 164, Assessment Techniques and the Clinical Setting, Copyright 2004, with permission from Elsevier.

4. To percuss, use both hands in the following manner:

   a. Place your nondominant hand lightly against the surface to be examined.

   b. Hyperextend the middle finger and apply firm pressure to the surface to be percussed.

   c. Use one or two fingertips of the dominant hand to strike the middle phalanx of the middle finger of the nondominant hand.

   d. Apply the same force over each area of the body to make an accurate comparison of sounds produced by percussion.

E. Auscultation

   1. Auscultation requires a stethoscope for listening to sounds created in body organs to detect variations from normal. It is important to learn the types of sounds normally heard at different sites because abnormal sounds can be recognized only in comparison with normal variations. It is also important to remove clothing or any other material from the area being examined to avoid extraneous sounds.

   2. Bowel sounds, breath sounds, and turbulence of blood flow are typically heard with the use of a stethoscope.

      a. By design, a stethoscope can only block out ambient sounds. It cannot magnify sounds, but does funnel sounds through the device to the examiner's ears.

      b. Various models of stethoscopes are available; some have a flat diaphragm on one side and a bell or cup-like piece on the opposite side. Others have both the diaphragm and bell on one side which eliminates turning of the endpiece. Pressure of the endpiece on the patient determines whether low- or high-pitched sounds will be heard.

      c. Bowel and lung sounds are high-pitched and best heard with the flat diaphragm.

      d. Extra heart sounds and sounds such as bruits in blood vessels are best heard with the cup-like bell.

      e. Characteristics of the sounds heard through auscultation are:

         1) Pitch: high to low sound frequency

         2) Amplitude: soft to loud

         3) Quality: gurgling, swishing

         4) Duration: short to medium length of time heard

      f. While auscultating at any site, consider the origin and cause of the sound, the exact site at which it is heard best, and the normal qualities of the sound to assess deviations from normal.

III. Specific Principles of Assessment

   A. Assessment of the head and neck

      1. During the head and neck assessment, inspection and palpation are the major skills used. Assessment of the head and neck is considered separately in any patient who has had a cervical stabilization device applied. These devices often obstruct access to the neck, therefore, the head is examined first followed by the neck. In order to assess the neck, in-line stabilization is maintained manually by another nurse while stabilization devices are removed or released. Manual stabilization must be maintained throughout the assessment of the neck. Once the assessment is complete, the stabilization devices should be re-applied and manual stabilization discontinued. In patients where no cervical stabilization devices have been applied or are indicated, the assessment of the head and neck may be performed concurrently.

      2. Inspect the head and neck for lacerations, abrasions, contusions, avulsions, puncture wounds, impaled objects, ecchymosis, and edema. Also look for loose teeth or other material in the mouth and drainage from the nose or ears. If there is drainage from the nose or ears, it may be cerebrospinal fluid. Do not pack the nose or ears and do not insert a nasogastric tube.

      3. The position of the trachea should be observed and palpated to ensure it is centrally located. The position of the trachea is located by gently placing a finger in the suprasternal notch. Deviation of the trachea to any side indicates an abnormal finding (e.g., tension pneumothorax).

      4. Palpate soft tissues for the presence of

crepitus/subcutaneous emphysema. The presence of subcutaneous emphysema in the neck often occurs where air from a pneumothorax or pneumomediastinum has tracked up into the neck.

5. Gently palpate the cervical vertebrae assessing for tenderness, swelling, muscle spasm, or deformities which may indicate a potential cervical spine injury. Any patient who has positive findings on palpation of the neck should have a stabilization device applied if one has not previously been applied.

B. Assessment of pupils and extraocular eye muscles (EOMs)

1. Assess pupils for size, shape, equality, and reactivity to light.

2. Ask the patient to follow your index finger with his or her eyes as you move it in the six directions to check EOMs (see **Figure 6-6**). Entrapment of eye muscles or damage to any one of the three cranial nerves that innervate the six muscles may be responsible for inability of the eye to move. The patient should be told to hold his or her head still during this assessment.

C. Assessment of the chest

1. Inspect the chest for general rise and fall with respirations, any open wounds, ecchymotic areas, surgical scars, or paradoxical movement. Palpate for bony crepitus, crepitus/subcutaneous emphysema, and pain.

2. During the primary assessment, auscultation will involve a rapid assessment and identification of the presence, reduction, or absence of breath sounds. The most convenient site to assess breath sounds during the primary assessment is on the anterior chest wall bilaterally. By placing the stethoscope at approximately the 2nd intercostal space in the midclavicular line, a gross assessment of breath sounds can be determined. Detailed auscultation requires a systematic bilateral approach (see **Figure PA-1** Specific Sequence for Auscultation of Breath Sounds, **Table PA-2** Significance of Types of Breath Sounds and Muffled Heart Sounds).

3. During the primary assessment, auscultation of heart sounds may be indicated in patients with no palpable pulse, penetrating wounds to the left chest, distended neck veins, or hypotension. Heart sounds can be auscultated by placing the stethoscope over the apex of the myocardium at the fifth intercostal space in the midclavicular line. The presence of muffled heart sounds should be excluded.

a. The first heart sound (S_1) indicates the beginning of systole because of the closure of the tricuspid and mitral valves. It is best detected with the diaphragm of the stethoscope held over the apex of the heart at the midclavicular line of the 5th intercostal space.

b. The second heart sound (S_2) indicates the beginning of diastole because of the closure of the pulmonic and aortic valves. It is best detected with the diaphragm of the

Table PA-2 Significance of Types of Breath Sounds and Muffled Heart Sounds

Sound Auscultated	Significance
Normal breath sounds	• Proceed with assessment
Diminished or absent breath sounds	
• Unilateral • Bilateral	• Loss of integrity to chest wall because of rib fractures or open wounds • Splinting because of pain • Pneumothorax, hemothorax, pulmonary contusion, foreign body in lower bronchus (differentiated by percussion and radiographic investigation) • Upper airway obstruction • Altered respiratory effort because of the effects of central nervous system depression or pain
Abnormal sounds in the chest	
• Bowel sounds • Muffled heart sounds	• Rupture of the diaphragm resulting in the presence of gastrointestinal contents in the chest • Produced by the presence of fluid in the pericardial sac

stethoscope held over the base of the heart at the anterior clavicular line 2nd intercostal space to the right and left of the sternum.

c. Remember, both S_1 and S_2 can be heard over the entire precordium (area of the chest that is over the heart). To hear them more loudly, auscultate over the apex to hear S_1 and over the base to hear S_2. The bell may also be used to auscultate because valvular sounds are low-pitched. Identifying the timing and the loudness is basic. In a more advanced

Figure PA-1 Specific Sequence for Auscultation of Breath Sounds

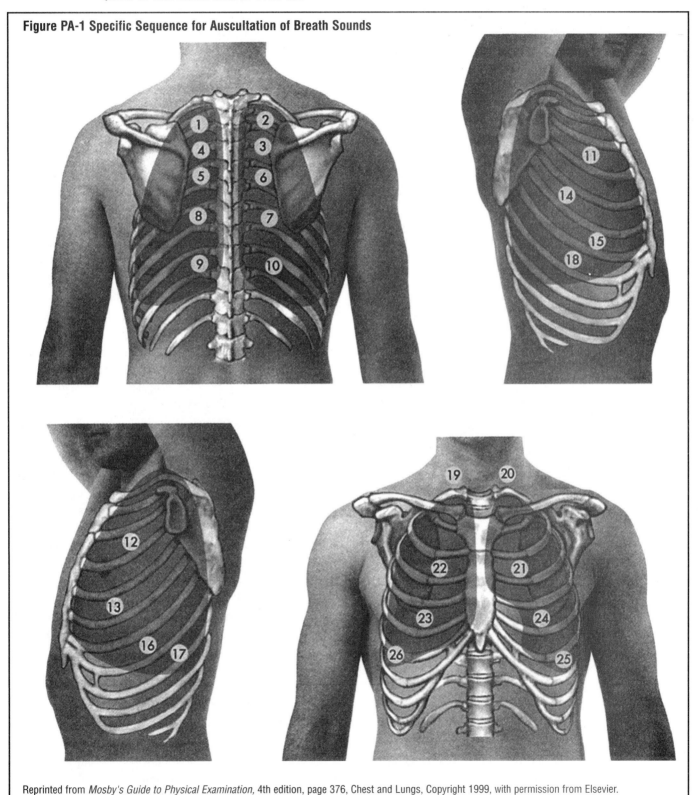

Reprinted from *Mosby's Guide to Physical Examination,* 4th edition, page 376, Chest and Lungs, Copyright 1999, with permission from Elsevier.

assessment, murmurs, clicks, friction rubs, and S_3 and S_4 sounds can be auscultated.

D. Assessment of the abdomen

1. The abdominal assessment includes an assessment of the liver, spleen, stomach, kidneys, and bladder. Injuries to the abdominal contents can often be detected early in the trauma assessment. Assessment of the abdomen is directed toward detecting the presence of masses, tenderness, rigidity, injury, enlargement of organs, and the presence or absence of peristaltic activity.

2. When assessing the abdomen, use a series of landmarks to map out the regions examined. The abdomen is divided into four quadrants with the tip of the xiphoid process marking the upper boundary and the symphysis pubis marking the lower boundary. Two imaginary lines cross the umbilicus to form the quadrants. The location of an abnormal assessment finding is described by the specific quadrant area. For example, a splenic injury may produce left upper quadrant pain.

3. The order of abdominal assessment differs from that of other body systems. The assessment should begin with a rapid inspection, followed by auscultation, palpation, and percussion. The reason behind changing the order is to ensure the accuracy of bowel sounds prior to palpation.

4. Stand at the patient's side and inspect the abdomen to detect abnormal shadows and movement. Inspect the abdomen from an angled position to detect abnormal protuberances such as lumps or swelling. Inspect the skin of the abdomen for scars (from previous surgery which may indicate altered anatomy), bruising patterns, lesions, and wounds.

5. Inspect the abdomen for:

   a. Shape and symmetry and note any masses, discoloration, swelling/edema/distension, wounds, or scars

   b. Normal movement during respiration

   c. Position of the umbilicus including shape, color, and any discharge or protruding mass

   d. Presence of peristaltic movement or aortic pulsation

6. Place the diaphragm of a stethoscope over each of the four quadrants. Listen for bowel sounds. It normally takes 5 to 20 seconds to hear bowel sounds. To describe bowel sounds as truly absent, the examiner should listen for at least five minutes. Patient's bowel sounds should be recorded as normal or audible, absent, hyperactive, or hypoactive.

7. When palpating the abdomen of the injured patient, always begin with a light palpation technique in an uninjured quadrant to avoid unnecessary discomfort. Palpate over each of the four quadrants. Depress the skin 1 cm.

E. Assessment of the pelvis and external genitalia

1. Inspect the pelvis and external genitalia for lacerations, abrasions, contusions, avulsions, puncture wounds, impaled objects, ecchymosis, edema, and scars. Look for blood at the urethral meatus, vagina, and rectum. Inspect the penis for priapism.

2. Palpation is utilized to assess the pelvis for the presence of tenderness and pelvic instability. A cautious and gentle approach should be taken to avoid severe pain and worsening bleeding associated with an underlying injury.

3. Locate the iliac crests and the symphysis pubis. The iliac crests should be compressed gently observing for the presence of pain, the feeling of instability, or crepitus. Do not "rock" the pelvis back and forth. The symphysis pubis should be assessed by placing one hand over the bony area and applying gentle pressure; once again the presence of pain, the feeling of instability, or crepitus should be assessed.

4. The physical assessment of pelvic injury is difficult and often unreliable when using the above methods and signs. The presence of any pelvic symptoms should always be fully investigated radiographically.

F. Assessment of the extremities

1. Assessment of the extremities involves the skills of inspection and palpation along with some active and passive limb movements. It is important to use a sys-

tematic approach, assessing the upper limbs first and then the lower limbs. Compare each limb with the same limb on the opposite side.

2. Inspect each extremity for lacerations, abrasions, contusions, avulsions, puncture wounds, impaled objects, ecchymosis, edema, deformities, and any open wounds. Assess for spontaneous movement. Inspect previously applied splints for correct application and adjust if necessary.

3. Palpate each limb from the most proximal aspect of the limb and progress toward the periphery in a systematic fashion.

4. Assess range of movement (ROM). If the patient is conscious, use active ROM where the patient controls the movement of the joint which may be limited by pain or injury involving the joint. If the patient is unconscious, passively assess the ROM of each joint. Note any abnormality which may indicate an injury to the bones or soft tissues such as bony crepitus, restricted ROM, or a particularly lax (floppy) joint.

5. Assess for any gross alteration in sensation. Any alteration in sensation should be reported to the physician/medical officer and may require more specific neurologic examination.

6. During palpation, perform a neurovascular assessment. The neurovascular assessment of an injured limb should occur distal to the site of the suspected injury. The neurovascular examination will involve the assessment of sensation, movement, warmth, color, and perfusion (pulse/capillary refill).

7. Pay particular attention to all joints and bones, especially those of the hands and feet, because injuries to these finer structures are occasionally missed during a preliminary trauma assessment.

G. Examination of the posterior surfaces

1. In most trauma patients, the assessment of the posterior surfaces will need to be performed while the patient is logrolled from a supine position into a lateral position with the alignment of the spine being maintained. To perform a safe and effective logroll, five people are required. One person controls the head and maintains the cervical spine in alignment throughout the

roll. Three other people roll the patient toward them controlling the shoulders, hips, and lower limbs. The last person is the examiner. The person controlling the head and cervical spine coordinates the timing of the logrolling. The examiner explains the procedure to the patient prior to commencing the examination. Where possible, the patient should not be rolled onto the side of a painful injury since this pain may distract him or her from identifying other areas of tenderness. Once the patient is in the lateral position, the assessment of the back involves the skills of inspection and palpation.

2. It is important at this time to remember to assess the occiput of the head during this part of the assessment.

This section highlighted some specific principles for identifying injuries in the trauma patient. The following section is a step-by-step performance of the secondary assessment which learners may choose to practice.

IV. Steps In Skill Performance

A. Assessment of the head, ears, eyes, face, and neck

1. Maintain cervical spine protection during assessment

2. Inspect and palpate the head for (assess the occipital area during the inspection of posterior surfaces):

   a. Lacerations, abrasions, avulsions, contusions, puncture wounds

   b. Bleeding, swelling/edema, ecchymosis, pain/tenderness, bony crepitus

   c. Foreign bodies/impaled objects

3. Inspect the nose for any drainage of fluid (rhinorrhea) or blood

4. Palpate the nose for position of septum

5. Ask the patient to open his or her eyes and inspect for:

   a. Ptosis of the eyelids

   b. Abnormalities of the globe (e.g., sub-conjunctival hematoma, hyphema)

   c. Foreign bodies/impaled objects

   d. Contact lenses

6. Inspect pupils for size, shape, equality, and reactivity to light

7. Inspect extraocular eye muscles (EOM)

8. Determine gross visual acuity

9. Inspect for facial symmetry by asking the patient to:

    a. Open and close mouth

    b. Smile and grimace

    c. Raise eyebrows

10. Inspect the ears for:

    a. Lacerations, abrasions, avulsions, contusions, puncture wounds

    b. Bleeding or fluid (otorrhea), swelling/edema, ecchymosis behind the ear at the mastoid process (Battle's sign), pain/tenderness

    c. Foreign bodies/impaled objects

11. Determine gross hearing function

12. Inspect the mouth, tongue, oral cavity, and lips for:

    a. Lacerations, abrasions, avulsions, contusions, puncture wounds, missing or malocclusion of the teeth

    b. Bleeding, swelling/edema, ecchymosis, pain/tenderness, pallor or cyanosis of the lips

    c. Presence of foreign bodies/foreign material/impaled objects

13. Remove the anterior portion of the cervical collar and while another trauma team member holds the patient's head in alignment, inspect and palpate the neck for:

    a. Lacerations, abrasions, avulsions, contusions, puncture wounds

    b. Bleeding, swelling/edema, ecchymosis, pain/tenderness, crepitus/subcutaneous emphysema, jugular veins for flattening or distension, tracheal deviation

    c. Foreign bodies/impaled objects

14. Inspect and palpate the cervical spine gently for:

    a. Lacerations, abrasions, avulsions, contusions, puncture wounds

    b. Bleeding, swelling/edema, ecchymosis, pain/tenderness, bony crepitus or step-off, crepitus/subcutaneous emphysema

    c. Foreign bodies/impaled objects

15. Replace the anterior portion of the cervical collar

B. Assessment of the chest

1. Repeat breathing assessment, as indicated (Refer to Chapter 3, Initial Assessment, for primary assessment)

2. Inspect and palpate the chest (anterior and lateral surfaces including the sternum, ribs, and clavicles) and axillae for:

    a. Lacerations, abrasions, avulsions, contusions, puncture wounds

    b. Bleeding, swelling/edema, ecchymosis, pain/tenderness, bony crepitus over the ribs or sternum, crepitus/subcutaneous emphysema

    c. Foreign bodies/impaled objects

3. Auscultate for breath sounds bilaterally for presence, absence, diminished sounds, and adventitious sounds (rales, crackles, rhonchi, or wheezes)

4. Auscultate S_1 and S_2 heart sounds noticing any muffled or abnormal sounds

5. Percuss the chest

C. Assessment of the abdomen

1. Inspect the abdomen for:

    a. Overall contour/shape/symmetry

    b. Lacerations, abrasions, avulsions, contusions, puncture wounds

    c. Bleeding, swelling/edema/distension, ecchymosis

    d. Foreign bodies/impaled objects

    e. Scars

2. Auscultate for bowel sounds in all four quadrants

3. Palpate the abdomen in all four quadrants for:

    a. Rigidity

    b. Guarding

    c. Masses

    d. Pain, tenderness

D. Assessment of the pelvic area and external genitalia

1. Inspect and palpate the pelvic area and external genitalia for:

    a. Lacerations, abrasions, avulsions, contusions, puncture wounds

    b. Bleeding, drainage or incontinence, swelling/edema, ecchymosis, pain/tenderness, bony crepitus over pelvis

    c. Foreign bodies/impaled objects

2. Inspect the urethral meatus for blood

3. Inspect the penis for priapism

4. Palpate the pelvis gently

E. Assessment of the extremities

1. Inspect and palpate all four extremities including the joints for:

   a. Shape and symmetry with opposite extremity

   b. Joint range of motion

   c. Lacerations, abrasions, avulsions, contusions, puncture wounds or protruding bond, deformities

   d. Bleeding, swelling/edema, ecchymosis, pain/tenderness

   e. Foreign bodies/impaled objects

2. Determine and grade muscle strength (**Table 3-4**)

3. Determine overall neurovascular status including:

   a. Vascular: pulses, color, temperature, capillary refill

   b. Palpate: femoral, popliteal, dorsalis pedis, brachial, and radial pulses

   c. Sensory: patient's ability to sense touch, pain, pressure

   d. Motor: patient's ability to wiggle toes, fingers

F. Assessment of posterior surfaces (including occiput)

1. Logroll the patient away from the person performing the assessment

2. Maintain cervical spine protection and immobilization during the logroll

3. Avoid rolling the patient onto an injured side

4. Inspect the posterior chest, buttocks, and posterior thighs for:

   a. Lacerations, abrasions, avulsions, contusions, puncture wounds

   b. Bleeding, swelling/edema, ecchymosis, pain/tenderness, deformity or misalignment

   c. Foreign bodies/impaled objects

6. Palpate the vertebral bodies and costovertebral angles (CVA) for pain, deformity, and areas of tenderness

7. Palpate the back, buttocks, and posterior thighs for pain or tenderness

8. Palpate the anal sphincter noticing presence or absence of tone (anal wink)

VII. Summary

Physical assessment utilizes the skills of inspection, palpation, percussion, and auscultation. These skills are the foundation of the assessment of the injured patient; they provide the nurse with the data to form nursing diagnoses and plan interventions. Physical assessment is undertaken with a focused systematic approach as described in the Initial Assessment chapter. During the initial management of the trauma patient, physical assessment and treatment may occur simultaneously.

A significant part of a nurse's practice is the ongoing assessment and evaluation of the patient's condition in collaboration with other health care professionals.

References

1. Fuller, J. & Schaller-Ayers,, J. (1994). *Health assessment: A nursing approach* (2nd ed.). Philadelphia: Lippincott.

2. Jarvis, C. (2004). *Physical examination and health assessment* (4th ed.). St. Louis, MO: W. B. Saunders.

Index

Bleeding. *See also* Fluid volume deficits; Hemorrhage
  with abdominal trauma, 153
  autotransfusion preparations, 143, 343
  of face and neck injuries, 119–20
  initial interventions, 37, 53–54
  with musculoskeletal trauma, 186–88
  in pregnant patients, 226
Blind nasotracheal intubation, 64
Blindness, 120
Blister agents, 252
Blisters, debridement in burn patients, 215
Blood agents, 253, 254
Blood alcohol concentration, 9
Blood glucose levels, 214
Blood oxygen saturation. *See* Oxygen saturation (SpO_2)
Blood pressure. *See also* Hypotension; Shock
  components of, 76–77
  obtaining for patients in shock, 82
  Revised Trauma Score values, 51
  with spinal injuries, 178
Blood product replacement for shock patients, 84
Blood substitutes, 85
Blood supply. *See* Circulation; Fluid volume deficits
Blood testing/typing, 40
Blood vessels, electrical injury to, 210
Blood viscosity, increases with burn trauma, 207
Blood volume, 76, 226, 231. *See also* Bleeding; Fluid volume deficits
Blunt cardiac injury, 139
Blunt trauma, 13, 152, 157
Blurred vision, 120
Boating fatalities, 13
Body surface area of burn injuries, 211–12
Bones. *See also* Musculoskeletal injuries
  facial, 115–16
  resistance to mechanical forces, 13
  of skull, 92
  types and structure, 184–85
Botulism, 257, 259
Bowel function loss, 176
Bowel sounds
  assessing for shock patients, 82
  indicating abdominal injuries, 157
  initial assessment, 44–45, 299, 364
Brachial plexus, 117, 171
Bradycardia, 176, 178, 232
Bradykinin release, 207
Brain
  anatomy, 93–94
  preferential blood flow during shock, 80
  protection from mechanical forces, 13, 92
Brain injuries
  assessing for, 101–4

indicating need for early transfer, 288
interventions, 104–6, 109–11
overview, 96–97
pathophysiologic responses, 97–98
selected types, 98–101
Brainstem, 93
Breathing. *See also* Airway; Ventilation
  assessing for chest injuries, 141, 146
  assessing for shock patients, 82
  burn trauma complications, 206, 210, 221
  effects of chemical attacks on, 252–54, 255, 256
  in infants and children, 230–31, 239
  interventions, 52–53, 64–68, 69–71, 74, 88, 336–41
  long-bone fracture complications for, 192
  maintaining for patients in transport, 290
  in older adults, 234, 239
  of pregnant patients, 227, 239
  primary assessment, 35–36, 44, 68–69, 298, 299
  respiratory anatomy, 134
  Revised Trauma Score values, 51
  spinal cord injuries compromising, 173
Breath sounds, 35, 361, 362, 363
Brown-Séquard syndrome, 176
Bubonic plague, 257
Bullets, 17, 18
Burns
  assessment, 210–13
  epidemiology and mechanisms of injury, 205–6
  interventions, 214–17
  pathophysiologic responses, 206–9
  types, 199, 201, 209–10, 211
BZ, 253

C

Calcaneus fractures, 186
Canada, trauma epidemiology, 24–28
Canadian Agricultural Injury Surveillance Program, 24
Canadian Hospitals Injury Reporting and Prevention Program, 24
Canadian Institute for Health Information, 24
Canadian Surveillance System for Water-Related Fatalities, 24–25
Cannabis use, 25
Capillaries, 198, 199, 207
Capillary refill, 36
Capnometry, 339
Car accidents. *See* Motor vehicle crashes
Carbon dioxide, 94, 338–39
Carbon monoxide poisoning, 208, 215
Carboxyhemoglobin, 339
Cardiac dysrhythmias, 211
Cardiac enzyme tests, 142
Cardiac output decrease
  with abdominal trauma, 163

Flat nose bullets, 18

Floods, 251

Fluid dynamics, 198, 199

Fluid resuscitation. *See* Intravenous fluid replacement

Fluid volume deficits
    with abdominal trauma, 163
    with burn trauma, 207, 211–12, 214, 221
    with chest injuries, 147
    in children, 243
    interventions and expected outcomes, 53
    with musculoskeletal trauma, 194
    in older adults, 246
    in pregnant trauma patients, 241
    with shock patients, 88
    with spinal injuries, 181

Fluorescein staining, 125

Focal brain injury, 99

Focused adjuncts, 39–40, 299

Focused assessments, 46

Focused assessment sonography for trauma (FAST)
    for abdominal trauma, 158, 159
    for chest trauma, 142
    screening for pregnancy with, 229
    for shock patients, 83
    use during initial assessments, 40
    use with children, 233

Fontanelles, 232

Fossae, 92

Fourth-degree burns, 211

Fracture types, 187, 188

Frontal impacts to vehicles, 15

Full-thickness burns, 199, 211, 213

Full vital signs, 39–41, 299

Fundal height, 228–29

G

Gamma rays, 259

Gas exchange impairments
    with airway and ventilation problems, 74
    with brain injuries, 110
    with burn injuries, 220
    with chest injuries, 146
    with face or neck injuries, 129
    initial assessment, 53
    in older adults, 246
    in pregnant trauma patients, 240
    with shock patients, 88
    with spinal injuries, 181

Gastric injuries, 155

Gastric motility in pregnant patients, 227

Gastric tubes, 40, 85, 160, 215

Gender, trauma incidence and, 8, 9, 25, 28–29, 30

General adaptation syndrome, 274

General appearance, assessing, 43–44

Genitalia, 364

Geriatric trauma patients. *See* Older adults

Giving comfort, 41–43, 299

Glasgow Coma Scale
    classifying head trauma by, 98, 102–3
    pediatric version, 232, 233
    use in primary assessment, 37–38, 51

Globe of eye, 114, 121. *See also* Eye injuries; Eyes

Glossopharyngeal nerve, 118

Glucose levels, 214

Government agencies, 27–28

Gray matter, 167, 168

Great vessels, 134–35

Grey Turner's sign, 156, 157

Grieving, 242, 277–79, 284

Ground ambulances, 289

G-series agents, 252

Guidelines for Essential Trauma Care, 285, 286

Gunshot wounds. *See* Firearm injuries

H

Hair clipping, 203

Halo devices, 178

Halo sign, 102

Hand burns, 213

Handguns, 17

Hands, palpation with, 359–60

Hangman's fracture, 175

Hazard detection, 263

Head and face. *See also* Maxillofacial injuries; Skull
    diagnostic studies, 300
    initial assessment, 44, 299, 361–62

Head-to-toe assessment, 43–45, 299

Health maintenance changes for children, 244

Heart
    anatomy, 76, 134
    contusions, 139
    pericardial tamponade, 78, 137, 139–40, 144
    rates in children versus adults, 231
    sounds, 82, 361, 362–63

Helicopters, 289

Helmet removal, 353, 354–55

Helplessness, 276

Hematomas, 100–101, 201

Hematuria, 156, 160

Hemoglobin
    carbon monoxide binding, 208
    levels as transfusion triggers, 84
    measuring oxygen saturation, 70, 83, 339

Hemoglobin-based oxygen carriers, 85

Hemorrhage. *See also* Bleeding; Fluid volume deficits
    common with abdominal trauma, 153

Inspection skills, 359. *See also* Assessments

Inspiration, 60, 61

Institutional-based disasters, 250

Integumentary system, 200–204. *See also* Burns

Intentional self-harm. *See* Suicides

Intentional trauma, 7, 8. *See also* Violence

Intercostal muscles, 60

Interfacility transfers, 39, 285–90

Internal disasters, 250

Internal mechanical forces, 12–13

Interstitial edema, 136

Interstitial fluid osmotic pressure, 199

Interstitial free fluid pressure, 199

Interventions. *See also* Skill stations
  for abdominal trauma, 160, 163–64
  airway, 34–35, 52, 63–68, 73–74
  for anxiety/fear, 54
  for brain injuries, 104–6, 109–11
  breathing, 36, 52–53, 88
  for burn injuries, 214–17
  for chest trauma, 142–44, 341–43
  circulation, 36–37, 53–54, 88–89
  for critical incident stress, 280, 281
  eye, face, and neck injuries, 125–26, 128–31
  for feelings of powerlessness, 55
  hypothermia, 38, 54, 89
  during intrafacility transport, 291
  for musculoskeletal trauma, 190–92, 194–95
  for older adults, 238–39, 245–47
  pain management, 42–43, 54
  for pediatric trauma patients, 238–39, 243–44
  for pregnant trauma patients, 238–42
  for psychosocial effects of trauma, 276–80, 281, 283–84
  for shock patients, 83–85, 88–89
  for skin and soft-tissue trauma, 203–4
  for spinal injuries, 178, 180–82
  for unconscious patients, 38
  ventilation, 69–71, 73–74
  for violence victims, 48
  for violent patients, 49

Intervertebral discs, 167

Intimate partner violence, 8, 9, 46–48, 326–30

Intracellular fluid, 76

Intracerebral hematomas, 100–101

Intracranial pressure, 94, 97, 105

Intrafacility transport, 290–91

Intraocular pressure, 120

Intrapleural pressure, 60

Intravascular fluid loss, 207

Intravenous contrast, 158–59

Intravenous fluid replacement
  for brain injuries, 105
  with burn trauma, 214, 216

  initial interventions with, 37
  for shock patients, 84, 85
  with spinal injuries, 178

Intravenous pyelogram, 159

Intubating laryngeal mask airway, 66

Ionizing radiation, 259–60

Irradiation, 260

Irregular bones, 184

Irreversible shock, 79, 81–82

Irrigation, 125, 203–4, 216–17

Ischemia, 173. *See also* Blood supply; Circulation

Isotonic crystalloid solution
  basic guidelines for use, 36, 37
  for brain injuries, 105
  irrigating injured eyes with, 125
  for shock patients, 88, 89
  to support circulation, 53, 54

J

Jacketed bullets, 18

Jaw fractures, 122

Jaw thrust maneuver, 63, 336

Jefferson fracture, 175

Joints. *See also* Musculoskeletal injuries
  anatomy, 184–85
  effects of aging on, 235
  effects of pregnancy on, 227
  injuries to, 187

Jugular venous distention, 36, 69

Jumps, 16–17

K

Kehr's sign, 154

Kidneys
  anatomy, 150
  effects of aging on, 235
  injuries to, 156
  responses to shock, 80, 81

Kinematics, 10–11

Kinetic energy, 11

Kleihauer-Betke Test, 230

Knowledge deficits, 284

L

Labor, premature, 227

Laboratory studies
  for abdominal trauma, 159
  for brain injuries, 104
  for burn trauma, 213
  for chest trauma, 142
  for pregnant patients, 229–30
  for shock patients, 83
  for surface trauma, 203

effects on normal responses, 225, 234, 235
to facilitate intubation, 35, 64, 65
following secondary assessment, 46
pain management, 42, 125, 144, 191, 214–15
potential role in trauma, 9
psychiatric, 262
in sexual assault protocols, 48
for violent patients, 49
Medulla, 93, 94
Medullary cavities, 184
Meninges, 92, 93
Mesenteries, 150
Metabolic acidosis, 83
Metabolism, 76, 209, 232
Methemoglobin, 339
Microcirculation, 76
Mild concussion, 99
Military triage, 267
Minimal equipment for intrafacility transport, 291
Minor head trauma, 98
Missile features, 17
Mitochondria, 76
MIVT mnemonic, 43
Mnemonics
    chest tube function, 71, 143
    disaster management, 262–65
    initial assessment, 34, 296
    meninges, 92
    organophosphate exposure, 254
    prehospital information, 43
    rapid sequence intubation medications, 64
    responses to stimuli, 37
    scalp layers, 92
Mobility impairments, 194
Moderate head trauma, 98
Modes of transportation, 286, 289
Modified Trendelenburg position, 85
Monro-Kellie doctrine, 94
Mood changes, 276
Moral knowledge, 2
Motorcyclists, 15, 345–46
Motor functions, 45, 168, 176
Motor nerves, 170
Motor responses (Glasgow Coma Scale), 103, 104
Motor vehicle crashes
    alcohol related, 8–9
    as cause of brain injury, 96
    as cause of chest trauma, 136, 140
    as cause of death, 8
    deceleration forces in, 12
    injury prevention measures, 14–16, 23
    pregnant patients in, 226
    rates in selected countries, 21, 25
    skill station assessments, 331–35

Mouth anatomy, 58, 59
Multicasualty/disaster triage, 267
Multiple-casualty incidents, 251
Multiple-patient incidents, 250
Multiple-system injuries, 288
Muscle anatomy, 185
Muscle strength scale, 45
Musculoskeletal injuries, 184–89, 209–10, 288
Mustard gas, 253
Myoglobin, 208, 213, 216

N

Nasogastric tubes, 40, 105
Nasopharyngeal airways, 64, 337
Nasopharynx, 210
National Center for Injury Prevention and Control, 10
National Highway Traffic Safety Administration, 15–16
National Strategy for Injury Prevention (Canada), 26
National Trauma Registry (Canada), 24
Native Americans, trauma-related death rates, 8
Natural disasters, 250, 251
Near drowning, 13
Neck
    anatomy, 58–59, 116–17
    diagnostic studies, 300
    distended veins in, 138, 140, 141
    initial assessment, 44, 299
Neck injuries
    assessing for, 123–25
    cervical collar contraindications with, 354
    interventions for, 125–26, 128–31
    overview and concurrent injuries, 119
    selected types, 123
Needle cricothyrotomy, 66–67, 340
Needle thoracentesis, 70, 142, 143, 297, 341
Needs, psychosocial, 274–75
Nerve agents, 252, 253
Nerve plexes, 171
Nervous system
    brachial plexus, 117, 171
    for circulatory controls, 77
    cranial nerves, 94, 117, 118
    spinal cord and spinal nerves, 167–71
Neurogenic shock
    basic features, 79
    intravenous fluid replacement with, 84
    with spinal injuries, 174, 177, 178
Neurologic assessments, 37–38, 51, 365
Neurologic deficits, 173, 187
Neuromuscular blocking agents, 65
Neutron particles, 259
Newton's Laws of Motion, 10–11

W

Warm zones, 266
Waterless drainage systems, 70, 341
Water-related injuries, 13. *See also* Drownings
Water seal chest drainage units, 143
White matter, 167, 168
Wildfires, 251
Word-graphic rating scale, 42
Work-related injuries. *See* Occupational injuries
Wound care interventions, 203–4, 215
Wound cleansing, 203
Wound closure, 204
Wound cultures, 204
Wound healing, 200, 202
Wound preparation, 203–4

X

X-rays, 259

Y

Yaw of projectiles, 17
Yersinia pestis, 257

Z

Zones of burn trauma, 206–7
Zones of decontamination, 265, 266
Zones of neck, 117